OXFORD MEDICAL PUBLICATIONS

Oxford Handbook of
Clinical and Laboratory Investigation

Published and forthcoming Oxford Handbooks

Oxford Handbook for the Foundation Programme 2e
Oxford Handbook of Acute Medicine 3e
Oxford Handbook of Anaesthesia 2e
Oxford Handbook of Applied Dental Sciences
Oxford Handbook of Cardiology
Oxford Handbook of Clinical and Laboratory Investigation 2e
Oxford Handbook of Clinical Dentistry 4e
Oxford Handbook of Clinical Diagnosis 2e
Oxford Handbook of Clinical Examination and Practical Skills
Oxford Handbook of Clinical Haematology 3e
Oxford Handbook of Clinical Immunology and Allergy 2e
Oxford Handbook of Clinical Medicine—Mini Edition 7e
Oxford Handbook of Clinical Medicine 7e
Oxford Handbook of Clinical Pharmacy
Oxford Handbook of Clinical Rehabilitation 2e
Oxford Handbook of Clinical Specialties 8e
Oxford Handbook of Clinical Surgery 3e
Oxford Handbook of Complementary Medicine
Oxford Handbook of Critical Care 3e
Oxford Handbook of Dental Patient Care 2e
Oxford Handbook of Dialysis 3e
Oxford Handbook of Emergency Medicine 3e
Oxford Handbook of Endocrinology and Diabetes 2e
Oxford Handbook of ENT and Head and Neck Surgery
Oxford Handbook of Expedition and Wilderness Medicine
Oxford Handbook of Gastroenterology & Hepatology
Oxford Handbook of General Practice 3e
Oxford Handbook of Genitourinary Medicine, HIV and AIDS
Oxford Handbook of Geriatric Medicine
Oxford Handbook of Infectious Diseases and Microbiology
Oxford Handbook of Key Clinical Evidence
Oxford Handbook of Medical Sciences
Oxford Handbook of Nephrology and Hypertension
Oxford Handbook of Neurology
Oxford Handbook of Nutrition and Dietetics
Oxford Handbook of Obstetrics and Gynaecology 2e
Oxford Handbook of Occupational Health
Oxford Handbook of Oncology 2e
Oxford Handbook of Ophthalmology
Oxford Handbook of Paediatrics
Oxford Handbook of Palliative Care 2e
Oxford Handbook of Practical Drug Therapy 2e
Oxford Handbook of Pre-Hospital Care
Oxford Handbook of Psychiatry 2e
Oxford Handbook of Public Health Practice 2e
Oxford Handbook of Reproductive Medicine & Family Planning
Oxford Handbook of Respiratory Medicine 2e
Oxford Handbook of Rheumatology 2e
Oxford Handbook of Sport and Exercise Medicine
Oxford Handbook of Tropical Medicine 3e
Oxford Handbook of Urology 2e

Oxford Handbook of
Clinical and Laboratory Investigation

Third Edition

Edited by

Drew Provan

Senior Lecturer in Haematology
St Barts and The London School of Medicine
and Dentistry
London, UK

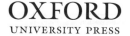

OXFORD
UNIVERSITY PRESS

OXFORD
UNIVERSITY PRESS

Great Clarendon Street, Oxford OX2 6DP

Oxford University Press is a department of the University of Oxford.
It furthers the University's objective of excellence in research, scholarship,
and education by publishing worldwide in

Oxford New York

Auckland Cape Town Dar es Salaam Hong Kong Karachi
Kuala Lumpur Madrid Melbourne Mexico City Nairobi
New Delhi Shanghai Taipei Toronto

With offices in

Argentina Austria Brazil Chile Czech Republic France Greece
Guatemala Hungary Italy Japan Poland Portugal Singapore
South Korea Switzerland Thailand Turkey Ukraine Vietnam

Oxford is a registered trade mark of Oxford University Press
in the UK and in certain other countries

Published in the United States
by Oxford University Press Inc., New York

First edition published 2002
Second edition published 2005
Third edition published 2010

British Library Cataloguing in Publication Data
Data available

Library of Congress Cataloging in Publication Data
Data available

Typeset by Glyph International (P) Ltd., India
Printed in China
on acid-free paper through
Asia Pacific Offset

ISBN 978–0–19–923371–7

10 9 8 7 6 5 4 3 2 1

To Val and Fraser with much love.

Foreword

This book fills an obvious gap in the Handbook series and, indeed, a major lacuna in the medical literature. Too often investigations of a particular condition are lost in the welter of other text. Alternatively, they appear as specialist books in pathology and radiology. One unique feature of this book is the inclusion of all clinical investigative techniques, i.e. both truly clinical tests in the shape of symptoms and signs and then laboratory-based investigations. This stops what is often an artificial separation. Each section is clearly put together with the intent of easing rapid reference. This is essential if the book is to have (and I believe it does have) real usefulness for bedside medicine. There are many other useful aspects of the text. These include a comprehensive list of abbreviations—the bugbear of medicine, as well as reference ranges that some laboratories still do not append to results. Overall, the Handbook should be of benefit to not just clinical students and junior doctors in training, but all who have patient contact. With this in one pocket, and Longmore in the other, there should be little excuse for errors in diagnosis and investigation, with the added benefit that the balance between the two will allow the upright posture to be maintained.

Professor Sir George Alberti
President of The Royal College of Physicians of London
July 2002

Preface to the third edition

Advances in modern medicine continue to improve the diagnostic and care pathways for patients. Keeping track of developments within one's own specialty can sometimes be difficult and, considering internal medicine as a whole, it is virtually impossible for most of us to remember which tests are required and in which specific situations.

This new and updated version of the *Oxford Handbook of Clinical and Laboratory Investigation* reflects today's practice. Major updating has been carried out particularly in the Cardiology, Poisoning and Rheumatology chapters. Other chapters have been updated where necessary, bringing them in line with current guidelines.

In addition, new and better quality illustrations have been used, and the line art has been redrawn to provide extra clarity. We have also cross-referenced where possible to the *Oxford Handbook of Clinical Medicine*, 8th edn, Oxford University Press.

The OUP team have been patient with us and has kept the project moving along. The writing team has managed to deliver great content, which is no mean feat when considering how busy each of them is delivering care to their patients. I am indebted to them for making this book relevant and readable for clinicians of all grades.

As before, I take responsibility for errors or omissions in the book and welcome any comments readers may have. This book is meant to be used, rather than kept on a bookshelf, and its usability relies on feedback from readers, so please contact me at *a.provan@virgin.net* if there is anything you feel could be improved in the next edition.

Drew Provan
2010

Preface to the first edition

With the increasing complexity of modern medicine, we now have literally thousands of possible investigative techniques at our disposal. We are able to examine our patient's serum and every other body fluid down to the level of individual nucleotides, as well as being able to perform precise imaging through CT, MRI, and other imaging technologies. The problem we have all faced, especially as senior medical students or junior doctors is: Which test should we use in a given setting? What hazards are associated with the tests? Are there any situations where specific tests should not be used or are likely to produce erroneous results? As medical complexity increases, so too does cost; many assays available today are highly expensive and wherever possible we would ideally like to use a test that is cheap, reliable, reproducible, and right for a given situation.

Such knowledge takes many years to acquire and it is a fact of life that senior doctors (who have attained such knowledge) are not usually those who request the investigations. In this small volume, we have attempted to distil all that is known about modern tests, from blood, urine, and other body fluids, along with imaging and molecular tests. The book is divided into two principal parts: the first deals with symptoms and signs in *The patient* section, because that is how patients present. We have tried to cover as many topics as possible, discussing these in some detail and have provided differential diagnoses where possible. We also try to suggest tests that might be of value in determining the cause of the patient's symptom or sign. The second part of the book, *Investigations*, is specialty-specific, and is more relevant once you know roughly what type of disease the patient might have. For example, if the symptom section suggests a likely respiratory cause for the patient's symptoms, then the reader should look to the *Respiratory medicine* chapter in order to determine which tests to carry out, or how to interpret the results.

The entire book is written by active clinicians, rather than scientists, since we wanted to provide a strong clinical approach to investigation. We have tried, wherever possible, to cross-refer to the *Oxford Handbook of Clinical Medicine* 5th edn, Oxford University Press, which provides the clinical detail omitted from this handbook. The symbol 📖 is used to highlight a cross-reference to *OHCM*, in addition to cross-referencing within this book.

We would value feedback from readers since there will doubtless be tests omitted, errors in the text and many other improvements we could, and will, make in future editions. All contributors will be acknowledged individually in the next edition. We would suggest you e-mail us directly: *a.provan@virgin.net*.

Drew Provan
Andrew Krentz
2002

Acknowledgements

Even small books such as this rely on the input of many people, besides the main editors, and we are indebted to many of our colleagues for providing helpful suggestions and for proofreading the text. Dr Barbara Bain, St Mary's Hospital, London, kindly allowed us to peruse the proofs of *Practical Haematology*, 9th edn (Churchill Livingstone) to help make sure the Haematology section was up to date. Dr Debbie Lillington, Department of Cytogenetics, Barts & The London NHS Trust, London, provided invaluable cytogenetic advice. Our registrars have had input into many sections and we thank the London registrars: Simon Stanworth, Jude Gaffan, Leon Clark, and Nikki Curry, and the Southampton registrars: Fiona Clark, Michael Masding, Mayank Patel, Ruth Poole, and Catherine Talbot. Thanks to Dr SJ Harris (Nottingham) for alerting me to some omissions in the book.

Dr Murray Longmore, the undisputed Oxford Handbook king, has provided invaluable wisdom and has very kindly allowed us to use his specially designed *OHCM* typeface (OUP) for many of the symbols in our text. Murray also provided page proofs of *OHCM*, which was invaluable for cross-referencing this handbook.

The team at Oxford University Press have, as ever, been a joy to work with and I especially extend my warmest thanks to Anna Winstanley, assistant commissioning editor, for her immense patience and forbearance in the face of delays and technical glitches.

I am grateful to Dr Andrew Krentz, who co-edited the first edition of this book. Dr Krentz's sections on diabetes, hyperlipidaemias, and others remain a valuable component of the book, and have been updated by Dr Colin Dayan.

Contents

Detailed contents

8 Respiratory medicine 499

14 Nuclear medicine   793

Contributors

Brian Angus
Reader in Infectious Diseases,
Nuffield Department of Clinical
Medicine, John Radcliffe Hospital,
Oxford, UK
Infectious and tropical diseases

James Ballinger
Department of Nuclear Medicine,
Guy's and St Thomas' Hospital,
London, UK
Nuclear medicine

R Martyn Bracewell
Senior Lecturer and
Consultant Neurologist,
University of Bangor,
Gwynedd, UK
Neurology

Joanna L Brown
Clinical Lead, Acute Medicine
Respiratory and GIM Physician,
Respiratory Department,
Imperial College Health-Care
NHS Trust,
London, UK
Respiratory medicine

Kuntal Chakravarty
Professor of Rheumatology (Hon),
London University of Southbank,
London, UK
Rheumatology

Tanya Chawla
Assistant Professor,
University Health Network &
Mount Sinai, Department of
Medical Imaging, Toronto, Canada
Radiology

Colin Dayan
Consultant Senior Lecturer in
Medicine,
Division of Medicine Laboratories,
Bristol Royal Infirmary, Bristol, UK
Endocrinology and metabolism

David Gray
Reader in Medicine and
Consultant Cardiologist,
Queen's Medical Centre,
University Hospital NHS Trust,
Nottingham, UK
Cardiology

Emma Greig
Consultant Gastroenterologist,
Taunton & Somerset NHS Trust,
Taunton, UK
Gastroenterology

Andrew R Houghton
Consultant Physician and
Cardiologist,
Grantham & District Hospital,
Grantham, UK
Cardiology

Alison Jones
Dean, School of Medicine,
University of Western Sydney &
Conjoint Professor of
Medicine and Clinical
Toxicology, University of
Newcastle, Australia
Poisoning and overdose

Suzanne Lane,
Consultant Rheumatologist,
Ipswich Hospital, Ipswich, UK
Rheumotology

James Moriarty
SpR Renal Medicine, Richard Bright Renal Unit, Southmead Hospital, Bristol, UK
Renal medicine

Drew Provan
Senior Lecturer in Haematology, Barts and The London School of Medicine and Dentistry, London, UK
Haematology, transfusion and cytogenetics

Gavin Spickett
Consultant Clinical Immunologist, Regional Department of Immunology, Royal Victoria Infirmary, Newcastle upon Tyne, UK
Immunology

Charlie Tomson
Consultant Nephrologist, The Richard Bright Renal Unit, Southmead Hospital, Westbury-on-Trym, Bristol, UK
Renal medicine

Ken Tung
Consultant Radiologist, Department of Radiology, Southampton University Hospitals NHS Trust, Southampton, UK
Radiology

Our registrars
We are indebted to our juniors for writing and checking various sections, in particular.

Symptoms & signs
Southampton University Hospitals:
Martin Taylor, Michael Masding, Mayank Patel, Ruth Poole, Tanay Sheth, and Catherine Talbot

St Bartholomew's & The Royal London School of Medicine & Dentistry:
Simon Stanworth, Jude Gaffan, Leon Clark and Nikki Curry

My thanks, also, to those who contributed to the first edition: John Axford, Keith Dawkins, and Praful Patel. Also to those who contributed to the second edition: James Dunbar, A Frew, Stephen T, Green, Val Lewington, Rommel Ravanan, Dr Penelope Sensky, Adrian Williams, Lorraine Wilson.

Symbols and abbreviations

~	approximately
Δ	differential diagnosis
γ	gamma
→	leading to
📖	cross-reference
↑	increased
↓	decreased
🖰	website
►	important
►►	very important
>>	much greater than
1°	primary
2°	secondary
♂	male
♀	female
↔	normal
↑↑	greatly increased
β-TG	β-thromboglobulin
γGT	γ-glutamyl transpeptidase
5HIAA	5-hydroxindole acetic acid
AA	aortic arch
AAA	abdominal aortic aneurysms
AAFB	acid and alcohol fast bacilli
ABG	arterial blood gas
ABO	ABO blood groups
ABPA	allergic bronchopulmonary aspergillosis
ACD	anaemia of chronic disease
ACE	angiotensin converting enyme
ACEI	angiotensin converting enzyme inhibitor
ACh	acetylcholine
AChE	red cell cholinesterase
ACL	anticardiolipin antibody
ACR	albumin:creatinine ratio
AChRAb	acetylcholine receptor antibodies
ACS	acute coronary syndrome
ACTH	adrenocorticotrophic hormone
ADA	American Diabetes Association
ADH	antidiuretic hormone
ADP	adenosine 5-diphosphate
AF	atrial fibrillation
AFP	α-fetoprotein
AIDS	acquired immunodeficiency syndrome
AIH	autoimmune hepatitis
AIHA	autoimmune haemolytic anaemia
AIP	autoimmune profile
ALD	adrenoleucodystrophy
ALL	acute lymphoblastic leukaemia
ALP	alkaline phosphatase
ALT	alanine transaminase
AMA	anti-mitochondrial antibodies
AML	acute myeloid leukaemia
ANA	antinuclear antibodies
ANAE	α-naphtholacetate esterase

ANCA	antineutrophil cytoplasmic antibody		BIPLED	bihemispheric periodic lateralized epileptiform discharges
ANNA	anti-neuronal nuclear antibodies		BJP	Bence–Jones protein
AP	anteroposterior		BM	bone marrow
APCR	activated protein C resistance		BMI	Body Mass Index
APS	antiphospholipid syndrome		BMT	bone marrow transplant
			BOLD	blood O_2 level
APTR	activated partial thromboplastin time ratio		BP	blood pressure
			BSG	British Society of Gastroenterology
APTT	activated partial thromboplastin time		C&S	culture & sensitivity
APVD	anomalous pulmonary venous drainage		CAD	computer assisted detection
ARF	acute renal failure		CAH	congenital adrenal hyperplasia
ARMS	amplification refractory mutation system		cANCA	cytoplasmic ANCA
ASCA	antibodies to *Saccharomyces cerevisiae*		CaSR	calcium sensing receptor
			CBC	complete blood count
ASMA	anti-smooth muscle antibodies		CBD	common bile duct
			CC	craniocaudal
ASO	anti-streptolysin		CCF	congestive cardiac failure
ASOT	anti-streptolysin O titre			
AST	aspartate transaminase		CCK	cholecystokinin
AT	antithrombin		CCP	cyclic citrullinated peptide
ATN	acute tubular necrosis			
AV	atrioventricular		CCU	coronary care unit
AVM	arteriovenous malformations		CD	cluster differentiation
			CEA	carcinoembryonic antigen
AVN	avascular necrosis			
AVP	arginine vasopressin		CF	complement fixation
AXR	abdominal X-ray		CFA	cryptogenic fibrosing alveolitis
BAEP	brainstem auditory evoked potential		CGMS	continuous glucose monitoring systems
BAER	brainstem auditory evoked response		CHD	coronary heart disease
BAL	bronchoalveolar lavage		ChVS	chorionic villus sampling
BC	blood cultures		CINCA	chronic infantite neurologic, cutaneous and articular syndrome
BCG	bacillus Calmette Guerin			
bd	bis die (twice daily)			

CJD	Creutzfeldt–Jakob disease	CTPA	computed tomography pulmonary angiography
CK	creatine kinase	CTU	computed tomography urography
CKD	chronic kidney disease	CVA	cerebrovascular accident (stroke)
CLL	chronic lymphocytic/lymphatic leukaemia	CVD	cardiovascular disease
CLO	*Campylobacter*-like organism	CVID	common variable immunodeficiency
CMAP	compound motor action potential	CVP	central venous pressure
CML	chronic myeloid leukaemia	CVS	cardiovascular system
CMR	cardiac magnetic resonance	CW	continuous wave
		CXR	chest X-ray
CMV	cytomegalovirus	CyF	cystic fibrosis
CNS	central nervous system	DAT	direct antibody test
CO	carbon monoxide	DBCE	double contrast barium enema
COHb	carboxyhaemoglobin	DCCT	Diabetes Control and Complications Trial
COPD	chronic obstructive pulmonary disease		
CPAP	continuous positive airway pressure	DDAVP	desamino D-arginyl vasopressin
CPK	creatinine phosphokinase	DEC	diethylcarbamazine
CPPD	calcium pyrophosphate disease	DEXA	dual-energy X-ray absorptiometry
CPS	complex partial seizure	DFa	direct fluorescein-labelled monoclonal antibody
CrC	creatinine clearance		
CREST	calcinosis, Raynaud's syndrome, oesophageal motility dysfunction, sclerodactyly, & telangiectasia	DFA	direct fluorescent antibody
		DHEAS	dehydroepi-androsterone sulphate
		DI	diabetes insipidus
CRH	corticotropin releasing hormone	DIC	disseminated intravascular coagulation
CRP	C-reactive protein	DIDMOAD	diabetes insipidus, diabetes mellitus, optic atrophy, and deafness
CSF	cerebrospinal fluid		
CSU	catheter specimen		
CT	computed tomography	DIF	direct immunofluorescence
CTC	computed tomography colonography	DIP	distal inter phalangear joint
CTLp	cytotoxic T lymphocyte precursor	DJ	duodendojejunal
		DKA	diabetic ketoacidosis

DLCO	diffusing lung capacity for carbon monoxide
DM	diabetes mellitus
DMSA	dimercaptosuccinic acid
DNA	deoxyribose nucleic acid
DPLD	diffuse parenchymal lung disease
dRVVT	dilute Russell viper venom test
DSA	digital subtraction angiography
Ds-DNA	double-stranded DNA
DSI	dimensionless severity index
DTPA	diethylenetri-aminepentaacetic acid
DU	duodenal ulcer
DVT	deep vein thrombosis
DXA	dual-energy X-ray absorptiometry
EBUS	endobronchial ultrasound
EBV	Epstein–Barr virus
ECG	electrocardiogram
EDH	extradural haemorrhage
EDTA	ethylenediamine tetra-acetic acid
EEG	electroencephalogram
EF	ejection fraction
EGFR	epidermal growth factor receptor
EIA	enzyme-linked assay
ELISA	enzyme-linked immunosorbant assay
EM	electron microscopy
EMA	endomysial antibody
EMG	electromyogram
EMU	early morning urines
ENA	extractable nuclear antigens

EOG	electro-oculography
EP	evoked potential
Epo	erythropoietin
EQA	external quality assurance
ER	evoked response
ERCP	endoscopic retrograde cholangiopan-creatography
ESR	erythrocyte sedimentation rate
ESS	Epworth sleepiness scale
ETT	endotracheal tube
FACS	fluorescence-activated cell sorter
FAP	familial polyposis syndrome
FBC	full blood count
FBHH	familial benign hypocalciuric hypercalcaemia
FCHL	familial combined hyperlipidaemia
FDG	fluorodeoxyglucose
FDP	fibrin degradation product
FEV	forced expiratory volume
FFP	fresh frozen plasma
FGF	fibroblast growth factor
FH	familial hypercholesterolaemia
FiO_2	inspired oxygen concentration
FISH	fluorescence *in situ* hybridization
FMRI	functional magnetic resonance imaging
FNA	fine needle aspirate
FOB	faecal occult blood
FPG	fasting plasma glucose
FSH	follicle stimulating hormone

FT4	free T4
FUO	fever of unknown origin
FVC	flow-volume curve
FVL	factor V Leiden
G&S	group & save serum
G6PD	glucose-6-phosphate dehydrogenase
GABA	γ-aminobutyric acid
GAD	glutamic acid decarboxylase
GAn	general anaesthetic
GBM	glomerular basement membrane
GBS	Guillain-Barre Syndrome
GC	gas chromatography
GCS	Glasgow Coma Scale
GFR	glomerular filtration rate
GGT	gamma glutamyl transferase
GH	growth hormone
GHRH	growth hormone releasing hormone
GI	gastrointestinal
GIT	gastrointestinal tract
GLC	gas–liquid chromatography
GM-CSF	granulocytic macrophage colony stimulating factor
GN	glomerulonephritis
GnU	genitourinary
GORD	gastro-oesophageal reflux disease
GPC	gastric parietal cell
GRA	glucocorticoid remediable aldosteronism
GT	glucose tolerance
GTT	glucose tolerance test
GU	gastric ulcer
GvHD	graft versus host disease

HAART	highly active anti-retroviral therapy
HAV	hepatitis A virus
Hb	haemoglobin
HbA_{1c}	haemoglobin A_{1c}
HbC	haemoglobin C
HbE	haemoglobin E
HbF	fetal haemoglobin
HbH	haemoglobin H
HbO	oxyhaemoglobin
HbS	sickle haemoglobin
HbSC	haemoglobin SC
HBV	hepatitis B virus
HC	haemoglobin content
hCG	human chorionic gonadotrophin
Hct	haematocrit
HCV	hepatitis C virus
HD	Hodgkin's disease
HDL	high-density lipoprotein
HDN	haemolytic disease of the newborn
HELLP	haemolysis, elevated liver enzymes, & low platelet count
HEMPAS	hereditary erythroblastin multinuclearity with positive acidified serum lysis test
HEV	hepatitis E
HHT	hereditary haemorrhagic telangiectasia
Hib	*Haemophilus influenzae* type B
HIV	human immunodeficiency virus
HLA	human leucocyte antigen
HNA	heparin neutralizing activity

HNPCC	hereditary non-polyposis colorectal carcinoma	IDA	iminodiacetic acid
		IDDM	insulin dependent (type 1) diabetes mellitus
HNPP	hereditary neuropathy with liability to pressure palsies	IEF	isoelectric focusing
		IF	intrinsic factor
HONK	hyperosmolar non-ketotic	IFA	intrinsic factor antibodies
Hp	haptoglobins	IFCC	International Federation of Clinical Chemistry
HPA	hybridization protection		
		IFG	impaired fasting glucose
HPFH	hereditary persistence of fetal haemoglobin	IFT	immunofluorescence test
HPLC	high-performance liquid chromatography	Ig	immunoglobulin
		IgA	immunoglobulin A
HPOA	hypertrophic pulmonary osteoarthropathy	IgD	immunoglobulin D
		IGE	idiopathic generalized epilepsy
HPV	human papiloma virus	IgE	immunoglobulin E
HRCT	high resolution computed tomography	IGF	insulin-like growth factor
HRT	hormone replacement therapy	IgG	immunoglobulin G
		IgM	immunoglobulin M
HUS	haemolytic-uraemic syndrome	IGT	impaired glucose tolerance
HUVS	hypocomple-mentaemic urticarial vasculitis syndrome	IHD	ischaemic heart disease
		IIH	intracranial hypertension
hx	history	ILR	implantable loop recorder
IABP	intra-aortic balloon pump	IM	intramuscular
IAT	indirect antiglobulin test	INR	international normalized ratio
IBD	inflammatory bowel disease	INR/PT	international normalized ratio/ prothrombin time
IBS	irritable/ bowel syndrome		
ICA	islet cell antibodies	iPRL	hyperprolactinaemia
ICD	internal cardioverter defibrillator	IPSS	inferior petrosal sinus sampling
ICP	intracranial pressure	IQ	intelligence quotient
ICPMS	inductively coupled plasma mass spectroscopy		
ICU	intensive care unit		

ITP	idiopathic thrombocytopenic purpura	LPL	lipoprotein lipase
		LSCC	lateral semicircular canal
ITT	insulin tolerance test		
ITU	intensive therapy unit	LTOT	long-term oxygen therapy
IUP	intrauterine pregnancy		
IV	intravenous	LUQ	left upper quadrent
IVC	inferior vena cava	LV	left ventricle
IVI	intravenous infusion	LVEDP	left ventricular end diastolic pressure
IVU	intravenous urogram		
JME	juvenile myoclonic epilepsy	LVF	left ventricular failure
		MAA	macroaggregatee albumin
JVP	jugular venous pressure		
		MAG	myelin associated glycoprotein
KCCT	kaolin cephalin clotting time		
		MAG3	mercaptoacetyl-triglycine
KCO	transfer coefficient		
KUB	kidney, ureter, bladder (X-ray)	MAHA	microangio pathic haemolytic anaemia
		MAIPA	monoclonal antibody immobilization of platelet antigens
LA	lactic acidosis		
LAn	local anaesthetic		
LAP	leucocyte alkaline phosphatase		
		MALT	mucosa-associated lymphoid tumour
LAt	left atrial		
LC	liver cytosol	MARS	Molecular Absorbance Recirculating Systems
LCM	left costal margin		
LDH	lactate dehydrogenase	MC&S	microscopy, culture, & sensitivity
LDL	low-density lipoprotein		
LDST	low dose dexamethasone suppression test	MCH	mean cell haemoglobin
		MCHC	mean corpuscular haemoglobin concentration
LEMS	Lambert–Eaton myasthenic syndrome		
		MCP	metacarpophalyngeal
LFT	liver function test	MCUG	micturating cystourethrogram
LH	luteinizing hormone		
LHRH	luteinizing hormone releasing hormone	MCV	mean cell volume
		MCVm	mutated citrullinated vimentin
LIF	left iliac fossa		
LKM	liver–kidney microsomal	MD	myotonic dystrophy
		MDMA	methylene dioxymethampetamine or Ecstasy
LMN	lower motor neurone		
LOC	loss of consciousness	MDR	multi-drug-resistant
LP	lumbar puncture	MDRD	Modification of Diet in Renal Disease

MDR-TB	multi-drug-resistant tuberculosis	MR	magnetic resonance
MDS	myelodysplastic syndrome	MRA	magnetic resonance angiogram
MELAS	mitochondrial myopathy, lactic acidosis and stroke-like	MRC	Medical Research Council
		MRCP	magnetic resonance cholangiopan-creatography
MEN	multiple endocrine neoplasia	MRD	minimal residual disease
MEP	motor evoked potentials	MRI	magnetic resonance imaging
MERRF	myoclonic epilepsy and ragged red fibres	mRNA	messenger ribonucleic acid
MetHb	methaemoglobin	MRSA	methicillin-resistant *Staphylococcus aureus*
MG	myasthenia gravis	MS	multiple sclerosis
MGUS	monoclonal gammopathy of undetermined significance	MSD	mean sac diameter
		MSK	musculoskeletal imaging
MHC	major histocompatibility complex	MSp	mass spectroscopy
		MSU	mid-stream urine
MI	myocardial infarction	MTP	metatarsophalangeal
MIBG	nuclear medicine iodine-131-meta-iodoben zylguanide	MUGA	multigated radionuclide angiography
		MUP	motor unit potential
MIC	minimum inhibitory concentration	MUSK	muscle specific kinase
MLC	mixed lymphocyte culture	NAG	N-acetyl-D-glucosaminidase
MLO	mediolateral oblique	NAP	neutrophil alkaline phosphatase
MND	motor neurone disease	NASBA	nucleic acid sequence-based amplification
MoAb	monoclonal antibody	NCS	nerve conduction studies
MODY	maturity onset diabetes of the young		
MP	metacarpophalyngeal	NCSE	non-convulsive status epilepticus
MPA	milli Pascals	NEC	necrotizing enterocolitis
MPD	myeloproliferative disease		
MPHR	max predicted heart rate	NET	neuroendocrine tumour
MPO	myeloperoxidase	NHL	non-Hodgkin's lymphoma
MPV	mean platelet volume		

NHS	National Health Service
NICE	National Institute for Health and Clinical Excellence
NIDDM	non-insulin dependent diabetes mellitus
NK	natural killer
NMS	neuroleptic malignant syndrome
NO	nitric oxide
NPA	nasopharyngeal aspirate
NPH	normal pressure hydrocephalus
NSAID	non-steroidal anti-inflammatory drugs
NSF	nephrogenic systemic fibrosis
NSTEMI	non-ST elevation myocardial infraction
OA	osteoarthritis
OCB	oligoclonal bands
OCP	oral contraceptive pill
OGD	oesophagogas-troduodenoscopy
OGTT	oral glucose tolerance test
OSA	obstructive sleep apnoea
OTC	over the counter
PA	pernicious anaemia
P-A	posteroanterior
PABA	para-amino benzoic acid
$P_aCO_2.$	partial pressure of CO_2 in arterial blood
PACS	picture archiving and communication systems
PAD	peripheral arterial disease
PAN	polyarteritis nodosa

pANCA	perinuclear antineutrophil cytoplasmic antibodies
PAS	periodic acid-Schiff
PB	peripheral blood
PBC	primary biliary cirrhosis
PC	protein C
PCH	paroxysmal cold haemoglobinuria
PCI	percutaneous coronary intervention
PCNA	proliferating cell nuclear antigen
PCO_2	partial passure of CO_2
PCP	*Pneumocystis jirovecii* pneumonia
PCR	polymerase chain reaction
PCrR	protein: creatinine ratio
PCT	procalcitonin
PCV	packed cell volume
PD	Parkinson's disease
PDW	platelet distribution width
PE	pulmonary embolism
PEFR	peak expiratory flow rate
PEG	percutaneous endoscopic gastrostomy
PET	positron emission tomography
PFR	peak flow rate
PICC	peripherally inserted central catheters
PIFT	platelet immunofluorescence tests
PK	pyruvate kinase
PkS	Parkinson's syndrome
PLED	periodic lateralized epileptiform discharges

PLMD	paroxysmal leg movement disorder		qds	*quarter die sumendus* (four times daily)
PmA	pulmonary artery		RA	refractory anaemia
PNH	paroxysmal nocturnal haemoglobinuria		RAPA	rheumatoid arthritis particle agglutination test
PNS	peripheral nervous system		RAS	renal artery stenosis
po	*per os* (by mouth)		RAST	radioallergosorbent test
PO_2	partial pressure of oxygen		RAt	right atrial
PP	pancreatic polypeptide		RBC	red blood cell
ppb	parts per billion		RBP	retinol binding protein
ppd	purified protein derivative		RCC	red cell count
PR	per rectum		RDW	red cell distribution width
P-R	PR interval???		REM	rapid eye movement
PR3	proteinase 3		RES	reticuloendothelial system
PRA	plasma renin activity		RF	rheumatoid factor
PrC	provocation concentration		RFLP	restriction fragment length polymorphisms
PRL	prolactin		RhA	rheumatoid arthritis
PRV	polycythemia rubra vera		RhMK	Rhesus monkey kidney
PS	protein S		RIA	radioimmunoassay
PSA	prostate specific antigen		RiCoF	Ristocetin Cofactor
PT	prothrombin time		RID	radial immunodiffusion
PTC	percutaneous transhepatic cholangiogram		RIF	right iliac fossa
			RIPA	ristocetin-induced platelet aggregation
PTH	parathyroid hormone		RNP	ribonucleoprotein
PTTK	partial thromboplastin time with kaolin		RNV	radionuclide ventriculography
PUO	pyrexia of unknown origin		RSV	respiratory syncytial virus
PV	plasma volume		RTA	renal tubular acidosis
PvC	provocation concentration		rTMS	repetitive transcranial magnetic stimulation
PW	pulse wave		RUQ	right upper quadrant
PWI	perfusion weighted imaging		RV	right ventricle
			Rx	treatment
PxCT	proximal convoluted tubule		SAA	serum amyloid A
			SAAG	serum ascites albumin gradient

SAH	subarachnoid haemorrhage		SSPE	subacute sclerosing panencephalilits
SaO_2	arterial oxygen saturation		SSR	somatostatin receptor
SARS	severe acute repiratory syndrome		STD	sexually transmitted diseases
SB	Sudan black		STEMI	ST-elevation myocardial infarction
SBE	subacute bacterial endocarditis		sTfR	serum transferrin receptor
SBO	small bowel obstruction		StFR	soluble transferrin receptor assay
SBP	spontaneous bacterial peritonitis		SUV	standardized uptake value
sbt	serum bactericidal test		SVC	superior vena cava
SC	subcutaneous		SWS	slow wave sleep
SCID	severe combined immunodeficiency		SXR	skull X-ray
SCLC	small cell lung cancer		T1W	T1-weighted
SDH	subdural haemorrhage		T2W	T2-weighted
SeHCAT	^{75}selenium homotaurocholate		TA	temporal arteritis
SG	specific gravity		TB	tuberculosis
SHBG	sex-hormone-binding globulin		TCR	T cell receptor
SI	Systeme International		TCT	thrombin clotting time
SIADH	syndrome of inappropriate antidiuretic hormone		tds	*ter die sumendus* (three times daily)
SLA	soluble liver antigen		TfR	transferrin receptor
SLE	systemic lupus erythematosus		TFT	thyroid function test
SMA	smooth muscle antibody		Tg	thyroglobulin
SNAP	sensory nerve action potential		TIA	transient ischaemic attack
SOB	short of breath		TIBC	total iron binding capacity
SOD	sphincter of Oddi dysfunction		TIPS	transjugular intrahepatic portosystemic stent shunt
SOL	space-occupying lesion		TLC	thin layer chromatography
SPECT	single photon emission computed tomography		TMS	transcranial magnetic stimulation
SSP	Single strand polymorphism		TN	trigeminal neuralgia
			tPA	tissue plasminogen activator

TPHA	treponema palidum haemagglutination assay		vCJD	variant Creutzfeldt–Jakob disease
TPN	total parenteral nutrition		VDRL	Venereas Disease Research Laboratory
TPO	thyroid peroxidise		VEP	visual evoked potential
TRALI	transfusion-related acute lung injury		VHF	viral haemorrhagic fever
TRAP	tartrate-resistant acid phosphatase		VHL	von Hippel–Lindau
			VIII	factor VIII
TRH	thyrotropin releasing hormone		VIP	vasoactive intestinal peptide
TRP	tubular reabsorption of phosphate		VLCFA	very long chain fatty acid
TSE	transmissible spongiform encephalopathy		VLDL	very low density lipoprotein
			VO_2	oxygen uptake
TSH	thyroid stimulating hormone		VP	vasoactive peptide
TTE	transthoracic echocardiogram		VSD	ventricular septal defect
tTG	tissue transglutaminase		VTE	venous thromboembolism
TTP	thrombotic thrombocytopenic purpura		vWD	von Willebrand's disease
U&E	urea & electrolytes		vWF Ag	vonWillebrand factor antigen
UCTD	undifferentiated connective tissue disease		WBC	white blood count/cells
UFC	urinary-free cortisol		WCE	wireless capsule endoscopy
UMN	upper motor neurone		WHO	World Health Organization
US	ultrasound		XDP	cross-linked fibrin degradation products
USS	ultrasound scan		XLA	X-linked agammaglobulinaemia
UTI	urinary tract infection			
UV	ultraviolet		ZN	Ziehl–Neelsen
V/Q	ventilation/perfusion		ZPP	zinc protoporphyrin
VATS	video-assisted thoracic surgery			

Approach to investigations

Why do tests?

Patients seldom present to their doctors with *diagnoses*—rather, they have symptoms or signs. The major challenge of medicine is being able to talk to the patient and obtain a history, then carry out a physical examination looking for pointers to their likely underlying problem. Our elders and, some would argue, betters in medicine had fewer tests available to them than we have today, and their diagnoses were often made solely from the history and examination. Of course, they would claim that their clinical acumen and skills were greater than ours, and that we rely too heavily on the huge armoury of laboratory and other investigations available today. This, in part, is probably true, but we cannot ignore the fact that advances in science and technology have spawned a bewildering array of very useful and sophisticated tests that help us to confirm our diagnostic suspicions.

By 'test' we mean the measurement of a component of blood, marrow or other body fluid or physiological parameter to determine whether the patient's value falls within or outside the normal range, either suggesting the diagnosis or, in some cases, actually making the diagnosis for us.

Factors affecting variable parameters in health

Many measurable body constituents vary throughout life. For example, a newborn baby has an extremely high haemoglobin concentration, which falls after delivery. This is completely normal and is *physiological*, rather than *pathological*. A haemoglobin level this high in an adult would be pathological, since it is far outside the normal range for the adult population.

Factors affecting measurable variables

- Age.
- Sex.
- Ethnicity.
- Altitude.
- Build.
- Physiological conditions (e.g. at rest, after exercise, standing, lying).
- Sampling methods (e.g. with or without using tourniquet).
- Storage and age of sample.
- Container used, e.g. for blood sample, as well as anticoagulant.
- Method of analysis.

Reference ranges (normal values)

These are published for most measurable components of blood and other tissue, and we have included the normal ranges for most blood and CSF analytes at the end of the book.

What makes a test useful?

A really good test, and one that would make us appear to be outstanding doctors, would be one that would *always* be positive in the presence of a disease and would be *totally* specific for that disease alone; such a test would never be positive in patients who did not have the disorder. What we mean is that what we are looking for are *sensitive* tests that are *specific* for a given disease. Sadly, most tests are neither 100% sensitive nor 100% specific, but some do come very close.

How to use tests and the laboratory

Rather than request tests in a shotgun or knee-jerk fashion, where every box on a request form is ticked, it is far better to use the laboratory selectively. Even with the major advances in automation where tests are batched and are cheaper, the hospital budget is finite and sloppy requesting should be discouraged.

Outline your differential diagnoses: what are the likeliest diseases given the patient's history, examination findings, and population the patient comes from?

Decide which test(s) will help you make the diagnosis: request these and review the diagnosis in the light of the test results. Review the patient and arrange further investigations as necessary.

The downside of tests

It is important to remember that tests may often give 'normal' results even in the presence of disease. For example, a normal ECG in the presence of chest pain does *not* exclude the occurrence of myocardial infarction with 100% certainty. Conversely, the presence of an abnormality does not necessarily imply that a disease is present. This, of course, is where clinical experience comes into its own—the more experienced clinician will be able to balance the likelihood of disease with the results available even if some of the test results give unexpected answers.

Sensitivity & specificity	
Sensitivity	% of patients with the disease and in whom the test is positive
Specificity	% of people without the disease in whom the test is negative

Quick-fix clinical experience

This simply does not exist. Talking to patients and examining them for physical signs and assimilating knowledge gained in medical school are absolute requirements for attainment of sound clinical judgement. Those students and doctors who work from books alone do not survive effectively at the coal face! It is a constant source of irritation to medical students and junior doctors, when a senior doctor asks for the results of an investigation on the ward round and you find this test is the one that clinches the diagnosis. How *do* they do it? Like appreciating good wine—they develop a nose for it. You can learn a great deal by watching your registrar or consultant make decisions. This forms of basis of your *own* clinical experience.

Laboratory errors and how to avoid them

It is a fact of life that the sophisticated automated analysers in current use are not 100% accurate 100% of the time, but they come pretty close. In order to keep errors to a minimum, precautions need to be taken when sampling biological material, e.g. blood.

Minimizing spurious results using blood samples

- Use correct bottle.
- Fill to line (if anticoagulant used). This is less of a worry when vacuum sample bottles are used since these should take in exactly the correct amount of blood, ensuring the correct blood:anticoagulant ratio. This is critical for coagulation tests.
- Try to get the sample to the laboratory as quickly as possible. Blood samples left lying around on warm windowsills, or even overnight at room temperature, will produce bizarre results, e.g. crenated RBCs and abnormal-looking WBCs in old EDTA samples.
- Try to avoid rupturing red cells when taking the sample (e.g. using narrow gauge needle, prolonged time to collect whole sample) otherwise a 'haemolysed' sample will be received by the laboratory. This may cause spurious results for some parameters (e.g. $[K^+]$).
- Remember to mix (not shake) samples containing anticoagulant.

Variations in normal ranges in health

As discussed earlier, most of the normal ranges for blood parameters discussed in this book are for non-pregnant adults. The reason for this is that blood values, e.g. Hb, RCC, are high in the newborn and many FBC, coagulation, and other parameters undergo changes in pregnancy.

Part I

The patient

Chapter 1

Symptoms & signs

Abdominal distension

Patients may describe generalized abdominal swelling or localized fullness in a specific area of the abdomen.

In the history enquire specifically about
- Change in bowel habit.
- Weight loss.
- Associated pain.

Generalized swelling

Consider
- Fat.
- Fluid.
- Faeces.
- Flatus.
- Fetus.
- Full bladder.

Ascites

Fluid in the peritoneal cavity. Look for shifting dullness and fluid thrill on percussion, stigmata of chronic liver disease, lymphadenopathy, oedema and assess jugular venous pressure (JVP).

Causes
- Malignancy.
- Cirrhosis/portal hypertension.
- Hypoproteinaemia.
- Right heart failure.

Investigations
- Urea & electrolytes (U&E).
- Liver function test (LFTs).
- Serum albumin.
- Ascitic tap for cytology, microscopy, culture, & sensitivity (MC&S).
- Serum-ascites albumin gradient.
- Ultrasound scan (USS) abdomen.
(See Fig. 1.1).

Flatus

Gaseous distension. Need to exclude bowel obstruction. Assess for colicky abdominal pain, bowel habit, flatus, and vomiting. Look for resonant distension on percussion, altered or absent bowel sounds, focal tenderness with rebound and guarding. Always check for herniae and perform PR examination in suspected obstruction.

Causes
- **Intraluminal**: faecal impaction, gallstone ileus.
- **Luminal**: inflammatory stricture (e.g. Crohn's), tumour, abscess.
- **Extraluminal**: herniae, adhesions, pelvic mass, lymphadenopathy, volvulus, intussusception.
- **Paralytic ileus**: drug-induced, electrolyte disturbances.

- **Age-related causes of obstruction**.
- **Neonatal**: congenital atresia, imperforate anus, volvulus, Hirschsprung's disease, meconium ileus.
- **Infants**: intussusception, Hirschsprung's, herniae, Meckel's diverticulum.
- **Young/middle age adults**: herniae, adhesions, Crohn's.
- **Elderly**: herniae, carcinoma, diverticulitis, faecal impaction.

Investigations
- Full blood count (FBC).
- U&E.
- Abdominal X-ray (AXR; erect and supine).
- Consider barium enema, barium follow-through, sigmoidoscopy, surgical intervention for complete acute obstruction.

Localized swelling/masses: common causes according to site

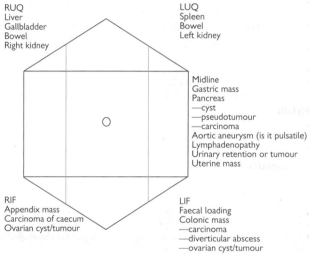

RUQ
Liver
Gallbladder
Bowel
Right kidney

LUQ
Spleen
Bowel
Left kidney

Midline
Gastric mass
Pancreas
—cyst
—pseudotumour
—carcinoma
Aortic aneurysm (is it pulsatile)
Lymphadenopathy
Urinary retention or tumour
Uterine mass

RIF
Appendix mass
Carcinoma of caecum
Ovarian cyst/tumour

LIF
Faecal loading
Colonic mass
—carcinoma
—diverticular abscess
—ovarian cyst/tumour

Fig. 1.1 Main causes of abdominal swelling according to site.

Investigate according to site
- Consider USS abdomen and pelvis.
- Computed tomography (CT) scanning.
- Barium studies.
- IVU.

📖 *OHCM* 8e, p57, p606.

Abdominal pain

Abdominal pain may be acute or chronic. Severe, acute pain may indicate a surgical emergency, including perforation, peritonitis, or obstruction. Assess nature and radiation of pain, clinical status of patient, including fever, tachycardia, and hypotension.

Common causes of abdominal pain according to site

- **Epigastric pain**: peptic ulcer disease, gastritis or duodenal erosions, cholecystitis, pancreatitis. early appendicitis.
- **Periumbilical**: pancreatitis, mesenteric artery ischaemia (older patient with vascular disease).
- **Right upper quadrant (RUQ) pain**: biliary colic, cholecystitis, hepatitis, peptic ulcer.
- **Left upper quadrant (LUQ) pain**: splenic, peptic ulcer.
- **Loin pain**: renal colic (colicky radiating loin → groin), pyelonephritis, renal pathology.
- **Left iliac fossa (LIF) pain**: constipation, diverticular disease, irritable bowel syndrome, pelvic referred pain, inflammatory bowel disease.
- **Right iliac fossa (RIF) pain**: appendicitis, pelvic referred pain, inflammatory bowel disease (e.g. Crohn's of terminal ileum).
- **Suprapubic**: urinary tract infection (UTI), cystitis, salpingitis.
- **Generalized**: gastroenteritis, irritable bowel, constipation, generalized peritonitis. mesenteric adenitis (in children, aka abdominal migraine).

Pitfalls

- **Metabolic causes**: e.g. diabetic ketoacidosis, hypercalcaemia, Addison's disease, porphyria, lead poisoning.
- **Atypical referred pain**: e.g. myocardial infarction, pneumonia.

Investigations

- FBC.
- U&E, e.g. deranged electrolytes following vomiting, diarrhoea, or bowel obstruction.
- Plasma glucose.
- Serum amylase (↑ in pancreatitis and bowel obstruction).
- Urinalysis and mid-stream urine (MSU), e.g. haematuria, proteinuria, glucose.
- LFTs (consider obstructive vs. hepatitic picture).
- Plain AXR (erect and supine to assess for perforation and bowel obstruction).
- Kidney, ureter, bladder (KUB) X-ray for renal tract calculi.
- USS abdomen, particularly for biliary tract, gallbladder and renal tract.
- Intravenous urogram (IVU) to assess for renal tract calculi/pathology.

📖 *OHCM* 8e, p57, p608.

Alteration of behaviour

This is usually reported by a relative or friend, rather than by the patient. Often the patient will have little or no insight into the disease, and taking a history can be difficult. In addition, to a full general and neurological physical examination a mental state examination is required.

Find out if this is the first episode of altered behaviour or if the episodes are recurrent. Is there a gradual change in behaviour (and personality) over time?

Acute delirium

Causes
- Sepsis (common).
- Acute intracranial event, e.g. haemorrhage.
- Metabolic disturbance, e.g. uraemia, hypercalcaemia (common).
- Intracerebral tumour (including meningioma).
- Drugs, especially interactions in elderly.
- Alcohol (and withdrawal syndrome).
- Hypoxia (common).
- Hypoglycaemia (iatrogenic in diabetic patients receiving insulin treatment, or oral insulin secretagogues, or insulinoma and other causes).

Dementia

- Alzheimer's (common), Pick's (rare).
- Vascular, e.g. multi-infarct.
- Huntington's chorea.
- Vitamin B_{12} deficiency (severe).
- Hypothyroidism (severe).
- Wilson's disease.
- Alcoholism.
- Normal pressure hydrocephalus.

NB 'Frontal lobe syndrome' from space-occupying lesion (SOL), e.g. meningioma. Presents with disinhibition, impaired social functioning, primitive reflexes, e.g. grasp reflex.

Anxiety states

Usually psychogenic, but consider organic possibilities such as
- Phaeochromocytoma (rare).
- Hyperthyroidism (common).
- Paroxysmal atrial tachycardia (fairly common).
- Alcohol withdrawal (usually history of excessive alcohol intake).

Psychosis

- Schizophrenia.
- Bipolar disorder or pseudo-dementia in:
  - Systemic lupus erythematosus (SLE).
  - Cushing's syndrome.
  - Multiple sclerosis.
  - Thyrotoxicosis ('apathetic' thyrotoxicosis in the elderly).

Temporal lobe epilepsy
Temporary disturbance of content of consciousness.

Investigations: guided by history and examination
- U&E.
- Glucose (in non-diabetics take fasting venous plasma in fluoride oxalate tube with simultaneous serum or plasma for insulin concentration, e.g. suspected insulinoma).
- CXR.
- LFTs.
- Thyroid function tests (TFTs).
- FBC.
- Erythrocyte sedimentation rate (ESR).
- Urinalysis (protein, nitrites, glucose).
- Cranial CT scan.
- Serum vitamin B_{12}.
- Arterial blood gases (ABGs) ± carboxyhaemoglobin.
- Blood cultures.

Consider
- Syphilis serology.
- Human immunodeficiency virus (HIV) test.
- Urine drug screen (□ Chapter 11).
- Blood ethanol level (may be low in withdrawal state).
- Electroencephalogram (EEG).
- 24 h electrocardiogram (ECG).
- Sleep study.

Alteration in bowel habit

A change in bowel habit in an adult should always alert you to the possibility of bowel cancer. Ask about associated features—PR bleeding, tenesmus, weight loss, mucus, abdominal pain, or bloating.

Has the patient started any new medications, including 'over the counter'? Look for signs of systemic disease.

Consider
- Carcinoma of the colon.
- Diverticular disease.
- Irritable bowel syndrome (IBS).
- Constipation with overflow diarrhoea.
- All of the above may present with alternating diarrhoea and constipation.

Investigations
- Digital rectal examination.
- Proctoscopy.
- Sigmoidoscopy (rigid/flexible).
- Colonoscopy.
- Barium enema.
- CT colonography.

📖 Diarrhoea (p32), 📖 Constipation (p29), 📖 Incontinence: faecal (p61).

Anaemia

Reduced Hb, no specific cause implied (and *not a diagnosis in itself, so don't be complacent*): ♂ < 13.5g/dL, ♀ < 11.5g/dL. Often associated with non-specific symptoms, such as fatigue, poor concentration, shortness of breath and dizziness. Older patients may experience palpitations and exacerbation of angina, congestive cardiac failure, or claudication.

Signs

Pallor of conjunctivae and skin creases, nail pallor, and koilonychia (spoon-shaped nails, very rare finding in severe chronic iron deficiency), angular cheilitis, and glossitis. Most of these signs are unreliable and it is difficult to gauge anaemia from skin signs alone.

Causes

There are two common approaches to assess anaemia.

Red cell dynamics
- ↑ Red blood cell (RBC) loss/breakdown, e.g. haemolysis (congenital or acquired) or bleeding.
- ↓ RBC production, e.g. vitamin/mineral deficiency, marrow suppression/infiltration, myelodysplasia, haemoglobin disorders (e.g. thalassaemia), chronic disease, renal failure.

Red cell indices (Table 1.1)

Table 1.1 Some causes of anaemia based on the mean cell volume (MCV)

Microcytic/ hypochromic	↓ MCV, ↓ mean corpuscular haemoglobin concentration (MCHC), e.g. Fe deficiency, thalassaemia, anaemia of chronic disease
Macrocytic	↑ MCV Reticulocytosis (polychromasia on blood film), B_{12} or folate deficiency, chronic liver disease, hypothyroidism, alcohol, myelodysplasia
Normocytic, normochromic	↔ MCV & MCHC anaemia of chronic disease, e.g. chronic infection, inflammation, inflammatory disease or malignancy, acute blood loss, renal failure, myeloma

Investigations

FBC and film
Assessment of RBC indices helps direct investigation as above.

Microcytic
- Check iron stores (ferritin or soluble transferrin receptor assay).
  NB Ferritin is ↑ in acute inflammation and may be misleading. Iron/total iron binding capacity (TIBC) no longer used for assessment of iron deficiency (☐ Assessment of iron status, p226).
- Consider thalassaemia screening if not iron deficient (i.e. ↓ MCV ↔ ferritin).

- If iron deficient, assess dietary history (vegetarians) and look for risk factors for blood loss and increased demands.
- **Premenopausal women**: assess menstrual losses.
- **Pregnancy/infants/adolescence**: consider physiological ($\uparrow$ requirements).
- **All others**: look for source of blood loss. Gastrointestinal (GI) tract is most common source. Consider oesophagogastroduodenoscopy (OGD) and/or colonoscopy if clinically indicated by symptoms and barium studies.

Macrocytic
- Reticulocyte count.
- Serum B_{12} and red cell folate levels.
- If folate deficient: assess dietary history and physiological requirements.
- If B_{12} deficient: rarely dietary cause alone, usually an associated pathology. Pernicious anaemia (PA) is the most common cause: check parietal cell antibodies (90% patients with PA are +ve, but seen in other causes of gastric atrophy, especially in older individuals) and/or intrinsic factor antibodies (+ve in only 50% with PA, but specific). Consider ileal disease and malabsorption.
- LFTs.
- Thyroid function.

Normocytic
- Blood film.
- ESR.
- Renal function.
- Consider myeloma screen in older adults (immunoglobulins (Igs), protein electrophoresis, urine Bence–Jones protein (BJP). Skeletal survey of value if paraprotein or BJP).
- Autoimmune screen to exclude connective tissue disease.

Haemolysis screen
- FBC, MCV ($\uparrow$ due to reticulocytosis—these are larger than RBCs).
- Blood film (spherocytes, polychromasia, bite cells, red cell fragmentation).
- Reticulocyte count.
- Serum bilirubin and serum lactate dehydrogenase (LDH).
- Haptoglobins (absent in haemolysis).
- Direct antibody test (DAT; old term is direct Coombs' test).

Consider
- **Congenital haemolytic anaemias**: membrane defects, enzyme deficiencies (e.g. G6PD, pyruvate kinase).
- **Disseminated intravascular coagulation (DIC)/microangiopathic haemolysis**: DIC screen.

Anaphylaxis

Defined as a systemic reaction (local oral angioedema is *not* anaphylaxis), with any or all of the following:
- Stridor (laryngeal obstruction).
- Wheeze (bronchospasm).
- Generalized urticaria and/or angioedema.
- Hypotension ± loss of consciousness.
- Abdominal pain/cramps, vomiting, and diarrhoea.

NB. Not all patients have urticaria or rash—only 50% will do so.

Differentiate IgE-mediated reactions (*anaphylaxis*) from non-IgE mediated reactions (*anaphylactoid*)—due to direct mast cell degranulation).

Causes
- Drugs (especially antibiotics, muscle relaxants, anaesthetics).
- Foods (peanuts, sesame, nuts, fish, shellfish, egg, fruits, vegetables).
- Venoms (bee, wasp).
- Latex.
- Food-dependent, exercise-induced.
- Idiopathic.

Investigations
- If uncertain of nature of reaction, check mast cell tryptase (raised in any condition with mast cell activation) (📕 Mast cell tryptase, p346).
- Checking specific IgE ('RAST tests') acutely at time of reaction can give false negatives.
- Consider referral to nearest Allergy/Immunology Centre for further investigation and advice on management.

Angioedema

Angioedema is deep tissue swelling, which is non-itchy. May be premonitory tingling. May occur with or without urticaria. Caused by bradykinin not histamine.

Causes
- As for urticaria; also hereditary angioedema (rare).
- Also think of drugs—these are the commonest cause:
  - Angiotensin converting enyme (ACE) inhibitors (elevated bradykinin levels due to inhibition of breakdown).
  - AT-II receptor antagonists.
  - Statins.
  - Proton pump inhibitors.
  - Non-steroidal anti-inflammatory drugs (NSAIDs).

May also be seen in patients with autoimmune disease, such as lupus and RhA (antibodies against C1q) and in older patients in association with paraproteins (myeloma, lymphoma).
  Angioedema *with* urticaria is *not* due to hereditary angioedema.

Investigations
Check drug history first! If drugs are suspected, then stop drugs and wait! If no drugs involved, then investigate.

Angioedema WITH urticaria

Investigate as for urticaria.

Angioedema WITHOUT urticaria

- Complement C3 & C4.
- If C4 low check C1-esterase inhibitor (immunochemical and functional).
- Serum immunoglobulins and electrophoresis.
- Autoantibody screen.
- Full blood count and ESR.
- Thyroid function.
- Liver function.

Anorexia

This describes a loss of appetite for food and is associated with a wide range of disorders. In fact, anorexia is a fairly common consequence of underlying disease and represents a general undernourishment. Anorexia *per se* is associated with increased morbidity especially when present in patients undergoing surgery; post-operative infection is more common, as is prolongation of the hospital stay.

The extent to which it will be investigated depends on the general status of the patient, and the presence and duration of any symptoms or signs. Clinical judgement will help! Dieticians can be very helpful.

Causes

- Anorexia nervosa.
- Depressive illness.
- Stress.
- Cancers: any, including carcinoma of stomach, oesophagus, metastatic, leukaemia or lymphoma.
- Drugs, including chemotherapy.
- Radiotherapy.
- Renal failure.
- Hypercalcaemia.
- Infections.
- Cigarette smoking.

Investigations

- Full history and examination.
- **FBC**: looking for anaemia or non-specific changes seen in underlying disease.
- **ESR**: may be elevated in inflammatory disorders.
- U&E.
- LFTs.
- Serum Ca^{2+}.
- Chest X-ray (CXR), e.g. lung cancer, tuberculosis (TB), etc.
- Cultures of blood, sputum, urine, stool if pyrexial, and/or localizing symptoms or signs.

Anuria

Anuria denotes absent urine production. Oliguria (<400mL urine/24 h) is more common than anuria. A catheter must be passed to confirm an empty bladder.

Causes
- **Urinary retention**: prostatic hypertrophy, pelvic mass, drugs, e.g. tricyclic antidepressants, spinal cord lesions.
- Blocked in-dwelling urinary catheter.
- **Obstruction of the ureters**: tumour, stone, sloughed papillae (bilateral).
- **Intrinsic renal failure**: acute glomerulonephritis, acute interstitial nephritis, acute tubular necrosis, rhabdomyolysis.
- **Pre-renal failure**: dehydration, septic shock, cardiogenic shock.

An urgent ultrasound of the renal tract must be performed and any physical obstruction relieved as quickly as possible, directly (urethral catheter) or indirectly (nephrostomy).

▶▶*Renal function and serum electrolytes must be measured without delay.*

Further tests as clinically indicated
- FBC.
- Blood cultures.
- ABGs.
- Uric acid.
- Autoimmune profile.
- ESR.
- Creatine kinase (CK).
- Prostate specific antigen (PSA, prostatic carcinoma).
- Serum Ca^{2+} & PO_4^{3-}.
- 12-lead ECG.
- CXR.
- CVP measurement via central line (to guide IV fluids).
- MSU (urinary tract infection (UTI)).
- Urine microscopy (for casts).
- Urine osmolality, sodium, creatinine, urea concentrations.
- IVU (📖 p744).
- Urinary stone analysis, if available.
- CT pelvis.
- Renal biopsy (if intrinsic renal disease suspected, normal-sized kidneys).

📖 *OHCM* 8e, p298.

Ataxia

Ataxia is an impaired ability to co-ordinate limb movements. There must be no motor paresis (e.g. monoparesis) or involuntary movements (e.g. the characteristic cog-wheel tremor in Parkinson's disease is not ataxia).

Ataxia may be
- Cerebellar.
- Vestibular.
- Sensory.

Note: Many forms of ataxia are hereditary (but are uncommon).

Hereditary causes
- Friedreich's ataxia.
- Ataxia telangiectasia.
- Spinocerebellar ataxia.
- Corticocerebellar atrophy.
- Olivopontocerebellar atrophy.
- Hereditary spastic paraplegia.
- Xeroderma pigmentosa.

Investigations
- Family studies.
- Genetic analysis (discuss with regional genetics laboratory—counselling may be required).

Vestibular ataxia
- Acute alcohol intoxication.
- Labyrinthitis.

Sensory ataxia
- Loss of proprioception—peripheral neuropathy, dorsal column disease.
- Visual disturbance.

Investigations
- Venous plasma glucose (diabetic neuropathy).
- Serum vitamin B_{12} (subacute combined degeneration of the cord—rare, but serious).
- LFTs.
- Cryoglobulins.

Cerebellar ataxia
- Demyelinating diseases, e.g. multiple sclerosis (MS).
- Cerebellar infarct or haemorrhage.
- Alcoholic cerebellar degeneration.
- **Cerebellar tumour**: primary in children, metastases in adults.
  Note: Von Hippel–Lindau disease (📖 *OHCM* 8e, p726).
- Nutritional deficiency:
  - Vitamin E
  - Vitamin B_{12}.
  - Thiamine.
- Cerebellar abscess.

- Drugs (supratherapeutic blood levels):
  - Carbamazepine.
  - Phenytoin.
- Tuberculoma.
- Paraneoplastic syndrome.
- Developmental.
- Arnold–Chiari malformation.
- Dandy–Walker syndrome.
- Paget's disease of skull.
- Wilson's disease (hepatolenticular degeneration).
- Hypothyroidism.
- Creutzfeldt–Jakob disease and other chronic infections.
- Miller Fisher syndrome.
- Normal pressure hydrocephalus.

Ataxia should be distinguished from movement disorders, e.g.

- **Chorea**: Huntington's, Sydenham's, thyrotoxicosis (very rare).
- **Athetosis**:
  - *Hemiballismus*—characteristic movement disorder; rare.
  - *Tardive dyskinesia*—chronic phenothiazine therapy.

Investigations

- Cranial CT.
- Magnetic resonance imaging (MRI) brain (if demyelination suspected).
- CXR (cerebellar metastases from bronchogenic carcinoma; paraneoplastic syndrome).
- TFTs.
- Triple evoked potentials (demyelination). Not routinely used to diagnose MS now.
- Lumbar puncture (LP; 📖 Lumbar puncture, p546).
- LFTs.
- Serum drug concentrations esp. anticonvulsants.
- Serum vitamin B_{12}.
- Erythrocyte transketolase (↓ in thiamine deficiency, e.g. alcoholism).
- Isotope bone scan (Paget's, metastases).
- Serum alkaline phosphatase (ALP)—bone isoenzyme (Paget's, metastases).
- Urine hydroxyproline (Paget's disease—reflects bone turnover).
- Caeruloplasmin (Wilson's disease).
- Serum and urine copper (Wilson's disease).

Consider whether the movement disorder is psychogenic (uncommon), rather than due to neuropathology, but uncommon and should not be confidently assumed.

📖 *OHCM* 8e, p383.

Bradycardia

Bradycardia is defined as a heart rate < 60beats/min. It is a normal physiological response to fitness training, but should always be considered a marker of potential cardiac disease until proved otherwise.

Causes

A comprehensive history and thorough examination are important. A transient bradycardia can cause disabling symptoms of dizziness or blackouts in the elderly, whilst persistent bradycardia often heralds systemic disease, e.g.:

- **Iatrogenic**: cardiac drugs, e.g. β-blockers (including eye drops for glaucoma), amiodarone, and calcium channel blockers, e.g. diltiazem and verapamil, cause sinus bradycardia; digoxin (atrioventricular block). The likelihood of extreme bradycardia or heart block is increased with combination therapy.
- **Cardiac causes**: acute myocardial infarction (often transient in inferior myocardial infarction), coronary artery disease, sick sinus syndrome, myocardial disease (amyloid, Chagas' disease, sarcoid, myocarditis).
- Increased vagal tone associated with nausea and vomiting.
- Diminished sympathetic activity.
- **Physiological**: bradycardia is normal in sleep and in athletes.
- **Hypothyroidism**: associated with characteristic symptoms and signs.
- ↑ Intracranial pressure, e.g. cerebral tumour.
- **Hypothermia**: e.g. myxoedema coma.
- **Metabolic**: severe hyperkalaemia, anorexia.
- **Toxic**: severe jaundice.
- **Drug toxicity**: opiates.
- **Infective**: inappropriate bradycardia seen in diphtheria, typhoid.

Investigations

12-lead ECG to identify underlying rhythm.

If there are symptoms of chest pain
- Serum troponin and creatine kinase.
- Bedside ECG monitoring.
- Exercise ECG.

If there is a history of intermittent dizziness
24 h ambulatory ECG monitoring, patient-activated event recorder, or implantable loop recorder, depending on the frequency of symptoms.

If indicated by clinical presentation, consider
- Thyroid function tests (hypothyroidism).
- Low reading thermometer (hypothermia—check for J waves on ECG).
- CT brain scan (?intracranial pathology).
- U&E.
- LFTs (especially bilirubin).
- Toxicology screen.

📖 *OHCM* 8e, p68, p119.

Breathlessness

Breathlessness (dyspnoea) is the subjective awareness of difficulty in breathing. Almost universal during exercise, it is a common presenting symptom in a broad spectrum of disease. A comprehensive history and thorough examination are, therefore, essential. Speed of symptom onset, patient's age and occupation, and local disease prevalence are particularly helpful in devising a differential diagnosis and a guide to investigations.

Causes
- **Acute pulmonary disease**: pneumonia, acute asthma, pulmonary embolus, inhaled foreign body, pneumothorax, acute respiratory distress.
- **Chronic pulmonary disease**: emphysema, chronic bronchitis, ruptured bulla, interstitial disease (sarcoid, fibrosing alveolitis, extrinsic alveolitis, pneumoconiosis).
- **Carcinoma**: bronchogenic carcinoma, lymphangitis carcinomatosis, secondary (2°) carcinoma.
- **Acute cardiac disease**: acute myocardial infarction (and associated complications of pulmonary oedema, ventricular septal defect, mitral valve chordal rupture, and arrhythmias).
- **Chronic cardiac disease**: left ventricular dysfunction, valvular heart disease (mitral or aortic stenosis and regurgitation), ischaemic heart disease, pulmonary hypertension, pleural effusion, arrhythmias (especially atrial fibrillation).
- **Metabolic**: poisoning from salicylates, methanol and ethylene glycol, diabetic ketoacidosis, lactic acidosis, hepatic and renal failure.
- **Neuromuscular**: intercostal muscle/diaphragmatic weakness due to Guillain–Barré syndrome, muscular dystrophy.
- **Haematological**: anaemia.
- Anxiety and hyperventilation.
- **Morphological**: kyphoscoliosis, obesity.
- **Laryngeal obstruction**: extrinsic compression (retrosternal goitre), angioedema (often acute drug allergy), laryngeal spasm (hypocalcaemia).

Initial investigations
- FBC.
- U&E.
- Glucose.
- CXR.
- ABGs.
- Peak expiratory flow rate.
- 12-lead ECG.

Additional investigations (as indicated)

- Transthoracic echocardiography.
- 24h ambulatory ECG monitoring.
- Pulmonary function tests.
- CT chest.
- Bronchoscopy.
- V/Q scan/CTPA.
- LFTs.
- Ca^{2+}.
- ESR.
- Serum salicylate levels.
- Lactate.
- Lung biopsy.

📖 *OHCM* 8e, p5, p796.

Bruising

Easy bruising is a common complaint and warrants careful assessment of onset and nature. Recent onset of spontaneous and unusual bruising or bleeding may suggest a serious acquired defect. A lifelong history of bruising and bleeding (e.g. post-tonsillectomy, dental extraction, or surgery) may imply a congenital defect. Family history may be informative.

Examine: skin, mouth, dependent areas, and fundi for mucocutaneous bleeding and purpura (non-blanching haemorrhages into the skin).

Platelet causes

- Thrombocytopenia or platelet dysfunction (e.g. aspirin).
- Marrow failure, infiltration, idiopathic thrombocytopenic purpura (ITP), DIC, hypersplenism, drugs or alcohol.

Vascular causes

- **Congenital**: e.g. Osler–Weber–Rendu syndrome.
- **Acquired**: e.g. senile purpura, vasculitis (Henoch–Schönlein purpura, infection), diabetes, corticosteroid therapy, scurvy, connective tissue diseases.

Coagulopathy

- **Congenital**: mucocutaneous bruising is suggestive of a platelet-mediated defect (e.g. von Willebrand's disease, Glanzmann's thrombasthenia), rather than clotting factor deficiency (e.g. haemophilia A and B).
- **Acquired**: e.g. DIC, vitamin K deficiency.

Hyperviscosity

Myeloma, Waldenström's macroglobulinaemia (low grade lymphoma associated with ↑ IgM and ↑ plasma viscosity), ↑↑ WBC in leukaemia.

Investigations

- FBC and film.
- **Coagulation**: international normalized ratio (INR) and activated partial thromboplastin time ratio (APTR).
- **Bleeding time**: measures platelet and vascular phase.
- **DIC screen**: including fibrinogen, thrombin time, D-dimers or fibrin degradation products (FDPs).

Consider further tests and referral to haematology for

- Factor assays.
- Platelet aggregation studies to assess platelet function.

📖 *OHCM* 8e, p338.

Calf swelling

Assess whether swelling is bilateral or unilateral, precipitating factors, and duration of onset. Careful examination of the affected leg should be extended to a full examination, particularly of abdominal and cardiovascular systems.

Causes

Venous and lymphatic
- Deep vein thrombosis (DVT).
- Superficial thrombophlebitis.
- Varicose veins.
- Post-phlebitic limb (post-DVT).

Soft tissue/musculoskeletal
- Calf haematoma or trauma.
- Ruptured Baker's cyst (synovial effusion in the popliteal fossa associated with rheumatoid disease).
- Cellulitis (associated fever, sepsis, tachycardia).

Systemic
- Congestive cardiac failure (bilateral limb oedema, ↑ JVP and signs of LVF).
- Hepatic failure.
- Hypoalbuminaemia.
- Nephrotic syndrome.
- Pregnancy: increased dependent oedema, but note also an ↑ thrombotic risk and DVT should be excluded.

Deep vein thrombosis

Usually affects lower limb and can extend proximally into iliofemoral veins and inferior vena cava (IVC) with higher risk of associated pulmonary embolism (PE) and higher incidence of post-phlebitic limb. Occasionally seen affecting upper limb, but this is atypical.

Risk factors for DVT
- Age >60 yrs.
- Previous DVT or PE.
- Recent major surgery, especially orthopaedic lower limb, abdomen, and pelvic.
- Marked immobility.
- Malignancy.
- Pregnancy and post-partum.
- High dose oestrogen oral contraceptive pill.
- Family history of venous thrombo-embolism (VTE).

Investigation

USS Doppler studies, impedance plethysmography, venography, exclude PE. If any associated symptoms arrange V/Q scan, spiral CT, pulmonary angiography. Thrombophilia screening for younger patients (age <55 yrs), atypical site and extensive clots, spontaneous onset, family history.

Chest pain

Acute chest pain is a common symptom. A detailed history and a full physical examination should be performed in order to define the most likely cause and necessary investigation pathway.

History

Be sure to ask the following questions about the pain

- Site and radiation.
- Character.
- Onset and duration.
- Precipitating and relieving features.
- Associated symptoms.
- Response to pain relief, antacids or nitrates.
- Previous similar episodes

Most types of chest pain fall within one of these categories (Table 1.2).

Table 1.2 Chest pain categories

Pain source	Description of pain
Myocardial ischaemia	Retrosternal, heavy ache, can radiate → jaw, arms, precipitated by exertion, and relieved by rest or nitrates
Aortic dissection	Severe central tearing pain, radiates to back
Gastro-oesophageal disease	Burning central pain, can radiate to shoulders, throat or abdomen, exacerbated by meals, eased with antacids/milk
Pleuritic pain	Focal sharp pain, exacerbated by inspiration
Pericardial pain	Sharp pain, radiates to left shoulder tip, worse on lying flat, and during inspiration, eased by sitting forwards
Musculoskeletal pain	Sharp focal pain exacerbated by movement and palpation

Investigations (Table 1.3)

Table 1.3 Causes of chest pain

Suspected diagnosis	Investigations
Cardiovascular causes: all patients should have a 12-lead ECG and CXR	
Myocardial ischaemia/infarction	
Consider: coronary artery disease, aortic stenosis, hypertrophic obstructive cardiomyopathy	Serial electrocardiograms, cardiac markers of necrosis, FBC, thyroid function tests, echocardiogram, exercise electrocardiogram, stress cardiac imaging, coronary angiography
Thoracic aortic dissection	
Note: Myocardial ischaemia may also be present if it involves the coronary arteries, e.g. syphilitic aortitis	FBC, U&E, X-match, echocardiogram (TTE or TOE), computed tomography, magnetic resonance imaging, syphilis serology
Mitral valve prolapse	Echocardiogram (TTE or TOE)
Acute pericarditis	FBC, viral titres, ESR, echocardiogram
Pulmonary causes: all patients should have CXR ± ABGs	
Pneumonia/pleurisy	FBC, CRP
Acute bronchitis	Sputum and blood cultures
Pulmonary tuberculosis (TB)	Aspiration if empyema suspected, early morning urine (TB), Mantoux test (TB)
Pneumothorax	CXR
Pulmonary embolus	D-dimers, 12-lead ECG, V/Q scan, CT pulmonary angiography
Lung carcinoma	Sputum cytology
Pleural tumour e.g. mesothelioma	High resolution CT
Mediastinal tumour	Bronchoscopy, tissue biopsy
Gastro-oesophageal causes	
Oesophageal:	
Spasm, oesophagitis, candidiasis, reflux disease, Mallory–Weiss tear	FBC, G&S, *Helicobacter pylori*, Endoscopy, oesophageal manometry, oesophageal biopsy
Peptic ulcer disease	Endoscopy, gastrograffin swallow, barium swallow, meal or follow through, erect CXR (if performation suspected clinically)

Table 1.3 Causes of chest pain (*continued*)

Suspected diagnosis	Investigations
Acute pancreatitis	Amylase, abdominal ultrasound scan
Cholecystitis/biliary colic	FBC, CRP, LFTs, urinalysis, abdominal ultrasound scan, ERCP
Musculoskeletal & dermatological causes	
Muscular	
Bony structures	
Chest wall bony metastases, rib/sternal fractures, costochondritis (Tietze's syndrome), ankylosing spondylitis, cervical/thoracic spine disease, thoracic outlet syndrome	Chest X-ray, Bone scan, spinal X-rays, CT scan
Skin/soft tissue	
Acute shingles, post-herpetic neuralgia	Herpetic serology/smear (rarely)

Taken from ACC/AHA (2002).[1]

OHCM 8e, p88, p798.

1. ACC/AHA Guideline Update for the Management of Patients with Chronic Stable Angina 2002.
http://www.acc.org/clinical/guidelines/stable/stable_clean.pdf

Clubbing

Soft tissue hypertrophy under the nail bed distorts finger and toenail growth.

Characteristic features

- Increased lateral and longitudinal nail curvature.
- The skin at the base of the nail becomes spongy.
- The angle between nail and skin is obliterated.
- In extreme cases, the terminal phalanx becomes bulbous like a drum-stick.

Clubbing can be an important visual indicator of major disease, although it can also be congenital. Rarely, clubbing may accompany swollen wrists and ankles as part of a proliferative periostitis seen in hypertrophic pulmonary osteoarthropathy (HPOA). This is associated with squamous carcinoma of the lung.

Major causes

- **Lung disease**: cystic fibrosis, bronchiectasis, empyema, lung abscess, asbestosis, mesothelioma, pulmonary sarcoid.
- **Carcinoma**: bronchogenic (especially squamous cell), mediastinal, pleural, oesophageal, gastric, colonic, thoracic lymphoma, familial polyposis coli.
- **Infection**: infective endocarditis, colonic amoebiasis.
- **Vascular disease**: cyanotic congenital heart disease, atrial myxoma, arteriovenous malformation.
- **Liver disease**: primary (1°) biliary cirrhosis, chronic active hepatitis.
- **Gastrointestinal disease**: ulcerative colitis and Crohn's disease, malabsorption.
- **Rare causes**: thyrotoxicosis, polycythaemia, SLE.

Investigations

As guided by differential diagnosis and clinical suspicion:

- FBC.
- ESR.
- C-reactive protein (CRP).
- LFTs.
- TFTs.
- Serum ACE.
- Autoantibodies.
- Blood cultures (at least 3 sets if infective endocarditis suspected).
- Faecal occult blood (3 samples).
- CXR.
- Echocardiography (transthoracic echocardiogram (TTE) or transoesophageal echocardiogram (TOE)).
- OGD and biopsy.
- Colonoscopy and biopsy.
- Abdominal ultrasound scan.
- CT chest.
- Bronchoscopy, biopsy, washings.
- Liver biopsy.

📖 *OHCM* 8e, p33.

Coma

The Glasgow Coma Scale (GCS) is used to assess level of consciousness. Minimum score is 3, maximum 15.

Assess level of consciousness and determine whether this is stable, fluctuating, improving, or deteriorating on serial assessments.

Cerebral causes

- Intracranial haemorrhage (subarachnoid haemorrhage (SAH), subdural haemorrhage (SDH), extradural haemorrhage (EDH), intracerebral bleed).
- Large cerebral infarct.
- Pontine haemorrhage (pinpoint pupils).
- Cerebral venous sinus thrombosis.
- Hypertensive encephalopathy.
- Cerebral tumour (associated local cerebral oedema may respond to dexamethasone).
- Head injury.
- Cerebral infection—encephalitis, meningitis, cerebral malaria, brain abscess.
- Post-ictal state.
- Sub-clinical status epilepticus (**Note**: this is an EEG diagnosis).
- Cerebral vasculitis, e.g. SLE.
- End-stage multiple sclerosis.
- Leucodystrophy.
- Creutzfeldt–Jakob disease (including variant CJD).

Table 1.4 Glasgow Coma Scale

Eye opening	1	Nil
	2	To pain
	3	To voice
	4	Spontaneously
Motor response	1	Nil
	2	Extension
	3	Flexion
	4	Withdrawal from pain
	5	Localizing to pain
	6	Voluntary
Vocal response	1	Nil
	2	Groans
	3	Inappropriate words
	4	Disorientated speech
	5	Orientated speech

Metabolic causes

- Drugs (usually in deliberate overdose, 📖 Chapter 11, p653).
- Alcohol excess (**Note**: remember hypoglycaemia as a cause of coma in alcoholics, as well as extradural haematoma).
- Hypoglycaemia (iatrogenic, overdose of insulin or sulphonylureas, insulinoma, immunoglobulin F-2 (insulin-like growth factor-2 (IGF-2)-associated hypoglycaemia in certain tumours)).
- Diabetic ketoacidosis (coma in ~10% of cases—adverse prognostic sign).
- Hyperosmolar non-ketotic coma (may present as severe dehydration ± coma).
- Uraemia.
- Late stages of hepatic encephalopathy.
- Severe hyponatraemia (relatively common—esp. inappropriate in antidiuretic hormone (ADH) syndrome).
- Hypothyroidism (myxoedema coma—rare).
- Hypercalcaemia.
- Inborn error of metabolism, e.g. porphyria, urea cycle disorders.
- Type 2 respiratory failure (CO_2 narcosis).
- Hypothermia (severe).
- Hyperpyrexia (neuroleptic malignant syndrome (NMS) after anaesthesia).
- Severe nutritional deficiency—thiamine, pyridoxine, vitamin B_{12}.

Investigations

- Venous plasma glucose (exclude hypoglycaemia with fingerstick + reflectance meter, confirm with venous plasma fluoride-oxalate sample).
- U&E.
- LFTs.
- Serum Ca^{2+}.
- Serum osmolality.
- Urine Na^+.
- Blood cultures.
- Clotting screen.
- ABGs.
- Drug screen (serum, urine).
- Cranial CT scan.
- LP.
- CXR (bronchogenic carcinoma with cerebral metastases).
- 12-lead ECG.
- EEG.
- Erythrocyte transketolase (↓ in thiamine deficiency).
- Serum NH_3 (↑ in urea cycle disorders).
- Brain biopsy.

Always assess Airway, Breathing, Circulation before assessment of the cause of ↓ consciousness. Consider psychogenic unresponsiveness.

📖 *OHCM* 8e, p800, p802, p838.

Confusion

A reliable witness, family member, or carer may be vital in assessing a patient with confusion, and care must be taken to discriminate between acute and chronic symptoms. Acute confusional states carry a very broad differential diagnosis and require careful initial evaluation (see Table 1.5 for causes). Any systemic illness can precipitate a confusional state.

Table 1.5 Causes of confusion

Hypoxaemia	Acute infection, asthma, COPD, etc.
Head injury	Cerebral trauma
Vascular	CVA, TIA, intracerebral, subdural haemorrhage
Infection	Systemic
	Meningitis or encephalitis
Endocrine/metabolic	Diabetic ketoacidosis, hypoglycaemia, thyrotoxicosis or myxoedema, uraemia, hypercalcaemia, hyponatraemia
Alcohol and drug abuse	Acute intoxification and withdrawal. Also, consider overdose
Iatrogenic	Full and recent medication history (especially opiates, analgesia and sedatives)
Post-ictal state	
Cerebral tumour	
Psychiatric	
Wernicke's encephalopathy	

Investigations

- FBC, U&E, LFTs, serum Ca^{2+}, bone marrow (BM) stix and blood glucose.
- ABGs.
- MSU, blood cultures, sputum culture.
- CXR.
- ECG.
- Thyroid function.
- Drug/toxicology screen—blood and urine.
- CT scan.
- Lumbar puncture.

▶▶ Always look for MedicAlert™ bracelet, necklace, or card.

📖 *OHCM* 8e, p488, p526, p578.

Constipation

Patients may use the term constipation to mean infrequent, hard, small volume or difficult to pass faeces. Patients vary enormously in their threshold to seek medical advice about bowel habit.

Ask about
- Associated pain.
- PR bleeding.
- Tenesmus.
- Weight loss.

Causes
- Carcinoma of the colon.
- Diverticular disease.
- Anorectal disease—fissure or haemorrhoid.
- Benign stricture.
- Rectocoele.
- Sigmoid volvulus.
- Hernia.
- Drugs, especially analgesics.
- Poor fluid intake.
- Low fibre diet.
- Change in diet.
- Immobility.
- Irritable bowel syndrome.
- Megarectum.
- Hirschsprung's disease.
- Spinal cord lesion.
- Stroke.
- Jejunal diverticulosis.
- Hypothyroidism.
- Diabetic neuropathy.
- Hypercalcaemia, hyperparathyroidism, hypokalaemia.
- Uraemia.
- Porphyria.
- Pregnancy.
- Multiple sclerosis.
- Parkinson's disease.
- Dermatomyositis.
- Myotonic dystrophy.
- Scleroderma.
- Psychological.

Investigations
- Digital rectal examination.
- Proctoscopy.
- Sigmoidoscopy.
- Colonoscopy.
- Barium enema.
- U&E.
- Ca^{2+}.
- TFTs.
- FBC.
- Bowel transit time studies.
- Anorectal manometry.
- Electrophysiological studies.
- Defaecating proctography.

▶▶ Elderly patients are more prone to constipation.

📖 *OHCM* 8e, p248.

Cyanosis

Cyanosis is a blue/purple dusky discolouration of tissue caused by a rise in blood deoxygenated haemoglobin content (>5g/dL). Rarely it may be caused by ↑ sulphaemoglobin, methaemoglobin, or carboxyhaemoglobin. Cyanosis may be peripheral, affecting only cutaneous areas or central, when mucous membranes of the mouth and tongue are also discoloured.

Causes of peripheral cyanosis
- Central cyanosis.
- Shock.
- Hypothermia.
- Mitral stenosis.
- Raynaud's syndrome.
- Peripheral arterial disease.
- Patent ductus arteriosus (differential cyanosis, i.e. cyanosed toes but not fingers, is pathognomonic of this condition).

Causes of central cyanosis
Pulmonary disease with severely impaired oxygen transfer
- Pneumonia.
- Asthma.
- Chronic obstructive pulmonary disease.
- Pulmonary embolism.
- Fibrosing alveolitis.

Right to left shunt (Eisenmenger's syndrome)
- Atrial septal defect.
- Ventricular septal defect.
- Patent ductus arteriosus.
- Partial anomalous pulmonary venous drainage (APVD).
- Arteriovenous malformation.

Methaemoglobinaemia, sulphaemoglobinaemia, carboxyhaemoglobinaemia
- Congenital.
- Ingestion of oxidizing agents, e.g. phenacetin, inorganic nitrates, local anaesthetic.

Cyanosis arising from pulmonary disease can be reversed by administration of oxygen to improve alveolar oxygen uptake. Oxygen has no effect where right to left shunts are the cause. Central cyanosis may be underestimated with significant anaemia and is more apparent in patients with polycythaemia. In methaemoglobinaemia, the arterial concentration of oxygen is normal. This condition can be treated with intravenous methylene blue (see 📖 Chapter 11, p653).

Investigations
- FBC.
- ABGs.
- CXR.
- 12-lead ECG.
- Transthoracic echocardiogram (proceeding to transoesophageal echocardiogram if shunt is suspected).
- CT chest (if arteriovenous malformation is suspected).
- Cardiac MRI (if APVD suspected).

📖 *OHCM* 8e, p28, p144, p151.

Diarrhoea

Patients may use the term diarrhoea to describe loose stools, increased frequency of defecation, increased volume of stool, steatorrhoea, melaena, or faecal incontinence (□ Incontinence: faecal, p61).

Ask about

- Duration.
- Associated features (abdominal pain, vomiting, mucus, or blood per rectum (PR)).
- Systemic symptoms.
- Recent foreign travel.
- Suspect food.
- Is anyone else in the household affected?

Causes

- Infection (including 'traveller's diarrhoea').
- Inflammatory bowel disease.
- Diverticular disease.
- Colonic carcinoma.
- Other tumour, especially villous adenoma.
- Coeliac disease.
- Tropical sprue.
- Irritable bowel syndrome (IBS).
- Ischaemic colitis/bowel infarction.
- Laxative use!
- Other drugs, e.g. metformin, orlistat.
- Over indulgence in fruit, or vegetables or fat.
- Overflow secondary to constipation.
- Carcinoid syndrome (uncommon).
- Gastrinoma (rare).
- VIPoma (rare).
- Glucagonoma (very rare).
- Hyperthyroidism (common).
- Medullary carcinoma of the thyroid (uncommon).
- Bile salt diarrhoea (previous ileal disease or surgery).
- Dumping syndrome (previous gastric surgery).
- Gut motility disorders.
- Malabsorption (cf. pancreatitis, lymphangiectasia, coeliac).
- Lactose intolerance.
- Scleroderma.
- Amyloidosis.
- Whipple's disease.

Investigations

- Stool culture, hot stool for parasites.
- *Clostridium difficile* toxin in stool.
- High rectal swab for parasites (**Note**: giardiasis is diagnosed on duodenal biopsy).
- Rectal examination, proctoscopy, sigmoidoscopy ± biopsy.
- Colonoscopy.
- AXR.
- Barium enema.
- Small bowel follow-through contrast studies.
- Upper GI endoscopy.
- Small bowel biopsy.
- FBC and blood film.
- ESR.
- CRP.
- Serum ferritin and folate.
- U&E (exclude haemolytic uraemic syndrome especially in children).
- Urine screen for laxatives.
- Antigliadin, antiendomysial antibodies, and anti-tissue transglutaminase (coeliac disease).
- TFTs.
- Serum gut hormone profile (gastrin, VIP, glucagon—seek expert advice).
- 24 h urine for 5-hydroxyindole acetic acid (5HIAA).
- Serum calcitonin (medullary carcinoma of thyroid).
- Lactose hydrogen breath test (for lactose intolerance).
- ^{14}C–xylose breath test (bacterial overgrowth in small bowel).
- CT abdomen.
- Mesenteric angiography (ischaemia).

Investigation must be guided by history and examination findings. If the patient is an inpatient they should be isolated until infection is excluded. Consider HIV and other immune disorders if an unusual bowel organism is found.

Dizziness & syncope

Dizziness is a term that may be used to describe a variety of symptoms, e.g. spinning (rotatory vertigo), light-headedness, muzzy feeling or unsteadiness on walking. It is, therefore, important to establish precisely what the patient means by dizziness.

Loss of consciousness or 'blackout' may not be reported by the patient and an eyewitness account is important. Enquire about any awareness of abnormal heart beat (rhythm-induced syncope), chest pain (ischaemia), neurological symptoms (cerebrovascular disease), preceding micturition, change of posture or unusual sensations (prodromal epileptic symptoms, e.g. strange taste or smell) prior to the collapse.

Causes of dizziness

- Rotatory sensation lasting > 10s, and precipitated by movement or position—vestibular cause such as labyrinthitis, Menière's disease, cerebello-pontine angle tumour (acoustic neuroma).
- Rotatory sensation lasting 2 or 3s, and precipitated by movement—cervical spondylosis.
- Non-rotatory sensation lasting 2 or 3s and precipitated by movement, position or standing up—cervical spondylosis, cerebrovascular disease, postural hypotension, cardiac arrhythmia (usually back to normal in minutes), epilepsy (incontinence is common and return to normal may take hours).

Investigations

Suspected vestibular cause
- Hallpike manoeuvre.
- MRI or CT cerebello-pontine angle.
- Audiometry.

Suspected non-vestibular cause
- Blood glucose.
- 12-lead ECG.
- 24h ambulatory ECG monitoring.
- EEG.
- MRI or CT head.
- Tilt table test.

Causes of syncope

- **Vasovagal**: pain, fear, prolonged standing, excess heat, alcohol, or food.
- **Micturition** (often elderly men standing up during night to urinate).
- **Defecation** (often elderly women with constipation).
- **Coughing**: chronic airways disease.
- **Orthostatic hypotension**:
  - Autonomic dysfunction (diabetic neuropathy, Shy–Drager syndrome).
  - Drugs (anti-hypertensives, diuretics, nitrates, tricyclics) dehydration and sodium depletion.
- **Carotid sinus syndrome**.
- **Epilepsy**.

- **Drugs**: alcohol, illicit drugs.
- **Cardiac**: arrhythmias, outflow obstruction (aortic stenosis, hypertrophic obstructive cardiomyopathy, myxoma).
- **Hyperventilation and anxiety**.
- **Acute cerebrovascular disease**: transient ischaemic attack, stroke, subarachnoid haemorrhage. Rarely causes LOC.
- **Acute vascular obstruction**: pulmonary embolus, myocardial infarction.
- **Hypoglycaemia**: poorly-controlled diabetes.

Investigations[1]
- 12-lead ECG.
- 24 h Holter monitoring.
- Echocardiography.
- MRI or CT head.
- Tilt table test.
- Blood glucose, haemoglobin A_{1c} (HbA_{1c}).
- U&E.
- Cardiac markers.
- ABG.
- Toxicology screen.
- V/Q scan.

▶ Driving and dizziness/syncope
Guidance on driving in the UK is available at ♪ www.dvla.gov.uk

1. Guidelines on management (diagnosis and treatment) of syncope. *Eur Heart J* 2004; **25**: 2054–72.

Dysarthria & dysphasia

Dysarthria is difficulty in articulating words. The patient may complain of 'slurred speech'. Dysphasia is a difficulty in the formation of speech due to interference with higher mental function. These disturbances often occur together, most commonly in the context of a stroke.

Damage to Wernicke's area causes a receptive dysphasia. Speech may be fluent, but meaning is lost. Damage to Broca's area causes an expressive dyphasia. Speech is non-fluent and the patients are aware they are not using the right words.

Causes of dysphasia include stroke (usually with right hemiparesis, arm more affected than leg) or space-occupying lesion. Psychosis, especially schizophrenia, may cause a similar picture—so-called 'word salad'.

Causes of dysarthria

- Stroke (internal capsule or extensive lesion of motor cortex—acute).
- MND.
- Mid-brain or brainstem tumour.
- Parkinson's disease.
- Cerebellar disease (haemorrhage, infarct, multiple sclerosis, hereditary ataxia, alcoholic or paraneoplastic degeneration).
- Syringobulbia (chronic, progressive).
- Neuromuscular (myasthenia gravis, dermatomyositis, myotonic dystrophy).
- Acute alcohol or drug intoxication.

Dysarthria may be more obvious when the (English-speaking!) patient is invited to say 'Baby hippopotamus', 'British constitution', etc.

Investigations

- Cranial CT scan.
- Venous plasma glucose.
- ESR.
- Serum lipids.
- 12-lead ECG.
- Echocardiogram.
- Carotid Doppler studies (especially if bruit).
- CXR.
- LFTs.

Less commonly

- Serum muscle enzymes (polymyositis).
- Autoimmune profile.
- Electromyogram (EMG).
- Skeletal muscle biopsy.

  📖 *OHCM* 8e, p72.

Dysphagia

Dysphagia is difficulty in swallowing. The patient may have associated odynophagia (painful swallowing) or regurgitation of food (immediate or delayed?). Elicit whether the dysphagia is for liquid, solids, or both. Is it intermittent or progressive? Are there associated symptoms?

A careful physical examination is mandatory. Pay special attention to the lower cranial nerves; search for lymph nodes in the supraclavicular fossae. Palpate the thyroid and percuss for retrosternal enlargement.

Causes
- Oesophageal carcinoma.
- Benign oesophageal stricture secondary to chronic acid reflux.
- Barrett's oesophagus.
- Achalasia or diffuse spasm.
- Stroke (bilateral internal capsule cerebrovascular accident (stroke, CVAs)—pseudo-bulbar palsy).
- Oesophageal web (+ iron deficiency anaemia = Plummer Vinson (Patterson Kelly Brown) syndrome).
- Pharyngeal pouch.
- Muscular problem (myasthenia gravis, dermatomyositis, myotonic dystrophy).
- Bulbar palsy (MS, MND, poliomyelitis).
- Scleroderma (including CREST syndrome—📖 *OHCM* 8e, Chapter 12).
- Infection (usually acute pain on swallowing).
- Mediastinal mass (goitre, carcinoma of the bronchus, enlarged left atrium, aortic aneurysm).

Investigations
- FBC.
- ESR.
- Upper GI endoscopy.
- Barium swallow.
- CXR.
- Oesophageal manometry studies (📖 Gastrointestinal physiology, p487).
- Cranial CT or MRI (if neurological signs).
- Acetylcholine (ACh) receptor antibodies and Tensilon® (edrophonium). test if myasthenia gravis suspected (📖 Edrophonium (Tensilon®) test, p588).

Note: Consider HIV testing if there is oesophageal candida, herpes simplex, or cytomegalovirus infection in the oesophagus.

See 📖 *OHCM* 8e, p240, p453, p495.

Facial pain

Is the pain unilateral or bilateral? Is it constant or intermittent? Are there any precipitating factors or trigger points? A full examination of head and neck is required in addition to a detailed neurological and systemic examination.

Causes

- Trigeminal neuralgia (TN).
- Temporal arteritis (TA). ►► Risk of visual loss (🕮 *OHCM* 8e, Chapter 12).
- Herpes zoster (shingles or post-herpetic neuralgia).
- Dental caries, sepsis.
- Sinusitis.
- Temporomandibular joint dysfunction.
- Cluster headache.
- Glaucoma.
- Angina pectoris.
- Tonsillitis.
- Syringobulbia.
- Atypical facial neuralgia.
- Migraine.

Investigations

- ESR—urgent in suspected TA.
- Temporal artery biopsy if TA strongly suspected. ►►Must be performed rapidly—*within days*—if steroid treatment is commenced. However, do not withhold corticosteroid therapy for this reason!). Because of 'skip' lesions, false −ve biopsies may be encountered. Be guided by the full clinical picture, rather than reliance on a single test.
- Plain radiographs or CT imaging of frontal or maxillary sinuses.
- MRI to exclude MS, basilar aneurysm, trigeminal schwannoma, neuro-fibroma as causes of TN.
- MRI of cervical spinal cord to exclude syringobulbia if pain is accompanied by brainstem signs.

🕮 Headache, p49; 🕮 *OHCM* 8e, pp71–2.

Fever/pyrexia of unknown origin

Defined as temperature > 38.3°C on several occasions lasting 3 weeks or more despite 1 week of inpatient investigation. In nosocomial, neutropenic and HIV +ve pyrexia of unknown origin (PUO), patients need only 3 days of investigations to fulfil the definition. It is very important to take a full history and consider infectious contacts, recent travel abroad, recent surgery and dental treatment, sexual history, and risk factors for HIV. Possible causes are given in Table 1.6.

Signs

Examine for heart murmurs, splinter haemorrhages, splenomegaly, lymphadenopathy, and rashes/pruritus.

Table 1.6 Possible causes of FUO/PUO

Infection	Abscesses (e.g. subphrenic, pelvic, lung), osteomyelitis, TB, endocarditis, parasites, rheumatic fever, brucellosis, toxoplasmosis, Lyme disease, histoplasmosis, viral (esp. EBV, CMV, hepatitis, and HIV)
Malignancy	Lymphoma, leukaemia, hypernephroma, ovary, lung, hepatoma
Connective tissue	PAN, SLE, RA, Still's disease, temporal arteritis
Other	Sarcoidosis, atrial myxoma, drug fever, inflammatory bowel disease, factitious

Investigations

- Re-take the history and re-examine the patient (something might have been missed or new symptoms/signs may have developed).
- FBC, ESR, CRP.
- U&E, LFTs, Ca^{2+}.
- CXR.
- MSU, urinanalysis.
- Serology for *Brucella* and *Toxoplasma*.
- All biopsy material should be sent for culture, including TB.
- Blood cultures (serial may be necessary).
- Monospot/Paul Bunnell.
- Autoimmune profile (antinuclear antibodies (ANA), rheumatoid factor (RF), antineutrophil cytoplasmic antibody (ANCA), etc.).
- Bone marrow aspirate/trephine/culture for TB with Ziehl–Neelsen (ZN) stain.
- Abdominal USS (?masses).

Extend investigations according to symptoms and signs:

- Consult microbiology or infectious disease consultant for advice.
- Stool cultures and fresh stool for ova, cysts and parasites.
- Repeat serological investigation for changing titres (2–3 weeks).
- Thick and thin blood film for malaria and parasites.
- Mantoux test.
- TTE or TOE to exclude endocarditic vegetations.
- CT chest, abdomen, and pelvis.

▶▶ Always re-examine the patient for evolving new signs if cause remains unknown.

📖 *OHCM* 8e, p386.

First fit

▶▶ A first fit in an adult requires careful evaluation, since the probability of an underlying structural lesion increases with age.

Take a careful history, preferably from a witness, as well as the patient. Most lay persons will recognize a generalized tonic-clonic fit. However, the occurrence of a few 'epileptiform' movements in patients with syncopal episodes (📖 Dizziness & syncope, p34) may cause diagnostic uncertainty.

Be sure to ask about

- Aura preceding episode. ▶ Temporal lobe epilepsy—olfactory or gustatory auras (not necessarily followed by convulsions).
- Loss of consciousness—how long? Often overestimated by witnesses!
- Tongue biting.
- Focal or generalized convulsive movements. **Note**: A clear history of a tonic-clonic fit commencing in a limb and progressing to a more generalized convulsion is highly suggestive of a structural intracerebral lesion; cranial imaging is mandatory.
- Central cyanosis (tonic phase).
- Urinary incontinence.
- Injuries.
- Post-ictal confusion.
- History of trauma.
- Alcohol intake. *Remember*: alcohol withdrawal fits, as well as acute intoxication.
- Drug history—prescribed and recreational.
- History of insulin-treated diabetes or type 2 diabetes treated with oral secretagogues, i.e. sulphonylureas, repaglinide, nateglinide. **Note**: Metformin and thiazolidinediones as monotherapy do not cause significant hypoglycaemia.

A full general and neurological examination is needed, specifically including:
- Fever.
- Meningism, i.e. nuchal rigidity, +ve Kernig's sign (meningoencephalitis).
- Cutaneous rash or ecchymoses (?bleeding diathesis).
- Evidence of head trauma (preceding fit or as a consequence).
- Signs of chronic liver disease.
- Focal neurological deficit. ▶ Third nerve palsy in intracranial SOL, including aneurysm of the posterior communicating artery. Sixth nerve lesion may act as a 'false localizing sign' in ↑ ICP.
- MedicAlert™ bracelet (history of epilepsy or diabetes—search personal belongings).

Bilateral extensor plantar reflexes can occur after a generalized fit without a structural brain lesion and there may be a transient hemiparesis (Todd's paresis).

Causes

- Epilepsy (📖 *OHCM* 8e, Chapter 10).
- Hypoglycaemia (acute, severe, history of diabetes?).
- Hyponatraemia (usually <110mmol/L or rapid development).
- Hypocalcaemia (📖 *OHCM* 8e, Chapter 18).
- Hypomagnesaemia (may accompany hypocalcaemia).
- Hypophosphataemia (rare).
- Alcohol withdrawal. ▶▶ Risk of associated hypoglycaemia.
- Discontinuation of anticonvulsant medication.
- Infection—viral encephalitis or bacterial meningitis. ▶▶ Consider intracerebral abscess, tuberculoma in predisposed patients.
- Encephalopathy—hepatic, uraemic, hypertensive, thyrotoxic (rare—'thyroid storm').
- Eclampsia.
- Porphyria.
- Cerebral SLE.
- Head injury.
- Hypoxia.
- Cerebral tumour.
- Stroke—cerebral infarct, haemorrhage.

Investigations

- Venous plasma glucose (fingerprick test at bedside useful as a 'screen', but can be unreliable).
- U&E.
- Serum Ca^{2+}, Mg^{2+}, PO_4^{3-}
- Cranial CT or MRI scan.
- EEG.
- LP (📖 Lumbar puncture, p546).
- CXR.
- Serum prolactin (PRL; may be ↑ after generalized convulsions, but not pseudoseizures).
- ABGs—remember transient lactic acidosis following generalized tonic-clonic convulsion.
- Blood ethanol (may be undetectable in withdrawal state).
- Serum or urine drug screen.

'Pseudoseizures' may be encountered in patients with atypical recurrent fits (usually long history of epilepsy) and this is unlikely in an adult presenting with a first fit. Pseudoseizures usually present as a recurrent problem, the fits typically happen in front of witnesses, are not accompanied by incontinence or tongue biting and the post-ictal phase is short or absent.

▶ In UK, the National Driving License Authority prohibits driving for 12 months following a first fit.

📖 *OHCM* 8e, p494.

Galactorrhoea

Denotes inappropriate breast milk production, i.e. in the absence of pregnancy, most commonly caused by hyperprolactinaemia (↑ PRL) due to a pituitary microprolactinoma < 10mm diameter (📖 Precocious puberty, p168). Prolactinomas (usually macroadenomas) may cause galactorrhoea in men.

Note: Other disease in the pituitary region, certain drugs, and several systemic disorders may be associated with ↑ PRL (📖 *OHCM* 8e, Chapter 5).

Causes

Normoprolactinaemic galactorrhoea
- This has been described in premenopausal women occurring after the conclusion of:
  - Treatment with the combined contraceptive pill.
  - Breastfeeding (for >6 months afterwards).
- Increased sensitivity of lactogenic tissue PRL is postulated, but the mechanism remains uncertain. In part, this may reflect difficulties that can arise in determining whether PRL is persistently elevated. Menstrual disturbances have been described.

Hyperprolactinaemia
The differential diagnosis and investigation of hyperprolactinaemia is considered on (📖 Galactorrhoea (hyperprolactinaemia), p162).

Investigations

- Serum PRL (📖 Galactorrhoea (hyperprolactinaemia, p162).
- Repeated measurements under controlled conditions may be required since PRL is a 'stress' hormone and may be increased by venepuncture.

Note: If ↑ PRL is confirmed, further investigations to exclude causes other than prolactinoma are required.

- Pituitary imaging (CT or preferabl, MRI) and visual field testing (Goldmann) may also be indicated if a macroprolactinoma is suspected (PRL concentrations usually very high).

Note: If there is doubt about the nature of the nipple discharge further specialized investigations may be required on the fluid, including:
- Casein.
- Lactose.
- Microscopy.

Clear fluid may result from benign breast disease.

Note: Bloody discharge should prompt urgent specialist investigations to exclude carcinoma of the breast:
- Mammography.
- Biopsy.

📖 *OHCM* 8e, p228.

Further reading

Kleinberg DL, *et al.* Galactorrhoea: a study of 235 cases, including 48 with pituitary tumors. *N Engl J Med* 1977; **296**: 589–600.

Gout

Gout is caused by the deposition of monosodium urate monohydrate crystals in tissues and relates to hyperuricaemia. Hyperuricaemia is due to an imbalance between purine synthesis and uric acid excretion. Episodes of acute gout may be precipitated by alcohol, trauma, dietary changes, infection, chemotherapy, or surgery. More common in men and very rare in premenopausal women.

Clinical features

- Inflammatory arthritis, classically a monoarthritis or oligoarthritis affecting 1st metatarsophalangeal (MTP) joint of foot, but can affect any joint including the spine.
- Tenosynovitis.
- Bursitis or cellulitis.
- Tophi—urate deposits in tendons, ear pinna, and joints.
- Urolithiasis and renal disease.

Investigations

- ESR (may be ↑).
- Urate crystals demonstrated in synovial fluid or tissues—negatively birefringent on polarized light microscopy.
- Serum urate (not always ↑ in acute episode and normal urate level does not exclude the diagnosis).
- X-ray—soft tissue swelling and punched out bony erosions.
- AIP (to exclude rheumatoid).
- Microscopy of synovial fluid (Gram stain and culture).

Treatment

Acute episode
- NSAIDs, colchicine, intra-articular steroids or oral steroids.
- Avoid precipitating factors and purine-rich foods.
- Urate lowering therapy (avoid in acute attacks) indicated for tophi, recurrent attacks and urine/renal disease, e.g.
  - Allopurinol (xanthine oxidase inhibitor).
  - Probenecid (uricosuric).

NB: Asymptomatic hyperuricaemia is more common than gout and a high serum urate with co-existent arthritis is not necessarily due to crystal deposition. Consider important other causes especially infective arthritis and pseudo-gout.

Pseudo-gout

Calcium pyrophosphate crystal deposition causing acute arthritis or chondrocalcinosis. Crystals are weakly +ve birefringent on polarized light microscopy. Associations include old age, dehydration, hyperparathyroidism, hypothyroidism, haemochromatosis, acromegaly, rheumatoid arthritis, and osteoarthritis.

📖 *OHCM* 8e, p550.

Gynaecomastia

Gynaecomastia is benign bilateral hyperplasia of glandular and fatty breast tissue in the male. The balance between androgens and oestrogens is thought to be of importance in the pathogenesis; many conditions may influence this ratio. Most commonly, it appears transiently during normal puberty (detectable at some stage in ~50% cases). Gynaecomastia may also be caused by specific endocrine disease or be associated with certain chronic diseases. Treatment with certain drugs is a common cause (~30% of cases) and arises via several mechanisms. Investigations will be guided by the individual circumstances. A careful drug history and thorough physical examination are required, particularly in the post-adolescent period.

When indicated and after excluding causes such as congenital syndrome and drug therapy, investigations are principally directed at:
- Excluding endocrine carcinoma (rare).
- Identifying associated chronic diseases.

Note:
- Simple obesity is not usually a cause of true gynaecomastia, i.e. the glandular element is not increased.
- ↑ Serum PRL in isolation does not cause gynaecomastia.
- Unilateral, eccentric breast enlargement should prompt exclusion of breast carcinoma (rare).

Causes include
- Physiological states (transient):
  - Newborn.
  - Puberty.
  - Advanced age.
- Klinefelter's syndrome (47, XXY; mosaics).
- Secondary hypogonadism, e.g. mumps orchitis.
- Androgen resistance syndromes, e.g. testicular feminization.
- ↑ Tissue aromatase activity (converts androgens to oestrogens).
- Oestrogen-producing tumours:
  - Leydig cell tumour.
  - Sertoli cell tumour.
  - Adrenal carcinoma.
- Chronic liver disease.
- Chronic renal failure.
- Panhypopituitarism.
- Tumours producing human chorionic gonadotrophin (hCG).
- **Drugs**: oestrogens (prostatic carcinoma, trans-sexuals), spironolactone, cimetidine, digoxin, cytotoxic agents, marijuana.
- Hyperthyroidism (↑ serum sex-hormone-binding globulin, SHBG).
- Primary (1°) hypothyroidism.
- Cushing's syndrome.
- Carcinoma of bronchus.
- Idiopathic.

Investigations

- Testosterone.
- FSH.
- LH.
- LFTs.
- TFTs.
- Oestradiol.
- β-hCG.
- PRL.
- SHBG (affinity of SHBG is higher for testosterone than for oestrogens, therefore ↑ SHBG causes disproportionate ↓ in free testosterone levels).
- Dehydroepiandrosterone sulphate (DHEAS).
- Androstenedione.
- Testicular USS.
- CXR.
- Abdominal CT or MRI imaging (for suspected adrenal tumours).
- Pituitary imaging.
- Karyotype.
- Urinary 17-oxo-steroids.

If carcinoma of breast is suspected

- Mammogram.
- Fine needle aspiration.

📕 OHCM 8e, p222.

Further reading

Braunstein GD. Gynecomastia. N Engl J Med 1994; **328**: 490–5.

Haematemesis

This literally means vomiting blood and is often associated with melaena (passage of black tarry stools).

Causes

- Chronic peptic ulceration (e.g. duodenal ulcer (DU) or gastric ulcer (GU)) accounts for 50% of cases of bleeding from the upper GI tract.
- Acute gastric ulcers or erosions.
- Drugs (e.g. NSAIDs) or alcohol.
- Reflux oesophagitis.
- Mallory–Weiss tear.
- Oesophageal varices.
- Gastric carcinoma (uncommon).

Investigations after admission and stabilization of the patient

- Full history, including drugs, alcohol, past history, indigestion, etc.
- FBC (**Note**: Hb will take ~24 h to fall; initially may be normal).
- U&E.
- Cross-match blood.
- Urgent upper GI tract endoscopy.
- Check *Helicobacter pylori* serology ± urea breath test.

📖 *OHCM* 8e, p252, p254, p830.

Haematuria

In health adults pass between 500,000 and 2,000,000 red cells over a 24 h period. Haematuria implies the passage of excess blood that may be detectable using dipsticks (microscopic haematuria) or may be obvious to the naked eye (macroscopic haematuria).

Causes
- Many.
- Glomerular disease, e.g. 1° glomerulonephritis, 2° glomerulonephritis (SLE, vasculitis, infection).
- Vascular or interstitial disease due to hypersensitivity reactions, renal infarction, papillary necrosis or pyelonephritis.
- Trauma.
- Renal epithelial or vascular tumours.
- Lower renal tract disease, e.g. tumours, stones, infection, drug toxicity (e.g. cyclophosphamide), foreign bodies, or parasites.
- Systemic coagulation abnormalities, e.g. platelet or coagulation factor abnormalities, such as profound thrombocytopenia or DIC.

Investigations
- Urinalysis—dipstick, microscopic examination, culture.
- Radiology*, e.g. KUB or IVU.
- Specialist investigation*, e.g. angiography, CT, or MRI scanning.
- Cystoscopy*.

*Ideally, these tests should be arranged after discussion with either a nephrologist or urologist.

📖 OHCM 8e, p286.

Haemoptysis

This describes coughing up blood or blood-stained sputum, and can vary from faint traces of blood to frank bleeding. Before embarking on investigation it is essential to ensure that the blood is coughed up from the respiratory tract, and is not that of epistaxis or haematemesis (easily confused).

Causes

- Infective, e.g. acute respiratory infection, exacerbation of chronic obstructive pulmonary disease (COPD).
- Pulmonary infarction, e.g. PE.
- Lung cancer.
- Tuberculosis.
- Pulmonary oedema.
- Bronchiectasis.
- Uncommon causes, e.g. idiopathic pulmonary haemosiderosis, Goodpasture's syndrome, microscopic vasculitis, trauma, haematological disease (e.g. ITP or DIC).

Investigations

- Colour of blood provides clues (pink frothy in pulmonary oedema, rust-coloured in pneumonia).
- Check O_2 saturation.
- FBC (? ↓ platelets).
- ESR.
- Coagulation screen.
- Sputum culture.
- CXR.
- Arrange bronchoscopy after discussion with respiratory team.

📖 *OHCM* 8e, p49.

Headache

📖 Facial pain, p38.

Headache is an extremely common complaint. Most patients self-medicate and only a small proportion will seek medical advice. Headache may be acute or chronic, constant, recurrent, or gradually progressive. It may arise from structures within the cranial vault or from external causes.

Causes differ according to age, e.g. temporal arteritis is very uncommon in patients under ~55 years. Migraine may be associated with classic features. Remember to enquire about the combined oral contraceptive pill—may exacerbate migraine. 'Tension' headaches predominate.

Causes in adults include

- 'Tension' headache (very common; usually recurrent and stereotyped).
- Migraine. Although common, many patients who believe they have 'migraine' probably have 'tension' headaches. Migraine predominantly affects adolescents and young adults, but may occur for the first time or persist in the second half of the lifespan.
- As part of a generalized viral illness, e.g. 'flu'.
- Causes of ↑ ICP.
- Acute infective meningitis (bacterial, viral most commonly).
- Encephalitis (most commonly viral, e.g. herpes simplex).
- Intracerebral haemorrhage.
- Post-traumatic (common).
- Intracerebral tumour (1° or 2°, benign or malignant).
- Acute subarachnoid haemorrhage.
- Subdural haematoma.
- Acute glaucoma.
- Acute sinusitis.
- Rubeosis iridis (2° glaucoma in patients with advanced diabetic eye disease).
- Trigeminal neuralgia.
- Cluster headaches.
- Referred pain, e.g. from dental caries or sepsis.
- Arterial hypertension; malignant or accelerated phase; essential hypertension is rarely the cause of headache.
- Temporal arteritis (TA). ▶▶ Visual loss preventable with prompt high dose corticosteroid therapy.
- Venous sinus thrombosis.
- Benign intracranial hypertension (mimics intracerebral tumour).
- Pneumonia caused by *Mycoplasma pneumoniae* may be associated with headache (meningoencephalitis).
- Nocturnal hypoglycaemia (often unrecognized) may cause morning headaches in patients with insulin-treated diabetes mellitus (DM).
- Analgesia-withdrawal headache.
- Hangover following alcohol excess.
- Otitis media.
- Chronic hypercalcaemia (rare).

Investigations
- ESR (►► temporal arteritis—*exclude with urgency*).
- CRP.
- FBC.
- U&E.
- Throat swabs.
- Blood cultures (if febrile).
- LP (📖 Lumbar puncture, p546).
- SXR ± cervical spine X-ray.
- Sinus X-rays (may be local tenderness in sinusitis).
- Cranial CT (📖 Computed tomography, p560).
- CXR (cerebral metastases from bronchogenic carcinoma).
- Urinalysis.
- Intra-ocular pressure measurement and refraction.
- Cerebral angiography (if aneurysm or atrioventricular (AV) malformation).
- Serum Ca^{2+}.

📖 *OHCM* 8e, p460, p794.

Heart sounds & murmurs

Auscultation of the heart should be conducted over several cardiac cycles. Keep listening until you are certain you have heard everything. Heart sounds and murmurs are traditionally assessed at the apex, lower left sternal edge, aortic area, and pulmonary area, but may radiate into other regions, such as the axilla or carotid arteries. The carotid pulse should be palpated simultaneously in order to time cardiac events. The following should be identified:

- First (S1) and second (S2) heart sounds.
- Added heart sounds, such as third (S3) or fourth (S4) heart sounds, opening snaps, ejection clicks, prosthetic sounds.
- Murmurs, including location, intensity, and characteristics.

The first heart sound is produced by closure of the mitral and tricuspid valves. It is best heard at the apex and is timed just prior to the carotid pulse. The second heart sound is caused by closure of the aortic (A2) and pulmonary (P2) valves, and is heard just after carotid pulsation. Closure of the pulmonary valve is slightly delayed relative to the aortic valve and so the second heart sound is normally split. This split is exaggerated by inspiration (see Table 1.7).

Normal and abnormal heart sounds are shown in Table 1.7.

The third heart sound is heard just after S2 and arises as a consequence of rapid ventricular filling and volume overload. The fourth heart sound occurs just before S1, and is caused by atrial contraction against a stiff ventricle or pressure overload. Abnormal valves may cause extra heart sounds on opening, e.g. an opening snap or ejection click. The heart sounds generated by artificial valve closure are referred to as prosthetic heart sounds. These should be crisp, not muffled (see Table 1.8).

Murmurs may be graded according to the following criteria

1. Very soft (just audible in optimal conditions).
2. Soft.
3. Moderate (easily heard with a stethoscope).
4. Loud ± palpable thrill.
5. Very loud/palpable thrill.
6. Heard without stethoscope/palpable thrill.

Table 1.7 Normal and abnormal heart sounds

Description	Diagram		Differential diagnosis
Normal	S1	A2 P2	Normal
Loud S1	S1	A2P2	Hyperdynamic circulation – anaemia, fever, thyrotoxicosis Mitral stenosis Left atrial myxoma
Soft S1	S1	A2P2	Low cardiac output Heart failure Tachycardia Mitral regurgitation Chronic obstructive pulmonary syndrome Systemic hypertension Dilated aortic root
Loud S2 (A2)	S1	A2P2	Aortic stenosis Cardiac failure
Soft S2 (A2)	S1	A2P2	Pulmonary stenosis
Soft S2 (P2)	S1	A2 P2	Pulmonary hypertension
Loud S2 (P2)	S1	A2P2	Normal physiological splitting exaggerated in: right bundle branch block, pulmonary stenosis, pulmonary hypertension
Normal split S2	Expiration Inspiration S1	A2 P2	Atrial septal defect
Fixed splitting S2	Expiration Inspiration S1	A2 P2	Left bundle branch block Systemic hypertension Aortic stenosis
Reversed splitting S2	Expiration Inspiration S1	P2 A2	

Innocent murmurs are generated by turbulent flow, such as in high cardiac output states, e.g. pregnancy, fever, anaemia, and thyrotoxicosis. They have the following characteristics:
- No accompanying thrill.
- Never > grade 3.
- Systolic.
- Maximal at left sternal edge.
- Normal heart sounds.
- Normal pulses, ECG, and CXR.

Systolic murmurs are synchronous with the carotid pulse and caused by
- Abnormal regurgitation through a structure that is normally closed in systole, e.g. atrioventricular valve, septum (pansystolic).
- Normal systolic flow through a narrowed or stenosed valve, e.g. aortic valve, pulmonary valve (ejection systolic).

Diastolic murmurs are audible after the carotid pulse and arise from
- Incompetence of the cardiac outflow valves, e.g. aortic or pulmonary valves.
- Narrowing of the cardiac inflow valves, e.g. mitral or tricuspid valves.

Mixed murmurs (systolic and diastolic) arise from
- Mixed valvular disease (stenosis and regurgitation).
- Patent ductus arteriosus.

Murmurs arising from the left heart structures are accentuated in expiration, whereas right heart murmurs are augmented in inspiration (see Table 1.9).

Table 1.8 Heart murmurs

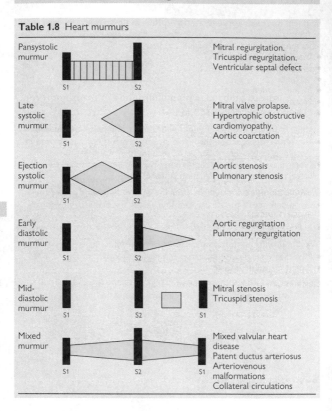

Pansystolic murmur	Mitral regurgitation. Tricuspid regurgitation. Ventricular septal defect
Late systolic murmur	Mitral valve prolapse. Hypertrophic obstructive cardiomyopathy. Aortic coarctation
Ejection systolic murmur	Aortic stenosis Pulmonary stenosis
Early diastolic murmur	Aortic regurgitation Pulmonary regurgitation
Mid-diastolic murmur	Mitral stenosis Tricuspid stenosis
Mixed murmur	Mixed valvular heart disease Patent ductus arteriosus Arteriovenous malformations Collateral circulations

Table 1.9 Added heart sounds

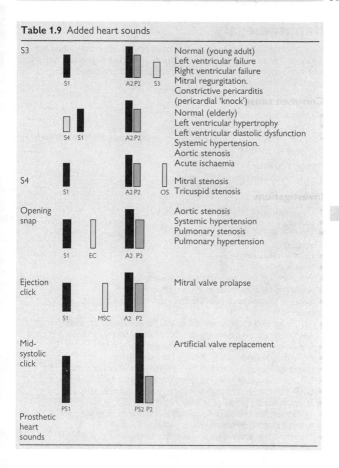

S3	Normal (young adult) Left ventricular failure Right ventricular failure Mitral regurgitation. Constrictive pericarditis (pericardial 'knock')
	Normal (elderly) Left ventricular hypertrophy Left ventricular diastolic dysfunction Systemic hypertension. Aortic stenosis Acute ischaemia
S4	Mitral stenosis Tricuspid stenosis
Opening snap	Aortic stenosis Systemic hypertension Pulmonary stenosis Pulmonary hypertension
Ejection click	Mitral valve prolapse
Mid-systolic click	Artificial valve replacement
Prosthetic heart sounds	

Hepatomegaly

Measure liver edge below the (R) costal margin after percussing out the upper and lower borders. Bruits may be heard in hepatoma and a friction rub may occur with malignant deposits. Other signs may suggest the underlying diagnosis.

Common causes

- Congestive cardiac failure (CCF).
- Malignant deposits.
- Hepatitis/cirrhosis (usually alcoholic or infectious, e.g. Epstein–Barr virus (EBV), viral hepatitis).

Foreign residence? or travel

If so, consider amoebic and hydatid cysts, schistosomiasis, malaria.

Investigations

- FBC, film, LDH (leukaemia, lymphoma).
- ESR.
- Virology (EBV, cytomegalovirus (CMV), hepatitis A, B, C antibody serology).
- LFTs—transaminases.
- Serum albumin.
- Prothrombin time (hepatocellular damage).
- γ-glutamyl transpeptidase, MCV (alcohol).
- Alkaline phosphatase (obstructive causes; malignant deposits if isolated↑).
- Serum Igs may be polyclonal ↑ in IgG (autoimmune hepatitis), IgA (alcoholic liver disease) or IgM (primary biliary cirrhosis (PBC)).
- Serum protein electrophoresis (myeloma, amyloid).
- Reticulocytes, bilirubin (if ↑ suggests haemolysis).
- Haemoglobinopathy screen (thalassaemia/sickle disorders).
- USS to assess liver texture, splenomegaly, lymphadenopathy.
- CXR and cardiac investigations (cardiomyopathies, sarcoid).
- α-fetoprotein (1° hepatocellular carcinoma).
- Serum ferritin, transferrin saturation, deoxyribose nucleic acid (DNA) analysis (haemochromatosis).
- Mitochondrial antibodies and autoimmune markers, e.g. ANA (autoimmune hepatitis), ANCA (1° sclerosing cholangitis).
- Caeruloplasmin, urinary copper (Wilson's disease).
- α1-antitrypsin (α1-antitrypsin deficiency).
- Porphyria screen.
- Pitfalls.
- Hepatomegaly is a common sign but may not necessarily implicate liver pathology.
- End-stage cirrhosis may commonly present with a small, shrunken liver.

📖 *OHCM* 8e, p63, p606.

Herpes zoster

The pattern of the eruption varies from mild to dense with the involvement of several dermatomes. Complications may occur if involvement of the eye, motor nerves, autonomic nerves (bladder), or when disease presents as an encephalomyelitis or purpura fulminans.

▶▶ In the immunocompromised host, zoster is both more likely to occur and to disseminate.

Investigations

- Confirm diagnosis by isolation of virus from vesicular fluid.
- Consider underlying disorders if recurrent or severe attacks.
- Look for lymphadenopathy (Hodgkin's or other lymphoma).
- FBC, blood film, LDH (↑ in lymphoma).
- Serum protein electrophoresis (myeloma, amyloid).
- Serology for HIV (zoster is common in adult HIV individuals).
- Immunodeficiency work-up.

Pitfalls

The rash is not always unilateral—it may be bilateral.

📖 *OHCM* 8e, p400.

Hyperlipidaemia

Abnormalities of lipid metabolism are common in Western societies. Populations with high levels of cholesterol have high rates of vascular morbidity, especially cardiovascular disease, and premature death. Vascular risk can be estimated from published risk tables or calculators.

Various classifications of hyperlipidaemia exist, each with a characteristic lipid profile. Many patients with lipid disorders have cutaneous markers, which identify to a certain extent the type of lipid abnormality.

Clinical features

Lipid abnormalities may cause dermatological manifestations

- Grey-yellow plaques or xanthomata in tendons, especially forearm and Achilles. Usually indicative of elevated LDL-cholesterol.
- Corneal arcus, a thin white rim around the iris—whilst this is common in the elderly, it is not a sign of ↑ LDL except in the under 40s.
- Yellow, fatty deposits or xanthelasmata around the eyelids—associated with elevated LDL, these painless, non-tender plaques are common in the elderly.
- Yellow streaks in palmar creases—palmar xanthomata are associated with IDL-cholesterol.
- Plaques over the tibial tuberosities and elbows—tubero-eruptive xanthomata. Often seen with hepatosplenomegaly with elevated triglycerides.
- Eruptive xanthomata—in severe triglyceridaemia associated with pancreatitis, hepatomegaly.

Hyperlipidaemia may be secondary to drugs, such as corticosteroids, oestrogens, and progestagens, as well as a range of conditions, such as hypothyroidism, myeloma, and alcoholism, each of which may be associated with specific clinical signs.

Hypertension

Blood pressure (BP) measurements are graded into a number of categories by the British Hypertension Society:

- **Optimal BP**: < 120/80.
- **Normal BP**: < 130/85.
- **High-normal BP**: 130–139/85–89.
- **Grade 1 hypertension (mild)**: 140–159/90–99.
- **Grade 2 hypertension (moderate)**: 160–179/100–109.
- **Grade 3 hypertension (severe)**: ≥ 180/110.

Hypertension should not be diagnosed on the basis of a single blood pressure reading. Unless urgent treatment is required, e.g. malignant hypertension, BP should be rechecked over a number of weeks to confirm the presence of sustained hypertension.

Causes

Remember that the cause of hypertension in most (95%) cases is unknown ('essential' hypertension). One of the following identifiable causes can be found in the remaining 5%:

- Renal disease, e.g. polycystic kidney disease.
- Renovascular disease, e.g. renal artery stenosis.
- Endocrine disease, e.g. Cushing's syndrome, Conn's syndrome, phaeochromocytoma, acromegaly.
- Coarctation of the aorta.
- Drugs, e.g. NSAIDs, oral contraceptive pill, steroids, erythropoietin, sympathomimetics, liquorice.
- Pregnancy, e.g. pre-eclampsia, eclampsia.

Routine investigation

The investigation of hypertensive patients has the following aims

- To confirm the presence and severity of hypertension.
- To assess overall cardiovascular risk.
- To identify target organ damage.
- To identify 2° causes (where present).

Routine investigations should include

- Urinalysis (protein, blood, glucose).
- U&E.
- Plasma glucose (ideally fasted).
- Lipid profile (ideally fasted).
- 12-lead ECG.

CXR, urine microscopy and culture and echocardiography are not required routinely but should be considered where indicated by your initial assessment and investigation of the patient. The use of 24 h ambulatory BP monitoring is often useful where clinic readings are thought to be unreliable because of 'white coat' hypertension.

Further investigation

Where more detailed assessment is required (for instance, to rule out a 2° cause or to identify end-organ damage), the following investigations may be appropriate:

Renal investigations
- Renal ultrasound scan (to assess overall renal morphology).
- Renal artery Doppler studies (for renal artery stenosis).
- Renal artery MRI (for renal artery stenosis).
- Captopril renogram (for renal artery stenosis).
- Renal angiography (for renal artery stenosis).
- Renal vein renin measurements (for Conn's syndrome).

Endocrine investigations
- Renin & aldosterone studies for Conn's syndrome (consult your local endocrine laboratory).
- Investigations for Cushing's syndrome.
- Investigations for acromegaly.
- Urinary catecholamine (& metabolite) excretion.

Further reading

Williams B, *et al.* Guidelines for management of hypertension: report of the fourth working party of the British Hypertension Society, 2004—BHS IV. *J Human Hypertension* 2004; **18**: 139–85.

Incontinence: faecal

📖 Alteration in bowel habit, p9; 📖 Constipation, p29; 📖 Diarrhoea p32.

Causes include

- Any cause of diarrhoea (📖 *OHCM* 8e, Chapter 6).
- Overflow diarrhoea from severe constipation.
- Inflammatory bowel disease (acute or chronic).
- Coeliac disease (diarrhoea is a variable feature).
- Infectious diarrhoea (📖 *OHCM* 8e, Chapter 6).
- Hyperthyroidism (may cause diarrhoea, rare cause of incontinence).
- Carcinoma of colon (stricture).
- Diverticular disease of colon (acute attack, chronic stricture).
- Neurological (multiple CVAs, MS, spina bifida, post-childbirth neuropathy) may often be associated with sphincter disturbances.
- Drugs, e.g. laxatives, orlistat (causes fat malabsorption).
- Causes of steatorrhoea (📖 *OHCM* 8e, Chapter 6).
- Intestinal hurry, e.g. post-gastrectomy (📖 *OHCM* 8e, Chapter 6).
- Diabetic diarrhoea (autonomic neuropathy—rare; diagnosis of exclusion, but may cause nocturnal faecal incontinence).
- Vasoactive intestinal peptide (VIP)oma (very rare).

Investigations

Non-invasive tests

- Stool cultures (ova cysts, parasites). **Note**: *Clostridium difficile*—relatively common in patients who have received recent antibiotic therapy.
- FBC (anaemia, especially iron deficiency).
- CRP.
- ESR.
- U&E.
- TFTs.

Imaging

- Pelvic/abdominal X-ray.
- Barium enema.
- CT abdomen.

Procedures

- Colonoscopy.
- Sigmoidoscopy ± biopsy.

📖 *OHCM* 8e, p58, p237.

Incontinence: urinary

📖 Anuria, p14.

Consider

- Common causes of polyuria (📖 *OHCM* 8e, Chapter 2); these may present as or aggravate urinary incontinence.
- Acute or chronic confusional state (common; loss of voluntary sphincter control).
- Urinary tract infection (very common—always exclude).
- Drug-induced, e.g. thiazide or loop diuretics; α-adrenergic blockade, e.g. doxazosin (uncommon).
- Psychological, e.g. severe depression.
- Immobility, e.g. Parkinson's disease (Shy–Drager syndrome is uncommon).
- Other causes of autonomic neuropathy (📖 *OHCM* 8e, Chapter 9).
- Detrusor muscle instability.
- Urethral incompetence.
- Stool impaction.
- Spinal cord compression.
- Tabes dorsalis (rare in the UK).

Investigations

- U&E.
- Urinalysis for blood, protein, glucose, nitrates, nitrites.
- MSU for C&S.
- Plasma glucose (if glycosuria).
- Serum Ca^{2+}.

In selected patients, consider referral to urology or gynaecology services for consideration of:
- Bladder manometry studies.
- Post-voiding USS of bladder.
- Pelvic imaging, e.g. CT scan.

📖 *OHCM* 8e, p650.

Indigestion

This term is often loosely used by patients to describe a variety of symptoms. These are often regarded as representing relatively minor and usually intermittent pathology. However, serious pathology, e.g. carcinoma of the stomach, may present as a vague complaint of 'indigestion'. The symptoms may be retrosternal or abdominal. A detailed history is essential, focusing on features that raise the probability of serious pathology, e.g. dysphagia and weight loss.

Examination

Examination should include a search for the following signs, particularly in the middle-aged and elderly patients:

- Anaemia (especially iron deficiency—common).
- Ascites.
- Troissier's sign (malignant involvement of left supraclavicular lymph nodes due to carcinoma of the stomach—rare).

Note: The presence of associated pathologies, e.g. pernicious anaemia—↑ risk of stomach cancer—will alter the threshold for more detailed, expert investigation. Carcinoma of stomach is more common in Japanese.

Peptic ulceration may have classic elements that point to the diagnosis. Non-ulcer dyspepsia is very common and is often treated empirically with antacids, H_2 receptor antagonists, or H^+ pump inhibitor drugs. The clinical challenge is to identify the patient for whom more detailed and often invasive investigation is indicated.

Alternative causes, e.g. cardiac ischaemia, should be considered in the differential diagnosis; similarities of the symptoms between cardiac and upper gastrointestinal disorders are well recognized, and sometimes pose considerable diagnostic difficulties.

Causes include

- Oesophageal acid reflux.
- Hiatus hernia.
- Inflammatory disease.
- Peptic ulcer disease of duodenum or stomach.
- Biliary colic (usually distinctive clinical features).
- Malignancy of oesophagus, stomach, or rarely small intestine.
- Cardiac symptoms, usually ischaemia.
- Irritable bowel syndrome.
- Symptoms arising from other structures within the chest or abdomen.

Investigations

- FBC.
- U&E.
- ESR.
- Upper GI endoscopy ± tissue biopsy.
- LFTs.
- Creatine kinase (CK) if MI/ACS suspected.
- Troponin (T or I) if myocardial infarction (MI)/acute coronary syndrome (ACS) suspected.

- Serum amylase (normal in chronic pancreatitis; may be ↑ by duodenal ulcer eroding posterior wall).
- Barium swallow and meal (for oesophageal disease).
- *Campylobacter*-like organism (CLO) test for *Helicobacter pylori*.
- Urea ^{13}C breath test for *H. pylori*.
- USS of biliary tract (📖 Ultrasound, p751).
- Cholecystogram.

If diagnosis remains uncertain consider
- CT abdomen (discuss with radiologist).
- Serum gastrin (Zollinger–Ellison syndrome, 📖 *OHCM* 8e, p730).
- 24 h ambulatory oesophageal pH monitoring.
- Oesophageal manometry (oesophageal motility disorders).

Infective endocarditis signs

Infective endocarditis is characterized by infection of the endocardial surface of the heart. The left heart valves are the most commonly affected, but the right heart valves and congenital heart lesions, such as ventricular septal defects may also become infected. Vegetations (composed of the organism, white cells, platelets, and fibrous tissue) are formed at the site of infection. They give rise to periodic septicaemia and may embolize to other parts of the body. There is gradual destruction of the valve with increasing valvular dysfunction, regurgitation, and heart failure.

Clinical features
- Pyrexia (low-grade or swinging).
- Pale conjunctivae suggestive of anaemia (of chronic disease).
- Clubbing (chronic low-grade infection).
- Cardiac murmur (new or changing).
- Left or right heart failure.
- Splenomegaly (friction rub if splenic infarction is present).
- Microscopic haematuria (on urinalysis).

Embolic phenomena
Embolic phenomena are common and produce clinical signs classically associated with infective endocarditis:
- Splinter haemorrhages (>5, sited in the proximal finger and toenail beds).
- Janeway lesions (palmar macular spots).
- Osler's nodes (painful nodules on palmar surface of the fingers or toes).
- Roth spots (retinal haemorrhages).
- Conjunctival haemorrhages.
- Microvascular infarction (in the distal limbs).

Further reading
Prendergast BD. Diagnostic criteria and problems in infective endocarditis. *Heart* 2004; **90**: 611–13.
Task Force on Infective Endocarditis of the ESC. Guidelines on prevention, diagnosis and treatment of infective endocarditis. *Eur Heart J* 2004; **25**: 267–76.

Irregular pulse

In health, the pulse is usually regular, although a minor degree of variation in heart rate with respiration (sinus arrhythmia) is common, particularly in children and young adults. In sinus arrhythmia, the heart rate increases with inspiration and decreases with expiration. This is a benign phenomenon.

An irregular pulse can present as a symptom (with the patient complaining of an awareness of irregular or 'missed'/'extra' heartbeats) or as a sign (incidental finding on clinical examination).

Pulse irregularities are traditionally classified into two groups

- Regular irregularities.
- Irregular irregularities.

A regular irregular pulse

Most commonly the result of ventricular or supraventricular ectopic activity. Ectopic beats often occur after a certain number of sinus beats, thus in ventricular bigeminy, every other beat will be a ventricular ectopic beat, and thus occur prematurely with reduced volume. In trigeminy, every third beat will be early.

Can also be evident in 2nd degree atrioventricular block (Mobitz type I or II).

An irregularly irregular pulse

Most commonly the result of:
- Multiple ectopic beats (supraventricular or ventricular).
- Atrial fibrillation.
- Atrial flutter with variable atrioventricular block.

Investigations

The key to diagnosis is to record an ECG, while the pulse irregularity is present. If the paroxysmal irregularity is infrequent, this can prove challenging. A 12-lead ECG is mandatory and may provide an immediate diagnosis. If not, a number of ambulatory ECG monitoring techniques are available:
- 24 h ambulatory ECG monitoring.
- Cardiac event monitoring.
- Implantable loop recorder.

The choice of technique should be guided by how frequently the irregularity is thought to occur.

Additional investigations depend upon the nature of the suspected arrhythmia:
- FBC.
- U&E.
- TFTs.

One may also consider
- CXR (to assess heart size and valvular calcification).
- Echocardiogram (if structural heart disease suspected).
- Exercise treadmill test (if ischaemic heart disease (IHD) suspected, or to provoke arrhythmias thought to be exercise-related).

Jaundice

This defines the yellow discoloration of the sclerae, mucous membranes and skin that occurs when bilirubin accumulates. Bilirubin is the major bile pigment in humans, and is produced as an end-product of haem catabolism. Jaundice usually only becomes noticeable when the serum bilirubin > 30–60µmol/L.

Causes (Table 1.10)

- Can be pre-hepatic, hepatic, or post-hepatic.
- Haemolysis.
- Hepatitis (viral, drugs, alcohol).
- Pregnancy.
- Recurrent cholestasis.
- Hepatic infiltration.
- Stones in the common bile duct.
- Carcinoma of the bile duct, head of pancreas, or ampulla.
- Biliary strictures.
- Sclerosing cholangitis.
- Pancreatitis.

Investigations (Fig. 1.2)

- FBC (?haemolysis).
- Clotting screen (often deranged in liver disease).
- LFTs.
- Viral serology for HAV, HBV, and HCV.
- USS abdomen.
- Consider ERCP.
- Liver biopsy may be indicated depending on history, examination and laboratory findings. Discuss with gastroenterology team before embarking on this.

Table 1.10 Common causes of jaundice

Pre-hepatic	Cholestatic	
	Intra-hepatic	**Post-hepatic**
Haemolysis	Viral hepatitis	Gallstones
Gilbert's syndrome	Drugs	Carcinoma (biliary tree, head of pancreas, ampulla)
Crigler-Najjar syndrome	Alcoholic hepatitis	
	Cirrhosis (any type)	Biliary stricture
Dubin-Johnson syndrome	Pregnancy	Sclerosing cholangitis
	Recurrent idiopathic cholestasis	Pancreatic pseudocyst
	Infiltration (e.g. amyloidosis etc)	

📖 *OHCM* 8e, p250, p388.

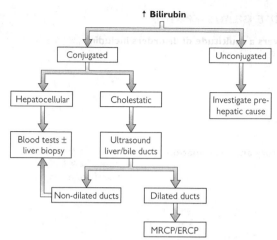

Fig. 1.2 Investigation of jaundice.

Joint pain/swelling

Covers a multitude of disorders including

- Osteoarthritis.
- Rheumatoid arthritis.
- Tendinitis.
- Bursitis.
- Trigger finger.
- Mechanical low back pain.
- Fibromyalgia.
- Other arthropathies.

History and examination

- Ask about affected joints, site of origin, mono- or polyarticular, oligo-articular (e.g. 2–4 joints involved), migratory features, arthralgia (joint pain without swelling).
- Is pain constant or intermittent?
- Aggravating or precipitating factors?
- Any associated neurological features?
- Is there swelling?
- Associated redness or excessive warmth?
- Drug history (e.g. diuretic induced).
- Race (e.g. sickle).
- Past history.
- Family history.
- Occupational history.
- Social history.

Investigations

- **FBC**: a normochromic normocytic anaemia is common in chronic inflammatory disorders. May be microcytic if long-standing inflammation or associated iron deficiency (e.g. induced by NSAIDs).
- **ESR**: non-specific marker of inflammation.
- **CRP**: as for ESR.
- Biochemistry screen, especially looking at bone profile and LFTs.
- Consider serum Igs and protein electrophoresis (myeloma).
- Uric acid levels (gout).
- X-ray affected joint(s).
- Consider USS, especially if soft-tissue swelling.
- MRI can be useful to help visualize intra-articular structures.
- CT scan.
- Bone scintigraphy (helps identify abnormal bone turnover).
- DEXA scan (useful for diagnosis and monitoring of osteoporosis).
- Arthroscopy may help in selected cases.
- Joint aspiration (allows culture and examination of fluid for crystals).

Jugular venous pulse

The height and waveform of the internal jugular venous pulse (JVP) reflect right atrial pressure and haemodynamics. The JVP should be inspected with the patient positioned at 45° to the horizontal. The JVP may be distinguished from the carotid pulse by the following features:

- Pulsation is not palpable.
- It may be compressed and obliterated by pressure.
- It rises on compression of the right upper quadrant (hepatojugular reflux).
- It varies with posture.
- Height decreases with inspiration.

The height of the JVP is measured as the vertical distance between the manubriosternal angle and the top of the venous pulsation. Elevation is defined as >3cm.

There are several components of the jugular venous pulsation waveform. The a wave is produced by atrial systole. This is followed by the x descent at the end of atrial contraction. The x descent is interrupted by a small barely perceptible deflection called a c wave. This deflection is caused by the rapid increase in right ventricular pressure just before the tricuspid valve closes. A subsequent v wave results from the rise in right atrial pressure as it fills with venous return during ventricular systole and whilst the tricuspid valve remains closed. At the end of ventricular systole, the tricuspid valve opens and the pressure in the right atrium falls leading to the y descent (see Table 1.11).

Table 1.11 Examples of JVP

Description	Diagram	Diagnosis	Comment
Normal		Normal	
↑ JVP normal waveform		Right heart failure Fluid overload Pulmonary embolus Cardiac tamponade	↑ right atrial pressure
Absent *a* wave		Atrial fibrillation	Poor atrial contraction fails to generate a wave
Large *a* waves		Tricuspid stenosis Right ventricular hypertrophy	Resistance to right atrial emptying causes ↑ right atrial pressure
Large *v* waves		Tricuspid regurgitation	Reflux of blood into the great veins with right ventricular contraction
Cannon (*a*) waves		Complete heart block Ventricular tachycardia	RA contracts against closed tricuspid valve creating a cannon wave
Rapid *y* descent		Constrictive pericarditis Cardiac tamponade Tricuspid regurgitation Right heart failure	A steep y descent is caused by RV diastolic collapse (Freidrich's sign)
Absent pulsation ↑ JVP		Superior vena caval obstruction	No right atrial pressure can be transmitted to the JVP

Loin pain

Definition: pain located in the renal angle.

Causes
- Ureteric colic.
- Renal or ureteric obstruction.
- Acute pyelonephritis.
- Renal infarction or papillary necrosis.
- Acute nephritis (uncommon).
- IgA nephropathy—pain caused by extension of the renal capsule.
- Musculoskeletal causes.
- Shingles at T10–12 (obvious if a rash is seen on examination or should be suspected if pain is in a dermatomal distribution).
- Infection or bleeding into a cyst in polycystic kidneys.
- Vesico-ureteric reflux—pain occurs when the bladder is full, this worsens at the initiation of micturition and then is rapidly relieved on voiding.
- Loin pain-haematuria syndrome—this is recurrent pain which occurs in young women. Angiography reveals tortuous vessels.

Investigations
- U&E.
- Serum creatinine.
- Creatinine clearance (if renal impairment).
- FBC.
- ESR.
- Urine dipstick for protein, blood, nitrites, leucocytes.
- Urine microscopy (for casts).
- MSU for culture and sensitivity testing.
- Blood cultures (if bacteraemia suspected).
- Plain X-ray (KUB view).
- IVU (e.g. if +ve urine dipstick for haematuria).
- Renal USS (useful for rapid non-invasive exclusion of obstruction).
- CT of urinary tract.
- Angiogram (if suspicion of thrombus, embolus or loin pain-haematuria syndrome).
- Serum immunoglobulin A (IgA) concentration.
- Cystoscopy (specialist procedure).
- Retrograde pyelography.
- Renal biopsy (only after specialist advice).

Lymphadenopathy

Lymph node enlargement may be localized or generalized (Table 1.12).

Localized cervical lymphadenopathy

- Local causes in mouth (pharyngitis, dental abscess).
- Scalp (skin malignancies or disease).
- Nose (nasopharyngeal carcinoma).

Enlargement of left supraclavicular nodes

May suggest carcinoma of stomach.

Isolated posterior cervical node enlargement

Is less often due to malignancy.

Other causes

Some drugs may be associated with lymph node enlargement (phenytoin, antithyroid).

Table 1.12 Causes of lymphadenopathy

Infection	
Viral	Infectious hepatitis, EBV syndromes, HIV, rubella, varicella, herpes zoster
Bacterial	Streptococcal, staphylococcal, salmonella, brucellosis, *Listeria*, cat-scratch (*Bartonella*)
Fungal	Histoplasmosis, coccidioidomycosis
Chlamydial	
Mycobacterial	
Parasites	Trypanosomiasis, microfilaria, toxoplasmosis
Spirochaetes	Syphilis, yaws, leptospirosis
Connective tissue	Rheumatoid arthritis, SLE, dermatomyositis, serum sickness
Drugs	E.g. phenytoin
Malignancy	
Haematological	Hodgkin's lymphoma, non-Hodgkin's lymphoma, acute and chronic lymphoid malignancies (CLL, ALL), AML
Non-haematological	Metastases from carcinomas (breast, bowel, lung, prostate, kidney, head, & neck)
Endocrine	Thyrotoxicosis
Miscellaneous	Sarcoidosis, amyloidosis

Investigations
- FBC, blood film, LDH (leukaemia, lymphoma, Hodgkin's).
- Serology/virology/microbiology/other antigen detection tests:
  - Viral (EBV, hepatitis, CMV, HIV).
  - Bacterial (tuberculosis, bacterial endocarditis, syphilis).
  - Fungal (histoplasmosis).
  - Protozoal (toxoplasmosis).
- ANA (collagen disorder, systemic lupus).
- TFTs (hyperthyroidism).
- CXR (sarcoid, tuberculosis).
- USS/CT scan (to assess intra-abdominal, mediastinal/hilar lymphadenopathy).
- LFTs/hepatomegaly (↑ alkaline phosphatase suggests malignant deposits).
- Lymph node biopsy (groin nodes should usually be avoided because commonly enlarged due to skin and infectious disorder).
- BM (may confirm haematological malignancy).

Note: Fine-needle aspiration, although easier to perform, may not be diagnostic and lymph node biopsy should be considered for microbiology and histology.

📖 *OHCM* 8e, p408.

Although we have provided a large list of possibilities, common sense should be used in determining the cause. For example, an 80-year-old woman with axillary lymphadenopathy is unlikely to have cat-scratch disease! Common things are common.

Nausea

The so-called vomiting centre is located in the medulla oblongata and is stimulated by the chemoreceptor trigger zone in the 4th ventricle. There are many causes of acute and chronic nausea. These can be divided into gastrointestinal (GI) causes and non-GI causes.

GI causes of nausea

- Food poisoning (viral, bacterial—common).
- Acute and chronic gastritis (remember *Helicobacter pylori*).
- Peptic ulceration.
- Biliary and renal colic.
- Inflammatory bowel disease.
- Cholecystitis.
- Appendicitis.
- Pancreatitis.
- Gastric outflow obstruction.
- Post-gastrectomy syndrome.
- Acute liver failure.
- Pseudo-obstruction of bowel.

Investigations

- U&E.
- LFTs.
- ESR.
- CRP.
- Serum or urinary amylase.
- Abdominal X-ray (erect and supine—*beware* perforated viscus).
- Abdominal ultrasound.

Consider

- OGD.
- Barium swallow and meal.
- Isotopic gastric emptying studies.
- Oesophageal manometry.
- Oesophageal muscle biopsy (rarely indicated).

Non-GI causes

- Acute infections, e.g. UTI.
- Metabolic disorders including:
  - Hypercalcaemia.
  - Ketoacidosis (diabetic, alcoholic).
  - Uraemia.
- Pregnancy. **NB**: hyperemesis gravidarum may be associated with ↑ FT4, ↓ TSH.
- Many drugs, notably opiates and digoxin toxicity (check serum levels).
- MI (nausea common; exacerbated by opiates).
- Acute glaucoma.
- Migraine.
- Raised intracranial pressure.

Investigations
- FBC.
- ESR.
- Venous plasma glucose.
- Urine dipstick (UTI).
- Serum Ca^{2+}.
- Serum drug levels, e.g. digoxin, theophylline.
- 12-lead ECG.
- CK.
- Troponin I.

Neurological causes
- Acute migraine.
- ↑ Intracranial pressure.
- Acute labyrinthine lesions.
- Menière's disease.
- Cerebellar lesions (e.g. infarct, haemorrhage, metastases, demyelination).

Investigations
- Cranial CT.
- MRI if cerebellar lesion suspected.
- Tilt table test (🕮 Tilt table testing, p461).
- Audiometry (specialist technique).

🕮 *OHCM* 8e, p450.

Neck stiffness

The main concern in a patient with neck stiffness is that s/he may have meningitis, which may result from infection or may reflect infiltration by a disease such as acute leukaemia. Distinguish neck stiffness (common) from meningism (rare, but serious).

Causes
- Bacterial infection.
- Viral infection.
- Fungal infection.
- Tuberculosis.
- Infiltration by malignancy (e.g. acute lymphoblastic leukaemia, high grade lymphoma, or sometimes acute myeloid leukaemia).
- Drug-induced.
- Contrast media (myelogram).
- Blood (e.g. post-subarachnoid haemorrhage).
- Mechanical/trauma.
- Connective tissue disease, e.g. rheumatoid arthritis.

Investigations
- CT scan of brain ± contrast.
- Lumbar puncture if no ↑ intracranial pressure:
  - Glucose.
  - Protein.
  - MC&S ± TB culture.
  - Xanthochromia if SAH suspected.
- If patient immunocompromised consider:
  - PCR for viruses, e.g. HSV.
  - Toxoplasma serology.
  - India ink stain for *Cryptococcus*.
- If considering malignancy, send cerebrospinal fluid (CSF) for cytospin.

📖 *OHCM* 8e, p460, p832.

Nystagmus

An involuntary oscillatory or (more commonly) rapid jerking movement of the eyes that is rhythmic and repetitive. It results from acute or chronic lesions of the eight cranial nerves, brainstem, or cerebellum. The 'slow' phase is pathological, the rapid rhythmic jerking phase (used arbitrarily to define the direction of nystagmus) being a corrective response. Nystagmus 'to the right' describes the direction of the quick phase. Such 'saw tooth' nystagmus may be evident in the horizontal or vertical plane (including 'downbeat' nystagmus of foramen magnum lesions) or as oscillations around a central point (e.g. in albinism).

Jerk nystagmus: May be graded in severity depending on whether it occurs:
- Only in the direction of directed gaze.
- When eyes are in the midline *or*
- Is present even on looking in direction contralateral to the rapid movement.

Note: Nystagmus (or more correctly, nystagmoid jerks) may be induced by inappropriate testing, often being present at the extremes of gaze. Do not ask patient to follow visual target beyond ~30° of midline when testing at the bedside. They are also a feature when drunk due to cerebellar dysfunction.

In unilateral causes

Cerebellar nystagmus
Greatest when gaze directed towards the side of the destructive lesion.

Vestibular nystagmus
Greatest away from the side of the lesion.

Pathological nystagmus
May be due to labyrinthine and vestibular lesions—occurs in one direction only. If visual fixation is removed, nystagmus becomes worse.

Central lesions
Including brainstem lesions caused by, e.g. tumour, MS; cerebellar lesions or medial longitudinal fasciculus lesions leading to internuclear ophthalmoplegia with ataxic nystagmus. Typically, 'central' nystagmus reverses direction in different directions of gaze, and may be complex (i.e. not in a single plane).

Investigations
- Positional nystagmus may be investigated by using the Hallpike manoeuvre. Abrupt alteration of the spatial position of the head (from supine, with head below the bed, rapidly to a sitting position) will induce nystagmus. This will demonstrate benign positional vertigo (common), vestibular disorders, or brainstem lesions.
- Audiometry (specialized investigation).
- Auditory and visual evoked potentials (VEPS) may be pathologically reduced in MS. Examination of CSF may reveal oligoclonal bands. (as noted above, EPs have a less important role in the modern diagnosis of MS than MRI and CSF).
- MRI to include brainstem. (Upbeat nystagmus may suggest a midbrain lesion and downbeat nystagmus will suggest a foramen magnum lesion.) MRI is superior to CT for demonstrating cerebellopontine angle lesions. Gadolinium enhancement is used to investigate acoustic neuromas.
- Ototoxicity can be caused by some drugs such as gentamicin and phenytoin. Acute poisoning with alcohol or barbiturates may cause transient nystagmus. Chronic alcoholism can lead to permanent cerebellar damage. Excessive doses of anticonvulsant drugs, e.g. phenytoin, are a common cause—measure serum concentrations of drug.

📖 OHCM 8e, p76.

Obesity

The World Health Organization defines obesity as a body mass index (BMI) greater than 30kg/m^2 (Table 1.13).

Table 1.13 Body Mass Index

	BMI (kg/m^2)
Underweight	<18.5
Normal	18.5–24.9
Overweight	>25.0–29.9
Obesity	
Class I	30.0–34.9
Class II	35.0–39.3
Class III	>40

Note: Central (abdominal) fat distribution—more common in men—is associated with greater health risks. Waist to hip ratio or simply waist girth can be used to identify levels at which long-term health risks warrant intervention:
- **Men**: > 102cm.
- **Women**: > 88cm.

Aetiology

The great majority of obese subjects have no identifiable metabolic or hormonal defects, and detailed investigation is rarely indicated. A chronic imbalance of the equation with energy intake (dietary calories) on the one hand and expenditure (resting metabolic rate + physical activity) on the other is thought to be responsible. Reduced levels of habitual activity allied to an abundance of energy-dense foods appears to account for the current pandemic of obesity and related disorders:
- Impaired glucose regulation.
- Type 2 DM.
- Dyslipidaemia.
- Hypertension.
- Cardiovascular disease (CVD).
- Osteoarthritis.
- Impaired physical functioning.
- Gout.
- ↑ Surgical risk.
- Depression.
- Certain cancers, e.g. bowel, breast.

Weight gain tends to occur in middle age; ♀ are more at risk than ♂. Socio-economic factors are also important.

Specific causes
- **Genetic**: e.g. Prader–Willi syndrome, Laurence–Moon (Biedl–Bardet) syndrome.
- **Single gene defects**: e.g. mutations of leptin (provides feedback from adipocytes to hypothalamus about body fat stores) or its hypothalamic receptor (very rare).
- **Hypothalamic lesions**: lesions that damage the ventromedial nucleus (the 'satiety' area) may lead to obesity.
- **Lesions include**:
  - *Trauma.*
  - *Tumours*—craniopharyngiomas and astrocytomas.
  - *Inflammation*—e.g. TB and meningitis.
  - *Infiltration*—histiocytosis and sarcoidosis.
- **Cushing's syndrome**: with 'buffalo' hump and central obesity.
- **Hypothyroidism**: disputed unless severe myxoedema, but hyperthyroidism is associated with non-physiological weight loss.
- **Insulinoma**: often associated with moderate weight gain; rare.
- **Marked ↓ motor inactivity**: e.g. severe mental retardation or physical disability.

Investigations
- Weight (calibrated scales).
- Height (stadiometer).
- Waist circumference (maximal).
- BP (large cuff required).
- Venous plasma glucose (or oral glucose tolerance test (OGTT)).
- TFTs.
- LFTs (↑ non-alcoholic steatohepatitis in obese subjects).
- Fasting lipid profile (📖 Investigation of hyperlipidaemia, p197).
- Serum urate.

Additional investigations
These may occasionally be indicated if clinical features give cause for suspicion of organic cause:
- Cranial CT or MRI of pituitary and hypothalamus.
- Investigations for Cushing's syndrome (📖 Obesity/hypercortisolism, p135).
- Genetic testing (seek advice of genetics service).

Further reading
Lean MEJ, Han TS, Seidell JC. Impairment of health and quality of life in men and women with a larger waist. *Lancet* 1998; **351**: 853–6.

Oliguria

Causes

Acute renal failure: distinguish pre-renal from renal and post-renal causes.

Pre-renal

- Severe sepsis.
- Hypovolaemia, e.g. GI haemorrhage, diuretics.
- Burn injury.
- CCF.
- Addison's disease.
- Acute pancreatitis.

Renal

- Acute tubular necrosis (ATN, e.g. 2° to nephrotoxins, such as aminoglycosides and radiological contrast media).
- Acute cortical necrosis.
- Renal infarction.
- Accelerated hypertension.
- Salicylate overdose.
- Hepatorenal syndrome.

Post-renal

- Renal calculi.
- Retroperitoneal calcinosis.
- Papillary necrosis.
- Bladder, prostate, and cervical tumours.
- Blocked urinary catheter (common!).

Investigations

- U&E.
- Serum creatinine.
- Creatinine clearance.
- FBC.
- ESR.
- Autoimmune profile.
- LFTs.
- Urinary Na^+ excretion (<20 pre-renal, >40 ATN).
- Urine osmolality (> 500mOsmol/L = re-renal, < 350mOsmol/L = ATN).
- Urine dipstick for blood, protein, nitrites, leucocytes.
- Urine microscopy for casts.
- Renal ultrasound (± biopsy in selected cases).
- Intravenous (IV) urogram.
- CT pelvis.
- Investigation of renal stones:
  - Serum calcium, phosphorus.
  - 24h excretion of oxalate, calcium, creatinine.

📖 *OHCM* 8e, p65, p285, p299, p578.

Palpitations

Patients generally use the term palpitations to refer to an awareness of an abnormally fast, forceful, or irregular heart rhythm. Palpitations can be physiological, as in the fast and/or forceful heart rhythm felt with exercise or anxiety, or pathological.

Common arrhythmias

Supraventricular arrhythmias
- Sinus tachycardia (📖 Tachycardia, p108).
- Atrial fibrillation.
- Atrial flutter.
- Atrial tachycardia.
- AV re-entry tachycardias.
- Supraventricular ectopics.

Ventricular arrhythmias
- Ventricular tachycardia.
- Torsades de pointes.
- Ventricular ectopics.

Investigations

The key to diagnosis is to record a 12-lead ECG while the palpitations are present. Although simple in principle, infrequent paroxysmal palpitations can make this very challenging. A 12-lead ECG is mandatory and may provide an immediate diagnosis if the patient is experiencing palpitations as it is performed. As well as assessing the heart rhythm, it is important to check for evidence of abnormal atrioventricular conduction (short P-R interval, pre-excitation) or abnormal repolarization (long QT interval). Check also for evidence of underlying structural heart disease, e.g. pathological Q waves indicative of previous myocardial infarction. If the patient's palpitations are paroxysmal, a number of ambulatory ECG monitoring techniques are available depending on how frequently the palpitations occur:
- 24h ambulatory ECG monitoring.
- Cardiac event monitoring.
- Implantable loop recorder.

Additional investigations depend upon the nature of the suspected arrhythmia. It is generally prudent to check:
- FBC.
- U&E.
- TFTs.
- One may also consider:
  - *CXR*—to assess heart size and valvular calcification.
  - *Echocardiogram*—if structural heart disease suspected.
  - *Exercise treadmill test*—if IHD suspected, or to provoke arrhythmias thought to be exercise-related.

📖 *OHCM* 8e, p35.

Pancytopenia

Pancytopenia (↓haemaglobin (Hb), ↓ white blood count (WBC) and ↓ platelets) may occur because of bone marrow failure (hypoplasia) or inefficient production (MDS), or peripheral destruction of cells or sequestration (splenomegaly/hypersplenism).

▶▶ Pancytopenia usually means something is seriously wrong.

Bone marrow assessment is necessary to establish whether the marrow is hypocellular or hypercellular in the face of peripheral blood pancytopenia. If hypercellular, the cause may be an infiltrative process (due to leukaemia/carcinoma, granulomatous disease, fibrosis–myelofibrosis, osteosclerotic–osteopetrosis, increased macrophages–haemophagocytic syndromes due to viral infections). Causes of hypoplastic bone marrow failure may be hereditary (e.g. Fanconi's anaemia) or acquired (e.g. drugs). Critically ill patients may develop pancytopenia for multiple reasons (sepsis, haemorrhage, DIC).

Investigations

- FBC, film (aplastic anaemia usually presents with ↓ lymphocyte count, but minor morphological changes).
- Reticulocytes (↓ if production failure).
- Serum vitamin B_{12}, folate (megaloblastic anaemia can be associated with pancytopenia).
- Serology for EBV, hepatitis A, B, C, HIV (associated with aplastic anaemia).
- Serology for parvovirus infection (if pure red cell aplasia also consider lymphoma, thymoma).
- ANA (lupus).
- Neutrophil alkaline phosphatase (NAP) score (↑ in aplastic anaemia).
- Check for lymphadenopathy, hepatomegaly, splenomegaly.
- CXR (bronchial carcinoma, sarcoid, tuberculosis, lymphoma).
- USS/CT to assess lymphadenopathy/splenomegaly (pancytopenia may be due to hypersplenism and portal hypertension).
- Ham's test for paroxysmal nocturnal haemoglobinuria (PNH) or cell marker analysis of CD55 and CD59.
- BM aspirate and cytogenetics (myelodysplasia is a clonal disorder).

📖 *OHCM* 8e, p358.

Paraesthesiae

This may be described by the patient as an abnormal sensation of aching, pricking, tickling, or tingling, commonly in the extremities or face. Often described as feeling like 'pins and needles'.

The selection of investigations will be determined largely by the history (transient? chronic?), the surface anatomical site of the abnormal sensation and associated symptoms or precipitating factors (e.g. clear history of hyperventilation).

The common causes include the numbness or tingling associated with pressure on the peripheral nerves such as caused by sleeping awkwardly on an arm ('Saturday night palsy' of the radial nerve), or chronic or recurrent pressure, e.g. on the ulnar nerve at the elbow.

If paraesthesiae is persistent, consider the following conditions, depending on the distribution of the symptoms:
- Carpal tunnel syndrome (with radiation proximally along forearm; worse at night).
- Peripheral neuropathy (DM, alcohol, drug-induced).
- Sciatica (reduced straight leg raising).
- Meralgia paraesthetica (lateral cutaneous nerve of the thigh).
- Lateral popliteal palsy (common peroneal nerve).

Other less common causes

Peripheral neuropathy
Due to:
- DM.
- Vitamin B_1 or B_{12} deficiencies.
- Chronic renal failure.
- Chronic hepatic failure.
- Malignancy.
- Neurotoxic drugs:
  - Vinca alkaloids.
  - Metronidazole.
  - Nitrofurantoin.
  - Isoniazid (pyridoxine-dependent).
- Environmental toxins.
- Hypothyroidism.
- Guillain–Barré syndrome (acute).
- Certain porphyrias.
- Multiple sclerosis.

Acute hypocalcaemia causes a characteristic perioral paraesthesia and can be due to many causes, including 1° and 2° hypoparathyroidism and alkalosis.

General investigations
- ABGs (acute or chronic acid-base disturbances leading to alterations in ionized Ca^{2+}).
- Serum calcium (not all laboratories measure ionized Ca^{2+}).
- Serum PTH (uncuffed sample).
- Serum magnesium (see next section).
- Venous plasma glucose.
- Vitamin B_{12} (and other investigations in suspected chronic peripheral neuropathy).

If serum calcium or magnesium concentration is low
Identify cause:
- Chronic GI loss (fistula, excessive diarrhoea, bowel obstruction).
- Chronic renal loss (diuretic drugs, intrinsic renal disease).
- Diabetic ketoacidosis (DKA)—total body magnesium may be low but this very rarely causes symptoms.

Additional investigations
Urinary (Mg^{2+}).

Consider
- USS abdomen/renal tract and subsequent GI investigations.
- U&E.
- Nerve conduction studies.
- TFTs.
- IGF-1, growth hormone (GH) response during 75g OGTT (if features of acromegaly present; 📖 Acromegaly (growth hormone excess), p128).

Peripheral neuropathy

The patient may complain of numbness in hands and feet that progresses proximally in a distribution classically termed 'glove and stocking'. Different aetiologies lead to motor, sensory, or mixed sensorimotor picture.

Common causes

- Idiopathic (50%, most common).
- Diabetes mellitus.
- Vitamin B_{12} deficiency (may occur in absence of anaemia).
- Vitamin B deficiency (e.g. alcoholics).
- Vitamin E deficiency.
- Carcinomatous neuropathy.
- Drugs, e.g. isoniazid, vinca alkaloids, cisplatin, dapsone, gold, metronidazole.
- Paraproteinaemias (e.g. MGUS or myeloma).

Rarer causes

- Amyloidosis.
- Uraemia.
- Collagen vascular diseases, e.g. rheumatoid, SLE, PAN.
- Endocrine disease, e.g. myxoedema, acromegaly.
- Guillain–Barré syndrome.
- Infections, e.g. tetanus, leprosy, diphtheria, botulism.
- Sarcoidosis.
- Hereditary, e.g. Charcot–Marie–Tooth disease.
- Acute intermittent porphyria.
- Toxins, e.g. lead (predominantly motor), arsenic (mixed sensory and motor), mercury (sensory), and thallium (mixed sensory and motor).
- Chronic inflammatory demyelinating polyneuropathy.
- Hereditary motor and sensory neuropathy types I or II.

Investigations

Nerve conduction studies to confirm the diagnosis.

Further investigations

- In order to determine the underlying cause.
- Discuss with neurology staff.

📖 *OHCM* 8e, p456, p506.

Peripheral oedema

Swelling of the legs or peripheral oedema is a common presenting symptom, which occurs when excess tissue fluid is redistributed by gravity. Severe oedema is usually pathological. Swelling of the ankles may progress to ascites, and even pleural and pericardial effusion.

Causes of generalized swelling

- **Cardiac failure**: congestive heart failure, dilated cardiomyopathy, constrictive pericarditis, cor pulmonale.
- **Hypoalbuminaemia**: liver failure (hepatic cirrhosis), renal failure (nephrotic syndrome), protein-losing enteropathy, malnutrition (malabsorption or starvation).

Causes of localized swelling

- **Immobility**: common in old age, long distance travel.
- **Infection**: cellulitis.
- Deep vein thrombosis and/or subsequent venous insufficiency.
- **Drugs**: calcium channel blockers (nifedipine, amlodipine), NSAIDs.
- **Malignancy**: compression of deep vein, enlarged lymph nodes or lymphatics.
- **Lymphatic obstruction**: congenital, infiltrative (filariasis).
- **Milroy's disease**.
- **Pregnancy**.
- **Wet beri-beri**.
- **Idiopathic**.

Patients at special risk

- Pregnancy.
- Prolonged bed rest.
- Following removal of lower limb plaster cast.
- Relative immobility: long-distance travel.
- Congestive cardiac failure.

Investigations

These should be guided by the history and examination.
- FBC.
- U&E.
- Albumin.
- ESR.
- Blood cultures.
- ECG.
- Echocardiography.
- Doppler studies of leg veins/contrast venography (according to local availability).
- Abdominal ultrasound.
- Malignancy screen for common cancers.
- Urine dipstick for proteinuria.
- 24 h urinary protein excretion or urine protein/creatinine ratio.
- Small bowel biopsy.
- Xylose breath test.

Petechiae & thrombocytopenia

Spontaneous bleeding in the absence of trauma is uncommon with platelet counts > 20 × 10^9/L. However, bleeding is much more likely if the thrombocytopenia is not immune in origin (e.g. aplastic anaemia, acute leukaemia, drug-induced, chemotherapy, myelodysplasia).

Thrombocytopenia may be inherited or acquired (e.g. DIC). As for pancytopenia, these may be classified as due to a failure of production, increased consumption in the peripheries (DIC, ITP) or due to abnormal tissue distribution (splenomegaly).

ITP may be 1° or 2° (e.g. lymphoma, lupus, HIV).

Drugs (e.g. heparin) and blood transfusion (post-transfusion purpura) may cause severe thrombocytopenia.

Investigations
- FBC, film:
  - Inherited causes may be associated with giant platelets.
  - Morphological abnormalities may suggest MDS.
  - Red cell fragments suggest thrombotic microangiopathies, e.g. thrombotic thrombocytopenic purpura (TTP).
- LDH (↑ in TTP and lymphoproliferative disorders).
- Serum vitamin B_{12}, folate (megaloblastic anaemia can be associated with ↓ platelets).
- ANA, autoimmune screen, immunoglobulins (lupus, hyperthyroidism).
- Virology (HIV, EBV, viral hepatitis, CMV).
- Clotting screen (DIC).
- Lupus anticoagulant, cardiolipin antibodies (antiphospholipid antibody syndromes).
- Platelet serology for drug- or transfusion-related causes.
- Bone marrow assessment to establish whether thrombocytopenia is due to a bone marrow production problem or due to peripheral consumption (discuss with haematology team: depending on degree of thrombocytopenia, other haematological findings and age of patient, a marrow may not be required).

Pitfalls
Thrombocytopenia due to HIV infection must be considered especially in all younger adults. Not worth checking platelet-associated immunoglobulin G (IgG) or immunoglobulin M (IgM), since these are elevated in thrombocytopenia caused by immune and non-immune mechanisms, so add no useful information.

Plethora

A plethoric appearance is typically seen in association with polycythaemia, but may also be mistaken for a normal outdoors complexion or cyanosis. Patients with haematocrits above the normal reference range may or may not have an increased red cell mass (real or relative polycythaemia, respectively; Table 1.14).

Investigations

- FBC, film (repeat FBC as sampling errors can falsely cause elevations of Hb; PRV may be associated with neutrophilia, basophilia, or ↑ platelets).
- Measurement of red cell mass may be necessary to confirm true polycythaemia. Investigations are then aimed at establishing whether real polycythaemia, if documented, is due to a 1° bone marrow abnormality (polycythemia rubra vera (PRV)) or a 2° disorder (e.g. respiratory disease).
- Neutrophil alkaline phosphatase score (may be raised in PRV). Seldom used now (□ Neutrophil alkaline phosphatase, p278).
- Vitamin B_{12} and urate (may be ↑ in PRV).
- ESR/CRP (acute phase reactants may suggest 2° causes).
- Blood gas analysis, oxygen saturation, carboxyhaemoglobin levels (2° polycythaemia due to respiratory disease, smoking).
- Biochemistry (urea, creatinine; renal disease).
- Erythropoietin (↑ in 2° causes).
- USS abdomen (renal cysts, liver disease, uterine fibroids, and other malignancies may 'inappropriately' secrete erythropoietin; also check for splenomegaly in PRV).
- Sleep studies (obstructive sleep apnoea, supine desaturation).
- O_2-dissociation studies (polycythaemia due to abnormal, high affinity Hb variant).
- Bone marrow aspirate and chromosomal studies/cytogenetics (PRV is a clonal disorder).

Table 1.14 Polycythaemia		
↑ Red cell count	>6.0 × 10¹²/L	♂
	>5.5 × 10¹²/L	♀
↑ PCV	>50%	♂
	>45%	♀
↑ Hb	>18.0g/dL	♂
	>16.0g/dL	♀

Polyuria

Polyuria (the passage of an excessive volume of urine, which may be associated with frequency of micturition and nocturia) must be differentiated from urinary symptoms associated with prostatic disease and urinary infections. The latter are also characterized by frequency, urgency, and nocturia, but usually small amounts of urine are passed at each void.

Causes

- DM.
- Cranial DI:
  - Familial (autosomal dominant).
  - 2° to posterior pituitary or hypothalamic disease, e.g. surgery, tumours, especially metastases, neurosarcoidosis.
- Nephrogenic DI:
  - Familial (X-linked recessive).
  - Chronic intrinsic renal disease, e.g. pyelonephritis.
  - Hypokalaemia.
  - Hypercalcaemia.
  - Sickle cell crisis.
  - Lithium, colchicine, amphotericin B.
  - Post-obstructive uropathy.
- 1° polydipsia (psychogenic).

Investigations

- 24 h urinary volume.
- Venous plasma glucose.
- U&E.
- TFTs.
- LH.
- FSH (?panhypopituitarism).
- Serum calcium and PTH.
- Sickle cell test.
- CXR (?mediastinal lymphadenopathy in TB, sarcoidosis).

If no obvious cause found consider detailed investigations for cranial or nephrogenic DI (📖 Polydipsia & polyuria: diabetes insipidus, p129).

📖 OHCM 8e, p65.

Pruritus

Implies generalized itching and may be associated with many disorders including:
- Iron deficiency.
- Malignant disease, e.g. lymphoma.
- Diabetes mellitus.
- Chronic renal failure.
- Liver disease, e.g. 1° biliary cirrhosis.
- Thyroid disease.
- Polycythaemia rubra vera.
- HIV infection.

Investigations
- Aim to exclude the above diseases.
- FBC.
- Biochemistry screen, including LFTs and renal function.
- Glucose.
- TFTs.

📖 *OHCM* 8e, p26, p532.

Ptosis

Ptosis can be unilateral and bilateral. Bilateral ptosis can be more difficult to recognize. Ptosis must be considered in association with other signs and symptoms. Ptosis may be long-standing, of recent onset, progressive or intermittent, especially at the end of the day—myasthenia gravis (MG).

Unilateral ptosis

Causes
- Constitutional (congenital).
- Oculomotor (III) nerve palsy—levator palpebrae. 'Down and out' pupil with loss of light reflex (e.g. DM, SOL, demyelination).
- Aneurysm (basilar or posterior communicating arteries).
- Cavernous sinus disease.
- Meningitis.
- Horner's syndrome—superior tarsal muscle (brainstem infarction, syringobulbia, SOL, MS).
- Encephalitis.

Abnormal (reduced) sweating on ipsilateral side face (damage to cervical sympathetic chain): Pancoast's tumour
- Aortic arch aneurysm.
- Cervical injuries.

No disorder of sweating
- Cluster headache.
- Parasellar tumours.
- Carotid artery aneurysm or dissection.
- Nasopharyngeal tumours.

Investigations
- Venous plasma glucose.
- CXR (Pancoast's syndrome).
- Cranial CT or MRI.
- Cerebral angiography (aneurysm).

Bilateral ptosis

Causes
- Guillain–Barré syndrome.
- Miller–Fisher syndrome.
- Myotonic dystrophy (MD).
- MG.
- Neurosyphilis (bilateral; Argyll Robertson pupils).

Investigations
- Syphilis serology.
- EMG ('dive-bomber' in MD).
- Serum anti-acetylcholine receptor antibodies (MG).
- Intravenous edrophonium (Tensilon) test (MG, 📖 Edrophonium (Tensilon®) test, p588; 📖 *OHCM* 8e, p78.

Pulmonary embolism

Occurs when thrombus in systemic veins or the right side of the heart embolizes into the pulmonary arterial system. Impaired gas exchange occurs because of a mismatch between ventilation and perfusion.

Investigations
- FBC (may be leucocytosis, neutrophilia most likely).
- ESR (often ↑).
- **Plasma D-dimers**: ↑ with fresh thrombus.
- **ABGs**: hypoxia and hypocapnia.
- **ECG**: look for atrial fibrillation (AF). Usually sinus tachycardia, may be evidence of RV 'strain'. In massive PE there may be $S_1Q_3T_3$.
- **CXR**: often normal, but may show signs of pulmonary infarction or effusion.
- **V/Q scan**: may be useful for detection of areas of the lungs that are being ventilated, but not perfused.
- **Spiral CT scan**: useful for detection of medium-sized pulmonary emboli but does not exclude small PEs.
- CT pulmonary angiogram.

📖 *OHCM* 8e, p182, p828.

Pulse character

Rate and heart rhythm can be determined from palpation of the radial pulse. The arm should then be elevated to check for a collapsing pulse. Pulse volume and additional characteristics are assessed from palpation of the brachial or carotid pulse (see Table 1.15).

Table 1.15 Examples of different pulse characters

Description	Diagram	Diagnosis	Comment
Normal		Normal	Normal volume and character
Slow rising		Aortic stenosis	Reduced volume pulse with delayed peak pulsation
Collapsing		Aortic regurgitation High cardiac output – Thyrotoxicosis – Anaemia – Fever Patent ductus arteriosus	Increased volume pulse with rapid rise and fall
Pulsus alternans		Severe heart failure	Pulse is regular, but alternate beats are weak and strong
Pulsus bisferiens		Hypertrophic cardiomyopathy Mixed aortic valve disease	Palpable double pulse
Pulsus bigeminus		Bigeminy	An ectopic beat occurs after every normal sinus beat
Pulsus paradoxus		Severe asthma Cardiac tamponade Constrictive pericarditis	There is exaggeration of the usual fall in blood pressure during inspiration >10mmHg)

Purpura

Implies bleeding of varying degrees into the skin. Includes petechial haemorrhages (pinpoint) and ecchymoses (bruises). There are many causes, including disorders of platelets and blood vessels.

Causes

- Congenital, e.g. Osler–Weber–Rendu syndrome (= hereditary haemorrhagic telangiectasia), connective tissue (Ehlers–Danlos), osteogenesis imperfecta, Marfan's.
- Severe infection (septic, meningococcal, measles, typhoid).
- Allergic, e.g. Henoch–Schönlein purpura.
- Drugs, e.g. steroids.
- Miscellaneous, e.g. senile purpura, scurvy, factitious.
- Thrombocytopenia—any cause (immune, marrow infiltration, deficiency of vitamin B_{12} or folate, myelofibrosis, DIC, TTP/ haemolytic-uraemic syndrome (HUS)).

Investigations

- FBC (looking for platelet abnormalities and presence of leukaemic cells or other signs of infiltration).
- Coagulation screen (looking for clotting factor deficiencies, DIC, etc.).
- Bleeding time using template device (previously used as test of platelet function, but largely abandoned now because of poor reproducibility).

📖 *OHCM* 8e, p308, p338, p716.

Recurrent thrombosis

The pathogenesis (and, hence, causes) of thrombosis reflect abnormalities in the dynamics of the circulation, the blood vessel walls, or the blood constituents (Virchow's triad). A hypercoagulable or thrombophilic risk factor is an inherited or acquired disorder of the haemostatic mechanisms, which may be associated with an increased likelihood of a thrombotic event (venous or arterial) or recurrent thrombosis (Table 1.16). This concept of risk factors for thrombosis is analogous to that for heart disease, and similarly for most patients *multiple causal factors operate*.

Hereditary thrombotic disease may be suggested by a positive family history but should be tested for if the venous thrombotic events occur in the absence of acquired causes, at a younger age, at unusual sites (e.g. mesenteric) or as recurrent thromboses.

Investigations in recurrent thrombosis

Inherited thrombophilia screening

- Deficiency of factors, e.g. protein C, protein S, or antithrombin.
- Abnormal protein (factor V Leiden (FVL)).
- Increased procoagulant (prothrombin time (PT, VIII)); others (homocysteinuria).
- Consider occult malignancy (PSA in ♂, pelvic USS in ♀).
- FBC (myeloproliferative disorder, PNH).
- Biochemistry (cardiac disease, liver disease, nephrotic syndrome).
- ESR/CRP (ulcerative colitis).

- ANA/lupus anticoagulant/cardiolipin antibodies (antiphospholipid antibody syndromes, lupus).

Pitfalls

Thrombophilia testing may be complicated if the patient is on warfarin/ heparin. Discuss with laboratory before sending samples.

📖 *OHCM* 8e, p368.

Table 1.16 Thromboembolic risk factors

Acquired	
Cardiac disease	MI, AF, cardiomyopathy, CCF
Post-operative	Especially abdominal, pelvic or orthopaedic surgery
Pregnancy	
Malignancy	Any
Polycythaemia	
Immobilisationization	Prolonged
Fractures	Especially hip and pelvis
Obesity	
Varicose veins	
Drugs	E.g. oestrogen-containing oral contraceptive
Inherited	Activated protein C resistance, e.g. factor V Leiden, mutation, protein C or S deficiency, dysfibrinogenaemias

Retinal haemorrhage

May be

- Flame-shaped (e.g. hypertension).
- Dot & blot (e.g. diabetes mellitus, vein occlusion, or haematological disease).
- Pre-retinal haemorrhage, suggests new vessel formation, e.g. diabetes or post-retinal vascular occlusion.
- Hyperviscosity syndromes.
- Severe anaemia.
- Severe thrombocytopenia.
- Haemoglobinopathy, e.g. HbSC.

Investigations

- Check BP.
- Renal function.
- FBC (↑↑ Hb or platelets).
- ESR or plasma viscosity (hyperviscosity syndromes such as myeloma or Waldenström's macroglobulinaemia).
- Serum Igs and protein electrophoresis.
- Hb electrophoresis.

Rigors

Fever is due to a resetting of the anterior hypothalamic thermostat, is mediated by prostaglandins (hence, aspirin is beneficial) and is most commonly caused by infection. Large variations in temperature may be accompanied by sweats, chills, and rigors. An undulant fever may suggest Hodgkin's disease or brucellosis. 'B' symptoms define fever (> 38°C), night sweats (drenching), weight loss (> 10%), and suggest a diagnosis of lymphoma. (Fever is unusual in CLL in the absence of infection.)

Investigations

- FBC, film (Hodgkin's disease is associated with anaemia, neutrophilia, eosinophilia, lymphopenia).
- LDH (↑ in lymphoma, non-specific test).
- Microbiological tests, blood/urine cultures (also consider pyogenic infection and abscesses in more unusual sites, e.g. renal).
- Antigen detection tests for specific pathogens.
- CXR (tuberculosis, lymphoma).
- ANA (connective tissue disease).
- BM aspirate/trephine may be necessary as part of leukaemia and lymphoma work-up.

Pitfalls

Not all fever is caused by infection.

📖 *OHCM* 8e, p27, p388, p394.

Short stature

The assessment of short stature can be a long and difficult process. Constitutional short stature is the most common cause. Psychosocial disease must be considered, but extensive investigation is required to rule out organic disease. If no cause is found, a period of observation may make the underlying cause apparent. Specialist evaluation should be undertaken in all cases.

Causes

Endocrine
- GH deficiency.
- GH resistance (very rare).
- Hypothyroidism (readily treatable).
- Cushing's syndrome (rare in children—**Note**: corticosteroid treatment for chronic asthma).
- Rickets.
- Pseudohypoparathyroidism.
- Type 1 DM—Mauriac's syndrome, now rare.

Non-endocrine
- Constitutional short stature (short parents).
- Emotional deprivation.
- Intra-uterine growth retardation.

- Achondroplasia.
- Mucopolysaccharidoses (rare).
- Turner's syndrome (46 XO and variants).
- Noonan's syndrome (46 XY, but features of Turner's in a male).
- Congenital cardiac disease, e.g. left-to-right shunt, cardiac failure.
- Cystic fibrosis.
- Other causes of malabsorption, e.g. coeliac disease, Crohn's colitis.
- Chronic liver disease.
- Haematological disease, e.g. sickle cell disease.
- Chronic renal disease.

Investigations

- Current height + weight (compare with any previous data available; plot on growth charts).
- Growth velocity—normal if prior problem, e.g. intra-uterine growth retardation.
- Physical stigmata of physical disease. **Note**: CNS examination mandatory.
- FBC.
- ESR.
- U&E.
- LFTs.
- TFTs.
- Serum albumin (?nutritional status).
- Venous plasma glucose.
- Serum calcium.
- Serum alkaline phosphatase (bone isoenzyme).
- Serum phosphate (reduced in rickets).
- X-ray pelvis (Looser's zones), epiphyses (wide, irregular in rickets), ribs (multiple fractures).
- Serum antigliadin and antiendomysial antibodies (coeliac).
- Testosterone or oestradiol, LH, FSH, PRL (if puberty delayed— panhypopituitarism?).
- X-ray of wrist for bone age. If delayed, measure serum IGF-1 (if IGF-1 normal, then GH deficiency unlikely; if IGF-1 low, consider nutritional and general health status before diagnosing GH deficiency—stimulation tests required, ∏ Endocrinology and metabolism, Short stature, p168). If normal—constitutional short stature.
- Karyotype (Turner's and Noonan's syndromes).
- 24 h urinary free cortisol (as screen for Cushing's syndrome, ∏ Obesity/hypercortisolism, p135).
- CT or MRI of pituitary (if GH deficiency or panhypopituitarism).

Skin pigmentation

Skin pigmentation can be due to increased melanin deposition, e.g. racial differences in skin pigmentation or due to ↑ melanin deposition seen in sun exposure. Lentigines and freckles are common. Haemosiderin and other substances can ↑ skin pigmentation. Increased pigmentation can be seen in various dermatological conditions; chronic inflammation, and fungal infection can result in increased skin pigmentation. Lichen planus and fixed drug eruptions are associated with increased pigmentation.

Increased pigmentation may also be found in association with chronic systemic disease:

- Addison's disease (palmar creases, buccal pigmentation, recent scars).
- Porphyria cutanea tarda (especially exposed areas—dorsum of hands).
- Chronic malabsorption syndromes.
- Drugs, e.g. amiodarone, psoralens, mepacrine, minocycline, chloroquine.
- Chronic uraemia.
- Haemochromatosis (so-called 'bronzed diabetes').
- 1° biliary cirrhosis (deep green-yellow jaundice, chronic pruritus).
- Ectopic ACTH syndrome, e.g. bronchial carcinoma.
- Nelson's syndrome (excessive ACTH secretion from pituitary basophil adenoma in Cushing's disease treated by bilateral adrenalectomy).
- Carotenaemia (orange discoloration does not involve sclerae *cf.* jaundice).
- Chloasma (pregnancy, oestrogen-containing oral contraceptive pill).
- Acanthosis nigricans—most often a marker of insulin resistance in obese patients with type 2 DM. Rarely in association with underlying carcinoma.
- Peutz–Jegher's syndrome (fingers, lips in association with small intestine polyposis).

Contrast with hypopigmentation

- Localized acquired depigmentation (vitiligo) is a marker of auto-immune disease.
- Oculocutaneous albinism (autosomal recessive).
- Chronic hypopituitarism (📖 Hypothalamus/pituitary function, p125).
- Phenylketonuria.

Investigations

- FBC.
- U&E.
- Venous plasma glucose.
- Antigliadin and antiendomysial antibodies.
- Short Synacthen test (if 1° hypoadrenalism suspected, 📖 Short Synacthen® test, p209).
- Urinary porphyrins.
- LFTs, serum albumin and prothrombin time (INR).
- Fe/TIBC/ferritin + genetic markers for haemochromatosis + liver biopsy.
- ESR and/or CRP.

- Autoimmune profile (📖 Chapter 4).
- Testosterone (or oestradiol) + LH, FSH.
- Antimitochondrial antibodies, liver Bx (1° biliary cirrhosis).
- Investigations for Cushing's syndrome (📖 Obesity/hypercortisolism, p135).
- Investigations for causes of chronic renal failure.

Splenomegaly

A palpable spleen is at least twice its normal size, when its length > 14cm. Enlargement may represent changes in the white pulp (lymphoid tissue expansion, inflammation), red pulp (blood congestion, extramedullary haemopoiesis), or occasionally supporting structures (cysts).

Causes in Western societies

- Leukaemias.
- Lymphomas.
- Myeloproliferative disorders.
- Haemolytic anaemias.
- Portal hypertension.
- Infections, e.g. infective endocarditis, typhoid, TB, brucellosis, viral (EBV, viral hepatitis).

Less common causes

- Storage disorders (e.g. Gaucher's).
- Collagen diseases.
- Sarcoid.
- Amyloid.

If foreign residence/travel, consider infectious causes (malaria, leishmaniasis, schistosomiasis) and haemoglobinopathies (HbC, HbE, thalassaemia).

Massive splenomegaly (> 8cm palpable below left costal margin (LCM))

- Myelofibrosis.
- Chronic myeloid leukaemia (CML).
- Gaucher's.
- Malaria.
- Leishmaniasis.

Investigations

Thorough history and physical examination.

- FBC, blood film, LDH (leukaemia, lymphoma, pernicious anaemia).
- Reticulocytes, bilirubin (if ↑ suggests haemolysis).
- Virology/microbiology (sepsis, bacterial endocarditis, EBV, CMV).
- Serum protein electrophoresis (myeloma, amyloid).
- Autoantibody screen, ANA (collagen disease, lupus, RhA).
- Haemoglobinopathy screen.
- LFTs (splenomegaly may be associated with hepatomegaly, or due to portal hypertension).

- Peripheral blood cell markers (immunophenotype—may show leukaemia or lymphoma).
- BM aspirate/trephine/cell markers/cytogenetics.
- Leucocyte glucocerebrosidase activity (Gaucher's disease).
- USS to assess liver texture, splenomegaly, lymphadenopathy.

 OHCM 8e, p582, p336, p367.

Steatorrhoea

Implies that the patient is passing pale, bulky stools that are offensive (contain fat and tend to float), and are difficult to flush away.

Causes

- Any disorder that prevents absorption of micellar fat from the small bowel.
- Ileal disease.
- Ileal resection.
- Parenchymal liver disease.
- Obstructive jaundice.
- Pancreatic disease, including cystic fibrosis.
- ↓ Bile salt concentration.
- Bile salt deconjugation by bacteria.
- Cholestyramine.
- β-lipoprotein deficiency.
- Lymphatic obstruction.

Investigations

Blood tests
- LFTs.
- Bone profile.
- Vitamin B_{12} and serum (or red cell) folate.
- Autoantibody profile.
- Serum amylase.

Pancreatic investigations
- Pancreatic function tests.
- CT scan.

Small bowel
- Small bowel follow-through.
- Jejunal biopsy (?villus atrophy).
- Bacterial overgrowth (^{14}C glycocholate breath test).

Parasites
Stool culture (e.g. *Giardia*).

Ileal disease
Consider Crohn's.

📖 *OHCM* 8e, p246.

Stridor

Stridor denotes a harsh respiratory added sound during inspiration. It may be a high-pitched musical sound similar to wheeze, but arises from constriction of the larynx or trachea. Stridor may be aggravated by coughing.

▶▶ Progressive breathlessness accompanied by indrawing of intercostal spaces and cyanosis indicates severe laryngeal obstruction with risk of sudden death.

In young children

Because of the smaller size of the larynx and trachea in children, stridor may occur in a variety of conditions:

- Postural stridor (laryngomalacia).
- Allergy, e.g. nut allergy, insect stings—common. **Note**: emergency Rx with intramuscular (IM) or subcutaneous (SC) adrenaline (epinephrine)—self-administered or by parent, and parenteral hydrocortisone.
- Vocal cord palsy.
- Croup (acute laryngitis—often coryza).
- Acute epiglottitis.
- Inhaled foreign body, e.g. peanut (common—inhalation further down the respiratory tract, usually into the right main bronchus, may produce localized wheeze or distal collapse, 🕮 Patterns of lobar collapse, pp717–8).

Investigations
- Pulse oximetry (non-invasive measurement of PO_2).
- Plain lateral X-ray of neck (for radio-opaque foreign body).
- Endoscopic nasolaryngoscopy.

Adults

- Infection especially *Haemophilus influenzae*.
- Inflammatory or allergic laryngeal oedema, e.g. penicillin allergy may be accompanied by anaphylactic shock.
- Pharyngeal pouch (may be recurrent lower respiratory tract infection).
- Inhaled vomitus or blood in unconscious patient.
- Tetany (due to low serum calcium or alkalosis).
- Large multinodular goitre, carcinoma or lymphoma of thyroid (uncommon).
- Laryngeal tumours.
- Bronchogenic tumour with bilateral cord paralysis (subcarinal and paratracheal gland involvement. **Note**: 'Bovine' cough of right recurrent laryngeal nerve palsy).
- Shy–Drager syndrome (of autonomic neuropathy).

Investigations
- CXR.
- Lateral X-ray of neck.
- Ultrasound of thyroid.
- Endoscopic nasolaryngoscopy.
- Bronchoscopy.
- Barium swallow (pharyngeal pouch).
- CT neck and mediastinum.
  🕮 *OHCM* 8e, p48.

Suspected bleeding disorder

Bleeding problems present a considerable challenge. Patients may present with simple easy bruising—a common problem—or catastrophic post-traumatic bleeding. The best predictors of bleeding risk are found in taking an accurate history, focusing on past haemostatic challenges (e.g. tonsillectomy, teeth extraction, menses—especially at time of menarche) and current drug history (e.g. aspirin). The history may also help delineate the type of defect. Platelet bleeding (e.g. thrombocytopenia) starts at the time of the (even minor) haemostatic insult, but if controlled by local pressure tends not to recur. Bleeding due to coagulation factor deficiency tends to be associated with internal/deep muscle haematomas as the bleeding typically occurs in a delayed fashion after initial trauma and then persists.

Inappropriate bleeding or bruising may be due to a local factor, or an underlying systemic haemostatic abnormality.

▶ Acquired causes of bleeding are much more common than inherited causes.

Causes of bleeding include
- Surgical.
- Trauma.
- Non-accidental injury.
- Coagulation disorders.
- Platelet dysfunction.
- Vascular disorders.

Clinical features
History and presenting complaint. Is this an isolated symptom? What type of bleeding does the patient have, e.g. mucocutaneous, easy bruising, spontaneous, post-traumatic. Duration and time of onset—?recent or present in childhood. Menstrual and obstetrical history are important.

Systemic enquiry
Do the patient's symptoms suggest a systemic disorder, bone marrow failure, infection, liver disease, renal disease?

Past medical history
Previous episodes of bleeding, recurrent—?ITP, congenital disorder. Exposure to trauma, surgery, dental extraction, or pregnancies.

Family history
First degree relatives. Pattern of inheritance (e.g. autosomal, sex-linked). If family history is negative this could be a new mutation (one-third of new haemophilia is due to new mutations).

Drugs

All drugs cause some side effects in some patients. Bleeding may result from thrombocytopenia, platelet dysfunction. Don't forget to ask about aspirin and warfarin.

Physical examination

Signs of systemic disease

Is there any evidence of septicaemia, anaemia, lymphadenopathy ± hepatosplenomegaly?

Assess bleeding site

Check palate and fundi. Could this be self-inflicted? Check size—petechiae (pin head); purpura (larger, but ≤1cm); bruises (ecchymoses; ≥1cm).

Joints

Swelling or other signs of chronic arthritis.

Vascular lesions

Purpura—allergic, Henoch–Schönlein, senile, steroid-related, hypergamma-globulinaemic, HHT—capillary dilatations (blanches on pressure), vasculitic lesions, autoimmune disorders, hypersensitivity reactions.

Investigations

- FBC, film, platelet count, biochemistry screen, ESR, coagulation screen.
- Special tests, e.g. BM for 1° haematological disorders; radiology, USS.
- Family studies.

Suspected stroke

A stroke denotes an acute neurological deficit. Strokes may vary in presentation, e.g. rapidly resolving neurological deficit to a severe permanent or progressive neurological defect (e.g. multi-infarct disease). Neurological deficits persisting >24 h termed 'completed stroke' *cf.* transient ischaemic attack (TIA). With suspected stroke, a full history and general physical examination are mandatory. Risk factors for cerebrovascular disease should be sought, including a history of hypertension (common—major risk factor), DM (common—major risk factor), and dyslipidaemia. Ask about recent falls or trauma. Hemiparesis can occur as a post-ictal phenomenon, or a result of migraine or hypoglycaemia. Hysterical or functional paralysis is also seen, but should not be confidently assumed at presentation. Neuroanatomical localization of the deficit and the nature of the lesion(s) requires appropriate imaging. *Note*: the post-ictal state may be associated with temporary (<24 h) limb paresis (Todd's paralysis) in focal epilepsy (suggests structural lesion—cranial imaging is mandatory).

General investigations

- FBC (polycythaemia, anaemia).
- U&E.
- ESR.
- Protein electrophoresis (if hyperviscosity syndrome suspected, e.g. ↑↑ ESR).
- ECG (atrial fibrillation, IHD—statins reduce risk of stroke in patients with previous MI).
- CXR (cerebral metastases from bronchogenic carcinoma?).

Specific risk factors

- Venous plasma glucose. NB: severe hypoglycaemia, e.g. insulin-induced or 2° to sulphonylureas, may mimic acute stroke. Always check capillary fingerprick glucose concentration to exclude this possibility—even if there is no history of DM. Take venous sample in fluoride-oxalate tube (+ serum for insulin concentration) if hypoglycaemia confirmed. (See 📖 Diabetes mellitus, p181 for further details of investigation and treatment.) Hyperosmolar non-ketotic diabetic coma may also be misdiagnosed as stroke (plasma glucose usually >50mmol/L with pre-renal uraemia.
- Thrombophilia screen (if indicated by clinical or haematological features).
- Lipid profile (not an immediate investigation; 2° prevention, *see above*).
- Blood cultures (if SBE or other sepsis suspected. *Note*: cerebral abscess).

Imaging

- Cranial CT scan (± IV contrast).
- Echocardiogram (if mural thrombus, endocarditis suspected—rarely a cause of ischaemic stroke).
- Carotid Doppler studies—may not be indicated if surgical intervention (endarterectomy) is unlikely because of poor prognosis, e.g. dense hemiplegia or coma.

Consider alternative diagnoses including
- 1° or 2° brain tumour (may present as acute stroke—search for primary).
- Cerebral abscess (usually clear evidence of sepsis).
- Cerebral lupus (ESR, autoantibodies).

📖 *OHCM* 8e, p474, p478.

Sweating

Fairly non-specific symptom, but one that may indicate serious underlying disease.

Causes
- Excess heat (physiological).
- Exercise (physiological).
- Fever—any cause.
- Anxiety.
- Thyrotoxicosis.
- Acromegaly.
- Diabetes mellitus.
- Lymphoproliferative disease, e.g. lymphomas.
- Cancer (any).
- Hypoglycaemia.
- Alcohol.
- Nausea.
- Gustatory.
- Neurological disease, e.g. lesions of sympathetic nervous system, cortex, basal ganglia, or spinal cord.

Investigations
- FBC.
- ESR.
- Biochemistry screen including LFTs.
- Glucose.
- TFTs.
- Urinalysis and culture.
- Blood cultures.
- CXR.
- Further investigation depending on results of above.

Tachycardia

Tachycardia is arbitrarily defined as a heart rate above 100 beats/min. It is a normal physiological response to exercise and to emotional stress, but can also herald a cardiac rhythm disorder. One should always begin by assessing the nature of the tachycardia, and identifying any underlying cause or contributing factor.

Assessment begins with a 12-lead ECG, performed, whilst the patient is tachycardic. This will enable the immediate identification of the heart rhythm. One must then differentiate between sinus tachycardia (which may or may not have a pathological cause) and tachycardias due to other (abnormal) cardiac rhythms.

Causes of sinus tachycardia
- Sympathetic stimulation, e.g. anxiety, pain, fear, fever, exercise.
- Drugs, e.g. adrenaline, atropine, salbutamol.
- Stimulants, e.g. caffeine, alcohol, amphetamines.
- Thyrotoxicosis.
- Heart failure.
- Pulmonary embolism.
- IHD, acute myocardial infarction.
- Anaemia.
- Blood or fluid loss, e.g. post-operative.
- Inappropriate sinus tachycardia (a persistent resting sinus tachycardia, diagnosed when all other possible causes have been excluded).

In assessing abnormal heart rhythms causing tachycardia, it is helpful to divide them into narrow-complex tachycardia (QRS duration < 120ms) and broad-complex tachycardia (QRS duration > 120ms).

Narrow-complex tachycardias
- Sinus tachycardia (see previous section).
- Atrial tachycardia.
- Atrial flutter.
- Atrial fibrillation.
- AV re-entry tachycardias.

Broad-complex tachycardias
- Narrow-complex tachycardia with aberrant conduction.
- Ventricular tachycardia.
- Accelerated idioventricular rhythm.
- Torsades de pointes.

Investigations

- 12-lead ECG to identify the underlying rhythm.
- Consider bedside monitoring on CCU, particularly if the patient is compromised or ventricular arrhythmias are suspected.
- Other investigations depend upon the underlying cause, but may include:
  - FBC.
  - U&E.
  - TFTs.
  - Cardiac markers.
  - CXR.
  - ABGs.
  - V/Q scan/CTPA.
  - Echocardiogram.
  - Exercise treadmill test.
  - Cardiac catheter.
  - Electrophysiological studies.

It can be useful to perform carotid sinus massage (▶ Exclude carotid bruits first) or to give IV adenosine (▶ Do not use in asthma/COPD), while the patient is on a bedside ECG monitor. Supraventricular tachycardias will usually slow transiently, allowing clearer identification of underlying atrial activity, and re-entry tachycardias may terminate altogether. Ventricular tachycardias will be unaffected.

📖 *OHCM* 8e, p88, p120, p122, p816, p818.

Tinnitus

Tinnitus is a common symptom in which the patient perceives a sound, often chronic and distressing, in the absence of aural stimulation. It usually manifests as a 'ringing' or 'buzzing' in the ears. Tinnitus may occur as a symptom of nearly all disorders of the auditory apparatus. Psychological stresses may be relevant in some cases.

Causes include

- Acoustic trauma (prolonged exposure to loud noise, e.g. gun shots, amplified music).
- Barotrauma (blast injury, perforated tympanic membrane).
- Obstruction of the external auditory meatus (wax, foreign body, infection).
- Otosclerosis.
- Menière's disease.
- Drug-induced ototoxicity.
- Gentamicin—may be irreversible.
- Acute salicylate toxicity.
- Quinine toxicity.
- Acute alcohol poisoning.
- Hypothyroidism.
- Hypertension (rare symptom).
- Intra- or extracranial aneurysm (typically or cause 'pulsatile' tinnitus).
- Glomus jugulare tumours.

Note: Consider acoustic neuroma in unilateral tinnitus.

Investigations

- FBC.
- Serum concentrations of e.g. salicylates, gentamicin (▶ Mandatory during systemic therapy).
- TFTs.
- BP.

Audiological assessment

Specialist investigations
- Assess air and bone conduction thresholds.
- Tympanometry and acoustic reflex testing.
- Speech perception thresholds.

Consider
- CT temporal bone (acoustic neuroma).
- Cranial MRI (following specialist advice).

📖 *OHCM* 8e, p468.

Tiredness

Tiredness is a common presenting complaint in association with many diseases, including endocrine, hepatic, renal, and cardiorespiratory disease. Where no cause is identified consider chronic fatigue syndrome (ME). Important diagnoses to exclude are hypo/hyperthyroidism, hypoadrenalism, hypercalaemia, diabetes mellitus. A U&E is useful to exclude hyponatraemia or hypokalaemia (muscle weakness) as well as renal failure.

Recommended investigations for tiredness in the absence of an obvious cause from history and examination

- TSH.
- FT4.
- Synacthen test.
- Serum Ca^{2+}.
- Glucose.
- U&E, creatinine.
- FBC.
- ESR (or CRP).
- LFTs.
- Anti-tissue transglutaminase or endomysial antibody (to exclude coeliac disease).

Urgency of micturition

Urgency of micturition denotes a strong desire to void and the patient often has to rush to the toilet because of an acute call to micturate. Urinary incontinence may result, especially if physical mobility is impaired. Urgency forms part of a cluster of symptoms which include frequency of micturition (📖 Polyuria, p91), nocturia, and hesitancy of micturition.

Men

- Prostatic disease.
- Urinary tract infection.
- Bladder irritability.
- Urethritis.
- States of polyuria (📖 Polyuria, p91); may lead to urinary incontinence (📖 Incontinence: urinary, p62).

Investigations to consider

- Urinalysis—stick test for glucose, protein, blood, nitrites.
- MSU for microscopy and culture.
- FBC.
- U&E.
- Venous plasma glucose.
- ESR.
- Serum PSA.
- PSA is increased in 30–50% of patients with benign prostatic hyperplasia, and in 25–92% of those with prostate cancer (depending on tumour volume), i.e. a normal PSA does not exclude prostatic disease. Check reference range with local laboratory.
- Transrectal USS of prostate.
- Prostatic biopsy (specialist procedure).

Women

- Urinary tract infection.
- Gynaecological disease, e.g. pelvic floor instability, uterine prolapse.
- Bladder irritability.
- Urethritis.
- States of polyuria; may lead to urinary incontinence (📖 Incontinence: urinary, p62).

Investigations to consider

- FBC.
- U&E.
- MSU for microscopy and culture.
- Urodynamic studies.

📖 *OHCM* 8e, p22, pp650–1.

Urticaria

Itchy superficial wheals; may be giant. Distinguish acute from chronic: chronic is rarely allergic in origin. If persists > 24 h and fade with brown staining consider urticarial vasculitis.

Causes
- **Allergic**: drugs, foods, additives, acute infection, e.g. HBV, *Mycoplasma*.
- **Physical**: sunlight, heat, cold, pressure, vibration.
- Stress.
- **Thyroid disease**: hypo- or hyperthyroidism.
- **Occult infection**: gallbladder, dental, sinus, *Helicobacter*.
- **Vitamin deficiency**: B_{12}, folic acid, iron.
- **Autoimmune**: antibodies against IgE receptor on mast cells—very rare.

Investigations
Based on history, but should include as baseline
- FBC (with eosinophil count).
- Thyroid function.
- Infection marker (CRP).
- Liver function.

Further tests may include
- B_{12} and red cell folate.
- Serum ferritin.
- Antibodies to *Helicobacter pylori* (and/or Urea Breath Test)

Allergy tests are of little value unless there is a clearly identified trigger.

Vasculitis

Definition
Disease caused by inflammatory destructive changes of blood vessel walls.

Presentation
Wide variety of clinical presentations affecting one or more organ systems:
- **Skin**: splinter haemorrhages, nail-fold infarcts, petechiae, purpura, livedo reticularis.
- **Respiratory**: cough, haemoptysis, breathlessness, pulmonary infiltration, sinusitis.
- **Renal**: haematuria, proteinuria, hypertension, acute renal failure.
- **Neurological**: multiple mononeuropathy, sensorimotor polyneuropathy, confusion, fits, hemiplegia, meningoencephalitis.
- **Musculoskeletal**: arthralgia, arthritis, myalgia.
- **Generalized**: pyrexia of unknown origin, weight loss, malaise.

Causes of primary vasculitis (Table 1.17)

Table 1.17 Causes of 1° vasculitis

	Granulomatous	Non-granulomatous
Large vessel	Giant cell arteritis	Takayasu's arteritis
Medium vessel	Churg–Strauss disease	Polyarteritis nodosa
Small vessel	Wegener's arteritis	Microscopic arteritis

Causes of secondary vasculitis
- Infective endocarditis.
- Meningococcal septicaemia.
- Malignancy.
- Rheumatoid arthritis (RhA).
- Henoch–Schönlein purpura.
- SLE.
- Cryoglobulinaemia.
- Drug reaction.

Investigations
- FBC.
- U&E.
- LFTs.
- ESR.
- CRP.
- Serum immunoglobulins and protein electrophoresis.
- Cryoglobulins.
- ANA, ENA, ds-DNA.
- Rheumatoid factor.
- ANCA.
- CXR.
- Biopsy of artery and/or skin lesions.
- Urine dipstick and microscopy.

📖 *OHCM* 8e, p314, p555, p558.

Visual loss

Total loss of vision may be bilateral or unilateral. Unilateral blindness is due to a lesion either of the eye itself, or between the eye and the optic chiasm. Determine whether the visual loss is gradual or sudden. Gradual loss of vision occurs in conditions, such as optic atrophy or glaucoma. In the elderly, cataract and macular degeneration are common. Remember tobacco amblyopia and methanol toxicity. Trachoma is a common cause worldwide.

Causes of sudden blindness include

- Optic neuritis, e.g. MS. (not sudden, usually gradual over days and incomplete).
- Central retinal artery occlusion.
- Central retinal vein occlusion.
- Vitreous haemorrhage (**Note**: proliferative diabetic retinopathy).
- Acute glaucoma.
- Retinal detachment.
- Temporal (giant cell) cell arteritis (TA). **Note**: visual loss is potentially preventable with early high-dose corticosteroid therapy.
- Migraine (scotomata).
- Occipital cortex infarction.
- Acute severe quinine poisoning (consider stellate ganglion block).
- Hysteria (rare), e.g. blindness:
  - *Complete?*—no pupil response or optikokinetic nystagmus.
  - *Cortical?*—normal papillary light reflex, no optikokinetic nystagmus.
  - *Hysterical?*—normal papillary light reflex, normal optikokinetic nystagmus.
- HELLP syndrome (haemolysis, elevated liver enzymes and low platelet count syndrome) complicating pre-eclampsia—rare.

Investigations will be determined by history and examination findings. A specialist opinion should be sought without delay.

If TA suspected

- ESR/CRP.
- Autoimmune profile including cANCA/pANCA.
- Temporal artery biopsy (within days ▶▶ Do not withhold steroid therapy).

Investigations in sudden onset of visual loss

- Visual acuity (Snellen chart).
- Goldmann perimetry.
- Intra-ocular pressure measurement (tonometry).
- Fluorescein angiography (specialist investigation—may delineate diabetic retinopathy in more detail. ▶▶ Risk of anaphylaxis).
- Cranial CT scan.
- Cranial MRI scan.
- LP (CSF protein and oligoclonal bands if MS suspected).

Screen for risk factors and causes of cerebrovascular thromboembolic disease

- Venous plasma glucose.
- Serum lipid profile.
- Carotid Doppler studies.
- 12-lead ECG.
- Echocardiogram.

Wasting of the small hand muscles

Wasting of the small muscles of the hand may be found in isolation or may be associated with other neurological signs. If found in isolation this suggests a spinal lesion at the level of C8/T1 or distally in the brachial plexus, or upper limb motor nerves.

Unilateral wasting of the small muscles of the hand may occur in association with

- Cervical rib.
- Brachial plexus trauma (Klumpke's palsy).
- Pancoast's tumour (may be associated with a Horner's syndrome).
- Cervical cord tumour.
- Malignant infiltration of brachial plexus.

Bilateral wasting of the small muscles of the hand occurs in

- Carpal tunnel syndrome (common).
- Rheumatoid arthritis (common).
- Cervical spondylosis (common).
- Bilateral cervical ribs.
- Motor neurone disease.
- Syringomyelia.
- Charcot–Marie–Tooth disease.
- Guillain–Barré syndrome.
- Combined median and ulnar nerve lesions.
- Cachexia.
- Advanced age.
- Peripheral neuropathies.

Investigations

- ESR.
- C-reactive protein.
- Rheumatoid factor.
- CXR.
- X-ray cervical spine.
- Nerve conduction studies (☐ Nerve conduction studies, p566).
- Electromyography (☐ Electromyogram, p570).
- LP, CSF protein, etc. (☐ Lumbar puncture, p546).
- CT thorax.
- MRI of cervical cord/brachial plexus.

Weight loss

Causes
- Diet.
- Anorexia. (□ Anorexia, p13).
- DM.
- Malnutrition.
- Small intestinal disease (coeliac, bacterial overgrowth).
- Malignant disease (carcinoma and haematological malignancies).
- HIV/aquired immunodeficiency syndrome (AIDS).
- Chronic pancreatitis.
- Chronic respiratory failure.
- Cirrhosis.
- Diuretic therapy.
- Hyperthyroidism.
- Addison's disease.

Investigations
May well need extensive investigation before determining the cause, but start with:
- FBC.
- ESR or CRP.
- Biochemistry screen.
- TFTs.
- MSU including culture & sensitivity (C&S).
- CXR.
- Stool culture (if appropriate).
- Blood culture.
- Other endocrine tests as appropriate.
- Consider HIV testing.

□ *OHCM* 8e, p29.

Wheeze

Wheezes (rhonchi) are continuous high-, medium-, or low-pitched added sounds audible during respiration. Typically, they are loudest on expiration in asthma and may, on occasion, be heard without a stethoscope. The implication is reversible or irreversible airway obstruction. If wheeze is audible only during inspiration this is termed stridor, implying upper respiratory obstruction. An important distinction must be made between monophonic and polyphonic wheezes and whether wheeze is localized to a single area or is heard throughout the thorax.

Polyphonic wheeze

Wheezes with multiple tones and pitch. The most common causes of wheeze (usually recurrent) are:
- Asthma.
- COPD (often audible during both phases of respiration).

Fixed monophonic wheeze

A wheeze with a single constant pitch. Implies local bronchial obstruction, usually due to:
- Bronchogenic carcinoma.
- Foreign body.

Note: stridor is a harsh form of monophonic wheeze arising from upper airway obstruction (📖 Stridor, p103).

Investigations

- ABGs (**Note**: inspired O_2 concentration should be recorded).
- Pulse oximetry at bedside (does not provide information about PCO_2).
- Spirometry (PFR, pre- and post-bronchodilator therapy).
- Pulmonary function tests (FEV_1, flow-volume curve (FVC), total lung capacity; 📖 Flow volume loops/maximum expiratory flow-volume curve, p518).
- CXR (postero-anterior (P-A) and lateral).
- Sputum cytology (if tumour suspected).
- CT thorax.
- Bronchoscopy and biopsy (specialist procedure—especially if foreign body or suspected tumour).

📖 *OHCM* 8e, p52.

Part II

Endocrinology & metabolism

Guiding principles of endocrine investigation

Investigations for endocrine disease have caused a lot of confusion in the minds of clinicians (many still do!). Tests have come and gone over the years and have been adopted with varying degrees of enthusiasm by specialist centres. In particular, there is often confusion over which tests to do, what procedures to follow and how to interpret the results. In some areas (e.g. Cushing's syndrome), controversy persists among the experts. In others, a clear consensus approach exists.

Some useful general principles

1 **Use dynamic tests**, rather than random (untimed) sampling where the hormone under investigation is secreted in infrequent pulses (e.g. growth hormone, GH) or levels are easily influenced by other factors (e.g. cortisol varies markedly with stress levels and has a marked circadian rhythm; see Table 2.1).

In general

- If you are suspecting a LOW level—do a **STIMULATION** test (*to see if it stays LOW*)
- If you are suspecting a HIGH level—do a **SUPPRESSION** test (*to see if it stays HIGH*)

2 **Use the correct collection method**, e.g. ACTH or insulin levels require rapid separation of the sample and prompt freezing (–20°C). Urinary catecholamines require a specific acid preservative in the collection container. Timing of sampling may also be critical. Label samples carefully, including time of collection! Check procedures with the local laboratory. Many units will have protocols for endocrine investigations.
3 **Do tests in the correct sequence**, e.g. ACTH levels can only be interpreted once the cortisol status is known. In many cases, simultaneous samples are required for interpretation, e.g. PTH with calcium for hypo/hyperparathyroidism, glucose with insulin for insulinoma.
4 **'Normal' results may be 'abnormal'** depending on the activity of the hormone axis under investigation. Interpretation of the absolute levels of hormones in isolation may be highly misleading. For example, a serum PTH within the normal range in the presence of hypocalcaemia suggests hypoparathyroidism; 'normal' LH and FSH levels in the presence of a very low serum testosterone concentration suggest pituitary failure. In both instances, the regulatory hormone concentration is inappropriately low. Thus, the level of the regulatory hormone (or releasing factor) must be considered in the light of the simultaneous level of the 'target' hormone or metabolite.
5 **Results may vary according to the laboratory assay**. Reference ranges vary between laboratories—it is especially important with endocrine tests to interpret your results according to your lab's 'normal range'. Also, interfering factors may differ between assays, e.g. different PRL

assays cross-react very differently with macroprolactin (📖 Galactorrhoea (hyperprolactinaemia), p162). Some individuals have a heterophile interfering antibody that affects the results of many radioimmunoassays. Resist 'discarding clinical evidence in favour of a numerical value'.

6 **Beware of interfering medication**, e.g. inhaled beclomethasone can suppress serum cortisol levels, administered hydrocortisone (cortisol) is detected by the cortisol assay, synthetic androgens, and oestrogens can appear to cause low serum testosterone/oestrogen (as they are not detected in the testosterone/oestrogen assay), some anti-emetics and antipsychotics can raise circulating PRL levels, carbenoxolone or liquorice may cause hypokalaemia. Always ask patients for a full medication list (including herbal remedies and other self-medication).

7. **Take a family history**: familial forms of many common endocrine problems exist that require important changes in management approach, e.g. familial hypercalcaemia may suggest multiple endocrine neoplasia (MEN)-1 or MEN-2 requiring a different form of parathyroid surgery and a risk of phaeochromocytoma (MEN-2).

Endocrine tests are generally expensive and should not be performed unnecessarily or outside standard protocols. Dynamic tests may have cautions and contraindications and *can be hazardous* if used inappropriately (Table 2.1). A high degree of organization and close liaison with the laboratory is required to perform these tests in a way that can be clearly interpreted. Dynamic tests should ideally be performed in an endocrine investigation unit. Chemical pathologists (clinical biochemists) and other laboratory staff generally have great experience with performing and interpreting endocrine tests—*seek their advice wherever possible*—*before* embarking on tests with which you are unfamiliar. Tests in children should be performed and interpreted under expert paediatric guidance.

Table 2.1 Random sampling vs. dynamic testing

Hormone	Random or dynamic sampling?
GH	*Dynamic*: glucose tolerance test for excess; insulin stress test or GHRH arginine stimulation test for deficiency
IGF-1	Random
LH, FSH	Random in ♂, post-menopausal Timed with menstrual cycle in pre-menopausal ♂ Random or stimulated in pre-pubertal children
Testosterone	Random
Oestrogen (oestradiol)	Random in ♂, post-menopausal ♂ Timed with menstrual cycle in pre-menopausal
ACTH	Random
Cortisol	*Dynamic*: dexamethasone suppression test for excess Synacthen stimulation test if suspect deficiency
TSH	Random
T4 & T3	Random
Prolactin (PRL)	Random
ADH/vasopressin	Don't normally measure directly
Osmolality	*Dynamic*: water deprivation test if suspect DI
Parathyroid hormone	Random, but need simultaneous calcium value
Insulin	Fasting, plus simultaneous glucose value
Calcitonin	Random
Renin/aldosterone	Upright usually, off medication
Catecholamines	Measure in urine, 24 h sample
5HIAAs	Measure in urine, 24 h sample

Further reading

AACE. American Association of Clinical Endocrinologists Clinical Guidelines. ✍ www.aace.com/pyb/guidelines/

Endocrine Society. *Endocrine Society Guidelines*. ✍ www.endo-society.org/guidelines

Ismail AAA, Bart JH. Wrong biochemistry results. *Br Med J* 2001; **232**: 705–6.

Hypothalamus/pituitary function

Hypothalamic dysfunction

Causes

- Familial syndromes (Laurence–Moon–Biedl, Prader–Willi).
- Tumours (especially craniopharyngiomas, dysgerminomas, optic gliomas, meningioma—rarely pituitary tumours).
- Pituitary surgery.
- Infiltration (histiocytosis X, sarcoidosis).
- Trauma.
- Meningitis.
- Encephalitis.
- Tuberculosis (TB).

Symptoms & signs

- Obesity/hyperphagia.
- Somnolence.
- Thermodysregulation.
- Diabetes insipidus.
- Hypogonadism.
- Precocious puberty.

Investigations

- MRI.
- Water deprivation test for diabetes insipidus (DI; 📖 Polydipsia & polyuria: diabetes insipidus, p129, tests of pituitary function).

Hypopituitarism

Definition

Failure of one or more pituitary hormones (usually multiple).

Causes

- Congenital.
- Pituitary tumour (including infarction of tumour 'apoplexy').
- Craniopharyngioma.
- Post-cranial irradiation.
- Following pituitary irradiation.
- Metastases to pituitary (especially breast).
- Post-surgery.
- Empty sella syndrome (occasionally).
- Sheehan's syndrome (infarction with post-partum haemorrhage).

Symptoms & signs

Often very vague, e.g. tiredness, normocytic anaemia (easily missed). Combined with impotence or amenorrhoea—very suggestive. Other clues include loss of body hair (especially axilliary), reduced shaving, hyponatraemia, and growth failure in children. Diabetes insipidus is not a feature (unless there is also hypothalamic damage) as ADH can be secreted directly from the hypothalamus. There may also be signs of space-occupying lesion—bi-temporal hemianopia (rarely optic nerve compression, homonymous hemianopia), headache (especially following apoplexy), III, IV, V_1, V_2 or VI cranial nerve lesions, CSF rhinorrhoea. Occasionally galactorrhoea following pituitary stalk compression by tumour ('disconnection'). **Note**: Generally GH is lost first, then luteinizing hormone (LH)/follicle stimulating hormone (FSH), and ACTH/thyroid stimulating hormone (TSH) last. If multiple pituitary hormones are deficient, GH deficiency can be assumed.

Investigations

See Fig. 2.1. Basal-free T4 (not TSH, which can be misleadingly normal), LH, FSH, prolactin (PRL) and oestrogen/testosterone are usually sufficient to test the thyroid and gonadal axes. Adrenal and growth hormone testing require dynamic tests (e.g. insulin tolerance test (ITT), but see below). Severe growth hormone deficiency = peak stimulated GH < 9mU/L (3ng/mL). Note that the short synacthen test (📖 Short Synacthen® test, p209) is only suitable for testing the hypothalamopituitary adrenal axis if pituitary failure is of long standing (> 6 weeks) allowing time for adrenal atrophy to occur.

Alternative investigations

- Growth hormone releasing hormone (GHRH) arginine stimulation test. Although the ITT (📖 Test protocols, p201) is the traditional gold standard test for GH and secondary adrenal insufficiency, the GHRH arginine test has equal sensitivity and specificity for GH deficiency. It is also safer and better tolerated and is gradually replacing the ITT.[1]
- Combined anterior pituitary testing—giving LHRH, TRH, ACTH, and GHRH (📖 Combined anterior pituitary function testing, p203)—no clear advantage of this approach has been demonstrated and the results of the LHRH test in particular are difficult to interpret in prepubertal children.
- Long (depot) Synacthen® test—rarely required (📖 Adrenal failure, p154; 📖 Long (depot) ACTH test, p209).

---

1 NICE. *UK NICE guidelines for GH replacement 2006.* ॐ http://www.nice.org.uk/guidance/index.jsp?action=download&o=32665

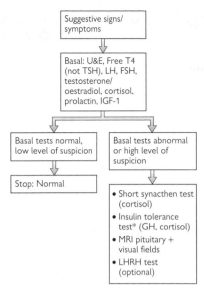

Fig. 2.1 Investigation of suspected hypopituitarism. *Note:* Specialist paediatric advice should be taken in children.
* See also note under alternative investigations, first paragraph.

Further reading

Endocrine Society. *Evaulation and Treatment of Adult Growth Hormone Defiency* Endocrine Society, 2006. 𝄞 www.endo-society.org.guidelines

Acromegaly (growth hormone excess)

For growth hormone deficiency see 📖 Hypothalamus/pituitary function, p125).

Clinical features

- Often insidious over many years.
- Enlarging hands and feet with rings having to be resized.
- Increase in shoe size.
- Coarsening of facial features especially enlargement and broadening of the nose.
- Sweating.
- Headache.
- Malocclusion (protuberance of lower jaw) and splaying of teeth.
- Skin tags.
- Hypertension.
- Cardiac failure.
- Renal stones.
- Arthritis.
- Colonic polyps.
- Sleep apnoea.
- Carpal tunnel syndrome.
- Diabetes mellitus.
- May be local symptoms from the pituitary tumour and symptoms/signs of loss of other pituitary hormones (📖 Hypothalamus/pituitary function, p125).
- Growth hormone excess commencing before puberty results in gigantism (tall stature).

Investigations

- A random growth hormone is not helpful—may be high in normal people.
- Perform a standard 75g oral GTT with glucose and growth hormone measurements at 0, 30, 60, 90, and 120 min.
- If no growth hormone values are < 2mU/L then the diagnosis of acromegaly is confirmed.
- A random insulin-like growth factor-1 (IGF-1) level should be measured and compared with laboratory normal ranges corrected for age. This can be used as a screening test, but IGF-1 assays vary in reliability. IGF-1 levels should be raised in all cases of acromegaly, but levels can be affected (reduced) by fasting and systemic illness.
- The vast majority (99%) of cases of acromegaly are due to pituitary tumours. If a pituitary tumour is not seen on MRI scanning yet acromegaly is confirmed, a GHRH level should be requested to exclude ectopic production of this polypeptide by non-pituitary tumours stimulating the release of growth hormone from the pituitary.
- For follow-up of treated cases of acromegaly, IGF-1 levels (more sensitive) and nadir of growth hormone in a series of 4 estimations over 2 h is a reasonable approach.
- Life expectancy appears to return to normality when the nadir of GH values is < 5mU/L.

Polydipsia & polyuria: diabetes insipidus

'First line tests'

It is relatively common for patients to report excess thirst or increased need to pass urine. Figure 2.2 and Table 2.2 summarize the causes. Prostatism and urge incontinence resulting in urinary frequency should be distinguished by history-taking as the patients do not have thirst. Then the first step is to identify straightforward causes, such as drugs (diuretics), diabetes mellitus (DM), hypercalcaemia, hypokalaemia and chronic renal failure with U&E, creatinine, glucose, and calcium. Measuring 24 h urine volume is also useful as volumes over 3L are likely to be pathological and volumes under 2L do not require further investigation. A glucose tolerance test should not be required to diagnose DM as the renal threshold for glucose needs to be exceeded (~10mmol/L) to cause polyuria and there should be glucose in the urine.

Table 2.2 Causes of polyuria/polydipsia
Diabetes mellitus
Diabetes insipidus (cranial or nephrogenic)
High Ca^{2+}
Low K^+
Chronic renal failure
Primary polydipsia (including dry mouth, e.g. Sjögren's)

'Second line tests'

Once other diagnoses have been excluded, subsequent tests aim to distinguish DI from primary polydipsia (compulsive water drinking). A carefully supervised water deprivation test should be performed (📖 Water deprivation test, p204). However, it is not always easy to arrive at a conclusive diagnosis. Serum sodium levels are helpful as DI is unlikely if Na^+ < 140mmol/L. Morning spot urine osmolality after overnight water restriction (not shown on chart) is occasionally useful: values > 600mOsmol/L make significant degrees of DI unlikely. Measuring 24 h urine volume is also useful as volumes over 3L are likely to be pathological. However, obligate urine volumes as low as 2L could still cause the patient to complain of polyuria. In such borderline cases, the distinction between partial DI, normality, and primary polydipsia can be very difficult. Guidance on interpretation of the second line tests including the water deprivation test is given in Table 2.3. Note that primary polydipsia may be a psychiatric condition, but can also occur in patients with a dry mouth (e.g. Sjögren's syndrome, anticholinergic drugs) or who have been previously encouraged to drink regularly 'to help their kidneys'.

Distinction between partial cranial DI and habitual (psychogenic) water drinking is complicated by the fact that drinking very high volumes over time may 'wash out' the renal medullary concentrating gradient. In this situation a plasma vasopressin level at the end of the water deprivation test may be very helpful to distinguish lack of vasopressin from a lack of vasopressin action. 24 h urine volume is also helpful as volumes of less than 3L/day are unlikely to cause renal 'wash-out'. Clues to primary poly-dipsia include an initial plasma osmolality (and serum Na$^+$) that is low, plasma osmolality rises to > 295mOsmol/L and thirst is not abolished by desmopressin (DDAVP), despite a rise in urine osmolality. Note that 'full blown' cranial DI results in urine volumes around 500mL/h (12L/day).

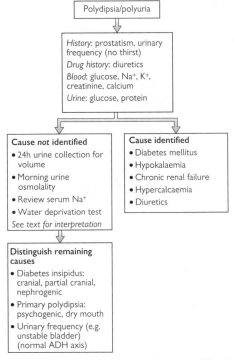

Fig. 2.2 Investigation of polydipsia/polyuria. **Note:** Once cranial DI is diag-nosed, further investigations into the underlying cause are required—see Hypothalamus/pituitary function, Hypothalamic dysfunction, p125.

Interpretation of second line tests for polyuria/polydipsia

Table 2.3 Interpretation of second line tests for polyuria/polydipsia

	Normal	Partial DI: cranial (C) or nephrogenic (N)	Primary polydipsia
Random serum Na$^+$	Normal	>140mmol/L	<140mmol/L
Random serum osmolality**	Variable	>290	<290
Morning urine mOsm**	Variable	Unlikely if >600 (C) Excluded if >600 (N)	
End of water deprivation test *before* DDAVP**	Urine >600 Plasma 280–295	Urine >600* Plasma >295	Urine <600 Plasma 280–295
Urine osmolality after DDAVP SC**	>600	Rises to >600 or >50% increase (C) Rises to <600 or <50% increase (N)	Rises to >600 or >than 50% increase
Plasma vasopressin at end of water deprivation test	Normal for plasma osmolality	Low for plasma osmolality (C) Normal for plasma osmolality (N)	Normal for plasma osmolality

*With longstanding large volume polyuria (>3L/day), these values may not be achieved due to wash-out of the renal medullary concentrating gradient—if results equivocal, see text.

**Osmolalities are all expressed in mOsmol/L.

'If all else fails'

In cases of doubt, a carefully supervised therapeutic trial of DDAVP (desmopressin) can be useful to distinguish DI from primary polydipsia (📖 Diagnostic trial of DDAVP, p206). This should be done as an in-patient as there is a risk of significant hyponatraemia in habitual water drinkers. The principle is that patients able to regulate water intake according to their thirst (DI) should not develop a hypo-osmolar plasma. In primary polydipsia, the urine volume will fall and the urine concentrating gradient will gradually recover. However, if the patient continues to drink due to their psychological drive, rather than their thirst, they will become water overloaded and hypo-osmolar.

An additional valuable test to distinguish partial DI from primary polydipsia is hypertonic saline infusion testing, which usually requires access to a plasma vasopressin assay, but has been used with urinary vasopressin levels.[1-] MRI scanning typically shows an increased signal in the posterior pituitary, which is lost in cranial DI. However, this sign is not helpful in distinguishing more subtle degree of DI from other causes.

1. Robertson GL. Diabetes insipidus. *Endocr Metab Clin N Am* 1995; **24**: 549–72.

2. Thompson CJ, Edwards CR, Baylis PH. (1991) Osmotic and non-osmotic regulation of thirst and vasopressin secretion in patients with compulsive water drinking. *Clin Endocrinol (Oxf)* 1991; **35**: 221–8.

3. Diederich S, et al. (2001) Differential diagnosis of polyuric/polydipsic syndromes with the aid of urinary vasopressin measurements in adults. *Clin Endocrinol (Oxf)* 2001; **54**: 665–71.

Hyponatraemia (including syndrome of inappropriate anti-diuretic hormone)

Hyponatraemia is a very common clinical problem. Figure 2.3 shows a flow chart for investigation. If patients are on diuretics, further evaluation is usually not possible. The diuretic will need to be discontinued. If this is not possible, the hyponatraemia is likely to be attributable to an under-lying condition (cardiac, renal, or liver failure). Pseudo- or dilutional hyponatraemia is important to exclude at an early stage (see Table 2.4). A careful clinical assessment should be made of volume status including identification of oedema, fluid loss (e.g. diarrhoea, fistula leakage), and signs of dehydration, including postural drop in blood pressure. A urine sodium and TSH estimation is useful at this stage (see Fig. 2.3). Note that the most important diagnosis not to miss is hypoadrenalism as this can be fatal if untreated. Clinicians should have a low threshold for performing a short synacthen test (📖 Short Synacthen® test, p209). Hypoadrenalism due to pituitary failure may not be accompanied by hyperkalaemia, hypotension or hyperpigmentation and can easily be missed. Cerebral salt wasting occurs within days of brain injury (e.g. subarachnoid haemorrhage (SAH), neurosurgery, or stroke) and is probably due to release of brain natiuretic peptides.

Table 2.4 Causes of pseudohyponatraemia

With normal serum osmolality
- Hyperproteinaemia (e.g. myeloma)
- Hyperlipidaemia (hypertriglyceridaemia)
- Glycine or sorbitol (from bladder irrigant)

With raised osmolality
- Hyperglycaemia
- Mannitol
- Glycerol

The syndrome of inappropriate anti-diuretic hormone (SIADH) is a diagnosis of exclusion (Table 2.5).

Table 2.5 Criteria for diagnosing SIADH

- Hyponatraemia present
- No diuretics
- No oedema
- Normal renal function
- Normal adrenal function
- Normal thyroid function
- Urine Na^+ >20mmol/L
- Euvolaemic

All the criteria in Table 2.5 should be met. A specific cause for SIADH is frequently not found or there may be a combination of precipitating factors (see Table 2.6). In the elderly, a state of chronic SIADH is relatively common and usually explains hyponatraemia persisting for many years without any other apparent cause. Affected individuals should be encouraged to drink less than a litre a day ('5 cups or less'), to only drink if they are thirsty and avoid exacerbating factors (see Table 2.6).

Table 2.6 Causes of SIADH

Cause	Examples
Drugs	Carbamazepine, chlorpropamide, opiates, psychotropics, cytotoxics
CNS disorders	Head trauma, post-pituitary surgery (transient), stroke, cerebral haemorrhage, Guillain–Barré, meningitis, encephalitis, fits
Malignancy	Small-cell lung cancer, pancreas, prostate
Chest disease	Pneumonia, TB, abscess, aspergillosis
General stimuli	Nausea, pain, smoking
Other	Acute intermittent porphyria

The following features of SIADH/hyponatraemia are often underappreciated

1. Other than a chest X-ray, there is no requirement to search for an underlying malignant cause. If there is underlying malignancy it is usually extensive, very apparent, and incurable (e.g. extensive small-cell carcinoma of the lung).
2. The urine osmolality does not have to be high. In individuals drinking large volumes of fluid, a urine osmolality as low as 250mOsmol/L (i.e. less than plasma) may be inappropriately concentrated reflecting true SIADH.
3. Conditions previously diagnosed as 'sick cell syndrome' are now thought to represent SIADH in ill patients.
4. 'Water intoxication' is usually the combination of SIADH and excessive fluid intake. Healthy patients drinking to excess can rarely exceed the renal capacity to excrete a water load (~12L/day) and, hence, do not become hyponatraemic. A degree of SIADH is required for potomaniacs (excess water drinkers) to become hyponatraemic.
5. The post-operative state contains many precipitants to SIADH (nausea, pain, opiates, pneumonia) and ADH secretion is promoted by hypovolaemia from blood loss. The administration of '3L of intravenous fluid a day' post-operatively frequently results in hyponatraemia.

6. Symptoms of hyponatraemia, such as drowsiness, coma, or fits, are dependent on the rate of fall of serum Na^+ not the absolute value. Patients who are alert with $Na^+ < 125mmol/L$ have clearly been chronically hyponatraemic and their serum sodium requires only gentle correction. However, a very rapid fall in serum Na^+ to $< 130mmol/L$ (typically due to massive infusion of hypotonic fluid into the bladder) may cause coma and needs to be corrected as a medical emergency with hypertonic saline.

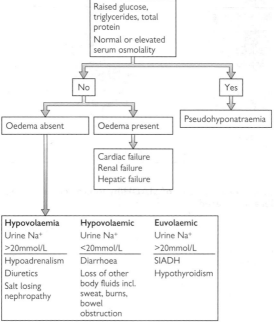

Fig. 2.3 Investigation of hyponatraemia.

Obesity/hypercortisolism

Endocrinologists are frequently asked to determine whether there is an underlying endocrine cause in patients who are obese. Secondary causes of obesity are listed in Table 2.7. A long history of obesity, typically going back to childhood, is characteristic of constitutional obesity and further investigation other than thyroid function is rarely necessary. However, simple obesity may result in effects suggestive of hypercortisolism, e.g. striae, bruising, central obesity, rounded facial features, mild hyperandrogenism in women, buffalo hump, hypertension, and hyperglycaemia. Rapidly progressive obesity, marked hypertension, hypokalaemia, proximal muscle weakness, poor sleep, osteoporosis/vertebral collapse, and marked hirsutism or acne are more suggestive of hypercortisolism and require further investigation. Hypothalamic damage is usually apparent from the history.

Table 2.7 Secondary causes of obesity

- Constitutional
- Hypothyroidism
- Cushing's syndrome
- Hypothalamic damage (extreme hyperphagia)
- Genetic, e.g. Prader–Willi
- Growth hormone deficiency
- Drugs, e.g, antidepressants

The optimal approach to the diagnosis of hypercortisolism (Cushing's syndrome) is probably the most controversial subject in endocrinology. Endocrinologists who have seen many cases of Cushing's syndrome have seen exceptions to every rule, and the episodic nature of ACTH and cortisol secretion means that low values can occur even in disease. True cyclical Cushing's disease also occurs, but is rare.

Diagnosis consists of two phases

1. Does the patient have hypercortisolism or not?
2. What is the cause of the hypercortisolism? Phase 1 must be completed first as phase 2 tests can only be interpreted if hypercortisolism is present.

Investigation of hypercortisolism phase 1

Does the patient have hypercortisolism?

Patients being investigated for hypercortisolism should look Cushingoid. Depression and alcoholism may cause abnormal tests for hypercortisolism without representing a true hypercortisolaemic state and, hence, are termed 'pseudo-Cushing's syndrome'. Such depressed patients often do not appear Cushingoid and alcoholism should be identifiable clinically and biochemically. If there is a high degree of suspicion of hypercortisolism in a depressed patient, midnight cortisol levels < 140nmol/L or a negative result on dexamethasone-CRH testing (📕 Low dose dexamethasone suppression test, p207) may be helpful in excluding the diagnosis. Note that iatrogenic or factitious Cushing's syndrome is usually due to a steroid other than hydrocortisone (not detected In the cortisol assay) and characteristically results in apparent suppression of the hypothalamopituitary-adrenal axis on testing.

Four tests are used to determine whether a patient does have hypercortisolism

1. **24 h urinary-free cortisol collections (UFC)**. Three collections with simultaneous creatinine excretion estimation are ideal. If the creatinine excretion varies > 10% between collections, the samples are not true 24 h collections and should be repeated. If two or more collections have a value > 3 times the laboratory upper limit of normal (e.g. > 800nmol/24 h), then the diagnosis of hypercortisolism is secure. Patients with intermediate values should have repeat sampling after several weeks or additional tests. Steroids, adrenal enzyme inhibitors, statins and carbamazepine must be discontinued prior to testing. False positives can be caused by pregnancy, anorexia, exercise, psychoses, alcohol, and alcohol withdrawal.

2. **Low dose dexamethasone suppression test (LDST)**. This can be preformed overnight or over 2 days (📖 Low dose dexamethasone suppression test, p207), the latter having less false-positives. Some authorities believe it adds little to UFCs as when cortisol secretion is high, the UFC is clearly raised, but in times when it is intermediate, the LDST may be normal. It is a useful out-patient screening test (📖 Low dose dexamethasone suppression test, Overnight dexamethasone suppression test p207) in individuals who cannot reliably collect 24 h urine samples.

3. **Midnight cortisol levels**. High serum cortisol levels (> 200nmol/L) measured between 23.00 and 01.00 h indicate loss of diurnal rhythm and, although inconvenient, are one of the best tests of hypercortisolism. Samples should be taken via an in-dwelling cannula in as relaxed state as possibly, preferably during sleep. Values <140nmol/L make hypercortisolism very unlikely. Late evening salivary cortisol levels in an outpatient setting can be used where the assay is available.

4. **Dexamethasone-suppressed CRH test** (📖 Low dose dexamethasone suppression test, p207). This is a modification of the LDST, which has been said to have a specificity of 100% for hypercortisolism. Experience suggests that exceptions still occur.

Summary

In patients who appear Cushingoid, 3 UFCs should be performed (note causes of false +ves). If these give equivocal results additional tests are required including further UFCs, midnight cortisols, and a formal 2-day LDST followed by CRH.

Investigation of hypercortisolism phase 2: what is the cause of the hypercortisolism?

The common and rare causes of hypercortisolism are summarized in Tables 2.8 and 2.9, along with useful clinical features. Approximately 65% of cases are due to a pituitary adenoma (Cushing's disease), 20% are due to an adrenal adenoma or carcinoma, and 10% to ectopic ACTH production.

These are the three main causes to be distinguished using a combination of the tests shown below. Distinction between a pituitary adenoma (which may not be visualizable on MRI) and a small indolent tumour (typically lung carcinoid) represents the greatest challenge. Despite extensive investigation, the cause will remain uncertain in some of these cases.

Investigations

1. **Plasma ACTH level** (separate and freeze immediately). Undetectable plasma ACTH levels are strongly suggestive of an adrenal tumour. However, ACTH secretion is intermittent and two suppressed values with simultaneous high cortisol levels (> 400nmol/L) are preferable and should prompt adrenal CT scanning.

2. **High dose dexamethasone suppression test** (📖 High dose dexamethasone suppression test, p208). Greater than 90% suppression of basal urine free cortisol (UFC) levels is strongly suggestive of a pituitary adenoma. Lesser degrees of suppression are seen with ectopic ACTH.

3. **Inferior petrosal sinus sampling (IPSS)**. This is an excellent diagnostic tool, but requires expert radiological support and should only be performed in tertiary referral centres. 100mg intravenous (IV) of CRH is also given via a peripheral vein while sampling to ensure active secretion of ACTH during the test. ACTH levels are compared between the inferior petrosal sinus on both sides, and a peripheral vein. Sampling is performed at −15, 0, +15, and +30min after CRH injection. Ratios > 2 (ideally > 3) post-CRH are strongly suggestive of pituitary-dependent disease. Risks include failure to enter the sinus, and sinus thrombosis.

4. **Imaging**. Pituitary and adrenal imaging should not be performed without biochemical testing as non-functioning tumours of the pituitary and adrenal are common (false +ves) and, conversely, functioning pituitary tumours are often be too small to be visualized by magnetic resonance imaging (MRI; false −ve). However, if the findings are consistent with the biochemical tests this is useful supportive evidence. Patients with findings suggestive of ectopic ACTH production should have thin-slice computed tomography (CTs) of the chest looking for a bronchial adenoma and MRI scanning of the pancreas for an islet tumour. [111]Indium-labelled octreotide scanning may also be useful in locating small tumours.

5. **Plasma CRH levels**. Very rarely 'ectopic ACTH' syndrome is actually due to ectopic CRH production stimulating ACTH from the pituitary (see Table 2.9). Raised plasma CRH levels may be diagnostic in this condition.

Additional tests include
- **Metryapone test**: here the adrenal enzyme blocker metyrapone is used to lower cortisol levels. Pituitary adenomas respond by increasing ACTH production, but ectopic sources of ACTH do not. The test can also be used to confirm that ACTH levels are truly suppressed in adrenal tumours (rarely necessary).
- **Peripheral CRH test**: ACTH levels are measured before (−30, −15 min) and +15 and +30 min after injection of 100mg IV of CRH into a peripheral vein. A rise in ACTH levels of >34% is suggestive of a pituitary adenoma. The addition of 5µg IV of desmopressin improves the response rate and reduces false negatives.

Table 2.8 Common causes of hypercortisolism (Cushing's syndrome)

Cause	Pathology	Characteristic features
ACTH-secreting pituitary adenoma (Cushing's disease)—65%	Pituitary adenoma	Typical features of hypercortisolism with little virilization
Ectopic ACTH secretion—10%	Malignant: small cell lung cancer, thymic carcinoid, medullary thyroid cancer	*Malignant*: rapid progression marked hypokalaemia, proximal muscle weakness, ↑ BP, tumour clinically apparent, few Cushingoid signs
	Indolent/benign: bronchial/pancreatic carcinoids, phaeochromocytoma	*Indolent*: indistinguishable from Cushing's disease, tumour not easily detected
Adrenal tumour—20%	Adrenal adenoma Adrenal carcinoma	*Adenomas*: typical Cushingoid signs, sometimes virilization *Carcinomas*: rapid progression (months) with virilization, poor prognosis

Summary

See Fig. 2.4.

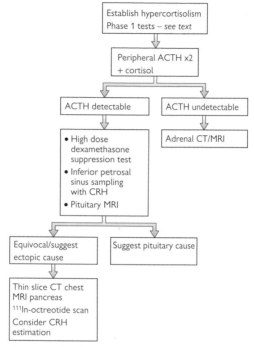

Fig. 2.4 Hypercortisolism. Flow chart for diagnosing the cause once hypercortisolism is established.

Table 2.9 Rare causes of hypercortisolism (Cushing's syndrome)

Cause	Pathology	Characteristic features
Ectopic CRH secretion	Variety of tumours, mostly carcinoids	Clinical features indistinguishable from Cushing's disease but no pituitary tumour, ↑ serum CRH and may fail to suppress with high dose dexamethasone
Ectopic gastrin-releasing peptide secretion	Medullary thyroid cancer	Very rare, resembles ectopic CRH
Factitious ACTH administration	Injections of ACTH	Very difficult to distinguish from ectopic CRH secretion or Cushing's disease, but if isolated from their ACTH source, become adrenally insufficient in days
Cyclical Cushing's disease	Cyclical secretion from pituitary adenoma	Cushing's disease with intermittently negative tests
Pseudo-Cushing's syndromes	Depression or alcoholism	Clinical evidence of Cushing's disease may be limited; evidence of depression or alcoholism
Bilateral micronodular adrenal hyperplasia	Often associated with Carney complex	Investigation suggestive of adrenal tumour (ACTH suppressed) but adrenals normal or slightly enlarged and contain pigmented nodules
Bilateral macronodular adrenal hyperplasia	Sporadic or familial	Investigation suggestive of adrenal tumour (ACTH suppressed), but marked or very marked bilateral nodular enlargement of adrenals on CT Scanning

Further reading

Armadli G, et al. Diagnosis and complications of Cushing's syndrome: a consensus statement. J Clin Endocrinol Metab 2003; **88**: 5593–602.

Boscaro M, Barzon L, Fallo F, Sonino N. Cushing's syndrome. Lancet 2001; **357**: 783–91.

Findling JW, Raff H. Diagnosis and differential diagnosis of Cushing's syndrome. Endocrinol Metab Clin North Am 2001; **30**: 729–47.

Yanovski JA, Cutler GB, Chrousos G, et al. Corticotrophin-releasing hormone stimulation following low-dose dexamethasone administration; a new test to distinguish Cushing's syndrome from pseudo-Cushing's syndrome from pseudo-Cushing's states. JAMA 1993; **269**: 2232–8.

⅏ http://www.endo-society.org/guidelines/Current-Clinical-Practice-Guidelines.cfm

Endocrine hypertension

95% of cases of hypertension are 'essential hypertension' with no specific underlying cause. If hypertension is very marked, occurring in younger patients, difficult to control with drugs, episodic/fluctuating, recent-onset, familial, associated with recurrent hypokalaemia or has associated features (see Table 2.10) then an underlying cause should be excluded.

History and examination should include features of conditions in Table 2.10, with particular attention to paroxysmal attacks, drugs (e.g. liquorice) and family history.

Table 2.10 Secondary causes of hypertension

Physical features	Notes
Absent	
Phaeochromocytoma	May be familial, e.g. in MEN-2 (may have mucosal neuromas), von Hippel–Lindau syndrome, neurofibromatosis; paroxysmal ↑ BP in only 60% cases with headache, sweating and palpitations
Hyperaldosteronism	Multiple syndromes including Conn's syndrome (see Table 2.11)
Renal artery stenosis	Congenital or acquired (atheroma)
Renal disease	Any cause, including polycystic kidneys
Hyper/hypothyroidism	Diastolic hypertension with hypothyroidism, systolic hypertension with hyperthyroidism
Hyperparathyroidism	Does not usually improve after surgical cure
Drugs	Erythropoietin, cyclosporin, cocaine, amphetamines, steroids, liquorice, oestrogens, and androgens
Physical features present:	
Coarctation of the aorta	
Cushing's syndrome	
Acromegaly	
Pregnancy-induced	

Fig. 2.5 provides a flow chart for further investigation. At least 3 separate blood pressure (BP) readings should be obtained—24 h BP monitoring may be useful where 'white coat hypertension' is suspected.

The majority of secondary causes of hypertension can be rapidly excluded by the investigations shown in the first box of Fig. 2.5. If the results are normal or the only abnormality is a low potassium, then the possibilities of hyperaldosteronism or renal artery stenosis remain to be distinguished from essential hypertension. Further investigation should be driven by the severity of the hypertension, the (young) age of the patient and the difficulty in obtaining control with drugs.

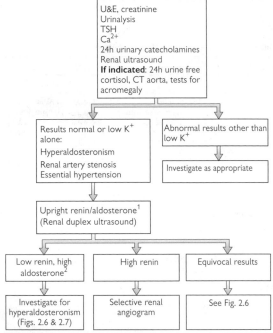

U&E, creatinine
Urinalysis
TSH
Ca^{2+}
24h urinary catecholamines
Renal ultrasound
If indicated: 24h urine free cortisol, CT aorta, tests for acromegaly

Results normal or low K^+ alone:

Hyperaldosteronism
Renal artery stenosis
Essential hypertension

Abnormal results other than low K^+

Investigate as appropriate

Upright renin/aldosterone[1]
(Renal duplex ultrasound)

Low renin, high aldosterone[2]

High renin

Equivocal results

Investigate for hyperaldosteronism (Figs. 2.6 & 2.7)

Selective renal angiogram

See Fig. 2.6

Notes
1 Ideally, this test should be performed off all antihypertensive drugs for 2 weeks (6weeks for spironolactone) except alpha blockers.
2 Low renin and very low aldosterone should prompt investigations for 'apparent mineralocorticoid excess'.

Fig. 2.5 Investigation of cause of hypertension.

Investigation of renal artery stenosis/high renin levels

Selective renal angiography remains the gold standard for diagnosing renal artery stenosis—other imaging methods can miss the diagnosis. 3D MR angiography is now considered a non-invasive alternative. High renin levels associated with hypertension (off drugs) in the absence of renal artery stenosis should prompt a search for juxtaglomerular cell tumour of one kidney. Note that the presence of hypertension is essential, as many conditions associated with low or normal blood pressure can result in 'appropriate' hyper-reninaemia (e.g. diuretics, cardiac, renal or liver failure, hypocortisolism, hypovolaemia). High renin levels can also occur in essential hypertension.

Investigation of hyperaldosteronism

Hypertension with persistent hypokalaemia, raises the possibility of hyperaldosteronism which may be due to a variety of causes (see Table 2.11). Note that investigation for hyperaldosteronism is also appropriate with K^+ levels in the normal range, if other investigations are negative and hypertension is marked, difficult to control or in a younger patient. The optimal approach to investigation remains controversial and equivocal cases frequently occur. If there is marked hypokalaemia of recent onset, a 24 h UFC (and review of medication) is indicated to exclude recent-onset hypercortisolism (usually due to ectopic ACTH production) in which Cushingoid features have not yet become apparent. True hyperaldosteronism is never due to a malignant lesion, so that if hypertension can be medically controlled, it is not always necessary to establish a definitive diagnosis of aetiology. A detailed scheme provided in Fig. 2.6.

Establishing hyperaldosteronism

The initial investigation is an upright renin/aldosterone ratio, performed when the patient has been upright or sitting (not lying) for at least 2 h. The sample needs to be taken to the laboratory and frozen immediately. Ideally, the patient should be on no antihypertensives other than α-blockers (e.g. doxazosin) as most drugs can affect interpretation of the test results (see Table 2.12). This is difficult to achieve in subjects with very marked hypertension. Combination antihypertensive therapy and spironolactone cause most confusion. An undetectable renin with an unequivocally high aldosterone level makes the diagnosis very likely. A normal or raised upright renin excludes hyperaldosteronism. Borderline results should be repeated off interfering medication and after potassium replacement (hypokalaemia can inappropriately lower aldosterone). A low renin with a normal aldosterone can be seen in essential ('low renin') hypertension. Refer to the laboratory for normal and diagnostic ranges. Additional tests (e.g. renin after sodium restriction/furosemide, aldosterone after captopril, sodium loading, or IV saline) are used in specialist centres, but their exact role in testing remains unresolved.

Table 2.11 Investigating established primary hyperaldosteronism

	Change in aldosterone with posture	CT findings	Adrenal venous sampling (ratio of aldosterone between sides)	Response to glucocorticoids*	Treatment of choice	Notes
Adenoma (Conn's)	None/fall	Unilateral nodule	>10:1	Absent	Surgery	
Renin-responsive adenoma	Rise	Unilateral	>10:1	Absent	Surgery	
Unilateral hyperplasia	None/fall	'Normal'	>10:1	Absent	Surgery	
Bilateral hyperplasia	Rise	'Normal'	No difference	Absent	Medical	
Glucocorticoid remediable aldosteronism (GRA)	None/fall	Normal	No difference	Present	Steroids	Very raised 18-oxo cortisols. Positive genetic screening**

* Dexamethasone 0.5mg 6-h for 2–4 days resulting in suppression of aldosterone levels to nearly undetectable levels (usually associated with a fall in blood pressure also).

** Positive for chimeric CYP11B1/CYP11B2 gene.

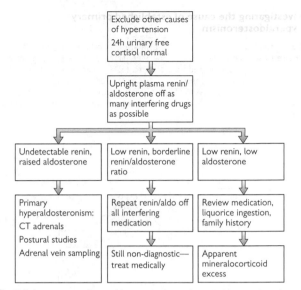

Fig. 2.6 Investigation of hyperaldosteronism/mineralocorticoid excess in patients with hypertension.

Table 2.12 Renin/aldosterone testing and drugs

Drug	Effect on PRA	Effect on aldosterone
Drugs that ↑ PRA		
Spironolactone	↑	Variable
Ca²⁺ channel blockers	May ↑	↓
ACE inhibitors*	↑	↓
Diuretics	↑	↑
Vasodilators	↑	↑
Drugs that ↓ PRA		
α-blockers	↓	↓
NSAIDs	↓	↓

PRA, plasma renin activity; *angiotensin II receptor antagonists are likely to have same effects.

Investigating the cause of established primary hyperaldosteronism

There are 5 causes of established primary hyperaldosteronism with suppressed renin and high aldosterone (see Table 2.13). Surgery (unilateral adrenalectomy) is indicated for adenoma (65% of cases), the unusual renin-responsive adenoma, and the rare cases of unilateral hyperplasia, but not for bilateral hyperplasia (idiopathic hyperaldosteronism, 30% of cases) or the rare, familial GRA. Tests to distinguish these are summarized in Table 2.13 and Fig. 2.7.

📖 *OHCM* 8e, p220.

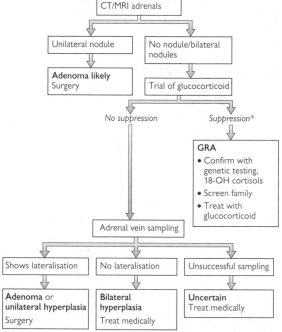

*See footnote to Table 2.9 for suppression protocol.

Fig. 2.7 Identifying the cause of established primary hyperaldosteronism.

Table 2.13 Causes of hyperaldosteronism/apparent mineralocorticoid excess

Primary hyperaldosteronism (↓ renin ↑ aldosterone)
- Aldosterone-producing adenoma (Conn's syndrome)
- Renin-responsive adenoma
- Idiopathic unilateral hyperplasia
- Idiopathic bilateral hyperplasia
- Glucocorticoid-remediable hyperaldosteronism

Apparent mineralocorticoid excess (↓ renin ↑ aldosterone)
- Liquorice ingestion, carbenoxolone, fludrocortisone
- Congenital 11β-hydroxysteroid dehydrogenase deficiency
- Liddle's syndrome
- Congenital adrenal hyperplasia (11β-hydroxylase or 17α-hydroxylase def.)
- Hypercortisolism

If hyperaldosteronism is established and a nodule is visible on CT/MRI imaging, it is reasonable to proceed to unilateral adrenalectomy/excision of the nodule. If no nodule or bilateral nodules are seen, then adrenal vein sampling is the most useful test to determine whether surgery should be performed. Aldosterone levels after glucocorticoid administration or genetic testing for the chimeric CYP11B1/CYP11B2 gene should be performed beforehand to exclude GRA (see Table 2.11, p135—family members may be only mildly hypertensive, making family histories unreliable). Unfortunately, the right adrenal vein cannot be catheterized in up to 25% of cases and there is a risk of precipitating adrenal haemorrhage. Postural studies identifying a >50% rise in aldosterone comparing recumbent and 2–4 h of standing/walking suggest idiopathic hyperplasia, but a small renin-responsive adenoma not visible on CT could give similar results.

Investigating the cause of apparent mineralocorticoid excess

Rarely, investigation reveals low renin and low aldosterone levels in the presence of hypertension, hypokalaemia, and alkalosis. There are 5 causes of this (see Table 2.13). A 24 h UFC estimation will rapidly exclude recent-onset, aggressive hypercortisolism. Repeated enquiry should be made for drug and liquorice product ingestion. The remaining causes may be diagnosed by urinary cortisol/cortisone ratio (11β-OH steroid dehydrogenase deficiency—often referred to alone as 'apparent mineralocorticoid excess') or other appropriate changes in urinary and plasma cortisol metabolites (e.g. raised DOC levels—11 β-hydroxylase or 17α-hydroxylase deficiency) or responsiveness to amiloride (Liddle's syndrome).

Phaeochromocytoma

1. **Clinical features**. Phaeochromocytoma is rare, but an important diagnosis not to miss—can result in fatal hypertensive crisis especially during surgery or after inadvertent adrenoreceptor blockade without blockade. It can be sporadic (90%) or be the first clue to a familial syndrome (see Table 2.10). Approximately 10% of cases are extra-adrenal, 10% multiple, and 10% malignant ('tumour of 10%'). 90% of cases have sustained or paroxysmal hypertension, but paroxysmal attacks of some nature are a feature of only 55% of cases. Pure adrenaline-secreting lesions can occasionally cause hypotension. They are always intra-adrenal. Phaeochromocytoma needs to be excluded in cases of incidentally found adrenal masses. Paragangliomas are non-secreting phaeos.

2. **Diagnostic Tests**. 24 h urinary catecholamine estimations (collect into an acidified container) have now replaced measures of catecholamine metabolites (VMAS) as they are more sensitive and specific. A single clearly positive estimation in the presence of hypertension is usually sufficient. If non-diagnostic, sampling initiated immediately after an 'attack' should provide the answer. Mild ↑ can be seen in anxiety states, and with very small lesions detected in the follow-up of familial, recurrent disease. Causes of false positive results include methyldopa, levodopa, labetalol, clonidine withdrawal, intracranial events (e.g. subarachnoid haemorrhage, posterior fossa tumour), or metabolic stress (e.g. hypoglycaemia, myocardial infarction). Measurement of plasma or urinary metanephrines has a higher sensitivity and specificity than urinary catecholamines and should be used if available.

3. **Finding the tumour**. Once the diagnosis is established, blockade (typically with increasing bd doses of phenoxybenzamine) should be established before invasive investigation. The tumours are usually large (>2cm) and bright on T2-weighted images. CT/MRI scanning therefore identifies virtually all adrenal lesions. Radionuclide scanning with ^{131}I-MIBG is useful to confirm activity if more than one adrenal nodule is present and to identify extra-adrenal lesions where no adrenal lesion is seen. Note that extra-adrenal phaeo-chromocytomas (paraganglionomas) are usually in the chest or abdomen, but can occur in the neck (including chemodoctomas of the carotid body), pelvis, and bladder. Biopsy of suspected phaeochromocytoma lesions is contraindicated.

4. **Malignant phaeos**. The only reliable indicator of malignancy in phaeos is the presence of distant metastases or local invasion on histology. The histological appearance of the tumour cells themselves surprisingly has no significance.

5. **Genetic testing**. Up to 25% of phaeos, especially if familial will have a genetic basis (see Table 2.14). Genetic testing is indicated in familial or recurrent cases.

📖 *OHCM* 8e, p220.

Table 2.14 Phaeochromocytomas: Genetic mutations associated with phaeochomocytomas or paragangliomas.

Gene	Syndrome	Associated features	Frequency
RET	MEN 2	Medullary carcinoma of thyroid, hyperparathyroidism	5%
VHL	Von Hippel–Lindau syndrome	Hemangioblastomata, renal, pancreatic tumours	8%
SDH B		Large, malignant, extra-adrenal paragangliomas	6%
SDH D		Often head and neck paragangliomas	4%
SDH C		Rare	0%
Neurofibrimatosis	Von Recklinghausens/ disease	Skin neurofibromata, *café-au-lait* spots	4%

SDH = succinate dehydrogenase

Further reading

Gimenez-Roqueplo New advances in the genetics of phaechromocytoma and paraganglimoa syndromes. *Ann NY Acad Sci* 2006; **1073**: 112–21.

Primary hyperaldosteronism. ♒ http://www.endo-society.org/guidelines/Current-Clinical-Practice-Guidelines.cfm

Pacak et al. Phaeochromocytoma:recommendations for clinical practice from the first international symposium. *Nature Clin Pract Endocrinol* 2007; **3**: 92–102.

Hypokalaemia

Persistent hypokalaemia (< 2.5mmol/L) can cause muscle weakness, cramps, tetany, polyuria, exacerbate digoxin toxicity, and predispose to cardiac arrhythmias. The majority of cases are due to the common causes (see Table 2.15) and are relatively easy to diagnose. However, puzzling cases where none of these features are present occur and prompt further investigation. A flow chart is shown Fig. 2.8.

Table 2.15 Common causes of hypokalaemia*

- Diuretics
- Vomiting/diarrhoea
- Intestinal fistula
- Laxative or diuretic abuse
- Steroids (including fludrocortisone), liquorice, ACTH therapy

*See text for investigation of rare causes.

Note in Fig. 2.8 the importance of identifying the presence of acidosis and hypertension. Occult diuretic and purgative use should always be borne in mind. The commonest cause of persistent hypokalaemia with no other cause presenting in adulthood is Gitelman's syndrome (NCCT-Na-Cl cotransporter defect), an asymptomatic congenital disorder, which can usually be separated from the rare, more severe Bartter's syndrome (which usually presents neonatally or in early childhood, and represents gene defects in the renal tubular proteins NKCC2, ROMK, or CLCNKB) by low serum Mg^{2+} levels.

📖 *OHCM* 8e, p688.

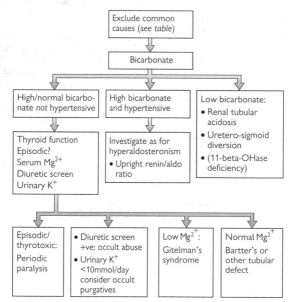

Fig. 2.8 Investigation of hypokalaemia.

Further reading

Shaer AJ. Inherited primary tubular hypokalemic alkalosis: a review of Gitelman and Bartter syndromes. *Am J Med Sci* 2001; **322**: 316–22.

Hyperkalaemia

Artefactual and common causes need to be excluded of which renal failure is the most important (see Table 2.16). If these fail to reveal a cause, then hypoadrenalism (which can be life-threatening), isolated mineralocorticoid deficiency and type IV renal tubular acidosis (RTA) need to be excluded.

Table 2.16 Causes of hyperkalaemia

Artefactual	Other	Rare, but important
Sample left unseparated overnight	Excess K^+ replacement	Hypoadrenalism
Sample haemolysed	K^+-sparing diuretics, ACE inhibitors	Type IV RTA
Myeloproliferative disease (leakage of K^+ from high cell counts)	Renal impairment, esp. acute and after trauma or surgery Metabolic acidosis (esp. DKA), rhabdomyolysis, burns, massive blood transfusion	Isolated mineralocorticoid deficiency

Hypoadrenalism is suggested by concomitant hyponatraemia, hypotension (including postural), malaise and skin pigmentation. Diagnosis is by short synacthen testing (📖 Adrenal failure, p154). Note that hyperkalaemia is not a feature of secondary (pituitary) hypo-adrenalism since aldosterone production is maintained by the renin–angiotensin system. Type IV renal tubular acidosis is common in patients with diabetes. It is associated with a renal tubular dysfunction, as well as mildly impaired glomerular function. Serum creatinine is usually at or above the upper limit of normal. It is a state of hyporeninaemic hypoaldosteronism. Renin/aldosterone testing is suggestive, but there is no definitive test. Isolated mineralocorticoid deficiency is usually congenital (e.g. due to aldosterone synthase deficiency), but can be acquired (e.g. HIV disease). High renin and low aldosterone levels would be expected. Aldosterone resistance (pseudohypoaldosteronism with high aldosterone levels but biochemical mineralocorticoid deficiency) has been described.

📖 OHCM 8e, p299, p849.

Adrenal failure

See Table 2.17

Hypoadrenalism is often insidious in clinical onset. However, it is an important diagnosis to make as it can be life-threatening, especially at times of stress. The key is to have a high index of suspicion. Primary adrenal failure is suggested by hyperkalaemia, hyponatraemia, hypotension (including postural), malaise, weight loss, nausea, abdominal pain, and skin pigmentation. In pituitary (secondary) adrenal failure, hyperkalaemia, hypotension, and pigmentation are absent, and malaise may be the only feature. Signs/symptoms of gonadal failure (e.g. loss of libido, reduced shaving, or amenorrhoea) if present mandate exclusion of pituitary failure. Random cortisol levels can be misleading as they may be high in the morning and low in the evening. Nonetheless, a random cortisol level >550nmol/L excludes the diagnosis and is a useful test in patients undergoing severe stress/illness (e.g. in intensive therapy unit (ITU)).

▶ **Do not delay treatment**. Where there is a strong suspicion of adrenal failure, treatment must not be delayed pending investigation. A short synacthen test or random cortisol should be performed immediately and treatment commenced with steroids awaiting results. Alternatively, treatment with dexamethasone, 0.5mg daily (which does not cross-react in the cortisol assay) can be used and then discontinued for the day of testing. Patients on other forms of glucocorticoid therapy should discontinue treatment on the morning of the test and ideally 24 h beforehand (12 h for hydrocortisone or cortisone acetate). Mineralocorticoid replacement need not be discontinued.

Short ACTH (Synacthen®) test

The standard test for adrenal failure is the short ACTH test. A low dose of synthetic ACTH (0.5 or 1.0 µg) test was previously in vogue but has not been confirmed to be useful.

For secondary (pituitary) adrenal failure, alternative tests include the insulin stress test (📖 Short Synacthen® test, p209) and the metyrapone test (📖 Obesity/hypercortisolism, Additional tests include, p135). However, these tests involve applying a stress and carry a risk in patients who are profoundly hypo-adrenal. They are only indicated in patients within 6 weeks of pituitary surgery or a pituitary insult, where hypotrophy of the adrenal cortices has yet to develop.

Test to distinguish primary vs. secondary adrenal failure

In the context of known pituitary disease and with failure of other pituitary hormones, adrenal failure can be assumed to be secondary (pituitary) in origin. Where isolated adrenal failure is identified, primary adrenal failure is most likely and suggested by increased skin pigmentation and hyperkalaemia.

Table 2.17 Causes of primary adrenal failure

Cause	Associated features	Diagnostic tests/notes
Autoimmune adrenalitis (> 90% cases in developed countries)	Autoimmune damage may be associated with polyglandular failure types 1 and 2	Anti-adrenal (21-OH-ase) antibodies
Drugs	Ketoconazole, mitotane, etomidate, rifampicin, phenytoin	Exacerbate pre-existing adrenal impairment
Tuberculosis	Extra-adrenal TB	Calcified or enlarged adrenals, extra-adrenal TB, but may only show shrunken glands
Other infections, e.g. histoplasmosis, syphilis	Seen in N and S America	Adrenal glands enlarged
Metastatic malignancy	Common with breast, lung, melanoma or GI cancer though does not always cause adrenal failure	Enlargement/deposits in adrenal glands on CT
Bilateral adrenal haemorrhage	Anticoagulation, adrenal vein sampling	Signs of haemorrhage on CT
AIDS	CMV/TB, cryptococcus adrenalitis	
Adrenaleukodystrophy	Especially in ♂ < 15 years, dementia, quadriplegia	
Adrenomyeloneuropathy	Neuropathy, blindness—may appear after adrenal failure	
Familial glucocorticoid deficiency	Defective melanocortin 2 receptors including Allgrove's syndrome, hypoadrenalism associated with seizures, achalasia and alacrima from childhood	
Defective cholesterol metabolism		
Congenital adrenal hypoplasia	Mutation on DAX1 or related genes causing failure of adrenal to develop. Adrenal insufficiency from birth	

Three additional tests can be used to confirm the level of adrenal failure

1. **Basal plasma ACTH**. This is usually the only additional test required. High levels are seen in primary adrenal failure, 'normal' or low levels are be seen in secondary adrenal insufficiency. Note that the sample must be taken and separated immediately at least 24 h after the last dose of a short-acting glucocorticoid (e.g. hydrocortisone) to avoid pharmacological suppression. Patients on longer acting steroid, may have to have the test repeated more than 24 h after cessation of the steroid if the result is equivocal.

2. **Anti-adrenal antibodies** (anti-21 hydroxylase antibodies). These antibodies are present in around 70% of patients with autoimmune adrenalitis (Addison's disease), the commonest cause of primary adrenal insufficiency. However, they can also be present without adrenal failure in patients with other autoimmune conditions.

3. **Long (depot) ACTH test**. Chronic stimulation with ACTH can recover function in adrenal glands that have failed because of lack of pituitary ACTH, but not in primary adrenal failure. This is given in the form of ACTH in oil on 2 consecutive days (📖 Long (depot) ACTH test, p209), or as an infusion over 48 h. With the advent of reliable ACTH assays, this test is rarely indicated.

Additional diagnostic tests—exclude adrenoleucodystrophy in males

While the majority of cases of primary hypoadrenalism are due in developed countries to autoimmune disease, there are multiple other rare causes. These should particularly be considered where adrenal failure occurs in childhood and/or is associated with neurological disease or hypogonadism (see Table 2.17). In particular, adrenoleucodystrophy (ALD) should be excluded. All males diagnosed with primary adrenal failure should have serum sent for very long chain fatty acids (VLCFAs—raised in ALD) as early bone marrow transplantation (and to a limited extent treatment with 'Lorenzo's oil') may prevent irreversible progressive neurological disease developing (e.g. spastic paraparesis).

Further reading

Spurek M, Taylor-Gjevre R, Van Uum S, *et al*. Adrenomyeloneuropathy as a cause of primary adrenal insufficiency and spastic paraparesis. *Canad Med Ass J* 2004; **171**: 1073–7.

Ten S, New M, Maclaren N. Clinical review 130: Addison's disease 2001. *J Clin Endocrinol Metab* 2001; **86**: 2909–22.

Vaidya B, Pearce S, Kendall-Taylor P. Recent advances in the molecular genetics of congenital and acquired primary adrenocortical failure. *Clin Endocrinol (Oxf)* 2000; **53**: 403–18.

Amenorrhoea

Amenorrhoea is often separated into primary (never menstruated) and secondary (cessation of periods after menarche) amenorrhoea, but many causes are shared between the two categories. Structural assessment of the genital tract should be performed earlier in investigation of primary amenorrhoea. Investigation of oligomenorrhoea is similar to secondary amenorrhoea. Menorrhagia and intermenstrual bleeding are due to different causes, often gynaecological in origin. 'Irregular periods' can fall into either category, depending on whether it actually refers to intermenstrual bleeding or variably spaced (anovulatory) periods. A plan of investigation is shown in Fig. 2.9.

In secondary amenorrhoea, it is helpful early on to identify primary ovarian failure (e.g. due to Turner's syndrome, premature ovarian failure, radiation, mumps orchitis, radiation, chemotherapy or non-45XO gonadal dysgenesis) characterized by high gonadotrophins (LH, FSH). Where the gonadotrophins are equivocal or low, amenorrhoea due to hyperprolactinaemia or thyrotoxicosis should be excluded, but the commonest diagnosis is chronic anovulation due to polycystic ovarian syndrome. In this condition, the ovaries still produce oestrogen resulting in a positive progesterone withdrawal test: 10mg of medroxyprogesterone is given daily for 5 days and the test is positive if any menstrual bleeding occurs in the following week. If the test is negative, a pituitary (e.g. pituitary tumour) or hypothalamic (e.g. stress, anorexia nervosa, systemic illness or weight loss) cause resulting in profound oestrogen deficiency must be considered.

Further reading

Azziz R. The evaluation and management of hirsutism. *Obstet Gynecol* 2003; **101**: 995–1007.

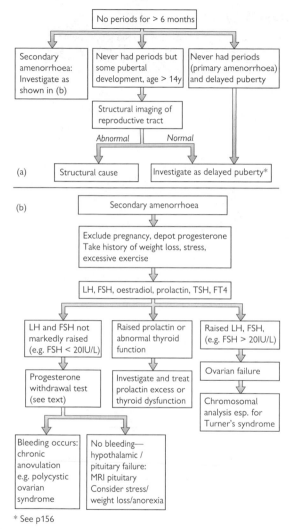

Fig. 2.9 Investigation of amenorrhoea: (a) primary and (b) secondary. See 🔲 p166 for investigation of delayed puberty.

Infertility

Detailed assessment of infertility is beyond the scope of this text and is best referred to a specialist in this area. However, the general physician can take the following basic steps, always remembering that the couple should be assessed together as the problem may lie with the man, the woman, or a combination of both:

1. Semen analysis of the male and where possible a post-coital test to confirm that live semen are delivered to the vaginal tract.
2. If amenorrhoea is present in the female, investigate as in Fig. 2.9.
3. If female is menstruating, determine if the cycles are ovulatory, e.g. by day 21 progesterone levels or home measurement urinary dipstick of the LH surge.

If live semen are delivered and ovulation is occurring, then structural damage or chlamydial infection in the female genital tract is likely, and will require gynaecological assessment.

Hirsutism/virilization (raised testosterone)

Hirsutism refers to an increase in androgen-dependent terminal hairs in the female, typically over the face/chin, lower abdomen, arms and legs, and around the areola of the breast. Virilization reflects much higher androgen levels and comprises the features shown in Table 2.18. Over 20% of women have more androgen-dependent hair than they consider to be normal. In > 95% of cases, this is associated with androgen levels in the female normal range or slightly elevated in association with polycystic ovarian syndrome. Some drugs such as ciclosporin, diazoxide, minoxidil, and androgenic steroids can also cause hirsutism. A history of recent onset (< 6 months), rapidly progressive hirsutism, particularly when associated with features of virilization and a testosterone level of > 5nmol/L, should prompt a search for alternative adrenal or ovarian causes (Fig. 2.10).

Table 2.18 Features of female virilization

- Clitoral enlargement
- Temporal hair loss
- Breast atrophy
- Deepening of voice

📖 OHCM 8e, p222.

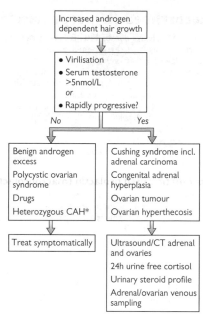

*CAH, congenital adrenal hyperpalsia

Fig. 2.10 Investigation of hirsutism.

Galactorrhoea (hyperprolactinaemia)

Galactorrhoea is always due to PRL. Rarely, it can occur with PRL levels in the normal range and regular menses, but usually is associated with mildly raised levels and amenorrhoea in females or very elevated levels in males. There is no link with breast size—gynaecomastia in males is associated with excess oestrogen. Once dopamine-blocking drugs (major tranquillizers and anti-emetics, but not antidepressants), depot progesterone administration and hypothyroidism have been excluded, all patients should have pituitary imaging to exclude a large tumour pressing on the pituitary stalk (Fig. 2.11). Very high PRL levels (> 10,000IU/L) are invariably associated with prolactinomas. Nipple manipulation (e.g. to check if galactorrhoea has ceased) and chest wall trauma (including shingles) can also stimulate PRL levels.

Asymptomatic raised prolactin (macroprolactin)

If PRL is found (accidentally) to be persistently raised (> 1000IU/L), but menstruation is normal and there is no galactorrhoea, consider the possibility of macroprolactin. This is a circulating complex of PRL and immunoglobulins of no biological importance, but gives a high reading in the PRL assay and the result often varies widely between assays. If the laboratory is alerted to a mismatch between PRL levels and clinical picture, they can easily screen for this with a percutaneous endoscopic gastrostomy precipitation. Stress and epileptic fits can result in transiently raised PRL levels insufficient to cause galactorrhoea.

📖 OHCM 8e, p228.

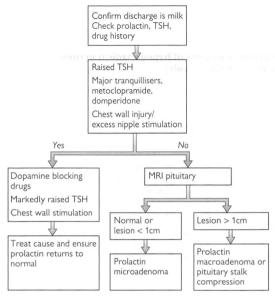

Fig. 2.11 Investigation of galactorrhoea.

Further reading

Fahie-Wilson MN, Ahlquist JA. Hyperprolactinaemia due to macroprolactins: some progress but still a problem. *Clin Endocrinol (Oxf)* 2003; **58**: 683–5.

Leslie H, Courtney CH, Bell PM *et al.* Laboratory and clinical experience in 55 patients with macroprolactinemia identified by a simple polyethylene glycol precipitation method. *J Clin Endocrinol Metab* 2001; **86**: 2743–6.

Impotence/loss of libido/male hypogonadism

Symptoms and signs of hypogonadism in men (low testosterone levels)

- Reduced shaving.
- Loss of libido.
- Impotence.
- Reduced energy/aggression levels.
- Loss of pubic, chest, and axilliary hair.
- Gynaecomastia often results due to a lower testosterone/oestrogen ratio.

Note that very low levels of testosterone (at least < 5nmol/L, typical normal range 10–30nmol/L) are required to result in symptoms. Mild reductions are common especially in the elderly and are rarely of importance. Impotence alone (without loss of libido) can also be caused by neurovascular and psychological causes (e.g. diabetes, spinal damage, urological surgery, atheroslerosis of the aorta, drugs, stress, and psychosexual dysfunction).

After history taking for conditions described above, investigation of suspected male hypogonadism requires

- Prolactin.
- Thyroid function.
- LH & FSH.
- Testosterone.

Hyperprolactinaemia or Thyrotoxicosis, if present, need to be treated on their own merits. If the testosterone level is clearly low, high gonadotrophins point to testicular failure (e.g. testicular surgery, irradiation, or trauma, chemotherapy, crypto-orchidism, previous orchitis, gonadal dysgenesis including Klinefelter's syndrome XXY). Low gonadotrophin levels with a clearly low testosterone point to a hypothalamic or pituitary cause (systemic illness, pituitary tumour). If no cause is found for hypogonadotrophic hypogonadism, the likely cause is Kallman's syndrome, especially if associated with anosmia.

📖 *OHCM* 8e, p222.

Further reading

Sato N *et al.* Clinical assessment and mutation analysis of Kallmann syndrome 1 (KAL1) and fibroblast growth factor receptor 1 (FGFR1, or KAL2) in five families and 18 sporadic patients. *J Clin Endocrinol Metab* 2004; **89**: 1079–88.

Gynaecomastia

Gynaecomastia results from an excessive effect of oestrogens or a raised oestrogen/testosterone ratio. Causes are summarized in Table 2.19. True gynaecomastia should be associated with palpable breast tissue and distinguished from apparent breast enlargement due to obesity. Though very rare, the most important diagnoses to exclude are hypogonadism, testicular and lung tumours.

Table 2.19 Causes of gynaecomastia

Physiological	Newborn, adolescent, elderly
Hypogonadism	e.g. Klinefelter's syndrome, testicular failure
Increased oestrogen	Testicular tumours, lung Ca producing hCG, liver disease, thyrotoxicosis
Drugs	Including oestrogens, spironolactone, cimetidine, digoxin, testosterone administration

Investigations should include

- LFTs.
- Thyroid function.
- LH & FSH.
- Testosterone.
- Oestradiol.
- hCG.
- AFP.
- Chest X-ray.
- Testicular ultrasound.
- Further review of drug history.

Physiological gynaecomastia should only be diagnosed if other causes have been excluded.

📖 *OHCM* 8e, p222.

Delayed puberty

Definition

Puberty is considered delayed in girls if there is no breast development by age 13 (or menses by age 15) and in boys if there is no testicular enlargement by age 14. Note that 3% of normal children will fall into these categories.

Clinical features & initial investigations

A detailed history and examination is required for overt systemic disease, psychosocial stress, anorexia nervosa, and to assess the child's height, pubertal features (pubic hair, testicular size, breast growth, menses), and any dysmorphic features (e.g. features of Turner's syndrome). Where possible growth rate should be calculated from sequential height measurements over at least 6 months.

If no obvious cause is identified, baseline investigations should include:
- LH & FSH.
- TSH, FT4, PRL.
- FBC, U&E, HCO_3^-, CRP, and antigliadin/endomysial antibodies for occult systemic disease.
- Bone age.

This should enable the child to be placed in one of 5 categories
1. **Raised LH/FSH (primary gonadal failure)**. *Causes*: Turner's syndrome, Kleinfelter's syndrome, ovarian/testicular injury. Proceed to karyotyping (should be performed in all girls with delayed puberty as Turner's syndrome may not be apparent).
2. **Short, low LH/FSH, overt systemic disease**. *Causes*: asthma, anorexia nervosa, social deprivation, generalized illness, treatment for cancer including cranial irradiation, dysmorphic (Noonan's syndrome and others).
3. **Short, low LH/FSH, occult systemic disease**. *Causes*: hypothyroidism, hyperprolactinaemia, renal failure, renal tubular acidosis, coeliac disease, Crohn's disease.
4. **Short, low LH/FSH, no systemic disease**. *Causes*: constitutional delay of puberty, hypothalamic/pituitary disease.
5. **Not short, low LH/FSH**. *Causes*: Kallman's syndrome (if anosmia present) or isolated gonadotrophin deficiency. Cannot reliably distinguish from constitutional delay of puberty. Observe.

The investigation of children who fall into the commonest category, 'short, low LH/FSH, no systemic disease', is summarized in Fig. 2.12. The onset of puberty after a period of observation is reassuring, but continued observation is required to ensure the process proceeds to completion including a growth spurt. If not, further investigation for disorders of steroidogenesis, androgen insensitivity, skeletal dysplasia, premature gonadal failure and, in the female, genital tract abnormalities and polycystic ovarian syndrome are indicated.

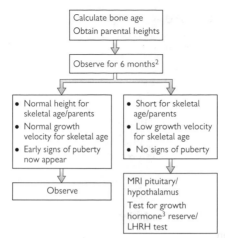

Fig. 2.12 Investigation of delayed puberty in children who are short, with no evidence of systemic disease[1] and low LH/FSH levels.

Notes

1 Including normal thyroid function and PRL.
2 If develops headache, vomiting or visual symptoms proceed immediately to MRI.
3 Refer to paediatric endocrinologist. Tests used vary, e.g. gonadotrophin response to LHRH after androgenic priming and insulin tolerance test for growth hormone response.

Short stature

Evaluation of children who are below the 3rd growth centile for age or particularly small for their family should include:
- Height for age (percentile).
- Mid-parental height (for girls mean of father's height minus 12.6cm + mother's; for boys add 12.6cm to mother's height).
- Bone age (to assess growth potential/height prediction).
- Observation over 3–6 months to determine growth velocity.

Children of short (but normal) parents, who are growing normally, can be observed. Dysmorphic children require further evaluation/specialist assessment. Children who are short for their parental heights (low predicted height), particularly if growing slowly, and short children of pubertal age who have not entered puberty should be investigated as for 'delayed puberty'. Referral for paediatric endocrinological assessment is advised.

Precocious puberty

Definition

Puberty is considered premature if multiple signs including accelerated growth rate and bone age appear by age 8 in girls or age 9 in boys. Note that isolated breast development (premature thelarche) or pubic hair (premature adrenarche) are benign conditions if no other evidence of puberty appears. True precocious puberty requires urgent investigation to determine the cause and avoid irreparable loss of final adult height. In girls, it is often idiopathic, but not in boys. The causes are given in Table 2.20.

Table 2.20 Causes of precocious puberty

Central	Gonadotrophin independent
Idiopathic (especially girls)	CAH (♂)
CNS hamartoma (esp. pinealoma)	Adrenal/ovarian/hCG-secreting tumour
Other CNS diseases, e.g. hydrocephalus, trauma	McCune–Albright syndrome, hypothyroidism, follicular cyst (♀) familial testitoxicosis (♂)

Investigations

Precocious puberty is confirmed by pubertal levels of sex steroids (oestradiol, testosterone). Testicular enlargement (or ovarian enlargement on ultrasound), and detectable LH/FSH levels suggest central precocious puberty and CT/MRI scan of the brain is indicated. Gonadal enlargement can also be seen with testitoxicosis, hCG-producing tumours, hypothyroidism and McCune–Albright syndrome. Further investigation should be performed in combination with a paediatric endocrinologist.

Thyroid function testing: general

In the majority of cases, thyroid function testing and interpretation are straightforward (see Fig. 2.13). However, the following points should be borne in mind.

1. **Which first line test?—TSH**. TSH levels are the most sensitive indicator of thyroid dysfunction except in patients with pituitary disease where they are uninterpretable. TSH used alone as a first line test will miss (levels 'normal') unsuspected cases of secondary hypothyroidism and some laboratories combine TSH and T4 as first line tests. TSH is also unreliable in patients with recently treated hyperthyroidism as it can remain suppressed (undetectable) for several weeks after FT4 or FT3 levels have normalized.

2. **Which tests?—T4/T3**. Free T3 and T4 tests (FT3, FT4) are now more reliable and preferred (although more expensive) to total T3 or T4 measurements. Interference in these assays does occur, but is increasingly rare. Total thyroid hormone levels are markedly influenced by changes in binding proteins (e.g. due to pregnancy, oestrogen-containing contraceptives).

3. **Thyroid autoantibodies**. These are markers of autoimmune thyroid disease. Anti-thyroid microsomal antibodies have been identified as anti-thyroid peroxidase (anti-TPO) antibodies. Anti-TPO antibodies are more sensitive than anti-thyroglobulin antibodies and are present in around 45–80% of Graves' disease and 80–95% of Hashimoto's disease/atrophic thyroiditis. Increasingly, laboratories are measuring anti-TPO directly as their only antibody test (sometimes just referred to as 'anti-thyroid antibodies'). Note that anti-TSH receptor antibodies—the cause of Graves' disease—are currently difficult to measure and not routinely assayed, although simpler tests are being developed. (for indications for testing, see anti-TSH receptor antibody testing 📖 p173).

4. **Tests should agree**. To confirm thyroid dysfunction at least two thyroid function tests and, in cases of doubt, all three (TSH, FT3, FT4) should be performed. The results of the tests should be in agreement—if not, assay interference (heterophile antibodies, anti-T4 or anti-T3 antibodies present in the serum) or unusual causes should be suspected.

5. **Avoid thyroid function testing in systemically unwell patients**. In very ill patients, especially in intensive care, a pattern of 'sick euthyroidism' is often seen, with low TSH levels, low free T3 levels, and sometimes low free T4 levels. Accurate interpretation of true thyroid status is impossible. A raised free T3 level in a very ill patient suggests significant hyperthyroidism and a very raised TSH (> 20mU/L) with undetectable free T4 levels suggests profound hypothyroidism. Other changes should be interpreted with extreme caution and the tests repeated after recovery.

📖 *OHCM* 8e, p208, p210.

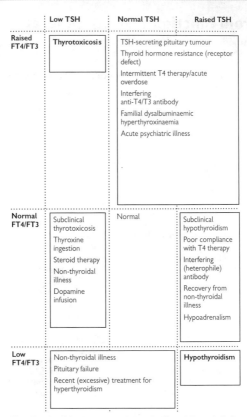

	Low TSH	Normal TSH	Raised TSH
Raised FT4/FT3	Thyrotoxicosis	TSH-secreting pituitary tumour Thyroid hormone resistance (receptor defect) Intermittent T4 therapy/acute overdose Interfering anti-T4/T3 antibody Familial dysalbuminaemic hyperthyroxinaemia Acute psychiatric illness	
Normal FT4/FT3	Subclinical thyrotoxicosis Thyroxine ingestion Steroid therapy Non-thyroidal illness Dopamine infusion	Normal	Subclinical hypothyroidism Poor compliance with T4 therapy Interfering (heterophile) antibody Recovery from non-thyroidal illness Hypoadrenalism
Low FT4/FT3	Non-thyroidal illness Pituitary failure Recent (excessive) treatment for hyperthyroidism		Hypothyroidism

Note: free thyroid hormone assays are assumed—effects of changes in binding proteins on total thyroid hormone assays are not included.
(Adapted from Dayan CM. (2001) Interpretation of thyroid function tests. *Lancet*, **357**, 619–624)

Fig. 2.13 Patterns of thyroid function tests. To use this table you need the results of both TSH and *either* free T4 (FT4) *or* free T3 (FT3) tests. If *either* FT4 or FT3 are outside the reference range, then FT4/FT3 are considered abnormal in this table. If FT4 and FT3 are abnormal in different directions (e.g. one is low and the other is high), see point 4, 'Test should agree', p169.

Dayan CM. Interpretation of thyroid function tests. *Lancet* 2001; **357**: 619–24.

Further reading

Association of Clinical Biochemists/British Thyroid Association. UK guidelines for the use to thyroid function tests. London: ACB/BTA, 2006. ℘ www.british-thyroid-association.org/info-for-patients/Docs/TFT_guideline_final_version_July_2006.pdf

National Academy of Clinical Biochemistry guidelines (2002). ℘ www.aacc.org/members/nacb/LMPG/Pages/default.aspx

Hyperthyroidism (thyrotoxicosis)

Clinical features

Hyperthyroidism is rare in childhood, but affects all adult age groups. Classic features include weight loss despite increased appetite, palpitations, atrial fibrillation, heat intolerance, anxiety, agitation, diarrhoea, tremor, and proximal weakness. Lid-retraction and lid-lag can be seen in any cause of hyperthyroidism, but proptosis, periorbital oedema, chemosis, diplopia, and optic nerve compression only occur in association with Graves' disease (thyroid eye disease), occasionally associated with pretibial myxoedema and thyroid acropachy. In the elderly, presentation with isolated weight loss or atrial fibrillation is common. Raised alkaline phosphatase and sex hormone-binding globulin, leucopenia, and rarely hypercalcaemia are recognized associations.

Thyroid function testing

An undetectable TSH level and a ↑ free T3 level are required to diagnose hyperthyroidism. In milder cases, T4 levels may be in the normal range ('T3 toxicosis'). Normal TSH levels with ↑ T4 and T3 are seen in TSH-secreting pituitary tumours (very rare) or in patients with thyroid hormone resistance (also very rare) – see Figure 2.13.

Investigation of cause (see Fig. 2.14)

Under the age of 40, Graves' disease is the commonest cause. After this age, Graves' disease, toxic nodular goitre, and toxic nodule all occur. However, a short history (≤1 month) of symptoms or absence of relevant symptoms (chance blood test finding) raises the possibility of self-resolving (transient) thyroiditis, a diagnosis supported by neck pain and raised ESR (viral/subacute/De Quervain's) or occurrence in the first 9 months post-partum (post-partum thyroiditis—painless). Transient thyrotoxicosis can also occur in patients with subclinical autoimmune thyroiditis ('silent thyroiditis'—painless) especially during cytokine therapy (e.g. interferon for hepatitis C). If self-resolving thyroiditis is suspected, withhold treatment and repeat the tests after 6 weeks. When thyroid eye disease is present, no further tests are required to diagnose Graves' disease. If not, anti-thyroid antibodies (e.g. anti-TPO antibodies) and isotope thyroid scanning can be useful to distinguish possible causes (see Fig. 2.14 and 📖 Chapter 14). No uptake is seen in transient thyroiditis. Excess thyroid hormone ingestion rarely causes very marked thyrotoxicosis unless the active form (T3) is taken (T3 tablets or desiccated thyroid extract).

Iodine

Iodine has multiple and conflicting effects on the thyroid. Potassium iodide inhibits release of thyroid hormones from the gland and thyroid hormone biosynthesis (Wolff–Chaikoff effect) promoting hypothyroidism. However, escape from these effects occurs in most individuals in a few weeks. In patients with a multinodular goitre, excess iodine (e.g. in amiodarone or radiographic contrast media) can result in thyrotoxicosis by excess provision of substrate (Jod–Basedow effect).

Amiodarone

Has 3 main effects on the thyroid hormone axis:

- Inhibits T4 → T3 conversion, which in the pituitary can result in an asymptomatic mild rise in TSH (reduced thyroid hormone action) and/ or a rise in FT4.
- Can induce true hypothyroidism, usually in the first year of treatment.
- Can induce true hyperthyroidism either via the Jod–Basedow effect in patients with multinodular goitre or by a destructive thyroiditis in healthy glands.

Thyrotoxicosis can occur at any time after commencing therapy and can be very difficult to treat. *Interpretation of thyroid function tests on amiodarone: a raised FT3 indicates true hyperthyroidism; a markedly raised TSH (e.g. >10mU/L), especially if the FT4 is low, indicates true hypothyroidism.*

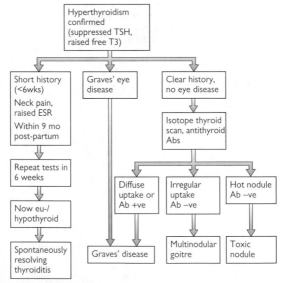

Fig. 2.14 Investigation of the cause of hyperthyroidism.

Hyperthyroidism in pregnancy

Significant hyperthyroidism in pregnancy is generally due to Graves' disease. Mild hyperthyroidism, particularly in association with hyperemesis gravidarum in the first trimester, is often due to a cross-reaction by the very high hCG levels with the TSH receptor ('gestational thyrotoxicosis'). In the post-partum period, thyrotoxicosis may be due to post-partum thyroiditis (self-resolving) or a recurrence of Graves' disease (requires treatment). Measurement of anti-TSH receptor antibody levels may be indicated to distinguish these possibilities.

Thyroid storm

This is defined as severe thyrotoxicosis with confusion/delirium not explained by other factors. There is no definitive test and levels of thyroid hormone are not higher than in other thyrotoxic individuals with no features of storm. Severe agitation, tachycardia and hyperpyrexia are usually seen. Usually precipitated by infection, trauma or surgery, especially to the thyroid gland. Very rare, but tends to occur in individuals who have been poorly compliant in the first few weeks of drug therapy for thyrotoxicosis.

Anti-TSH receptor antibody testing

This test is not routinely available in most laboratories. Although it is positive in > 90% of cases of Graves' disease, in most cases it does not alter clinical management. Indications include distinguishing gestational thyrotoxicosis or post-partum thyroiditis from Graves' disease, indicating the risk of neonatal thyrotoxicosis and (controversial) predicting recurrence after a course of thioamide drug therapy.

📖 OHCM 8e, p210.

Further reading

Association of Clinical Biochemists/British Thyroid Association: UK guidelines for the use to thyroid function tests (2006). 🔊 www.british-thyroid-association.org/info-for-patients/Docs/TFT_guideline_final_version_July_2006.pdf

NHS Library for Health. Clinical Knowledge Summaries (CKS): 🔊 http://cks.library.nhs.uk/hyperthyroidism

Hypothyroidism

Clinical features

Classic clinical features of hypothyroidism include weight gain, cold intolerance, dry skin, constipation, memory loss, lethargy/slow thought/'slowing up', menorrhagia, periorbital/facial oedema, loss of outer two-thirds of eye brows, deafness, chest pain, and coma. These are rarely seen nowadays as thyroid function tests are easy to perform and detect the disease usually at an earlier stage. Weight gain, dry skin, and lethargy are frequently reported, but even in biochemically hypothyroid individuals can only confidently be ascribed to thyroid status if they reverse on treatment.

Biochemical diagnosis

↑ TSH with T4 in the normal range is referred to as subclinical hypothyroidism. ↑ TSH with ↓ T4 is overt hypothyroidism. ↓ T4 with TSH in the normal range may also be due to pituitary failure (2° hypothyroidism) and if persistent requires pituitary function testing. See Fig. 2.13 for other patterns of thyroid function tests.

Differential diagnosis (causes)

In iodine sufficient countries, most spontaneous hypothyroidism is due to autoimmune thyroiditis (Hashimoto's disease if goitre present, atrophic thyroiditis if goitre absent)—anti-thyroid antibodies present in 80–90% of cases. Other common causes are post-thyroidectomy, post-radioiodine therapy, and side effects of amiodarone or lithium. Rarer causes include treatment with cytokines (e.g. interferons, GM-CSF, interleukin-2), vast excess iodine intake (iodine drops, water purifying tablets), congenital hypothyroidism (caused by a variety of genetic defects, should be detected by neonatal screening programme), iodine deficiency (urinary iodide excretion <45µg/day, commonest cause worldwide, esp. mountainous areas, S. Germany, Greece, Paraguay—'endemic goitre'), thyroid-blocking substances in the indigenous diet (goitrogens, esp. in brassicas and cassava, e.g. in Sheffield, Spain, Bohemia, Kentucky, Virginia, Tasmania—'endogenous goitre' without iodine deficiency), Pendred's syndrome (mild hypothyroidism with sensorineural deafness due to Mondini cochlear defect, positive perchlorate discharge test). For transient hypothyroidism, see below.

▶▶ Diagnostic catches ↑ TSH and ↓ T4 always represents hypothyroidism. If the TSH alone is ↑ and the T4 is not even slightly low, a heterophile antibody interfering in the TSH assay may be present in the patient's serum. This is especially likely if there is no change in TSH level after thyroxine treatment, but the T4 level rises (confirming compliance with tablets). For unusual patterns of thyroid function tests, see Fig. 2.14. Note that, within the first 1–3 months (or longer) after treatment of hyperthyroidism, profound hypothyroidism may develop with a ↓ T4, but the TSH may still be suppressed or only mildly raised due to the long period of TSH suppression prior to treatment. Raised TSH alone with disproportionate symptoms of lethargy may be seen in hypoadrenalism.

Transient hypothyroidism

Transient/self-resolving hypothyroidism, often preceded by hyperthyroidism, is seen in viral thyroiditis, after pregnancy (post-partum thyroiditis), and in some individuals with auto-immune thyroiditis. Treatment temporarily with thyroxine IS only required if the patient is very symptomatic. Thyroid function should return to normal within 6 months.

Subclinical hypothyroidism

A raised TSH (< 20mU/L) with normal T4/T3 is very common and seen in 5–10% of women and ~2% of males. It is usually due to subclinical autoimmune thyroid disease and is frequently discovered on routine testing. In randomized trials, ~20% of patients obtain psychological benefit from beginning T4 therapy, in many others it is probably truly asymptomatic. If anti-thyroid antibodies are detectable, the rate of progression to overt hypothyroidism is ~50% at 20 years, but higher than this with higher initial TSH levels. If the TSH alone is raised with negative antibodies (or the TSH is normal with raised antibodies alone), overt hypothyroidism develops in 25% at 20 years. A reasonable approach is a trial of thyroxine for 6 months in symptomatic patients with subclinical hypothyroidism or TSH >10mU/L, and observing the TSH level at 6–12-monthly intervals in asymptomatic patients with TSH <10mU/L.

Hypothyroidism and pregnancy

Overt hypothyroidism is associated with poor obstetric outcomes. Recent evidence suggests that subclinical hypothyroidism is associated with a slight reduction in the baby's IQ and should be treated. Some authorities advocate screening for hypothyroidism in all antenatal patients as early as possible in pregnancy. Patients on T4 need to increase their dose by 25–50µg from the first trimester of pregnancy. Maternal thyroxine can compensate for fetal thyroid failure *in utero*, but congenital hypothyroidism must be detected at birth (screening test) to avoid mental retardation developing. Where the mother and fetus are both hypothyroid—most commonly due to iodine deficiency—mental retardation can develop *in utero* (cretinism). Note that mothers with positive anti-thyroid antibodies and/or subclinical hypothyroidism have a 50% chance of developing (transient) post-partum thyroiditis.

📖 *OHCM* 8e, p210.

Further reading

National Academy of Clinical Biochemistry guidelines. ℰ www.nacb.org/lmpg/thyroid_lmpg_pub.stm

NHS Library for Health – Clinical Knowledge Summaries (CKS): ℰ http://cks.library.nhs.uk/hypothyroidism

Surks MI et al. Subclinical thyroid disease: scientific review and guidelines for diagnosis and management. *J Am Med Ass* 2004;**291**: 228–38.

Hypercalcaemia

Clinical features

Usually asymptomatic if Ca^{2+} < 3.0mmol/L. Typical symptoms include polydipsia/polyuria, constipation, indigestion, pancreatitis, hypertension, tiredness, drowsiness/confusion, abdominal pains, renal colic. Renal failure can occur due to dehydration (reversible), nephrocalcinosis and/or staghorn calculi. Osteitis fibrosa cystica in cases of hyperparathyroidism (with subperiosteal resorption of bone, particularly of the distal phalanges and bone cysts—brown tumours) is now rare, other than in renal failure, but can be associated with bone pain.

Investigation of the cause (Fig. 2.15)

95% of persistent hypercalcaemia is due to either hyperparathyroidism or malignancy. Asymptomatic primary hyperparathyroidism is common in 50–70-yr-old women and a parathyroid hormone level (PTH, sampled simultaneously with the ↑ calcium and measured in a highly sensitive assay), which is raised or in the upper normal range in the presence of hypercalcaemia confirms the diagnosis. Low normal or low levels of PTH should prompt a search for malignancy, especially breast, prostate, bronchus, kidney, thyroid, or myeloma. Bone-derived alkaline phosphatase levels may be raised in both malignancy and hyperparathyroidism. Bone scan may be useful in disseminated malignancy, but can be negative in cancers releasing PTH-related peptide (NOT detected in routine PTH assays) and in myeloma. If malignancy is not found, the conditions shown in Fig. 2.15 need to be considered. Markedly abnormal renal function is seen in milk-alkali syndrome, myeloma, and tertiary hyperparathyroidism. Sarcoid may be difficult to diagnose, but is suggested by a raised serum angiotensin converting enzyme level ((ACE)—not invariable), a dramatic response to steroids and a positive liver or other biopsy for granulomata.

Investigation of established hyperparathyroidism.

Familial benign hypocalciuric hypercalcaemia (FBHH) is a very rare condition caused by an inactivating mutation of the calcium-sensing receptor. This results in stable, lifelong hypercalcaemia with a raised PTH, which rarely causes complications. It is inherited in autosomal dominant fashion.

The hallmark is hypocalciuria—defined as:

Urine $[Ca^{2+}]$ × plasma creatinine/plasma $[Ca^{2+}]$ × urine creat < 0.01

All in units of mmol/L.

Although rare, it is important to recognize as parathyroidectomy is not required.

Further investigation of primary hyperparathyroidism should include serum creatinine, kidney-ureters-bladder plain abdominal X-ray (KUB) to exclude renal stones and a spot urine Ca^{2+}/creatinine to rule out FBHH.

In > 80% of cases, primary hyperparathyroidism is due to adenomatous change in one of the four parathyroid glands. In a minority of cases, and in familial hyperparathyroidism associated with multiple endocrine neoplasia type 1 (pituitary tumours, endocrine pancreatic tumours and hyperparathyroidism) or type 2 (medullary carcinoma of the thyroid, phaeochromocytoma and hyperparathyroidism) 4 gland hyperplasia occurs requiring resection of at least 3½ glands for treatment. Very rarely (< 1% of cases) parathyroid carcinoma is the cause. Lithium therapy may also be associated with (mild) hyperparathyroidism. Once a diagnosis of primary hyperthyroidism is made, ^{99m}technetium-sestamibi radionucleotide scaning is the most sensitive imaging technique and will show the location of the parathyroid adenoma. In difficult cases, local venous sampling may be required for localizing a parathyroid adenoma, especially if it is outside the neck.

Tertiary hyperparathyroidism
Refers to acquired autonomy of the parathyroid glands leading to hypercalcaemia following chronic vitamin D deficiency as seen in renal failure or with malabsorption. Secondary hyperparathyroidism is associated with hypocalcaemia and is the appropriate response to vitamin D deficiency.

Investigation of hypercalcaemia

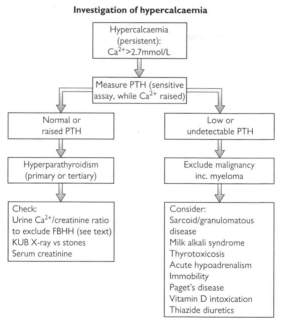

Fig. 2.15 Investigation of hypercalcaemia.

Hypocalcaemia/osteomalacia

Clinical features

Chronic hypocalcaemia is often surprisingly asymptomatic. Symptoms and signs, when present, include muscle spasms, parasthesiae especially around the mouth and in fingers, tetany, fits, positive Chvostek's (VIIth nerve hyperexcitability) and Trousseau's signs (tetany of the hand when BP cuff inflated). Chronic hypocalcaemia is also associated with papilloedema, abnormal dentition (if begins in childhood), cataract, and intracranial calcification (of no clinical consequence). Hypocalcaemia due to vitamin D deficiency is associated with muscle pains, proximal myopathy and osteomalacia. In some cases of pseudohypoparathyroidism (type 1a) there are phenotypic abnormalities (somatic features) including short 4th metacarpal, bone changes (Albright's hereditary osteodystrophy), mental retardation, short stature, obesity, and resistance to other hormones, e.g. TSH, glucagon, gonadotrophins (see below).

Investigation of cause

Persistent hypocalcaemia (corrected for serum albumin levels) with a normal serum creatinine is almost always due to either hypoparathyroidism or vitamin D deficiency (osteomalacia). Other causes and distinguishing features are shown in Table 2.21 and a scheme for diagnosis is shown in Fig. 2.16. In failure of PTH action, the calcium is very low (<1.8mmol/L), the phosphate is raised, but the alkaline phosphatase is not raised and there is no osteomalacia. If the PTH is found to be raised, then pseudohypoparathyroidism can be diagnosed, which is subclassified as type 1a (paternally inherited Gs-alpha defect with somatic features), type 1b ('renally selective' maternally inherited Gs alpha defect—no somatic features) or type II. The classic test is the Elsworth-Howard test—measuring the urine cAMP response to infused PTH (1–34) analogue—but PTH is currently difficult to obtain and this test is rarely required. Families with type 1a may also include patients with pseudopseudohypoparathyroidism, characterized by normocalcaemia, but somatic changes of pseudohypoparathyroidism. The mutations are in the same gene. The aetiology of type II pseudohypoparathyroidism (normal renal Ca^{2+} excretion and no other somatic features) remains unclear.

A low or normal PTH in the presence of a Ca^{2+} level < 1.8mmol/L makes hypoparathyroidism the likely diagnosis (see Table 2.21 for possible causes), but an attempt to rule out an activating calcium sensing receptor (CaSR) mutation with a urine Ca^{2+}/Creat ratio (see Fig. 2.15) should be made. In this rare genetic condition, Ca^{2+} levels are generally higher (around 1.75mmol/L). Importantly, calcium or vitamin D replacement has a high likelihood of causing nephrocalcinosis and is best avoided. Autoimmune hypoparathyroidism in children or young people is particularly seen in association with autoimmune polyglandular syndrome type 1 (chronic candidiasis, coeliac disease, adrenal insufficiency).

In failure of vitamin D action (Fig. 2.16, Table 2.21), there is a compensatory PTH rise, which partly corrects the calcium level, but causes a raised alkaline phosphatase. In addition, there is osteomalacia. In the presence of a significantly raised creatinine, renal osteodystrophy (impaired 25-OH vitamin D generation) is the most likely diagnosis, otherwise dietary vitamin D deficiency (low 25-OH vitamin D), or vitamin D resistance must be distinguished (Table 2.21).

Osteomalacia

Osteomalacia is strictly a histological diagnosis, but is suggested by Looser's zones and pseudo-fractures on X-ray (esp. pelvis and upper femur). If osteomalacia with muscle weakness occurs in the absence of hypocalcaemia or a raised alkaline phosphatase, hypophosphataemia ('vitamin D resistant rickets') is likely. Causes of a low phosphate include intrinsic renal disease, congenital phosphate leak, acquired phosphate leak, and oncogenic osteomalacia. This last condition is associated with very difficult to find tumours, often benign, typically haemangiopericytomas of the naso/oropharynx that may take years to become manifest. It is due to secretion of the cytokine FGF23 (fibroblast growth factor 23) by tumours causing a phosphaturic effect. If suspected, FGF23 levels can be assayed in specialized laboratories. Treatment is phosphate replacement until the tumour can be resected.

Investigation of hypocalcaemia

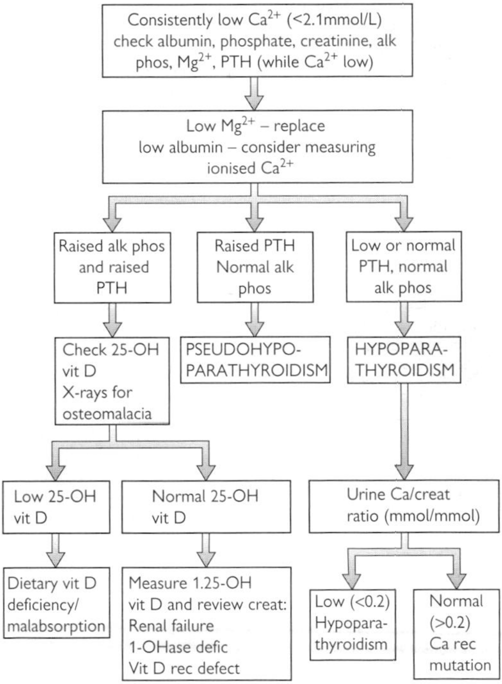

Fig. 2.16 Investigation of hypocalcaemia.

Table 2.21 Causes of hypocalcaemia

Cause	Features
Lack of parathyroid hormone action:	*Very low Ca^{2+}, high PO_4^{3-}, normal alkaline phosphatase*
Hypoparathyroidism	Autoimmune, post-neck surgery (may be transient), radioiodine, congenital (e.g. DiGeorge)
Pseudohypoparathyroidism	Type Ia (paternally inherited Gs alpha mutation plus somatic features), Type Ib (maternally inherited, no somatic features 'renally selective'), Type II (no somatic features, normal Ca^{2+} excretion
Hypomagnesaemia	Inhibits PTH release
Activating Ca^{2+} sensing rec mutation	Indistinguishable from 1° hypoparathyroidism except present from childhood and urinary Ca^{2+}/ creatinine ratio not low
Failure of vitamin D action:	*Ca^{2+} not v. low (> 1.8mmol/L), ↑ alkaline phosphatase, ↓ PO_4^{3-}, ↑, PTH, osteomalacia*
Vitamin D deficiency	Dietary/ ↓ sunlight, malabsorption, ↑ metabolism (phenytoin, rifampicin)
Renal failure	Failure of 1-hydroxylation of vitamin D
Inherited failure of 1-α hydroxylase (vitamin D-dependent rickets type I)	Normal 25-OH vit D, ↓ 1,25OH vitamin D levels
Vitamin D receptor defect (Vitamin D-dependent rickets type 2*)	Normal 25-OH, normal 1,25-OH vitamin D levels
Other:	
Acute pancreatitis	Transient
Hungry bone syndrome— immediately post- parathyroidectomy	Transient
Drugs e.g. foscarnet, bisphosphonates, EDTA, citrate in blood	Transient
Neonatal (with prematurity)	Transient

*'Vitamin D resistant rickets' is rickets with a normal Ca^{2+} and vitamin D due to X-linked hypophosphataemia.

Diabetes mellitus

Diagnosing diabetes mellitus

Diabetes is defined as a state of chronic hyperglycaemia at levels that if untreated would result in microvascular complications (e.g. retinopathy). However, since blood glucose levels vary through the day following meals, physical activity and stress, defining this level of glucose with a single test or a short dynamic test has proved difficult.

Fig. 2.17 provides a scheme for testing for diabetes. Table 2.22 provides the American Diabetes Association (ADA) and WHO criteria for the diagnosis of diabetes, which differ slightly. Oral glucose tolerance testing is rarely required (and only recommended in pregnancy by the ADA), but can sometimes be useful to make the diagnosis in borderline cases (see Fig. 2.17).

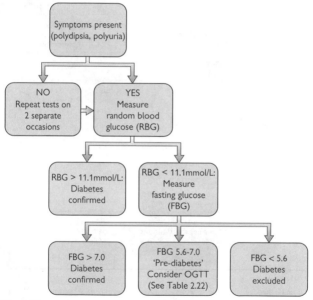

Fig. 2.17 Diagnosis of diabetes.

Table 2.22 American Diabetes Association and WHO criteria for the diagnosis of diabetes

	American Diabetes Association (2005)	WHO (2002)
Normoglycaemia	Fasting plasma glucose <5.6mmol/L (100mg/dL)*	Fasting plasma glucose <6.1mmol/L (110mg/dL)*
	OR 2hr post 75g load plasma glucose <7.8mmol/lL (140mg/dL)	**OR** 2h post 75g load plasma glucose <7.8mmol/L (140mg/dL)
Diabetes	Casual plasma glucose >11.1mmol/L (200mg/dL)[1]	Casual plasma glucose >11.1mmol/L 200mg/dL)[1]
	OR Fasting plasma glucose >7.0mmol/L (126mg/dL)[1]	**OR** Fasting plasma glucose ≥7.0mmol/L (126mg/dL)[1]
	OR 2 h post-75g load plasma glucose >11.1mmol/lL (200mg/dL)[2]	**OR** 2 h post-75g load plasma glucose >11.1mmol/L (200mg/dL)
Impaired fasting glucose ('pre-diabetes)	Fasting plasma glucose 5.6–6.9mmol/L*	Fasting plasma glucose 6.1–7.0mmol/L (126mg/dL)
		BUT not officially recognized—recommend progress to 2h 75g GTT*
Impaired glucose tolerance	Not routinely measured 2h post 75g load plasma glucose 7.8–11.1mmol/L (140–199mg/dL)	2 h post-75g glucose 7.8–11.1mmol/L (140–199mg/dL)
Gestational diabetes	Casual plasma glucose >11.1mmol/L (200mg/dL)	Casual plasma glucose 11.1mmol/L
	OR fasting plasma glucose ≥7.0mmol/L (126mg/dL)*	**OR** fasting plasma glucose ≥6.0mmol/L*
	OR 2 or more of the following plasma glucose values after 75g glucose load: fasting >5.3mmol/L; 1 h >10mmol/L; 2 h >8.6mmol/L (155mg/dL)*	**OR** 2h post 75g load plasma glucose >7.8mmol/L*

*ADA and WHO criteria differ.

[1]If patient does not have classic symptoms (polyuria, polydipsia, unexplained weight loss) then this test should be repeated on a different day.

[2]Not recommended by the ADA for routine clinical use.

Notes
- If symptoms are not present, tests must be repeated on two occasions, ideally more than a week apart, two confirm that levels are, indeed, chronically raised.
- Values are given for venous plasma glucose. Capillary blood glucose are approximately 1.0mmlo/L higher than venous plasma.
- HbA_{1c} is not used to diagnose diabetes
- If the patient has an intercurrent illness (e.g. infection or myocardial infarction) tests should be repeated once the patient has recovered.
- Different criteria are used to diagnose diabetes in pregnancy (gestational diabetes).

Blood samples for glucose testing. In unseparated whole blood, glycolysis by red cells reduces glucose levels by 10–15% per h at room temperature, leading to falsely low results. Clotted (serum) samples without preservative can be used for glucose measurements if the sample is separated rapidly; once separated, the glucose level is stable for 8 h at room temperature and 72 h at 4°C. Alternatively, a tube containing fluoride oxalate to inhibit glycolysis can be used if the sample is to be kept unseparated at room temperature for many hours.

False +ve diagnoses may arise if the subject has prepared inadequately (see Table 2.23).

Table 2.23 Preparation for a fasting blood test

Refrain from any food or drink from midnight before the morning of the test

Water only is permitted

Regular medication can generally be deferred until blood sample has been taken

The appropriate sample is taken between 0800–0900 h the following morning

This preparation is also required for a 75g oral glucose tolerance test (OGTT) or for measurement of fasting blood lipids. Fasting blood tests should be avoided in insulin-treated patients—risk of hypoglycaemia. Fasting is defined by the ADA as no caloric intake for at least 8h.

Normoglycaemic
The diagnostic criteria for normoglycaemia are given in Table 2.22 (note the difference between ADA and WHO for fasting plasma glucose cut-off). Note that there is NO defined random plasma glucose that confirms normoglycaemia, and this complicates the development of screening strategies for diabetes. However, if a random value is <5.6mmol/L, diabetes is unlikely.

Impaired glucose tolerance
This is the preferred diagnostic category for pre-diabetes used by the WHO. The diagnosis of impaired glucose tolerance (IGT) can only be made using a 75g oral glucose tolerance test; a random blood glucose measurement will often point to the diagnosis when other results are non-diagnostic.

This category denotes a stage intermediate between normal glucose levels and DM. By definition, plasma glucose levels are not raised to DM levels so typical osmotic symptoms are absent. Although subjects with IGT are not at direct risk of developing chronic microvascular tissue complications, the incidence of macrovascular complications (i.e. coronary heart disease (CHD), cerebrovascular disease, peripheral arterial disease (PAD)) is increased. Presentation with one of these conditions should therefore alert the clinician to the possibility of undiagnosed IGT (or type 2 DM). Note that up to 25% of individuals who are diagnosed with IGT by an OGTT may revert to normal on re-testing.

Impaired fasting glucose

This is the diagnostic category for pre-diabetes preferred by the ADA and depends on the fasting plasma glucose. Instructions for fasting blood test are shown in Table 2.23. The revised 2005 criteria lowered the lower limit for diagnosing impaired fasting glucose (IFG) so the range according to the ADA is 5.6–7.0mmol/L. This category is also usually asymptomatic. To date, cross-sectional studies suggest that IGT and IFG may not be synonymous in terms of pathophysiology and long-term implications, and a proportion of patients will fall into one category, but not the other. Also, some patients with fasting blood glucose < 7.0mmol/L may have 2 h blood glucoses on the OGTT of > 11.1mmo/L and, hence, would have diabetes by WHO criteria. If an OGTT is performed, the 2-h value takes precedence over the fasting value in the diagnosis of diabetes if the values do not agree.

Oral glucose tolerance test

The OGTT (see Table 2.24) continues to be regarded as the most relevant means for establishing the diagnosis of diabetes in equivocal cases, although its reproducibility is poor. In borderline cases, the WHO suggests that only when an OGTT cannot be performed the diagnosis rely on fasting plasma glucose (FPG). OGTTs should be carried out under controlled conditions after an overnight fast.

The interpretation of the 75g glucose tolerance test is shown in Table 2.25. These results apply to venous plasma. Marked carbohydrate depletion can impair glucose tolerance; the subject should have received adequate nutrition in the days preceding the test.

Table 2.24 Oral glucose tolerance test

Preparation: 3 d unrestricted CHO-intake, and activity. No medication on day of test. 8–14 h fast. No smoking

75g[1] of anhydrous glucose is dissolved in 250mL water; flavouring with sugar-free lemon and chilling increases palatability and may reduce nausea. The subject sits quietly throughout the test

Blood glucose is sampled before (time 0) and at 120 min after ingestion of the drink, which should be completed within 5 min

Urinalysis may also be performed every 30 min, although is only of interest if a significant alteration in renal threshold for glucose is suspected

[1] In children 1.75g/kg, up to 75g.

Effect of intercurrent illness on glycaemia

Patients under the physical stress associated with surgery, trauma, acute MI, acute pulmonary oedema, or stroke may have transient ↑ of plasma glucose—often settles rapidly without antidiabetic therapy. However, the hormonal stress response in such clinical situations is liable to unmask pre-existing DM or to precipitate DM in predisposed individuals. Blood glucose should be carefully monitored and urine tested for ketones. Sustained hyperglycaemia, particularly with ketonuria, demands vigorous treatment with insulin in an acutely ill patient. Re-testing is usually indicated following resolution of the acute illness—an OGTT at a 4–6-week interval is recommended if glucose levels are equivocal.

Table 2.25 Interpretation of the 75g oral glucose tolerance test (WHO)

	Venous plasma glucose (mmol/L)	
	Fasting	**120 min post-glucose load**
Normal	<6.0	<7.8
IFG	6.1–6.9	N/A
IGT	N/A	7.8–11.0
DM	>7.0	>11.1

1. In the absence of symptoms, a diagnosis of diabetes must be confirmed by a second diagnostic test on a separate day. 2. For capillary whole blood, the diagnostic cut-offs for diabetes are >6.1mmol/L (fasting) and 11.1mmol/L (120min). The range for impaired fasting glucose based on capillary whole blood is >5.6 and <6.1mmol/L. In the diagnosis of diabetes, the 2 h post-blood value predominates if values do not agree.

Further reading

American Diabetes Association (2005) Diagnosis and classification of diabetes mellitus. *Diabetes Care* **28**, S37–42.

Gabir M et al. The 1997 ADA and 1999 WHO criteria for hyperglycaemia in the diagnosis and prediction of diabetes. *Diabetes Care* 2000; **23**: 1108–12.

WHO 2006 Guidelines: ℘ http://www.who.int/diabetes/publications/Definition%20 and%20 diagnosis%20 of %20 diabetes_new.pdf

Diabetes websites

American Diabetes Association. ℘ www.diabetes.org

Diabetes UK. ℘ www.diabetes.org.uk

WHO. ℘ www.who.int/topics/diabetes_mellitus/en/

Which type of diabetes is it?

Table 2.26 shows the types and causes of diabetes. Type 2 diabetes due to insulin resistance is by far the most common (accounting for more than 90% of cases) and is increasing as the prevalence of obesity and low physical activity in our society rises. However, there are no definitive tests that can distinguish type 1 and type 2 diabetes. Instead, a collection of clinical and laboratory parameters are used (Table 2.27), but many cases are hard to catagorize (sometimes referred to as type 1.5 diabetes!).

Table 2.26 Types and causes of diabetes

Type of diabetes*	Comment
Type 1	Beta-cell destruction usually leading to absolute insulin deficiency: 1A—immune mediated; 1B—idiopathic (formerly known as juvenile onset or IDDM)
Type 2	Predominantly insulin resistant with relative insulin deficiency (formerly known as maturity-onset or NIDDM)
Gestational diabetes	Diabetes during pregnancy that resolves post-partum. Often an early manifestation of type 2 diabetes
Other specific types	Includes genetic (MODY, mitochondrial, insulin resistance syndromes), pancreatic disease, drug-induced, occurrence in other genetic syndromes, endocrinopathies (e.g. acromegaly)

*Abbreviated from the ADA classification.

Fig. 2.18 (guide to the type of diabetes) provides an algorithm for diagnosing the type of diabetes. Although type 2 diabetes remains the commonest diagnosis in adults and is increasingly common in children, **this is a diagnosis for the lifetime of the individuals** and care should be taken to diagnose any underlying conditions as accurately as possible. Note especially:

- **Unusual features**: if any of the unusual features listed in Table 2.28 are present, then the algorithm should not be pursued and an underlying cause for the diabetes investigated.
- **Type 1 diabetes**: it is important to always consider the possibility of Type 1 diabetes (see Fig. 2.18). Even in older people as early insulin treatment is essential to avoid the risk of ketoacidosis.
- **Pregnancy**: although the majority of diabetes diagnosed for the first time in pregnancy (gestational diabetes) is part of the spectrum of type 2 diabetes, diabetes due to other causes can occur. The algorithm in Fig. 2.18 should still be considered.

Table 2.27 Clinical features and laboratory tests used to distinguish type 1 and type 2 diabetes, and maturity onset diabetes of the young (MODY).

		Type 1	Type 2	MODY
Clinical features	Weight	Slim (BMI < 25) + weight loss at diagnosis	Over weight (BMI > 25)	Average weight (BMI < 30)
	Ketosis	Occurs	Rare	Rare
	Race	Caucasian	↑ risk in S. Asians and Afro-Caribbean	
	Acanthosis nigricans	Absent	May be present	Absent
	Parent with diabetes	Unusual	May occur	Common
Laboratory tests	Auto-Ab	Anti-GAD antibody +ve in around 80%	−ve	−ve
	Insulin c-peptide	Low (but still present for up to 5 yrs from diagnosis)	Present	Present
	HDL > 1.2	Usual	Rare	Usual

Maturity Onset Diabetes of the Young (MODY) Monogenic disorders resulting in diabetes (Tables 2.28 and 2.29). Although these account for less than 1% of cases, they are important to diagnose as they may be easily treated with sulphonylureas (MODY 3), associated with renal disease (MODY 5), or require no treatment (MODY 2). The diagnosis also has important implications for other family members diagnosed with diabetes. Note that it can be very difficult to distinguish type 2 diabetes from MODY without genetic testing and a high level of suspicion in young people is required (Fig. 2.18). If suspected, further advice from a genetic testing centre with experience in MODY should be sought (✆www.diabetesgenes.org).

'Flatbush' diabetes refers to patients who present in diabetic ketoacidosis, but subsequently have a course that is more like type 2 diabetes and are able to come off insulin. This is most commonly seen in African-Caribbeans.

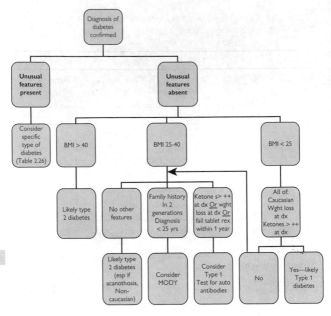

Fig. 2.18 Guide to the type of diabetes.

Table 2.28 Specific features suggestive of an unusual cause of diabetes

Feature	Possible diagnosis
Alcohol excess, hx of pancreatic disease	Chronic pancreatitis
Painless jaundice, weight loss in older person	Pancreatic cancer
Cystic fibrosis	Pancreatic disease
On steroids/cushingoid appearance	Steroid induced diabetes/Cushing's syndrome
Post organ transplant	Drug induced
Specific drugs, e.g. somatostatin analogues, diazoxide	Drug induced
Severe hypertension	Phaeochromocytoma
Acromegalic appearance	Acromegaly
'Muscular appearance' (lipodystrophy)	Partial lipodystrophy
Family history of diagnosis <25 in 2 or more generations	MODY
Renal cysts, urogenital dysplasia	HNF1beta MODY
Bilateral deafness (maternal inheritance)	Mitochondrial diabetes
Optic Atrophy, DI	Wolfram syndrome
Diagnosis < 6 months old	Kir 6.2 mutation
Megaloblastic anaemic	Roger's syndrome (thiamine)
Short stature, severe insulin deficiency (> 1000 units /day)	Insulin receptor defect (leprechaunism, Rabson-Mendenhall Syndrome)
Stiff legs/gait/falls	Stiff person syndrome

Table 2.29 Genetically inherited forms of diabetes including MODY

Gene	% of MODY cases	Comments
Glucokinase	20	MODY 2 'mild' complications rare
HNF-1α	60	MODY 3 diagnosed later ~35 yrs, progressive β cell failure, but very sensitive to sulphonylureas
HNF-4α	1	MODY 1
HNF-1β	1	MODY 5 renal cysts/abnormalities
IPF-1	1	MODY 4
NeuroD1	?<1	MODY 6
Unknown	15	'MODY X'
SUR1	<1%??	Hyperinsulinism in infancy and β cell failure as adult
Mitochondrial	Not MODY	Maternally inherited. May be associated with nerve deafness, lactic acidosis, or syndromes such as DIDMOAD
Lipodystrophy	Not MODY Lamin a/c and others	Associated with localized fat loss

Further reading

🕸 www.diabetesgenes.org

Monitoring diabetic control

Self-testing and near patient testing

Self-testing capillary blood glucose (or urine) can readily be performed by the majority of patients with results available in under 20 seconds Measurements of longer-term glycaemic control are typically laboratory-based, although increasingly near-patient testing equipment is available for use in clinics that can give results to patients within minutes

Urine testing

Glycosuria

Semi-quantitative testing for glucose using reagent-impregnated test strips is of limited value and although used to 'screen' for diabetes is not recommended for monitoring of glycaemic control. Urinalysis provides retrospective information over a limited period of time. Other limitations are:

- The renal threshold for the reabsorption of glucose in the proximal convoluted tubule (PxCT) is ~10mmol/L on average, but varies between individuals. Subjects with a low threshold will tend to show glycosuria more readily, even with normal glucose tolerance ('renal glycosuria'). Children are particularly liable to test positive for glucose. The renal threshold is effectively lowered in pregnancy. Conversely, a high threshold, common among the elderly, may give a misleadingly reassuring impression of satisfactory control. Fluid intake and urine concentration may affect glycosuria. Renal impairment may elevate the threshold for glucose reabsorption.
- Delayed bladder emptying, e.g. due to diabetic autonomic neuropathy, will reduce the accuracy of the measurements through dilution.
- Hypoglycaemia cannot be detected by urinalysis.

Ketonuria

Semi-quantitative test strips for acetoacetate (e.g. Ketostix®) are available for patients with type 1 DM. Useful when intercurrent illness leads to disturbance of metabolic control. The presence of ketonuria on dipstick testing (++ or +++) in association with hyperglycaemia indicates marked insulin deficiency. The patient may be developing ketoacidosis and urgent assessment for DKA is required (DKA, see below. Note that low level ketonuria ('+') can occur after a period of fasting especially in overweight patients and does not necessarily indicate DKA. Occasionally, patients with type 2 DM develop ketosis during severe intercurrent illness, e.g. major sepsis. Urine testing strips do not detect 3-hydroxybutyrate (although acetone is detected by Acetest®). Occasional underestimation of the degree of ketonaemia using these tests is a well-recognized, albeit uncommon caveat of alcoholic ketoacidosis. Testing for blood ketones is possible with newer reagent strips (e.g. Optimum® β-ketone test strips) and is increasingly replacing urine testing especially in emergency departments as a blood sample can be obtained more quickly.

Self-testing of blood glucose

Self-testing of capillary blood glucose obtained by fingerprick has become an established method for monitoring glycaemic control. Frequent testing is a prerequisite for adjusting insulin doses and for safe intensive insulin therapy such as that employed in the DCCT. Use in type 2 diabetes treated by diet or tablets only is not essential. Enzyme-impregnated dry strip methods are available, which are used in conjunction with meter devices and give results in less than 20 s with just 50 µL of blood. Adequate training and a system of quality control are important; even when trained health professionals use such systems in clinics or hospitals misleading results are possible, particularly in the lower range of blood glucose results. Where there is doubt, an appropriate sample (in a tube containing the glycolysis inhibitor fluoride oxalate) should be collected immediately for analysis by the clinical chemistry laboratory. However, acute treatment of hypoglycaemia, where indicated, should not be delayed.

Continuous glucose monitoring systems (CGMS)

Several systems are now available using electrical conductance or microdialysis to provide continuous monitoring of interstitial glucose. Sensors are inserted subcutaneously and need to be replaced every 3–7 days. Newer systems can display the results in real-time (if regularly calibrated against traditional finger stick readings) so that they can be reviewed by the patient, and linked to alarms indicating high and low levels. While these systems, although expensive, are proving increasingly valuable for patients with type 1 diabetes on complex insulin regimes and insulin pump therapy, it must be remembered that the interstitial glucose level is up to 30 min 'behind' the blood level and if glucose levels are changing rapidly, continuous monitors may 'miss' significant hypoglycaemic events.

Laboratory assessment of glycaemic control

Glycated haemoglobin

Measuring HbA$_{1c}$. HbA$_{1c}$ (comprises 60–80% total glycated haemoglobin, HbA$_1$) is formed by the slow, irreversible, post-translational non-enzymatic glycation of the N-terminal valine residue of the β chain of haemoglobin. The proportion of HbA$_{1c}$:total haemoglobin (normal non-diabetic reference range approximately 4–6%) provides a useful index of average glycaemia over the preceding 6–8 weeks. The result is disproportionately affected by the blood glucose levels during the final month before the test (~50% of value). Laboratory values have now been aligned to a standard from the Diabetes Control and Complications Trial (DCCT) trial (DCCT aligned) and values are generally consistent between laboratories. Recent recommendations suggest expressing HbA$_{1c}$ in new units (mmol/mol) against a new International Federation of Clinical Chemistry (IFCC) standard—see Table 2.30.

Table 2.30 Guide to HbA$_{1c}$ values in new and old units

DCCT-aligned HbA$_{1c}$ (%)	IFCC-HbA$_{1c}$ (nmol/mol)
6.0	42
6.5	48
7.0	53
7.5	59
8.0	64
9.0	75

Frequency of testing HbA$_{1c}$. It is suggested that HbA$_{1c}$ is measured every 6 months in stable patients, every 3 months in patients with unstable metabolic control and every month in pregnancy.

Interpreting HbA$_{1c}$ levels. Average HbA$_{1c}$ levels collected over a longer period (i.e. years) provide an estimate of the risk of microvascular complications. Sustained high concentrations identify patients in whom efforts should be made to improve long-term glycaemic control. Table 2.31 summarizes recent recommendations for target HbA$_{1c}$ levels and capillary glucose measurements in subjects with diabetes. Targets need to be modified in pregnancy (see footnote to Table 2.31), in patients with recurrent hypoglycaemia or difficulty complying with medication, and in patients with vascular (especially coronary artery) disease in whom hypoglycaemia may precipitate fatal arrhythmias.

Table 2.31 Target levels of HbA$_{1c}$ and capillary blood glucose values

	Pre-meal (mmol/L)	Post-meal (mmol/L)	HbA$_{1c}$ (nmol/mol)
Non-diabetic	3.5–5.5	<7.8	4–6% (20–42)
Ideal	4–7*	<10*	<7%** (<53)
Suboptimal control			7–10%
Poor control			>10%

*In pregnancy, NICE recommends 3.5–5.9 pre-meal, <7.8 post-meal (1 h), HBA$_{1c}$ aim for <6.1%.

**In Type 2 diabetes, NICE recommends a target of 6.5% in patients with out vascular disease.

Limitations of HbA$_{1c}$ measurements

Although glycated haemoglobin levels are a reliable indicator of recent average glycaemic control they do not provide information about the daily pattern of blood glucose levels or the frequency of hypoglycaemic episodes; this supplementary information required for logical adjustment of insulin doses is derived from frequent home blood glucose monitoring. More recent changes in glycaemia (i.e. within the preceding 4 weeks or so) will influence HbA_{1c} level more than glucose levels 12 or more weeks ago.

Spurious HbA_{1c} levels may arise in states of:
• Blood loss/haemolysis/reduced red cell survival (low HbA_{1c}).
• Haemoglobinopathy.
  • ↑ levels of HbS.(low levels of HbA_{1c})
  • ↑ levels of HbF (high HbA_{1c}).

Modern HbA_{1c} methods are likely to detect haemoglobinopathies without specific testing. Where haemoglobinopathy is present, the HbA_{1c} test is uninterpretable and capillary blood glucose levels or fructosamine must be used.

HbA_{1c} measurements are less reliable in pregnancy where rapid changes in blood glucose levels can occur (e.g. last trimester). They are still used as they are more reliable than other available methods or estimating overall control, but results should be interpreted with caution.

Uraemia due to advanced diabetic nephropathy is associated with anaemia and ↓ RBC survival thereby falsely lowering HbA_{1c} levels.

Fructosamine: refers to protein-ketoamine products resulting from the glycation of plasma proteins. The fructosamine assay measures glycated plasma proteins (mainly albumin) reflecting average glycaemia over the preceding 2–3 weeks. This is a shorter period than that assessed using glycated haemoglobin measurements and may be particularly useful when rapid changes in control need to be assessed, e.g. during pregnancy. Levels can be misleading in hypoalbuminaemic states, e.g. nephrotic syndrome. Some fructosamine assays are subject to interference by hyperuricaemia or hyperlipidaemia.

The main indications for fructosamine measurement are currently (a) presence of haemoglobinopathy or other interference with the HbA_{1c} assay (see above), and (b) rapidly changing blood glucose levels (e.g. pregnancy).

Further reading

American Diabetes Association (ADA). Clinical guidelines on pages of health professionals.
  ℘ www.diabetes.org
Standards of Medical Care in Diabetes. *Diabetes Care* 2009; **32**: S13–61.
℘ www.nice.org.uk—diabetes guidelines

Diabetic emergencies: diabetic keto-acidosis, hyperosmolar non-ketotic syndrome, & lactic acidosis

Diabetic keto-acidosis (DKA) should be considered in any unconscious or hyperventilating patient. The hyperosmolar non-ketotic (HONK) syndrome is characterized by marked hyperglycaemia (> 30mmol/L) and dehydration in the absence of significant ketosis or acidosis. Lactic acidosis (LA) associated with metformin is uncommon. A rapid clinical examination and bedside blood and urine tests should allow the diagnosis to be made. Treatment (IV rehydration, insulin, electrolyte replacement) of these metabolic emergencies should be commenced without delay (see reference for details).

Confirm diagnosis by bedside measurement of:

- Capillary blood glucose (📖 Diabetes mellitus, Reagent test strip; p181).
- Urinary dipstick for glucose and ketones (e.g. Ketostix®). **Note**: nitroprusside tests detect acetoacetate, but not 3-hydroxybutyrate. This may be relevant in some circumstances, e.g. alcoholic ketoacidosis (see below). Venous plasma may also be tested for ketones.
- Urine for nitrites and leucocytes (urinary tract infection (UTI)).

Venous blood for urgent laboratory measurement of:

- Plasma glucose (fluoride-oxalate; ▶ true 'euglycaemic' DKA is rare).
- Urea & electrolytes (U&E; arterial K^+ can be measured by some gas analysers). Plasma Na^+ may be depressed as a consequence of hyperglycaemia or marked hyperlipidaemia.
- Plasma creatinine (▶ may be falsely elevated in some assays by DKA).
- Plasma lactate (if indicated—can also be measured by some gas analysers). Indicated if acidosis without heavy ketonuria is present. LA is a complication of tissue hypoxia (type A) and is a rare complication of metformin treatment in patients with type 2 DM (type B).
- Plasma osmolality in HONK—either by freezing point depression or calculated:

  $2 \times$ [plasma Na^+] + [plasma K^+] + [plasma glucose] + [plasma urea].

- FBC (non-specific leucocytosis is common in DKA).
- Blood cultures (signs of infection, e.g. fever, may be absent in DKA).
- ABGs (corrected for hypothermia) for arterial pH, bicarbonate, PCO_2 and PO_2 (if shock or hypotension).

Repeat laboratory measurement of blood glucose, electrolytes, urea at 2, 4, and 6 h, and as indicated thereafter. Electrolyte disturbances, renal impairment or oliguria should prompt more frequent (1–2 h) measurements of plasma K^+. Capillary blood glucose is monitored hourly at the bedside. ▶ Avoidance of hypokalaemia and hypoglycaemia is most important during therapy.

Other investigations, as indicated

- Chest X-ray (CXR).
- Microbial culture of urine, sputum, etc.
- Electrocardiogram (ECG) acute myocardial infarction (MI) may precipitate metabolic decompensation; note that serum transaminases and creatine kinase (CK) may be non-specifically elevated in DKA.
- Sickle cell test (in selected patients).
- Venous plasma $PO^3_4{}^-$ (if there is respiratory depression).
- ► Performance of investigations should not delay initiation of treatment, and transfer to a high-dependency or intensive care unit.

A severe metabolic acidosis in the absence of hyperglycaemia (or other obvious cause of acidosis such as renal failure) raises the possibility of

- LA.
- **Alcoholic ketoacidosis**: this occurs in alcoholics following a binge. Alterations in hepatic redox state may result in a misleading negative or 'trace' Ketostix® reaction. A similar caveat may occasionally be encountered when significant LA co-exists with DKA. Venous plasma glucose may be normal or ↑.

► Anion gap > 15mmol/L. Normally, the anion gap (< 10mmol/L) results from plasma proteins, $SO^2_4{}^-$, $PO_4{}^{3-}$ and lactate ions. When the anion gap is increased, measurement of plasma ketones, lactate, etc. usually confirms the aetiology (Table 2.32).

Table 2.32 Causes of an anion gap acidosis

Ketoacidosis	Diabetic ketoacidosis
	Alcoholic ketoacidosis
	Lactic acidosis (► metformin)
Chronic renal failure	
Drug toxicity	Methanol (metabolized → formic acid)
	Ethylene glycol (metabolized → oxalic acid)
	Salicylate poisoning

Further reading

ADA position statement. Hyperglycaemic crises. *Diabetes Care* 2004; **27**: S94–102

Krentz AJ, Nattrass M. Acute metabolic complications of diabetes: diabetic ketoacidosis, hyperosmolar non-ketotic syndrome and lactic acidosis. In Pickup J, Williams G (eds) *Textbook of Diabetes*. Oxford: Blackwell Science, 1997.

Investigation of hyperlipidaemia

Primary dyslipidaemias are relatively common and contribute to an individual's risk of developing atheroma (e.g. CHD, CVD). Prominent examples include familial combined hyperlipidaemia (FCHL, ~2–3% of UK population) and heterozygous familial hypercholesterolaemia (FH, UK incidence 1 in 500). Major hypertriglyceridaemia also predisposes to pancreatitis. The key features of familial FH, FCHL, and diabetic dyslipidaemia are considered later.

Investigations

Although many subtle alterations in plasma lipids have been described, therapeutic decisions rest on measurement of some or all of the following in serum or plasma (plasma being preferred, since it can be cooled rapidly):

- Total cholesterol (may be measured in non-fasting state in first instance since levels are not greatly influenced by meals).
- Triglycerides (after 12 h fast).
- Low-density lipoprotein (LDL)-cholesterol (calculated using the Friedewald formula when triglycerides are < 4.5mmol/L):

    LDL-cholesterol = [(Total cholesterol − HDL-cholesterol) − Triglycerides] ÷ 2.19

- High-density lipoprotein (HDL)-cholesterol (regarded as the 'cardioprotective' subfraction)—HDL particles are synthesized in the gut and liver and thought to be involved in 'reverse transport' of cholesterol from peripheral tissues to the liver, where it can be excreted as bile salts.

Notes on sampling in relation to lipoprotein metabolism

- Triglycerides (triacylglycerols) are measured after a ~12 h overnight fast in order to clear diet-derived chylomicrons.
- Alcohol should be avoided the evening prior to measurement of triglycerides (can exacerbate hypertriglyceridaemia).
- A weight-maintaining diet is recommended for 2–3 weeks before testing.
- Lipid measurements should be deferred for 2–3 weeks after minor illness and 2–3 months after major illness, surgery or trauma since cholesterol levels may be reduced. Following acute myocardial infarction it is generally accepted that plasma cholesterol is reliable if measured within 24h of the onset of symptoms.
- The effects of certain drugs on lipids should be considered (see Table 2.33).
- Glycaemic control should be optimized wherever possible before measuring plasma lipids in patients with diabetes.

Important additional considerations are

- **Day-to-day variability**: generally, decisions to treat hyperlipidaemia should be based on more than one measurement over a period of 1–2 weeks. This is especially true for patients with mixed hyperlipidaemia (i.e. including hypertriglyceridaemia).
- Exclusion of secondary hyperlipidaemia—many common conditions, drugs and dietary factors can influence plasma lipids (see Table 2.33).
- Family members should also have their plasma lipids measured if a familial hyperlipidaemia is suspected in a proband.

Both cholesterol and triglycerides may be affected to some degree by these factors, but one often predominates. Pre-existing primary hyperlipidaemias may be exacerbated.

Clinical features

E.g. xanthelasma, tendon xanthomas, etc., should always be sought. A detailed family history, drug history, and medical history (for diabetes and other cardiovascular risk factors such as hypertension) should always be obtained. Certain endocrine disorders, impaired hepatic or renal function can influence circulating lipid composition and cardiovascular risk. A classification of the major familial dyslipidaemias is presented in Table 2.34.

Table 2.33 Causes of secondary hyperlipidaemia

Hypercholesterolaemia
- Hypothyroidism (even minor degrees of 1° hypothyroidism)
- Cholestasis (raised lipoprotein X levels)
- Nephrotic syndrome
- Anorexia nervosa
- Diuretics
- Immunosuppressive agents
- Hepatoma
- Dysglobulinaemias

Hypertriglyceridaemia
- Obesity
- Diabetes (esp. type 2 DM)
- Lipodystrophic syndromes (of diabetes and HIV-associated)
- Alcohol excess (*n.b.* moderate alcohol consumption may raise HDL-cholesterol)
- Renal failure
- Antiretroviral agents
- Oestrogens (esp. oral preparations in some women)
- Corticosteroids
- Beta-adrenergic blockers
- Retinoids

Recommended investigation for exclusion of 2° hyperlipidaemia: U&E; plasma creatinine; fasting venous glucose; LFTs; TFTs. For patients on statins check: LFTs; CK periodically (▶ measure urgently if myositis occurs—a rare but potentially fatal complication).

▶Specialist advice should be sought in the management of major or resistant hyperlipidaemias.

Table 2.34 Familial hyperlipoproteinaemias

Genetic disorder	Defect	Presentation	Cholesterol	Triglycerides	Phenotype
Familial LPL deficiency	Absence of LPL activity	Eruptive xanthomata hepatosplenomegaly	↑	↑↑↑	I
Familial apo C-II deficiency	Absence of apo C-II	Pancreatitis	↑	↑↑↑	I or V
Familial hypercholesterolaemia	LDL receptor deficiency	Tendon xanthomata premature atheroma	↑↑↑	↑ or N	IIa or IIb
Familial dysbeta-lipoproteinaemia	Abnormal apo E and defect in TG metabolism	Turbo-eruptive and palmar xanthoma; premature atheroma	↑↑↑	↑↑↑	III
Familial combined hyperlipidaemia	Uncertain	Premature atheroma	↑ or N	↑ or N	IIa, IIb or IV
Familial hypertriglyceridaemia	Uncertain eruptive xanthomata hepatosplenomegaly; pancreatitis		N	↑↑↑	IV
			↑	↑↑↑	V

↑, ↑↑, and ↑↑↑, mildly, moderately or severely raised; cholesterol and triglycerides refers to concentrations in plasma; phenotype refers to Fredrickson classification (I to V, see Table 2.35); apo, apoprotein; LPL, lipoprotein lipase; n, normal; TG, triglycerides.

Table 2.35 Phenotypic (Fredrickson) classification of hyperlipidaemias

Type	Cholesterol	Triglycerides	Particle excess	Usual underlying cause
I	↑	↑↑↑	Chylomicrons	LPL or apo C-II deficiency
IIa	↑↑	↑	LDL	LDL receptor defect, LDL overproduction
IIb	↑↑	↑↑	VLDL, LDL	VLDL or LDL overproduction or ↓ clearance
III	↑↑	↑↑	IDL* — dysbetali-poproteinaemia	Impaired remnant removal may be due to certain apo E phenotypes or apo E deficiency
IV	N or ↑	↑↑	VLDL	VLDL overproduction or ↓ clearance
V	↑	↑↑↑	Chylomicrons VLDL	Diabetes

i, ii, and iii, mildly, moderately or severely raised; LDL, low-density lipoprotein; VLDL, very-low-density lipoprotein; LPL, lipoprotein lipase; apo, apoprotein. IDL—intermediate density lipoproteins.

Further reading

Frayn KN. *Metabolic regulation—a human perspective.* London: Portland Press, 1996.

Jialal I. Dyslipidaemias and their investigation. In: Bouloux P-MG, Ree LH (eds) *Diagnostic Tests in Endocrinology and Diabetes.* London: Chapman & Hall Medical, 1994.

Joint British recommendations on prevention of coronary heart disease in clinical practice. *Heart* 1998; **80** (Suppl 2): S1–29.

National Cholesterol Education Program (NCEP) expert panel on detection, evaluation and treatment of high blood cholesterol in adults (adult treatment panel III). Executive summary of the 3rd report. *J Am Med Ass* 2001; **285**: 2486–97.

National Cholesterol Education Programme Guidelines. ℗ www.nhlbi.nih.gov/guidelines/cholesterol/

Test protocols

Insulin tolerance test (insulin stress test)

- **Indication**: suspected ACTH or GH deficiency.
- **Contraindications**: patients with epilepsy, coronary heart disease (check ECG).
- **Children**: use no more than 0.1U/kg. Considerable care should be exercised; the test should only be performed in a centre with expertise.
- **Alternatives**: short synacthen test for hypocortisolism; stimulation tests for growth hormone deficiency e.g. GHRH-arginine test (📖 Hypothalamus/pituitary function, p125).
- **Preparation**: patient fasting overnight. Bed required (although day case procedure). Patient must be accompanied home and may not drive. OMIT morning hydrocortisone or other steroid hormone replacement if patient is taking this and previous day's growth hormone. Physician must be present throughout the test. Requires written consent.
- *Procedure*: early morning outpatient test in fasting patient. In-dwelling venous cannula and constant medical supervision required throughout. Cannula is kept patent by running saline infusion with three-way tap for sampling. Discard initial 2–3mL when each sample is taken. Label all samples clearly with time and patient details. Near-patient testing glucometer required.
1. Take baseline blood for glucose, cortisol and GH. Check IV access working well. Review test with the patient and explain symptoms s/he is likely to experience (see point 5 below).
2. Draw up 25mL of 50% dextrose for immediate administration IF REQUIRED.
3. Give soluble (regular) insulin as an intravenous bolus in a dose of 0.15U/kg after an overnight fast. Consider 0.1U/kg (lower dose) if suspected profound hypocortisolism. ► This appears a very small dose, e.g. typically around 10U. CHECK DOSE CALCULATION CAREFULLY. Usually an insulin syringe is used to draw it up and then transfer it to a 2mL syringe containing saline.
4. Take blood at 15 min intervals (0, 15, 30, 45, 60 min) for glucose, cortisol, and GH.
5. Observe for symptoms and signs of hypoglycaemia. First sign is usually profuse sweating. Patient may then be aware of symptoms such as palpitations, hunger, paraesthesiae. This typically occurs 30–45min into the test. Check near-patient glucose to confirm < 3.5mmol/L. Continue to talk to and reassure patient. If patient becomes very drowsy or unrousable then give 25mL of 50% glucose. This does not invalidate the test as the hypoglycaemic stimulus has already occurred. Continue blood sampling at standard times.
6. If patient has not experienced hypoglycaemia by 45 min and near-patient glucose is > 4mmol/L, give a further intravenous bolus of 0.15 or 0.3U/kg if patient known to be very insulin resistant (e.g. acromegalic). Repeat sampling at 15-min intervals for 60 min after this second bolus.

7. At end of procedure (usually 60 min), give IV 25mL 50% dextrose if patient still has symptoms of hypoglycaemia.
8. Give patient a meal including complex carbohydrate (e.g. sandwiches or lunch) and observe for a minimum of 1 h further before accompanied discharge.

- **Unwanted effects**: severe hypoglycaemia with depressed level of consciousness or convulsion requires immediate termination of test with 25mL of 50% dextrose IV. Repeat if necessary and follow with 5 or 10% dextrose infusion. Continue to collect samples for hormone and glucose measurements.
- **Interpretation**: test is only interpretable if adequate hypoglycaemia is achieved (< 2.2mmol/L). Normal maximal cortisol response > 550nmol/L. Normal GH response > 20mU/L. Impaired responses (if hypoglycaemic stimulus adequate) denote corticotrophin (assuming adrenal glands are normal) or GH deficiency or both. Peak GH response < 10mU/L is sufficient to consider GH replacement; peak GH response < 5mU/L is severe growth hormone deficiency.

Combined arginine-growth hormone releasing hormone (GHRH) test

- **Indication**: GH deficiency. Now preferred to insulin tolerance test.
- **Contraindications**: previous reaction to stimulatory hormones. Administer with caution to patients with severe liver or renal disease.
- **Alternatives**: insulin tolerance test. Other stimulation tests now outdated (e.g. glucagon, exercise). Serum IGF-1 levels give an idea of GH status but are unreliable at low levels.
- **Preparation**: order GHRH and arginine from pharmacy. Omit growth hormone injections for a minumum of 24 h. Patient arrives in the morning after fasting for 10 h (overnight). Water is allowed and patients should take all their routine medication in the morning (but not growth hormone). Informed consent must be obtained and documented. Warn patients about possible side effects of IV GHRH, such as flushing lasting less than 5 min.
- **Procedure**:
  - Weigh patient.
  - Insert in-dwelling iv cannula for blood sampling, administration of bolus GHRH and arginine infusion (keep patent with heparinized saline).
  - Patients should rest throughout the test.
  - Take basal samples for GH at −30 and 0 min.
  - Give GHRH as IV bolus of 1μg/kg body weight at 0 min; at the same time start infusing 30g of 12.5% arginine solution over 30 min, preferably using an infusion pump. (children: 0.5 g/kg as 12.5% solution, to a maximum of 30 g).
  - Take blood samples for GH at 30, 45, 60, 75, 90, 105, and 120 min.
  - Patients are allowed home after a full lunch.
- **Interpretation**: the diagnosis of adult GHD is confirmed if the peak GH concentration is < 20mIU/L.Severe growth hormone deficiency (as defined by NICE) – peak < 9mIU/L.

Note: Conversion factor: μg/L × 3.0 = mIU/L.

Combined anterior pituitary function testing

- **Indication**: assessment for anterior pituitary hypofunction.
- **Contraindications**: previous reaction to stimulatory hormones.
- **Alternatives**: insulin tolerance testing for GH and adrenal axis; metyrapone test for adrenal axis. Other stimulation tests for GH, e.g. GHRH-arginine test.
- **Preparation**: test usually performed in morning for basal sampling.
- **Procedure**: IV cannula inserted. Basal blood samples taken for cortisol, oestradiol (♀) or testosterone (♂), free T4, and IGF-1. Hypothalamic hormones are given sequentially intravenously each as a bolus over around 20s: LHRH 100µg, TRH 200µg and ACTH 250µg. Additionally GHRH (1µg/kg body weight) may be given. (Reduce doses in children.) Samples are drawn at 0, 20, 30, 60, and 120min for LH, FSH, TSH cortisol, and PRL. If GHRH is given, samples are drawn at the same time points for GH.
- **Interpretation**: normal values as follows:
  - *TRH*—suspect secondary hypothyroidism if peak response (at 20 min) <20mU/L (**Note**: low levels also seen in hyperthyroidism—ensure free T4 or total T4 not raised).
  - *ACTH*—peak cortisol response >550nmol/L at 30 or 60 min.
  - *LHRH*—peak LH/FSH response 2–5 × basal value. LH, peak at 20 min, FSH later.
  - *GHRH*—normal GH peak response >15mU/L.

Water deprivation test

- **Indication**: diagnosis of DI, and to distinguish cranial and nephrogenic DI.
- **Contraindications**: none if carefully supervised. For correct interpretation, thyroid and adrenal deficiency should be replaced first. Interpretation in the presence of DM and uraemia can be difficult.
- **Alternatives**: morning urine osmolality of > 600mOsmol excludes significant degrees of DI. No other definitive test for DI.
- **Patient preparation**: usually an outpatient procedure. Correct thyroid and adrenal insufficiency in advance. Renal function and blood glucose should have been checked in advance. Steroid and thyroid hormone replacement should be taken as normal on the day of the test. If the patient is on desmopressin, omit the dose on the evening before the test (or, if not possible, halve this dose). Free fluids, but not to excess, up to 07.30 h on the day of the test. No alcohol on the night before the test or in the morning of the test. Light breakfast, but no tea, coffee, or smoking on the morning of the test. Empty bladder before attending for the test. If urine volume is < 3L/day ('mild cases'), ask patient to have no fluids or food from 18.00 h on the evening before the test ('prolonged water deprivation test').
- **Requirements for test**: accurate weighing scales. Supervision for the whole test (up to 8h). Desmopressin for injection (2μg). Immediate access to serum electrolyte, plasma and urinary osmolality assays. Access to a plasma AVP (ADH) assay desirable.
- **Procedure**: 07.30 h
  1 Weigh patient and calculate 97% of body weight.
  2 Mark this target on the chart.
  3 No food or fluid for next 8 h.
  4 Insert cannula for repeated blood sampling and flush.
- **Procedure**: 08.00 h
  5 Obtain plasma for Na^+ and osmolality, and urine for osmolality.
  6 Then collect urine hourly for volume and osmolality and plasma every 2 h for Na^+ and osmolarity.
  7 Weigh patient before and after passing urine if unobserved.
  8 If patient loses 3% body weight, order urgent plasma osmolality and Na^+.
  9 If plasma osmolality > 300mOsmol (Na^+ > 140mmol/L) stop test, allow patient to drink and give desmopressin (see below).
  10 If plasma osmolality < 300mOsmol, patient may have been fluid overloaded before test and water deprivation can continue.
  11 Stop test at 8 h (16.00 h) and take final recordings of urine and plasma.
  12 Save an aliquot of plasma for vasopressin levels in case of difficulties in test interpretation.
  13 Ideally urine osmolalities will have reached a plateau (< 30mOsmol rise between samples).
  14 Now give 2μg desmopressin IM (or 20μg intranasally) and collect urine samples only for a further 2 h. Allow free fluids at this stage.

- **Interpretation**: normal response: plasma osmolality remains in the range 280–295mmol, urine osmolality rises to > 2× plasma (> 600mOsmol). If urine volumes during water deprivation do not reduce and yet the plasma does not become more concentrated (rising osmolality) and weight does not fall, suspect surreptitious drinking during test. For interpretation of abnormal results see Table 2.3 (p131).

Diagnostic trial of desamino D-arginyl vasopressin

- **Indication**: distinction of partial DI from primary polydipsia.
- **Contraindications**: cardiac failure. Current diuretic use (test uninterpretable). Note that this test may precipitate severe hyponatraemia in primary polydipsia and should be preformed in an in-patient unit with clinical and biochemical regular review.
- **Preparation**: admission to assessment unit. First line tests for polydipsia/polyuria should have been performed (📖 Polydipsia & polyuria: diabetes insipidus, p129).
- **Procedure**:
  1 24 h urine volume, morning urine osmolality, weight, fluid intake (as far as possible), serum osmolality, Na^+, urea, and creatinine should all be performed daily and the results reviewed the same day.
  2 Subjects should have access to fluid *ad libitum*, but should be reminded that they should only drink if they are thirsty.
  3 After an initial 24 h period of observation, desmopressin (DDAVP) is administered at a dose of 2µg bd SC for 3 days.
  4 Stop test if serum Na^+ falls to <130mmol/L.
- **Interpretation**: reduction in urine volume to < 2L/day, in urine osmolality to > 600mOsmol/L without fall in serum Na^+ to < 140mmol/L suggests central DI. Reduction in urine volume with no increase in urine osmolality > 600mOsmol/L and without a fall in serum Na^+ suggests partial nephrogenic DI. Limited reduction in urine volume, with some increase in urine osmolarity, but a fall in serum Na^+ suggests primary polydipsia.

Low dose dexamethasone suppression test

- **Indication**: to distinguish hypercortisolism from normality. The dexamethasone suppressed CRH test is believed to have less false positives in cases of alcoholic or depressive pseudo—Cushing's syndrome.
- **Patient preparation**: patients should not be on oral steroids or drugs that increase steroid metabolism.
- **Overnight dexamethasone suppression test**: 1mg dexamethasone is taken po at midnight. Serum sample for cortisol is taken the following morning between 08.00 and 09.00 h.
- **Interpretation**: serum cortisol should suppress to < 140nmol/L (usually <50nmol/L). Values 140–175nmol/L are equivocal and suggest a 2-day test should be performed. 10–15% false +ve rate.
- 2-day low dose dexamethasone suppression test (preferred)
- Dexamethasone 0.5mg is given po every 6 h for 8 doses (2 days) starting in the early morning. Ideally tablets are taken strictly at 6-hourly intervals (06.00, 12.00, 18.00, 00.00 h), which may necessitate an in-patient stay. A 24 h collection for UFC is taken on the second day of the test and serum cortisol is measured at 06.00 h on the 3rd day, 6 h after the last dose. IV administration of dexamethasone can be used if there are concerns over absorption or compliance.
- **Interpretation**: serum cortisol 6 h after the last dose should be < 140nmol/L, usually < 50nmol/L. Urinary free cortisol on the second day should be < 70nmol/L, normally < 30nmol/L. The 2-day test strictly performed has less false +ves than the overnight test.
- **Dexamethasone suppressed CRH test**: dexamethasone 0.5mg is given po every 6 h for 9 doses (2 days), but starting at midnight and ending at 06.00 h. Tablets are taken strictly at 6-h intervals (00.00, 06.00, 12.00, 18.00 h), which may necessitate an in-patient stay. Last dose is taken at 06.00 h and an injection of CRH (100µg IV or 1µg/kg) |is given at 08.00 h. A blood sample for cortisol is taken at 08.15 h (i.e. 15 min later).
- **Interpretation**: serum cortisol level should be < 38nmol/L (normal).

Further reading

Yanovski JA, Cutler GB, Chrousos G, et al. Corticotrophin-releasing hormone stimulation following low-dose dexamethasone administration: a new test to distinguish Cushing's syndrome from pseudo-Cushing's states. J Am Med Ass 1993; **269**, 2232–8.

High dose dexamethasone suppression test

- **Indication**: to distinguish between patients with Cushing's disease (ACTH-secreting pituitary tumour) and ectopic ACTH production in patients with established hypercortisolism.
- **Patient preparation**: as low dose test except that the test can be performed immediately following the 2-day low dose test.
- **Procedure**:
  1 2 × 24 h UFC collections are made to calculate the mean basal 24 h UFC.
  2 Baseline serum cortisol measurement is also taken before the first dexamethasone dose, ideally at 06.00 h. If the low dose test is performed first, the baseline values (urine and blood) must be taken prior to the low dose test (i.e. any doses of dexamethasone).
  3 Dexamethasone 2mg is given po every 6 h for 8 doses (2 days) starting in the early morning. Ideally tablets are taken strictly at 6-h intervals (06.00, 12.00, 18.00, 00.00 h), which may necessitate an in-patient stay.
  4 A 24h urine collection for UFC (final) is taken on day 2 and a blood sample is taken for (final) cortisol 6h after the last dexamethasone dose (0600h on day 3). Creatinine excretion should be measured and compared between urine samples to confirm true 24h collections.
- **Interpretation**: % suppression of basal cortisol is calculated as:

  (basal cortisol − final cortisol)/basal cortisol × 100

The same calculation is made for basal and day 2 UFC. 50% suppression is suggestive of pituitary-dependent disease. 90% suppression increases the likelihood (strict criteria). Thymic carcinoids and phaeochromocytomas releasing ACTH are source of false positives.

Short Synacthen® test

- **Indication**: suspected adrenal insufficiency. Will not detect recent-onset 2° adrenal insufficiency.
- **Contraindication**: asthma/allergy to ACTH—risk of allergic reaction (can be performed with careful medication supervision of patient).
- **Preparation**: patient must not take hydrocortisone on the morning of the test as this will be detected in the cortisol assay. The test can be performed on low dose dexamethasone, but the morning dose should be omitted until after the test. May have some value in patients on higher dose steroid therapy to indicate the degree of suppression of adrenocortical function.
- **Procedure**: 250µg of synthetic ACTH (Synacthen®) given IM or IV. Blood taken at times 0, 30, and 60 min for serum cortisol.
- **Low dose test**: the test can be performed with a very low dose of ACTH (e.g. 1µg). This may detect more subtle degrees of hypoadrenalism but the clinical significance of these findings remains uncertain.
- **Interpretation**: a value at any time > 550nmol/L makes the diagnosis very unlikely.

Long (depot) ACTH test

- **Indication**: distinguishing 1° and 2° adrenal failure.
- **Patient preparation**: a short synacthen test should be performed prior to the test to diagnose adrenal failure. If patient is on steroid replacement, change to dexamethasone 0.5mg/day.
- **Procedure**: blood is taken at 09.00 h for basal cortisol. 1mg of depot synthetic ACTH (Synacthen®) is then given IM on 2 consecutive days and blood collected 5 h after each dose (14.00 h). A final cortisol sample is taken at 09.00 h on the 3rd day.
- **Interpretation**: serum cortisol should rise to > 1000nmol/L on the last day and, if adrenal failure previously indicated by a short synacthen test, such a rise indicates secondary adrenal failure (pituitary/hypothalamic cause incl. suppressive drugs).

Haematology

Full blood count

Called *complete blood count* (CBC) in the USA.

Before the advent of modern haematology blood analysers the blood count consisted of a haemoglobin (Hb) concentration (estimated using a manual colorimetric technique), a white cell count and manual platelet count. Other parameters such as mean cell volume (MCV) had to be mathematically calculated (*derived*) using the measured variables Hb, red cell count (RCC) and packed cell volume (PCV).

Modern analysers use a variety of methods to provide a huge range of full blood count (FBC) variables including electronic impedance, laser light scatter, light absorbance and staining characteristics. The resultant FBC provides measured variables such as Hb, PCV and RCC along with derived (mathematically) MCV, mean cell haemoglobin (MCH), and mean corpuscular Hb concentration (MCHC). These machines also provide automated platelet counts and a 5-part differential white blood count (WBC).

Sample: Peripheral blood ethylenediamine tetra-acetic acid (EDTA); the sample should be analysed in the laboratory within 4h, if possible.

Main parameters measured
- Hb concentration.
- RCC.
- MCV.
- MCH.
- MCHC.
- Haematocrit (Hct) or packed cell volume (PCV).
- Red cell distribution width (RDW).
- White cell count.
- WBC differential.
- Platelet count.

Some machines are even more sophisticated and will measure *reticulocyte counts* in addition to determination of reticulocyte Hb and MCV.

Role of the full blood count

Why ask for a full blood count (FBC)? How will this aid the diagnosis or management of the patient? The FBC assesses several different parameters and can provide a great deal of information. The red cell variables will determine whether or not the patient is anaemic. If anaemia is present the MCV is likely to provide clues as to the cause of the anaemia. The white cells are often raised in infection—neutrophilia in bacterial infections and lymphocytosis in viral (but not always so). Platelets (size or number) may be abnormal either as a direct effect of underlying blood disease or may simply reflect the presence of some other underlying pathology. Most of us take a somewhat cursory glance at the FBC when the report arrives on the ward or in clinic, but a more detailed look may reveal a great deal more!

Further reading
℗ http://www.bbc.co.uk/health/talking/tests/blood_full_blood_count.shtml
℗ http://www.rcpa.edu.au/pathman/full_blo.htm

Red cell parameters

Haemoglobin concentration
Units: g/dL or g/L (Europe uses SI units; the USA uses g/dL or grams%).

Defines anaemia (Hb < lower limit of normal adjusted for age and sex). Values differ between ♂ and ♀ since androgens drive RBC production and, hence, adult ♂ has higher Hb, PCV, and RCC than adult ♀.

Red cell count
Unit: $\times 10^{12}/L$.

Useful in the diagnosis of polycythaemic disorders (↑ production of microcytic, hypochromic erythrocytes) and thalassaemias.

Causes of a low red cell count include
- Hypoproliferative anaemias, e.g. iron, vitamin B_{12}, and folate deficiencies.
- Aplasias, e.g. idiopathic or drug-induced (don't forget chemotherapy).
- Parvovirus B_{19} infection-induced red cell aplasia resulting in transient marked anaemia.

Causes of high red cell count
- Polycythemia rubra vera (PRV).
- Thalassaemia.

Mean cell volume
Unit: Femtolitre (fL), $10^{-15}L$.

Provided as part of the derived variables or can be calculated if you know the PCV and RCC [PCV ÷ RCC, e.g. if PCV 0.45 and RCC $5 \times 10^{12}/L$ then mean cell volume (MCV) is 90fL].

This index provides a useful starting point for the evaluation of anaemia (see Table 3.1).

Table 3.1 MCV index

MCV ↓	MCV normal	MCV ↑
Iron deficiency	Blood loss	B_{12} or folate deficiency
β thalassaemia trait	Myelodysplasia	Myelodysplasia
Sideroblastic anaemia	Anaemia of chronic disease	

Mean cell haemoglobin
Unit: pg.
- **High** (for range see 📖 Normal ranges, p231): macrocytosis.
- **Low**: microcytosis, e.g. iron deficiency anaemia.

Mean cell haemoglobin concentration
Unit: g/dL or g/L.

Of value in evaluation of microcytic anaemias.

High
- Severe prolonged dehydration.
- Hereditary spherocytosis.
- Cold agglutinin disease.
- Low
- Iron deficiency anaemia.
- Thalassaemia.

Haematocrit or packed cell volume
These are not entirely synonymous terms (but they are, more-or-less). If blood is placed in a microcapillary tube and centrifuged the red cells are spun down to the bottom, leaving the plasma above. The RBCs will occupy about 40% of the blood in the tube—the blood will have a PCV of 0.4 (or 40%). The Hct is similar, but derived, using automated blood counters.

PCV unit: L/L (although the units are seldom cited on reports).
- **High PCV**: polycythaemia (any cause).
- **Low PCV**: anaemia (any cause).

Red cell distribution width
Measures the *range* of red cell size in a sample of blood, providing information about the degree of red cell anisocytosis, i.e. how much variation there is between the size of the red cells. Of value in some anaemias, e.g.:
- ↓ MCV with normal RDW suggests β thalassaemia trait.
- ↓ MCV with high RDW suggests iron deficiency.

(Probably noticed more by haematology staff than those in general medicine!)

White cells

The automated differential white cell count is provided as part of the FBC. The RBCs in the sample are lysed before WBCs are counted. A typical FBC will show the *total* WBC and the *5-part differential white cell count*, broken down into the 5 main white cell subtypes in peripheral blood which include:

- Neutrophils.
- Lymphocytes.
- Monocytes.
- Eosinophils.
- Basophils.

The printed FBC usually shows the % of each type of white cell, but unless the absolute WBC (as $\times 10^9$/L) is known this % count is of little value.

▶ As a general rule ignore the % count—you cannot detect abnormalities such as neutropenia unless you have the absolute values.

Abnormalities of the WBC, e.g. neutrophilia, neutropenia, etc., are discussed in 📖 *OHCM* 8e, p324.

Platelet count

Unit: $\times 10^9$/L.

Normal: 150–400 $\times 10^9$/L.

Platelets (*thrombocytes* in the USA) are the smallest cells in peripheral blood. Traditional counting methods with microscope and counting chamber have now been replaced by automated counting with haematology analysers.

Platelet distribution width

This is analogous to the RDW and provides information about the range of platelet size in a blood sample.

- The platelet distribution width (PDW) will be high if there are giant platelets in the presence of normal sized platelets, e.g. essential thrombocythaemia (one of the myeloproliferative disorders).
- The PDW will be normal in a reactive thrombocytosis (where the platelet count is increased, but they are all of normal size).

Platelet clumping

This is an *in vitro* artefact in some individuals. Platelets clump in EDTA and the blood analyser will report spurious thrombocytopenia. The actual *in vivo* count is normal and the platelets function normally. Taking the blood into citrate or heparin will show the patient's platelet count to be normal. The presence of even a small blood clot in an EDTA sample may also reduce the platelet count (the haematology technical staff will usually check to see whether the sample contains a small clot before sending out the report).

Peripheral blood film

Examining a stained peripheral blood smear under the microscope allows the examination of red cells, white cells, and platelets. In addition, the blood film will help detect parasites (e.g. malaria, trypanosomes) or abnormal cells in the blood.

When to request a blood film examination

The haematology laboratory will usually examine a peripheral blood film if the patient's indices are abnormal (unless there has been no major change from previous FBCs). If you suspect an underlying blood disorder you should request a film. *Note*: the laboratory staff may not make a film if the indices are completely normal.

Method

A finger prick blood sample may be spread onto a glass slide (the phlebotomists may do this for you), air-dried, fixed, and stained. Alternatively, a drop of EDTA blood may be treated in the same manner (the haematology laboratory staff will make the film). *Beware*: old EDTA samples produce strange artefacts such as extreme red cell crenation—if a film is required it should be made from a fresh blood sample.

Sample: EDTA (as fresh as possible).

Information from the blood film

Red cells
- Size.
- Shape (e.g. sickling).
- Membrane changes (e.g. oxidative membrane damage).
- Colour.
- Basophilic stippling.
- Inclusions, e.g. Howell–Jolly bodies, malarial parasites, HbC crystals, etc.

White cells
- Number.
- Morphology.
- Abnormalities, such as toxic granulation, dysplastic changes.
- Presence of abnormal cells, e.g. leukaemic blasts or lymphoma cells.

Platelets
- Number.
- Size.
- Shape.

Other features on the film
- Parasites.
- Red cell rouleaux (stacking effect, seen, e.g. when erythrocyte sedimentation rate (ESR) is ↑).
- Nucleated red cells.
- Plasma cells.
- Occasionally see circulating carcinoma cells.

📖 *OHCM* 8e, p322.

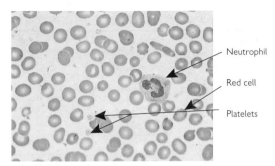

Neutrophil

Red cell

Platelets

Fig. 3.1 Normal peripheral blood film showing a neutrophil with its typical lobulated nucleus, numerous red cells, and a few platelets.

Red cell morphology

In health the normal RBC is a pink biconcave disc-shaped cell, and most red cells are roughly the same size, shape, and colour. They should be roughly the size of a small lymphocyte nucleus. Many diseases and deficiency disorders alter the RBC appearance by either reducing its Hb content, or altering the membrane such that characteristic morphological abnormalities are produced. Examples include target cells, sickle cells, bite cells, burr cells and many others (see Table 3.2). Most of the morphological features are not absolutely specific for one particular disorder, but rather they suggest a range of conditions that may be associated with the red blood cell (RBC) feature (Fig. 3.2). This should prompt you to look for conditions which might account for the abnormality.

▶Pay attention to the peripheral blood film comment (inserted on the report by the haematology laboratory staff, or automated blood counter)—it should help you decide which tests to carry out next. Conversely, cryptic laboratory comments like 'anisopoikilocytosis noted' do not help the clinician much. (**Note**: aniso = unequal, poikilo = varied.)

Table 3.2 Peripheral blood film in anaemias

Microcytic RBCs	Fe deficiency, thalassaemia trait, & syndromes, congenital sideroblastic anaemia, ACD (if longstanding)
Macrocytic RBCs	Alcohol/liver disease (round macrocytes), MDS, pregnancy and newborn, compensated haemolysis, B_{12}, or folate def., hydroxyurea and antimetabolites (oval macrocytes), acquired sideroblastic anaemia, hypothyroidism, chronic respiratory failure, aplastic anaemia
Dimorphic RBCs	Two populations, e.g. Fe deficiency responding to iron, mixed Fe and B_{12}/folate deficiency, sideroblastic anaemia, post-red cell transfusion
Hypochromic RBCs	Reduced Hb synthesis, e.g. iron deficiency, thalassaemia, sideroblastic anaemia
Polychromatic RBCs	Blood loss or haematinic treatment, haemolysis, marrow infiltration
Spherocytes	Hereditary spherocytosis, haemolysis, e.g. warm AIHA, delayed transfusion reaction, ABO, HDN, DIC, and MAHA, post-splenectomy
Pencil/rod cells	Fe deficiency anaemia, thalassaemia trait, & syndromes, PK deficiency
Elliptocytes	Hereditary elliptocytosis, MPD, and MDS
Fragmented RBCs	MAHA, DIC, renal failure, HUS, TTP
Teardrop RBCs	Myelofibrosis, metastatic marrow infiltration, MDS
Sickle cells	Sickle cell anaemia, other sickle syndromes (*not* sickle trait)
Target cells	Liver disease, Fe deficiency, thalassaemia, HbC syndromes
Crenated RBCs	Usually storage or EDTA artefact. Genuine RBC crenation may be seen post-splenectomy and in renal failure (→ burr cells)
Burr cells	Renal failure
Acanthocytes	Hereditary acanthocytosis, a-β-lipoproteinaemia, McLeod red cell phenotype, PK deficiency, chronic liver disease (esp. Zieve's syndrome)
Bite cells	G6PD deficiency, oxidative haemolysis
Basophilic stippling	Megaloblastic anaemia, lead poisoning, MDS, liver disease, haemoglobinopathies, e.g. thalassaemia
Rouleaux	Chronic inflammation, paraproteinaemia, myeloma
↑ Reticulocytes	Bleeding, haemolysis, marrow infiltration, severe hypoxia, response to haematinic therapy
Heinz bodies	Not seen in normals (removed by spleen), small numbers seen post-splenectomy, oxidant drugs, G6PD deficiency, sulphonamides, unstable Hb (Hb Zurich, Köln)

Table 3.2 (continued)

Howell–Jolly bodies	Composed of DNA, removed by the spleen, seen in dyserythropoietic states, e.g. B$_{12}$ deficiency, MDS, post-splenectomy, hyposplenism
H bodies	HbH inclusions, denatured HbH (β_4 tetramer), stain with methylene blue, seen in HbH disease (– ––/–α), less prominent in α thalassaemia trait, not present in normal subjects
Hyposplenic film	Howell–Jolly bodies, target cells, occasional nucleated RBCs, lymphocytosis, macrocytosis, acanthocytes. Infectious mononucleosis, any viral infection, toxoplasmosis, drug reactions

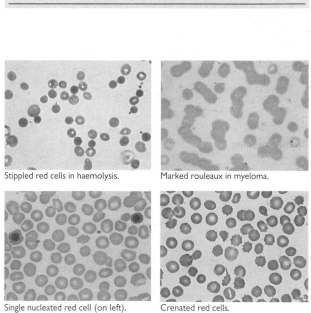

Stippled red cells in haemolysis.

Marked rouleaux in myeloma.

Single nucleated red cell (on left).

Crenated red cells.

Fig. 3.2 Red cell abnormalities in various disease states.

Parasites on the blood film & marrow

Blood film

Although there are now highly sensitive monoclonal antibody kits for the diagnosis of diseases, such as malaria, a well-stained blood film can often make the diagnosis more easily and more cheaply. Blood films are useful for confirming a diagnosis of:

- Malaria.
- Trypanosomiasis.
- Microfilaria.

Parasites in bone marrow

Some diseases, such as Leishmaniasis' require bone marrow aspiration and staining (in fact there are many infections that can be diagnosed using a bone marrow):

- *Leishmania donovani.*
- *Tuberculosis.*
- *Tropheryma whippelii* (Whipple's disease).
- *Cryptococcus neoformans.*
- *Penicillium.*
- *Histoplasma capsulatum.*
- *Candida albicans.*
- *Toxoplasma gondii.*

See Fig. 3.3 for examples.

Further reading

♪ http://health.allrefer.com/health/bone-marrow-transplant-formed-elements-of-blood.html
♪ http://www.nlm.nih.gov/medlineplus/ency/article/003642.htm
♪ http://www.bcshguidelines.com/pdf/CLH165.pdf

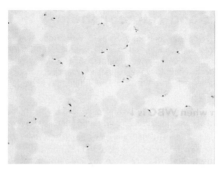

Falciparum malaria (blood film)

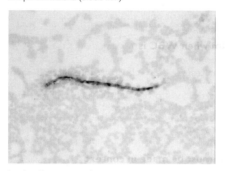

Loa loa (bone marrow)

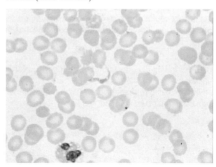

Trypanosome (blood film)

Fig. 3.3 Parasites such as malaria, loa loa, and trypanosomes may be seen on a stained blood film.

White blood cell morphology

In much the same way as RBC morphology provides clues about underlying disease, so too does microscopical examination of stained peripheral blood WBCs. Modern counters enumerate WBCs and our greater reliance on modern technology means that visual inspection of blood films is becoming a dying art. A well-stained blood film may provide the diagnosis much more cheaply.

Blood film when WBC is ↓

- Sometimes difficult to determine diagnosis since so few WBCs.
- May suggest B_{12} or folate deficiency (are the RBCs normal or large?).
- **Aplastic anaemia**: are the platelets and Hb normal?
- **Underlying leukaemia**: are there any leukaemic blasts* present?
- **Overwhelming infection**: may see toxic granulation (large dark granules in the cytoplasm—not diagnostic, but suggestive).
- **May be immune or post-viral**: atypical lymphocytes may be seen; other indices usually normal.

Blood film when WBC is ↑

What cell predominates?

- **Lymphocytes**: suggests viral, chronic lymphocytic/lymphatic leukaemia (CLL), acute leukaemia (lymphoblastic).
- **Granulocytic?** (neutrophils, eosinophils, basophils)—may be reactive or chronic myeloid leukaemia (CML).
- **Abnormal looking WBC?** Look for Auer rods (≡ acute myeloid leukaemia (AML)), smear cells (CLL), bilobed neutrophils (pseudo-Pelger cells seen in myelodysplastic syndrome (MDS)).

Diagnosis must be made in context

How old is the patient?

- Viral illnesses often produce bizarre films in children, but beware of complacency (acute leukaemia may be the cause).
- MDS, and malignancies like CLL and CML are diseases of older individuals.

Is the patient well?

- May be worth repeating FBC and film to see if abnormalities have resolved.
- If patient unwell or has lymphadenopathy or hepatosplenomegaly then underlying disease must be excluded.

---

* A blast is a primitive cell seen in the marrow in large numbers in leukaemia. We all have some blasts in our marrows, but these should be < 5% of the total nucleated bone marrow cells in health.

Table 3.3 Some WBC abnormalities seen on FBC reports

Atypical lymphocytes	Infectious mononucleosis, any viral infection, toxoplasmosis, drug reactions
Auer rods	Seen in myeloblasts; pathognomonic of AML Prominent in AML M3 subtype (acute promyelocytic leukaemia)
Pelger–Huët anomaly	Bilobed neutrophils. May be hereditary (neutrophils are functionally normal) or acquired, e.g. MDS (pseudo-Pelger cells)
Left shifted	Immature WBCs seen in peripheral blood. Seen in severe infections, inflammatory disorders, DKA, marrow 'stress', MPD, CML
Right shifted	Hypermature WBCs seen in, e.g. megaloblastic anaemia and iron deficiency
Toxic granulation	Coarse granules in neutrophils. Seen in severe infection, post-operatively and inflammatory disorders
Smear cells	Lymphocytes in which the cell membrane has ruptured when making the blood film—there are no smear cells *in vivo*! Seen in CLL

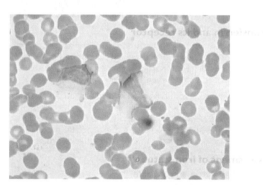

Fig. 3.4 Blood film: atypical white blood cells (this was from a patient with glandular fever, but these cells may be seen in any viral illness).

Further reading

Atlas of Haematology slides. 🔗 http://pathy.med.nagoya-u.ac.jp/atlas/doc/atlas.html

Assessment of iron status

The anaemia of iron deficiency is caused by defective synthesis of Hb resulting in red cells that are smaller than normal (microcytic) and contain reduced amounts of Hb (*hypochromic*). The diagnosis of iron deficiency anaemia is generally straightforward, but it may be confused with anaemia of chronic disease (ACD) or other hypochromic anaemias (see Table 3.4, Fig. 3.6).

Iron plays a pivotal role in many metabolic processes and the average adult contains between 3 and 5g of iron, of which two-thirds is present in the O_2-carrying molecule, Hb. Somewhat surprisingly, there is no specific excretion mechanism in humans. Iron balance is controlled at the level of gut absorption, and relies on two iron-sequestering proteins, *transferrin* (iron transport and recycling of iron) and *ferritin* (safeguards iron entry into the body, and maintains surplus iron in a safe and readily accessible form).

Ferritin

This is the 1° iron-storage protein consisting of 24 apoferritin subunits forming a hollow sphere (each can hold up to 4500 Fe atoms).

Haemosiderin

Haemosiderin, located predominantly in macrophages, is a water-soluble protein–iron complex with an amorphous structure.

Transferrin and its receptor

Transferrin contains only 4mg iron and is the principal iron transport protein with more than 30mg iron transported round the body daily. Synthesis of transferrin is inversely proportional to the body iron stores, with increased transferrin concentration when iron stores are reduced.

The transferrin receptor (TfR) is a disulphide-linked dimer composed of two identical 85kDa subunits. The serum TfR (sTfR) concentration is elevated in iron deficiency. However, sTfR may also increase in any condition in which there is increased erythropoiesis, e.g. haemolytic anaemias, thalassaemia, polycythaemia vera, and other myeloproliferative disorders.

Assessment of iron status

Several parameters are available
- Haemoglobin concentration.
- Serum ferritin.
- Serum iron and transferrin (as total iron binding capacity, TIBC).
- % hypochromic cells in peripheral blood.
- Red cell protoporphyrin assay (not widely available).
- Bone marrow aspirate (stained for iron)—the 'gold standard'.
- Soluble transferrin receptor assay (STfR).

Remember, iron deficiency is not an 'all-or-nothing' phenomenon. In progressive deficiency there is a gradual loss of iron with subtle alterations of iron-related parameters during which the red cells may look entirely normal. In the initial stages of developing iron deficiency macrophages become depleted of iron and the serum ferritin ↓ to the lower end of the normal range; during this 'latency' period the Hb is normal. As the deficiency progresses plasma iron levels ↓ and TIBC ↑. Free RBC protoporphyrin levels ↑ as it accumulates, and eventually hypochromic RBCs appear in the peripheral blood. At this stage a full blood count will usually show ↓ Hb, MCV, MCH and MCHC, and the peripheral blood film will show microcytic hypochromic red cells.

Confirmation of simple iron deficiency anaemia (Fig. 3.5)

● Hb ↓.
● Serum ferritin will be ↓.

> ►**Beware**: serum ferritin is an acute phase protein and may be normal or even ↑ in inflammatory, malignant or liver disease. During the inflammatory response the iron/TIBC are unlikely to be of any value (iron ↓ and TIBC will be ↓). If an inflammatory process is suspected, an alternative test is required, e.g. STfR, which is not affected by inflammatory disorders.

● Serum iron ↓ and TIBC ↑ (generally unhelpful and little used today).
● STfR ↑.
● MCV ↓.
● MCH & MCHC ↓.
● Microcytic & hypochromic RBCs on blood film.
● Absent marrow iron.

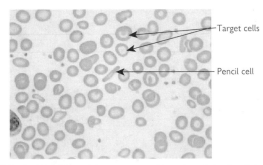

Target cells

Pencil cell

Fig. 3.5 Blood film of iron deficiency anaemia. Note the variation in cell size and shape.

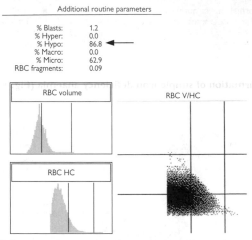

Additional routine parameters

% Blasts:	1.2
% Hyper:	0.0
% Hypo:	86.8 ←
% Macro:	0.0
% Micro:	62.9
RBC fragments:	0.09

RBC volume

RBC HC

RBC V/HC

Fig. 3.6 The % hypochromic red cells (provided by some automated counters) helps in the diagnosis of iron deficiency. Notice that the RBC volume and haemoglobin content (HC) are both shifted to the LEFT (=small pale red cells).

Table 3.4 Hypochromic anaemias—may be confused with iron deficiency

Disorder	Example
Disorders of Fe metabolism	Iron deficiency anaemia • Blood loss • Reduced iron intake • Impaired iron transport
Anaemia of chronic disorders	Chronic inflammatory diseases Malignant disease

Disorders of haem synthesis	Sideroblastic anaemias
	• Hereditary
	• Idiopathic
	• Secondary
	  • Drugs
	  • Alcohol
	  • Lead poisoning

Globin synthesis disorders	Thalassaemias • β-thalassaemia • α-thalassaemia

📖 *OHCM* 8e, p322.

Further reading

Provan D, Weatherall D. Acquired anaemias and polycythaemia. *Lancet* 2000; **355**: 1260–8.
ℛ http://www.ironpanel.org.au/AIS/AISdocs/adultdocs/Acontents.html
ℛ http://www.irondisorders.org/disorders/ida/

Assessment of vitamin B_{12} & folate status

Measurement of the serum B_{12} and red cell folate levels is necessary in the investigation of macrocytic anaemia and certain other situations (see below). Serum folate levels are an unreliable measurement of body stores of folate—the red cell folate level is probably more meaningful.

B_{12} unit: ng/L.

Serum & red cell folate units: µg/L.

Sample: Clotted blood sample (serum B_{12} and folate) and peripheral blood EDTA (red cell folate).

Deficiency of either vitamin leads to megaloblastic anaemia where there is disruption of cell division in all actively dividing cells (includes the bone marrow and gut). In the marrow there is nuclear:cytoplasmic asynchrony, where the nuclei are immature despite a mature well-haemoglobinized cytoplasm. In the peripheral blood there may be anaemia, often with pancytopenia; the red cells show oval macrocytic changes with basophilic stippling and, occasionally, nucleated red cells. Neutrophils typically become hypersegmented (they have > 5 lobes).

Until recently, B_{12} and folate assays were tedious microbiological assays, but these have now been replaced by automated techniques using radio-isotopic methods, which allow large numbers of samples to be batched and tested fairly cheaply.

Deficiencies of B_{12} or folate do not always cause macrocytic anaemia

In the past, deficiency of either B_{12} or folate was synonymous with macrocytic anaemia, but deficiency of either vitamin may present without anaemia or macrocytosis—*remember*, these are *late* features of the disease. However, in most cases of deficiency the marrow will show characteristic megaloblastic change (nuclear asynchrony with giant metamyelocytes). ▶ Deficiency of B_{12} may cause neurological problems in the absence of anaemia.

Whom should you test?

- Patients with GIT disease, glossitis, abnormalities of taste, previous surgery, or radiotherapy to stomach or small bowel.
- Neurological disease, e.g. peripheral neuropathy, demyelination.
- Psychiatric disturbance, e.g. confusion, dementia.
- Malnutrition, e.g. growth impairment in children; vegans.
- Alcohol abuse.
- Autoimmune disease of thyroid, parathyroid, or adrenals.
- Patients with family history of pernicious anaemia.
- Others, e.g. drugs that interfere with vitamin absorption or metabolism such as nitrous oxide, phenytoin, etc.

Look for blood film abnormalities

▶ B_{12} & folate deficiencies produce similar clinical and laboratory features:
- Oval macrocytes.
- Hypersegmented neutrophils (also seen in renal failure, iron deficiency, and MDS).

See Fig. 3.7.

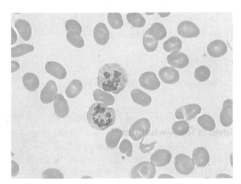

Fig. 3.7 Blood film of megaloblastic anaemia. There are large oval macrocytes and two hypersegmented neutrophils (the nucleus has > 5 lobes).

Which test next?

Make sure you have the following
- FBC.
- Blood film.
- Serum B_{12} level.
- Serum and red cell folate level.
- Intrinsic factor antibodies (IFA), +ve in 50–75% patients with pernicious anaemia (PA).
- Consider bone marrow (helps exclude MDS, myeloma, and other pathologies that give rise to macrocytic anaemia, but seldom performed today since it is easy to get a B_{12} and folate result back quickly).

Interpretation of results: vitamin B_{12}

Normal ranges are based on 2 standard deviations either side of the mean, so there will be 'normal' people who have 'abnormal' B_{12} (or folate) levels.
- B_{12} < normal
  - Deficiency.
  - Altered metabolism.
  - 'Normal'.

The *lowest levels are seen in those most deficient*. What matters is whether there is *tissue deficiency* (leads to marrow and neurological changes).

Mild ↓ in B₁₂ level?

Difficult, but common! Probably worth repeating the test, and reviewing the patient and other results. If no evidence of tissue deficiency, can probably observe the patient. If there is evidence of tissue deficiency then the patient will require treatment.

Detecting tissue deficiency

The most reliable method is probably the measurement of serum homocysteine (accumulates in vitamin B_{12} and folate deficiency).

Beware B₁₂ not associated with tissue deficiency

- Folate deficiency.
- Pregnancy.
- Myeloma.
- Transcobalamin I deficiency (very rare).

Folate

↓ Level seen in hospitalized patients due to negative folate balance.

The B₁₂ level is low—what next?

Available tests for the cause of B₁₂ deficiency include

- Parietal cell (+ve in serum of 90% patients with PA, but also found in other disorders and 15% of the normal elderly) and intrinsic factor antibodies (IFA better—if +ve confirms diagnosis of PA).
- Schilling test (urinary excretion method, where addition of IF restores B_{12} absorption in PA, but not in intestinal, e.g. ileal, disease) seldom performed now due to lack of required radioisotope, or
- Whole body B_{12} counting.
- Endoscopy with duodenal biopsy.
- Other gastroenterology tests for malabsorption (📖 Gastroenterology, p463).

The folate level is low—what next?

- Check dietary history.
- Endoscopy with duodenal biopsy.
- Other gastroenterology tests for malabsorption (📖 Gastroenterology, p463).

📖 *OHCM* 8e, p326.

Further reading

Provan D, Weatherall D. (2000) Acquired anaemias and polycythaemia. *Lancet* **355**, 1260–1268.
🔗 http://www.hlth.gov.bc.ca/msp/protoguides/gps/b12.pdf
🔗 http://www.med.utah.edu/healthinfo/adult/Hemat/folate.htm

Erythrocyte sedimentation rate

This simple, but very useful qualitative test measures how fast a patient's red cells fall through a column of blood. It is a sensitive, but non-specific index of plasma protein changes hat result from inflammation or tissue damage. The ESR is affected by haematocrit variations, red cell abnormalities (e.g. poikilocytosis, sickle cells) and delay in analysis, and is therefore less reliable than measurement of the plasma viscosity. The ESR is affected by age, sex, menstrual cycle, pregnancy, and drugs (e.g. oral contraceptive pill (OCP), steroids).

The ESR is widely used in clinical medicine and, despite attempts (by haematology departments) to replace the ESR with plasma viscosity, the ESR has remained in use, and appears to retain a valuable place in the armoury of disease diagnosis and monitoring.

Sample: Peripheral blood EDTA; the sample should be analysed in the laboratory within 4 h.

Table 3.5 Normal range (upper limits)

Age	Men	Women
17–50 years	10mm/h	12mm/h
51–60	12	19
>60	14	20

Many factors that influence the ESR, causing a high or low result:
- **High ESR (significant*—look for a cause)**:
  - Any inflammatory disorder, e.g. infection, rheumatoid, TB.
  - Myocardial infarction (the ESR ↑ as an early response).
  - Anaemia.
- **Low ESR (rarely important, but useful for exams)**:
  - Polycythaemia.
  - Hypofibrinogenaemia.
  - Congestive cardiac failure (CCF).
  - Poikilocytosis.
  - Spherocytosis.
  - Sickled cells.

▶▶ A normal ESR does not exclude organic disease.

📖 *OHCM* 8e, p366.

Further reading

Harris GJ. Plasma viscometry and ESR in the elderly. *Med Lab Technol* 1972; **29**: 405–10.
Lewis SM. Erythrocyte sedimentation rate and plasma viscosity. *Ass Clin Pathol Broadsheet* 1982; **94**: 1–6.
🔗 http://www.aafp.org/afp/991001ap/1443.html

---

* Depends exactly *how high*. An ESR of 30 probably means little but if > 100 is *highly significant* and indicates something seriously wrong.

Plasma viscosity

This test is a sensitive, but non-specific index of plasma protein changes, which result from inflammation or tissue damage. Provides much the same information as the ESR. The ESR and PV tend to rise in parallel but the PV is *unaffected* by haematocrit variations (e.g. severe anaemia or polycythaemia) and delay in analysis up to 24h, and is therefore more reliable than the ESR. It is not affected by sex but is affected by age, exercise and pregnancy. It is constant in health and shows no diurnal variation. There is a suggestion that the plasma volume (PV) may be a more sensitive indicator of disease severity than the ESR.

Sample: Peripheral blood EDTA. The sample is centrifuged and the plasma removed.

Normal range: 1.50–1.72CP (or MPA/s at 25°C).

High and low plasma viscosity

High PV generally signifies some underlying pathology, e.g. inflammatory states, paraproteinaemias, such as MGUS or myeloma; low PV can be ignored.

Note: Despite the advantages outlined the PV has not been adopted by all medical staff (who still prefer the ESR as a measure of inflammation). The PV is better for monitoring hyperviscosity syndromes, e.g. Waldenström's macroglobulinaemia. The fact that both tests are still used shows that there is a role for both.

📖 *OHCM* 8e, p366.

Further reading

Cooke BM, Stuart J. Automated measurement of plasma viscosity by capillary viscometer. *J Clin Pathol* 1988; **41**: 1213–16.

Tests for glandular fever

This infection is caused by Epstein–Barr virus (EBV). Infected cells produce so-called heterophile antibodies (these are IgM molecules that agglutinate horse and sheep RBCs but do not agglutinate ox RBCs and do not react at all with guinea-pig RBCs).

There are various kits available that can detect the presence of heterophile antibodies and in the right clinical context will confirm a diagnosis of EBV infection. The Monospot test is probably the commonest in current use. The Paul–Bunnell test was the first to demonstrate the presence of heterophile antibodies in patients with EBV infection.

Clinical features

Glandular fever often affects young adults (12–25 years) and results in malaise, fever, tonsillitis, petechial haemorrhages on palate and lymphadenopathy. Splenomegaly is fairly common. A similar clinical picture is seen in cytomegalovirus (CMV), *Toxoplasma*, and early human immunodeficiency virus (HIV) infections.

Sample: EDTA.

Positive monospot

EBV infection.

False positives

- Toxoplasmosis.
- CMV infection.
- Rheumatoid.
- Malaria.

Further reading

Hoff G, Bauer S. A new rapid slide test for infectious mononucleosis. *J Am Med Ass* 1996; **194**: 351–3.

Investigation of haemolytic anaemia

The normal red cell has a lifespan of ~120 days. Anaemia resulting from ↓ RBC lifespan is termed *haemolytic*. May be inherited or acquired and the basic underlying mechanisms may involve abnormalities of the RBC *membrane*, RBC *enzymes*, or *Hb*.

Extravascular vs. intravascular

Extravascular haemolysis implies RBC breakdown by the RES (e.g. liver, spleen, and macrophages at other sites), while intravascular haemolysis describes RBC breakdown in the circulation itself. There are many investigations available that will help determine the predominant site of destruction, which in turn will help define the underlying cause of haemolysis, which is why we do the tests in the first place.

Detection of haemolysis itself

The main question is whether the patient's anaemia is due to haemolysis or some other underlying mechanism, such as blood loss, marrow infiltration, etc.

📖 *OHCM* 8e, p330, p332.

General tests of haemolysis

Is haemolysis actually occurring? Suggestive features
- Evidence of ↑ red cell destruction.
- Evidence of ↑ red cell production (to compensate for red cell loss).
- Evidence of autoantibody in the patient's serum.

Evidence of RBC destruction
- ↑ Serum bilirubin.
- ↑ Serum lactate dehydrogenase (LDH; reflecting ↑ RBC turnover).
- Spherocytes or other abnormal RBCs, e.g. fragments on blood film.
- Plasma haptoglobins may be ↓ or absent.
- ↑ Faecal & urinary urobilinogen (faecal not measured).
- ↓ RBC lifespan (seldom measured nowadays).

Evidence of ↑ RBC production
- ↑ Reticulocytes (on film, manual, or automated count). Not absolutely specific, will ↑ in brisk acute bleed, e.g. gastrointestinal tract (GIT).
- ↑ MCV (reticulocytes are larger than mature RBCs and don't forget folate deficiency, which occurs in haemolytic disorders).

Is it mainly intravascular?
- ↑ Plasma Hb.
- Methaemalbuminaemia.
- Haemoglobinuria.
- Haemosiderinuria.

What is the cause?
Genetic
- RBC morphology (e.g. spherocytes, elliptocytes).
- Hb analysis.
- RBC enzyme assays.

Acquired
- Immune—check DAT.
- Non-immune: check RBC morphology (e.g. thrombotic thrombocytopenic purpura (TTP)/ haemolytic-uraemic syndrome (HUS)).
- Is there some other underlying disease?
- Consider PNH (rare).

Further reading
℘ http://www.umm.edu/blood/anehemol.htm
℘ http://www.emedicine.com/med/topic979.htm

HAEMOLYSIS

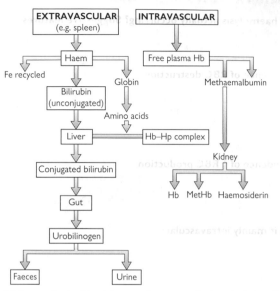

Fig. 3.8 Increased red cell breakdown may be extravascular (outside the circulation, predominantly spleen, liver and marrow) or intravascular (within the vessels).[1]

1. Modified from Lewis SM, Bain BJ & Bates I, eds. (2001) Dacie & Lewis *Practical Haematology*, 9th edition, Churchill Livingstone, Edinburgh.

Reticulocytes

These are immature RBCs formed in the marrow and found in small numbers in normal peripheral blood. They represent an intermediate maturation stage in marrow between the nucleated RBC and the mature RBC (the reticulocyte lacks a nucleus, but retains some nucleic acid). Measuring the number of reticulocytes in the blood may help determine whether the anaemia is due to ↓ RBC production. The reticulocyte count is also a useful measure of response to haematinic (iron, B₁₂ or folate) replacement therapy.

Detection and measurement

- Demonstrated by staining with supravital dye for the nucleic acid.
- Appear on blood film as larger than mature RBCs with fine lacy blue staining strands or dots.
- Some modern automated blood counters using laser technology can measure levels of reticulocytes directly.
- Usually expressed as a % of total red cells, e.g. 5%, though absolute numbers can be derived from this and total red cell count.

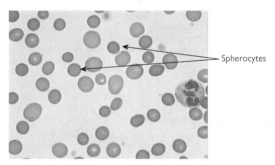

Spherocytes

Fig. 3.9 Blood film of numerous spherocytes (small darker red cells) and reticulocytes (larger red cells) in autoimmune haemolytic anaemia.

Sample: EDTA.

Normal range: 0.5–2.5% (50–100 × 10⁹/L).

Causes of ↑ reticulocyte counts

Marrow stimulation due to
- Bleeding.
- Haemolysis.
- Response to oral Fe therapy.
- Infection.
- Inflammation.
- Polycythaemia (any cause).
- Myeloproliferative disorders.
- Marrow recovery following chemotherapy or radiotherapy.
- Erythropoietin administration.

Causes of ↓ reticulocyte counts

Marrow infiltration due to
- Leukaemia.
- Myeloma.
- Lymphoma.
- Other malignancy.

Marrow underactivity (hypoplasia) due to
- Fe, folate, or B_{12} deficiency. **Note**: return of retics is earliest sign of response to replacement therapy.
- Immediately post-chemotherapy or radiotherapy.
- Autoimmune disease especially refractory anaemia (RA).
- Malnutrition.
- Uraemia.
- Drugs.
- Aplastic anaemia.
- Red cell aplasia.

Further reading

Howells MR, *et al.* Erythropoiesis in pregnancy. *Br J Haematol* 1986; **64**: 595–9.

Serum haptoglobins

Haptoglobins (Hp) are plasma proteins synthesized by the liver, whose function is the removal of free plasma Hb. Hp molecules bind free Hb and are taken up by the reticuloendothelial system for degradation. Hp–Hb complexes do not appear in the urine because their large size prevents them passing through the renal tubules.

The Hp–Hb complex is cleared by the reticuloendothelial system at a rate of 15mg/100mL/h, which means that even very mild haemolysis will cause the disappearance of Hp from the circulation. The serum Hp should be measured in patients with suspected intravascular haemolysis. However, the Hp level is frequently reduced in patients with extravascular haemolysis, and the Hp level cannot be used to determine whether the basic haemolytic process is intra- or extravascular. It should generally be accompanied by estimation of the serum methaemalbumin, free plasma Hb, and urinary haemosiderin.

Sample: Clotted blood.

Normal range (expressed as Hb-binding capacity): 30–250mg/dL.

Conditions with ↓ haptoglobins

Haemolysis including
- Incompatible blood transfusion.
- Autoimmune haemolytic anaemia.
- Sickle cell disease.
- Thalassaemia major.
- Paroxysmal nocturnal haemoglobinuria (PNH).

Others
- 1% population have genetic lack of Hp.
- Lower levels in infancy.

Note: it takes about 1 week after haemolysis has stopped for Hp levels to return to normal.

Conditions with ↑ haptoglobins (acute phase protein, like ferritin)

- Any disorder with ↑ ESR.
- Carcinoma especially if bony secondaries.
- Any inflammatory disorder.
- Trauma.
- Surgery.
- Steroid therapy.
- Androgen therapy.
- Diabetes mellitus.

Further reading

Rougemont A *et al.* Hypohaptoglobinaemia as an epidemiological and clinical indicator for malaria. Results of two studies in a hyperendemic region in West Africa. *Lancet* 1988; **2**: 709–12.

Serum bilirubin

Two forms are found: pre-hepatic bilirubin (unconjugated) and bilirubin conjugated to glucuronic acid (conjugated). Generally, serum bilirubin levels are 17–50µmol/L in haemolysis (mainly unconjugated).

▶**Beware**: serum bilirubin levels may be normal even if haemolysis is present; a level > 85µmol/L suggests liver disease.

The serum bilirubin may be modest ↑ (e.g. 20–30µmol/L) in dyserythropoietic disorders, such as vitamin B_{12} or folate deficiency, or myelodysplasia, due to ineffective erythropoiesis, where the RBCs are destroyed in the marrow before ever being released into the circulation.

Urobilin, urobilinogen, & urinary haemosiderin

Urobilinogen is the reduced form of urobilin, formed by bacterial action on bile pigments in the GIT. Faecal and urinary urobilinogen ↑ in haemolytic anaemias.

Urinary haemosiderin

Usage

The most widely used and reliable test for detection of chronic intravascular haemolysis. Results from the presence of Hb in the glomerular filtrate.

Principle

Free Hb is released into the plasma during intravascular haemolysis. The Hb-binding proteins become saturated resulting in passage of haem-containing compounds into the urinary tract of which haemosiderin is the most readily detectable.

Method

1 A clean catch sample of urine is obtained from the patient.
2 Sample is spun down in a cytocentrifuge to obtain a cytospin preparation of urothelial cells.
3 Staining and rinsing with Perl's reagent (Prussian blue) is performed on the glass slides.
4 Examine under oil-immersion lens of microscope.
5 Haemosiderin stains as blue dots within urothelial cells.
6 Ignore all excess stain, staining outside cells, or in debris, all of which are common.
7 True +ve only when clear detection within urothelial squames is seen.

Cautions

An iron-staining +ve control sample should be run alongside test case to ensure stain has worked satisfactorily. Haemosiderinuria may not be detected for up to 72 h after the initial onset of intravascular haemolysis so the test may miss haemolysis of very recent onset—repeat test in 3–7 days if −ve. Conversely, haemosiderinuria may persist for some time after a haemolytic process has stopped. Repeat in 7 days should confirm.

Causes of haemosiderinuria (Table 3.6)

Table 3.6 Causes of haemosiderinuria

Common causes	Red cell enzymopathies, e.g. G6PD and PK deficiency, but only during haemolytic episodes
	Mycoplasma pneumonia with anti-I cold haemagglutinin
	Sepsis
	Malaria
	Cold haemagglutinin disease
	TTP/HUS
	Severe extravascular haemolysis (may cause intravascular haemolysis)
Rarer causes	PNH
	Prosthetic heart valves
	Red cell incompatible transfusion reactions
	Unstable haemoglobins
	March haemoglobinuria

Plasma haemoglobin

In health, Hb is contained within RBCs, but during intravascular haemolysis excessive quantities of Hb may be released from ruptured RBCs. Normally Hps mop up free Hb. If there are insufficient Hps to cope with the free Hb, the kidneys clear the Hb leading to haemoglobinuria. Some Hb may be broken down in the circulation to haem and globin; haem can bind to albumin producing methaemalbumin (→ methaemalbuminaemia).

▶ The finding of free Hb in plasma is *highly suggestive* of intravascular haemolysis.

Sample: Sodium citrate (but discuss with haematology laboratory before sending sample).

Causes of ↑ plasma haemoglobin (Table 3.7)

Table 3.7 Causes of ↑ plasma haemoglobin

Mild ↑ (50–100mg/L)	Moderate↑ (100–250mg/L)	Severe↑ (>250mg/L)
Sickle/thalassaemia	AIHA	Incompatible blood transfusion
HbC disease	Sickle cell disease	PNH
	Thalassaemia major	PCH
	HbSC	Blackwater fever
	Prosthetic heart valve	
	March haemoglobinuria	

Normal range: 10–40mg/L (up to 6mg/L).

Pitfalls: any RBC damage occurring during blood sampling may result in an erroneously high reading. Great care must be taken during venepuncture.

Further reading

Crosby WH, Dameshek W. The significance of hemoglobinemia and associated hemosiderinuria, with particular reference to various types of hemolytic anemia. *J Clin Lab Med* 1951; **38**: 029.

Schumm's test

Use: Detection of methaemalbumin (seen after all haptoglobins used up in a haemolytic process, usually implies the haemolysis is predominantly intravascular).

This spectrophotometric test for methaemalbumin (which has a distinctive absorption band at 558nm) should be requested in patients with suspected intravascular haemolysis and may be abnormal in patients with significant extravascular (generally splenic) haemolysis. It should be accompanied by estimation of the serum Hp level, free plasma Hb, and urinary haemosiderin.

Sample: Heparinized or clotted blood.

Positive result in

- Intravascular haemolysis.
- Mismatched blood transfusion.
- RBC fragmentation syndromes.
- Glucose-6-phosphate dehydrogenase (G6PD) deficiency with oxidative haemolysis.
- PNH.
- March haemoglobinuria.
- Unstable Hbs.

Further reading

Hoffbrand AV, Lewis SM, Tuddenham EGD (eds). *Postgraduate Haematology*, 4th edition, Oxford: Butterworth-Heinemann, 2000.

Winstone NE. Methemalbumin in acute pancreatitis. *Br J Surg* 1965; **52**: 804–8.

Hereditary haemolytic anaemias

There are many inherited causes for haemolytic anaemia, which fall into 3 major groups shown in Table 3.8.

Table 3.8 Inherited causes for haemolytic anaemia

Mechanism	Example
Red cell membrane disorders	Hereditary spherocytosis Hereditary elliptocytosis
Red cell enzyme disorders	G6PD deficiency Pyruvate kinase deficiency
Haemoglobin disorders	Sickle cell anaemia Thalassaemia

Red cell membrane disorders

Hereditary spherocytosis
This is the best known inherited membrane abnormality leading to a reduced red cell lifespan and sometimes severe anaemia. Inheritance is usually autosomal dominant and there is often a positive family history.

Osmotic fragility test
Principle of the test
The test measures the ability of red cells to take up water before rupturing (lysing). This is determined by the volume:surface area ratio. Normal red cells can ↑ their volume by up to 70% before lysing (because they are disc-shaped, and have the capacity to take in extra water easily). Spherocytic red cells have an ↑ volume:surface area ratio and are able to take up less water than normal red cells before lysing (they are spheres and, as such, they are 'full' already).

Sample: EDTA (need normal control sample sent at the same time).

Method
- RBCs are incubated in saline at various concentrations. This results in cell expansion and eventually rupture.
- Normal RBCs can withstand greater volume increases than spherocytic RBCs.
- A positive result (confirming HS) seen when RBCs lyse in saline at near to isotonic concentration, i.e. 0.6–0.8g/dL (normal RBCs will simply show swelling with little lysis).
- Osmotic fragility is more marked in patients who have not undergone splenectomy and if the RBCs are incubated at 37°C for 24 h before performing the test.

Other supportive tests
- There will be a positive family history of HS in many cases.
- The blood film shows ↑↑ spherocytic RBCs.
- Anaemia, ↑ reticulocytes, ↑ LDH, unconjugated bilirubin, urinary urobilinogen with ↓ haptoglobins.
- DAT –ve.

▶ **Beware**: This test is not diagnostic of HS, but will be +ve in any condition in which there are increased numbers of spherocytic red cells. Use this test in conjunction with a history, blood film, and family studies (HS is inherited as an autosomal dominant, so one of the parents and some siblings should be affected).

Further reading
Parpart AK et al. The osmotic resistance (fragility) of human red cells. J Clin Invest 1947; **26**, 636.
Weatherall DJ, Provan AB. Red cells I: inherited anaemias. Lancet 2000; **355**: 1169–75.
♒ http://www.uq.edu.au/vdu/HDUAnaemiaHeridSphere.htm
♒ http://www.bcshguidelines.com/pdf/hereditaryspherocytosis.pdf

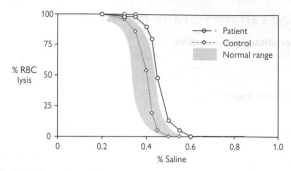

Fig. 3.10 Test and control samples subjected to varying concentrations of saline. The broad grey band represents the normal range. The red cells in the test sample (from a patient with hereditary spherocytosis) lyse at higher concentrations of saline than that seen in the normal control, which suggests that HS is a likely diagnosis.

Red cell enzyme assays

Numerous red cell enzymes are responsible for maintaining the integrity of the RBC in order to allow it to function efficiently in O_2 delivery and CO_2 removal. RBC enzyme defects lead to shortened RBC survival (i.e. haemolysis) and anaemia. Although there are numerous enzymopathies that may cause haemolysis, the most useful starting assays are for G6PD and pyruvate kinase.

Of course, one should start by taking a detailed history from the patient, asking about previous haemolytic episodes, family history, ethnic origin, and possible drug toxicities.

Sample: Fresh EDTA or heparin. The enzymes are stable for 6 days at 4°C and 24 h at 25°C.

Methods: These are too numerous and complex to list here.

Essentially there are 3 methods for analysis of G6PD
- Brilliant cresyl blue decolorization test.
- Methaemoglobin reduction test.
- UV spot test.

Normal range: Varies between laboratories (check with your local laboratory).

Pitfalls: During a haemolytic episode in patients with G6PD deficiency the oldest RBCs are destroyed first. Younger RBCs (and especially reticulocytes) have higher levels of the enzyme than older cells. It follows, therefore, that if the enzyme level is assayed during an acute episode the G6PD level obtained may be falsely normal. This will rise further as reticulocytes pour into the peripheral blood, as happens during recovery from the acute attack. It is better to wait until the acute attack is over and the patient is in steady-state.

Further reading

Arya R et al. Hereditary red cell enzymopathies. *Blood Rev* 1995; **9**: 165–75.

Beutler E. The molecular biology of G6PD variants and other red cell enzyme defects. *Annu Rev Med* 1992; **43**: 47–59.

World Health Organization Scientific Group. *Standardization of procedures for the study of glucose-6-phosphate dehydrogenase*, Technical Report Series, No. 366. Geneva: WHO, 1967.

℘ http://www.rcpa.edu.au/pathman/haemolys.htm

Haemoglobin abnormalities

There are 2 main classes of Hb abnormalities (Table 3.9).

Table 3.9 Main classes of Hb abnormalities

Abnormality	Example
Structural Hb variants	Sickle Hb, HbD, HbE
Imbalanced globin production	Thalassaemias (α, β, etc.)

Structural haemoglobin variants

If the amino acid change results in an electrical charge difference, this may be detected by protein electrophoresis (separates proteins on the basis of charge). Investigation requires full clinical history, FBC, blood film, and Hb electrophoresis.

Thalassaemias

β thalassaemia is diagnosed from the blood indices, blood film, HbA_2, and HbF levels. For α thalassaemia the investigation is more complex requiring deoxyribose nucleic acid (DNA) analysis to detect α-globin deletions. Globin chain synthesis, which examines the ratio of α:β-globin production, is performed less with the advent of DNA-based methods.

Further reading

Weatherall DJ, Provan AB. Red cells I: inherited anaemias. *Lancet* 2000; **355**: 1169–75.

Haemoglobin analysis

Haemoglobin electrophoresis

Electrophoresis is an electrical method for separating molecules on the basis of size (for DNA fragments) or overall electrical charge (for proteins). Hb electrophoresis allows the separation of different Hbs *providing* they have differing charges (Hb molecules with the same charge will move together on the gel and cannot be distinguished). The methods used take advantage of the fact that amino acid side chains on the globin molecules can be ionized. The net overall charge of a protein depends on the pH of the solution it is in and the pKs of the amino acids (the pK is the pH at which half the side chains are ionized).

> **Normal adult haemoglobins:**
> - **HbA**: 97% total.
> - **HbA$_2$**: 2.0–3.2%.
> - **HbF**: 0.5%.

Electrophoretic methods used

- Cellulose acetate (at pH 8.6).
- Citrate agar (at pH 6.0).
- Isoelectric focusing (IEF).
- High-performance liquid chromatography (HPLC).

Due to space limitations each of these methods will be discussed only briefly. Other texts deal with this topic in considerable detail.

Sample: Peripheral blood EDTA.

Cellulose acetate

This test is commonly performed in the diagnosis of abnormal Hb production (haemoglobinopathies or thalassaemia). Because some Hbs have the same net charge they will run together, e.g. HbS will run in the same band as HbD and HbG, and HbC will run with HbE. To resolve these bands electrophoresis is next carried out at acid pH.

Citrate agar

This is similar to cellulose acetate where Hbs are separated at an acid pH (pH 6.0) to separate out Hbs that run together at alkaline pH.

Isoelectric focusing

This is a high resolution method for separating different Hb molecules. The basic principle of the test relies on the fact that all proteins and amino acids have a pH at which their net charge is zero. This is termed the isoelectric point. At this pH there is no net movement in the presence of an externally applied electric field. The Hb molecules are subjected to a pH gradient. This method has the advantage of high resolution, but is more expensive than standard electrophoresis (Fig. 3.11).

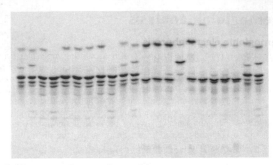

Fig. 3.11 Isoelectric focusing of haemoglobin.

High-performance liquid chromatography

This chromatographic technique has been around for 20 yrs or more, and is being increasingly used for analysis of Hb molecules. Haemoglobins are passed through a matrix column and eluted from the column at varying times, during which their absorbance is measured. Detection of standard Hb variants is simple; the advantage of HPLC is that novel Hb variants can also be detected, and HPLC can separate proteins that cannot be resolved using other means. HPLC is more expensive than all the techniques mentioned above (see Figs 3.12 and 3.13).

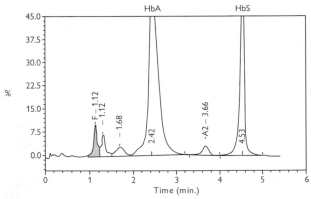

Fig. 3.12 HPLC analysis showing sickle trait (HbA + HbS).

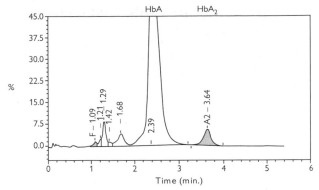

Fig. 3.13 HPLC analysis showing β-thalassaemia trait (elevated HbA$_2$).

When should you request these tests?

Haemoglobin analysis is usually carried out
- When the MCV is ↓↓, but Hb normal or slightly ↓.
- In patients from ethnic groups known to be associated with high levels of Hb disorder, e.g. sickle or thalassaemia.

Investigation of possible thalassaemia

1 Check FBC and look at MCV.
2 Is the MCV normal (> 76fL)? If so, thalassaemia is unlikely.
3 Does the FBC show anything else? ↑ RCC with ↓ MCV and MCH are likely in thalassaemia.
4 Measure the HbA$_2$: this is generally ↑ in β thalassaemia trait (carrier).
5 Carry out HPLC.
6 Measure HbF level.
7 Look at distribution of HbF in RBCs (HbF is present in *all* RBCs in African HPFH (hereditary persistence of fetal Hb), but not present in all cells in carrier for δβ thalassaemia.
8 Assess iron status (common cause of ↓ MCV—don't miss this!).
9 Look for RBC inclusions (e.g. H bodies in α thalassaemia or Heinz bodies in unstable Hb disorders).
10 Carry out DNA analysis, examining both α- and β-globin genes.

Further reading

📖 http://sickle.bwh.harvard.edu/menu_thal.html

Investigation of sickle haemoglobin

Sickle Hb is the result of a point mutation in the β-globin gene resulting in a glu → val switch at position 6 of the β globin protein. Sickle Hb (HbS) forms long filaments (tactoids) reducing its solubility when O_2 tension is reduced. This forms the basis of the sickle solubility test (Fig. 3.14).

Sample: Any anticoagulant.

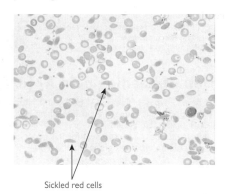

Sickled red cells

Fig. 3.14 Blood film of homozygous sickle cell anaemia (HbSS). Note the sickle-shaped (crescent) red cells.

The patient's blood is mixed with sodium dithionite solution and left to stand. A positive sickle sample should be used as a control. When the tubes are examined a clear solution implies that there is no sickle Hb; a turbid solution confirms the presence of HbSS in the patient's sample.

▶A positive result will be obtained for sickle carriers (HbAS) and sickle cell homozygotes (HbSS). If a positive result is obtained Hb electrophoresis must be carried out to determine whether the patient is a carrier or has homozygous sickle cell anaemia.

Molecular diagnosis of sickle cell disease

This is useful for prenatal diagnosis. The β-globin genes of the fetus are amplified using polymerase chain reaction ((PCR) cells are obtained by amniocentesis or chorionic villus sampling (CVS)) and digested with a bacterial restriction enzyme, e.g. Mst II. If the sickle mutation is present no digestion will occur (the mutation removes the restriction site).

Neonatal haemoglobin screening

- Obtain blood from neonate (e.g. heel prick) in babies at risk of sickle or β thalassaemia major (e.g. mother has gene for HbS, C, D^{Punjab}, E, O^{Arab}, β or δβ thalassaemia).
- Universal neonatal screening is generally used in areas where there is a high incidence of haemoglobinopathy.

📖 *OHCM* 8e, p334.

Further reading

Steinberg MH et al., (eds) *Disorders of Hemoglobin. Genetics, Pathophysiology, and Clinical Management.* Cambridge: Cambridge University Press, 2001.
🔗 http://sickle.bwh.harvard.edu/menu_sickle.html

Estimation of haemoglobin A$_2$ ($\alpha_2\delta_2$)

Normal adults have 3 types of Hb: HbA, HbA$_2$, and HbF. HbA ($\alpha_2\beta_2$) is the major Hb and HbA$_2$ is a minor adult Hb, which is very useful for the diagnosis of β thalassaemia trait. HbA$_2$ levels are ↑ in the heterozygote (carrier state) and this is a specific test for this genotype. The test is carried out using a column chromatography method.

Sample: EDTA.

Normal range: 2.0–3.2%.

Causes of ↑ HbA$_2$

β-thalassaemia trait (HbA$_2$ level is ~3.9–6.5%).

Causes of ↓ HbA$_2$

- Iron deficiency.
- δ-thalassaemia.

Estimation of fetal haemoglobin

Fetal haemoglobin HbF makes up > 50% of the total Hb at birth, but decreases to ~5% by 5 months of age (as γ chain production is replaced by β chains). HbF levels may be raised in some haemoglobinopathies.

Sample: EDTA.

↑ HbF found in

- β-thalassaemia trait.
- β-thalassaemia major.
- Hereditary persistence of fetal Hb.
- Homozygous sickle cell disease (HbSS).
- Sickle/β$^+$ thalassaemia (some cases).
- Sickle/β^0 thalassaemia (some cases).
- Juvenile chronic myeloid leukaemia.
- Multiple myeloma (uncommon and never measured).
- Acquired aplastic anaemia.

Haemoglobin H bodies (β_4)

HbH, consisting of a tetramer of β globins (β_4), is found in α-thalassaemia. The β chains form tetramers due to the relative lack of α-globins with which to pair. The demonstration of HbH allows the detection of α-thalassaemia trait (either $-\alpha/-\alpha$ or $--/\alpha\alpha$) and HbH disease ($--/-\alpha$).

Method

The HbH body test involves staining RBCs with brilliant cresyl blue; HbH bodies are seen as large dark inclusions in the red cells.

Sample: Fresh EDTA.

▶ **Note**: the presence of HbH confirms α-thalassaemia, but the *absence* of HbH bodies does not exclude the diagnosis.

Heinz bodies

These are red cell inclusions made up of insoluble denatured globin protein. Heinz bodies are seen when the RBCs are stained with methyl violet stain.

Sample: Fresh EDTA.

Interpretation: Heinz bodies are seen close to the RBC membrane. These are normally removed by the spleen and are, therefore, more frequent following splenectomy.

Causes of Heinz bodies

Oxidative haemolysis:
- Chlorates, phenacetin, other drugs.
- G6PD, pyruvate kinase (PK) deficiencies, and other enzymopathies.
- Unstable haemoglobins.

Further reading

Sevitt S *et al.* Acute Heinz-body anaemia in burned patients. *Lancet* 1973; **2**: 471–5.

Testing for unstable haemoglobins

Globin gene mutations may lead to amino acid substitutions that render the Hb molecule unstable, leading to haemolysis. Most mutations causing unstable Hb are autosomal dominant and > 80% affect the β chain. Affected individuals are heterozygotes. Heinz bodies in RBCs are intracellular Hb precipitates. Unstable Hbs can be detected electrophoretically or using the heat precipitation test, in which lysed RBCs are heated to 50°C for 1 h.

Sample: fresh EDTA.

Interpretation: normal fresh haemolysates should be stable for 1 h at 50°C. If there is an unstable Hb a precipitate will be seen in the tube.

Examples

- Hb Köln.
- Hb Gun Hill.

Molecular tests for diagnosis of thalassaemia

Although most haematology laboratories can diagnose β-thalassaemia trait and β-thalassaemia major, there are occasions when molecular tests are required, e.g. antenatal diagnosis where a couple are at risk of having a child with β-thalassaemia major or hydrops fetalis (absence of α-globin, usually lethal). In addition, the diagnosis of α-thalassaemia is difficult and requires DNA analysis, either using Southern blotting or PCR amplification of globin genes.

β-thalassaemia

There are > 100 β-globin mutations now known, but fortunately each population tends to have its own group of mutations (this avoids having to test for all known mutations). It is important that you include the ethnic group on the request form, since this will assist the laboratory who will then screen for mutations commonly found in the ethnic group of the patient. Details of these mutations can be found in the beta and delta thalassemia repository.

Methods used for molecular diagnosis of β thalassaemia

The methods used are complex and outwith the scope of this small book.[1-3]

How the ARMS PCR technique works

- This is amplification refractory mutation system PCR.
- Specific point mutations are known for the β-globin mutations.
- PCR primers are designed to bind with the mutated sequence.
- If the patient has the mutation there will be PCR amplification.
- If the patient lacks the mutation there is no binding of the primers to the patient's DNA and no amplification.
- So, a band on the gel means the mutation is present (and the reverse is true—if the band is absent then that particular mutation is absent).

Other techniques, including reverse dot blots and DNA sequencing, are sometimes needed if ARMS PCR fails.

Methods used for molecular diagnosis of α thalassaemia

Whereas β-thalassaemia is usually the result of point mutations (single base changes), the α-thalassaemias are usually the result of deletions of chunks of DNA in the region of the α-globin genes. Southern blotting is useful in detecting deletions, since the DNA band sizes after digestion with restriction enzymes will differ to the wild type (i.e. normal).

1 Bowden DK *et al.* A PCR-based strategy to detect the common severe determinants of a thalassaemia. *Br J Haem* 1992; **81**: 104–8.
2 Lewis SM, Bain BJ, Bates I (eds) *Dacie & Lewis Practical Haematology*, 9th edn, Edinburgh: Churchill Livingstone, 2001
3 Huisman TH, Carver MF. The beta- and delta-thalassemia repository. *Hemoglobin* 1988; **22**: 169–95.

UK Haemoglobinopathy Reference Laboratory

This is based at the John Radcliffe Hospital in Oxford (UK). Difficult cases (e.g. α-thalassaemia) can be sent to this laboratory (after discussing the case first); they will perform α-globin gene analysis and send a detailed report containing the genotype of the patient. See end of chapter for contact details (📖 Specialized haematology assays, pp306–7).

Acquired haemolytic anaemias

Determining the cause of haemolytic anaemia can be a complex process. Having excluded inherited disorders of Hb, RBC membrane, or enzymes we are left with a diverse group of disorders with a common phenotype of increased RBC destruction (and ↓ RBC lifespan; see Table 3.10).

Immune

- Autoimmune (1°, or 2° to systemic lupus erythematosus (SLE) or CLL).
- Alloimmune (e.g. transfusion reactions, haemolytic disease of the newborn).
- Antibody can be warm (IgG) or cold (IgM usually).

RBC damage

- Drugs.
- Poisons.
- Burns.

RBC fragmentation syndromes

- DIC.
- TTP/HUS.
- March haemoglobinuria.

Investigations

There is little point investigating the cause of haemolytic anaemia until you have shown that haemolysis is *actually* occurring.

Look for the acquired cause

- FBC and peripheral film:
  - Spherocytes (suggests warm antibody; also present in HS).
  - ↑ WBC, e.g. might suggest underlying lymphoproliferative disorder, such as CLL.
  - RBC fragments (suggests physical damage to the RBC, e.g. MAHA, TTP/HUS, burns, March haemoglobinuria, mechanical heart valves).
  - Parasites, e.g. malaria.
  - Infections, e.g. *Clostridium*, *Bartonella*, *Babesia*.
- Antiglobulin test (direct antibody test (DAT)):
  - IgG or IgG + complement (C3d) on RBC.
  - DAT is usually +ve in immune-mediated haemolysis.
- Renal function (abnormal in TTP/HUS).
- Coagulation screen (DIC with RBC fragmentation).
- Liver function test (LFTs—abnormal in Zieve's syndrome).
- USS for splenomegaly.
- **Cold agglutinins**: IgM, usually against I or i proteins, RBC membrane proteins.
- Ham's test or immunophenotype if suspect PNH.

Table 3.10 Acquired haemolytic anaemias: mechanisms

Mechanism	Examples
Autoimmune	**Warm antibody (IgG mainly)** Idiopathic haemolytic anaemia Secondary to other autoimmune diseases (e.g. SLE), lymphoid malignancies (e.g. CLL), infections, drugs (e.g. penicillins, methyldopa) **Cold antibodies (IgM mainly)** Cold agglutinin syndromes, cold haemagglutinin disease (CHAD), 2° to infection
Alloimmune	Haemolytic transfusion reactions, haemolytic disease of the newborn (HDN)
Infections	Many, including malaria, meningococcal, pneumococcal, viral
Chemical or physical	Drugs, burns, drowning
RBC fragmentation syndromes	Mechanical heart valves, microangiopathic haemolytic anaemia (MAHA, seen in DIC, HUS, TTP, pre-eclampsia, SLE, carcinoma)
Membrane disorders	Examples are liver disease, PNH

Ham's acid lysis test

This is a test for the rare acquired red cell membrane disorder called paroxysmal nocturnal haemoglobinuria (PNH). Its pathophysiology is complex and involves an abnormality of the red cell membrane in PNH making it prone to complement-mediated lysis and episodes of marked intravascular haemolysis leading to free Hb in the urine (haemoglobinuria).

Principle
- Abnormal sensitivity of RBCs from patients with PNH to the haemolytic action of complement.
- Complement is activated by acidification of the patient's serum to pH of 6.2, which induces lysis of PNH red cells, but not normal controls.

Sample: EDTA, heparin, citrate, oxalate.

Result: +ve result indicates PNH.

Specificity: High—similar reaction is produced only in the rare syndrome HEMPAS (a form of congenital dyserythropoietic anaemia type II), which should be easily distinguished morphologically.

Sensitivity: Low—as the reaction is crucially dependent on the concentration of magnesium in the serum.

Bleeding time

This is a test of 1° haemostasis, and mainly of platelet function *in vivo*, rather than a laboratory test. You will generally need to arrange this test through the Haematology Department who will carry out the test for you.

Procedure

A disposable spring-loaded blade is used to make 2 incisions of fixed depth into the skin of the forearm, whilst a sphygmomanometer is inflated to 40mmHg. Blood from the incisions is mopped up using circular filter paper (care needs to be taken to avoid disturbing the clot that forms on the cut surface).

Normal range: Up to 7 min (varies depending on method used; >9 min is abnormal). Longer in ♀.

Uses: Previously felt to be the best screen for acquired or congenital functional or structural platelet disorders. If bleeding time normal and history is negative (i.e. no major bleeding problems in past) this excludes an underlying platelet disorder.

Precautions

▶ Don't carry out bleeding time if platelet count is < 100 × 10⁹/L (will be prolonged). Aspirin will interfere with test—ask patients to stop aspirin 7 days before test carried out.

Causes of prolonged bleeding time
- Low platelet count.
- Platelet function defect (acquired, e.g. aspirin, paraprotein, MDS).
- von Willebrand's disease.
- Vascular abnormalities, e.g. Ehlers–Danlos.
- Occasionally low factor V or XI.
- Afibrinogenaemia.

Pitfalls

Highly operator-dependent, with low reproducibility. Because of this, the test is seldom used now.

📖 *OHCM* 8e, p338.

Further reading

Mielke CH Jr. Aspirin prolongation of the template bleeding time: influence of venostasis and direction of incision. *Blood* 1982; **60**: 1139–42.
Parkin JD, Smith IL. Sex and bleeding time. *Thromb Haemost* 1985; **54**: 731.

Prothrombin time

This tests the extrinsic coagulation pathway and is useful for detecting coagulation deficiencies, liver disease and disseminated intravascular coagulation (DIC). The prothrombin time (PT) is also the main monitor for coumarin therapy (e.g. warfarin), expressed as a ratio—the *international normalized ratio* (INR). The test measures the clotting time of plasma in the presence of a tissue extract, e.g. brain (thromboplastin). The test measures prothrombin but also factors V, VII, and X.

Sample: Citrate.

↑ Prothrombin time

- Oral anticoagulation therapy (vitamin K antagonists).
- Fibrinogen deficiency (factor I).
- Prothrombin deficiency (factor II).
- Deficiency of factors V, VII or X (in V or X deficiency the activated partial thromboplastin time APTT will be ↑).
- Liver disease especially obstructive.
- Vitamin K deficiency.
- DIC.

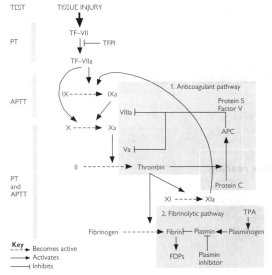

Fig. 3.15 Coagulation cascade showing the factors assayed using the various clotting tests. Modified from Provan D et al. (2004).[1]

Further reading

Provan D, et al. *Oxford Handbook of Clinical Haematology*, 2nd edn. Oxford: Oxford University Press, 2004.

Activated partial thromboplastin time

Other terms: Somewhat confusingly the APTT may be called kaolin cephalin clotting time (KCCT), partial thromboplastin time with kaolin (PTTK).

What is the APTT testing?

This is a test of the intrinsic coagulation system, and depends on contact factors + factors VIII, IX, and reactions with factors X, V, II, and I. The APTT is sensitive to circulating anticoagulants (e.g. lupus anticoagulant) and heparin.

Sample: Citrate.

Uses

• Heparin monitoring.
• Screening for haemophilia A and B (VIII and IX deficiency, respectively).
• Screening for coagulation inhibitors.

Normal range: 26.0–33.5 s (often expressed as activated partial thromboplastin time ratio (APTR)).

↑ Activated partial thromboplastin time

• DIC.
• Liver disease.
• Massive blood transfusion.
• Heparin treatment.
• Circulating anticoagulant.
• Modest ↑ in patients taking oral anticoagulants.
• Haemophilia.

Is there an inhibitor present?

The APTT will be long if there is an inhibitor such as the lupus anticoagulant present. This can be determined by mixing the patient's plasma with an equal volume of normal control plasma and repeating the APTT. If the APTT is long because of an inhibitor it will not fully correct when normal plasma is added. However, if the APTT is long because of a deficiency it will be corrected with the normal plasma.

Further reading

Denson KW. (1988) Thromboplastin—sensitivity, precision and other characteristics. *Clin Lab Haematol* 1988; **10**: 315–328;

Turi DC, Peerschke EI. Sensitivity of three activated partial thromboplastin time reagents to coagulation factor deficiencies. *Am J Clin Pathol* 1986; **85**: 43–9.

van den Besselaar AM *et al* (1987). Monitoring heparin therapy by the activated partial thromboplastin time—the effect of pre-analytical conditions. *Thromb Haemost* **57**: 226–31.

֍ http://www.labtestsonline.org/understanding/analytes/coag_cascade/coagulation_cascade.html

Thrombin clotting time

This is affected by the concentration of factor I (fibrinogen), and the presence of fibrin or fibrinogen degradation products and heparin.

Sample: Citrate.

↑ Thrombin clotting time

- Low fibrinogen, e.g. DIC.
- ↑ Fibrin degradation products (FDPs)/cross-linked fibrin degradation products (XDPs)/D-dimers.
- Heparin*.
- Dysfibrinogenaemia (inherited, mutation in fibrinogen gene leads to amino acid change and non-functional fibrinogen).

---

*If suspected, check reptilase time, similar to thrombin clotting time (TCT), but not affected by heparin.

D-dimers

D-dimers are produced during polymerization of fibrinogen as it forms fibrin. Measurement of D-dimer levels is more specific for this process than the older FDP test and is now being used to detect the presence of DIC and other coagulation disorders. The test measures fibrin lysis by plasmin and is a sensitive indicator of coagulation activation (e.g. such as that seen in DIC). The assay uses a monoclonal antibody specific for D-dimers; it will not cross-react with fibrinogen or fibrin.

Sample: citrate (clotting screen bottle).

↑ D-dimers seen in

- DIC.
- Deep vein thrombosis (DVT).
- Pulmonary embolism (PE).

Summary of clotting tests in a variety of disorders (Table 3.11)

Table 3.11 Summary of clotting tests in a variety of disorders

PT	APTT	TCT	Platelets	Diagnosis
N	N	N	N	Platelet function defect, XII deficiency, normal
↑	N	N	N	VII deficiency, early oral anticoagulation
N	↑	N	N	VIIIC/IX/XI/XII deficiency, vWD, circulating anticoagulant, e.g. lupus
↑	↑	N	N	Vitamin K deficiency, oralanticoagulant, V/VII/X/II deficiency
↑	↑	↑	N	Heparin, liver disease, fibrinogen deficiency
N	N	N	↓	Thrombocytopenia (any cause)
↑	↑	N	Low	Massive transfusion, liver disease
↑	↑	↑	Low	DIC, acute liver disease

Modified from Dacie & Lewis (1995).[1]

1 Dacie JV, Lewis SM. *Practical Haematology*, 8th edn. Edinburgh: Churchill Livingstone, 1995.

Laboratory diagnosis

▶▶ Disseminated intravascular coagulation

DIC is a medical and haematological emergency. It may be seen in a variety of situations and is characterized by generalized bruising and bleeding, usually from venepuncture sites, post-operatively, and spontaneously.

Diagnosis requires FBC, clotting screen, and evidence of rapid consumption of fibrinogen. Classic (acute) DIC, where the test results fit the bill, is easy to spot. The situation may be more subtle and you are strongly advised to discuss the case with a haematology registrar or consultant if you are in any doubt about the diagnosis of DIC.

▶▶ Laboratory diagnosis

FBC	↓ platelets ± red cell fragments seen on the blood film
PT	↑ In moderately severe DIC
APTT	Usually ↑
Fibrinogen	↓ (Falling levels significant—but remember this is an acute phase protein so level may be *normal*, even in florid DIC)
D-dimers	↑

Conditions associated with DIC (Table 3.12)

Table 3.12 Conditions associated with DIC

Disorder	Example
Infectious disease	Septicaemia
	Viraemia
Obstetric emergency	Placental abruption
	Eclampsia
	Amniotic fluid embolism
	Placenta praevia
	Septic abortion
Surgical	Cardiac bypass
Malignant disease	Metastatic cancer
	Acute leukaemia (esp. AML M3, i.e. acute promyelocytic leukaemia)
Shock	Trauma
	Severe burns
Transfusion	ABO mismatched transfusion
Miscellaneous	Snake bites (some)
	Liver cirrhosis

Further reading

ℜ http://www.emedicine.com/emerg/topic150.htm

Platelet function tests

These are specialized tests carried out by the coagulation laboratory for the investigation of patients with suspected platelet dysfunction. Because of their complexity, the platelet function tests will not be described in detail here.

Patients generally present with bleeding or bruising problems and have had normal coagulation results. Because of the labour-intensive nature and cost of these assays you will need to arrange these tests after discussion with your local haematology medical staff.

Sample: Blood collection needs to be optimal with non-traumatic venepuncture, rapid transport to the laboratory with storage at room temperature and testing within a maximum of 2–3 h.

Current tests
- Platelet count.
- Morphology.
- Adhesion.
- Aggregation.
- Platelet release.
- Bleeding time.

Platelet count

Normal range 150–400 × 10^9/L. Adequate function is maintained even when the count is <0.5 normal level, but progressively deteriorates as it drops. With platelet counts <20 × 10^9/L there is usually easy bruising and petechial haemorrhages (although more serious bleeding can occur).

Morphology

Large platelets are biochemically more active; ↑ mean platelet volume (MPV >6.5) is associated with less bleeding in patients with severe thrombocytopenia. Altered platelet size is seen in inherited platelet disorders.

Platelet adhesion

Adhesion to glass beads now rarely performed in routine laboratory practice, but potentially useful in vWD diagnosis.

Platelet aggregation

Most useful of the special tests is performed on fresh sample using aggregometer.

Aggregants used
- Adenosine 5-diphosphate (ADP) at low and high concentrations. Induces two aggregation waves: 1° wave may disaggregate at low concentrations of ADP; the second is irreversible.
- Collagen has a short lag phase followed by a single wave and is particularly affected by aspirin.
- Ristocetin-induced platelet aggregation (RIPA) is carried out at a high (1.2mg/mL) and lower concentrations and is mainly used to diagnose vWD.
- Arachidonic acid.
- Adrenaline (epinephrine), not uncommonly reduced in normal people.

Platelet release

Enzyme-linked immunosorbant assay (ELISA) or radioimmunoassay (RIA) are used to measure the granule proteins β-thromboglobulin (β-TG) and heparin neutralizing activity (HNA). These are sensitive markers of platelet hyper-reactivity and beyond the scope of the routine laboratory.

Practical application of tests

Their main role is in diagnosis of inherited platelet functional defects. In acquired platelet dysfunction 2° to causes such as renal and hepatic disease, DIC, and macroglobulinaemia, platelet function is rarely tested.

Further reading

Yardumian A, et al. Laboratory investigation of platelet function: a review of methodology. J Clin Pathol 1986; **39**: 701–12.

Thrombophilia screening

Thrombophilia describes acquired or inherited disorders that predispose to arterial or venous thrombo-embolism (VTE). Thrombophilia should be suspected when the blood clot affects an unusual site, patient is young, has recurrent thrombotic episodes, or a strong family history of VTE.

Causes: ⊞ Recurrent thrombosis, p95.

Which patients should be screened for possible thrombophilia?

- Arterial thrombosis, e.g. patients < 30 yrs, without obvious arterial disease.
- Venous thrombosis:
  - Patients < 40 years with no obvious risk factors.
  - Unexplained recurrent thrombosis.
  - VTE and family history of thrombosis in first degree relatives.
  - Unusual site, e.g. mesenteric, portal vein thrombosis.
  - Unexplained neonatal thrombosis.
  - Recurrent miscarriage (≥ 3).
  - VTE in pregnancy and the oral contraceptive pill (OCP).

Screen

- Exclude medical causes (check ESR, LFTs, AIP, fasting lipids).
- FBC (exclude thrombocytosis).
- Clotting screen for acquired defects (PT, APTT, lactic acidosis (LA)/ anticardiolipin antibody (ACL), ↑ fibrinogen).
- Screen for inherited thrombophilia:
  - First line protein C (PC), protein S (PS), antithrombin (AT), activated protein C resistance (APCR).
  - Check for presence of the factor V Leiden mutation in APCR +ve
  - patients (DNA analysis).
  - Consider testing plasminogen, factor XII, homocysteine levels, prothrombin variant.
- DNA analysis for prothrombin gene mutation.

Thrombophilia investigations are time-consuming and expensive and you should discuss with the local haematology medical or lab staff before sending samples. *Note*: some thrombophilia tests cannot be carried out in the 'acute' phase of a VTE event or while the patient is taking warfarin.

Further reading

Cattaneo M *et al.* Interrelation of hyperhomocyst(e)inemia, factor V Leiden, and risk of future venous thrombo-embolism. *Circulation* 1998; **97**: 295–6.

Dahlback B. Resistance to activated protein C as risk factor for thrombosis: molecular mechanisms, laboratory investigation, and clinical management. *Semin Hematol* 1997; **34**: 217–34.

Lane DA *et al.* Inherited thrombophilia: Part 1. *Thromb Haemost* 1996a; **76**: 651–62.

Lane DA *et al.* Inherited thrombophilia: Part 2. *Thromb Haemost* 1996b; **76**: 824–34.

↗ http://peir.path.uab.edu/coag/article_208.shtml

↗ http://www.bcshguidelines.com/pdf/BJH512.pdf

Antithrombin, proteins C&S

These proteins are the body's *natural anticoagulants*; hence, deficiencies may lead to thromboembolic disease.

Antithrombin

Used to be called ATIII, but there was never an ATI or ATII so now abbreviated to AT. A useful measure in thrombophilia screening since low levels of AT are found in 4.5% patients with unexplained VTE.

↓ Antithrombin levels

- Hereditary (40–60% normal level), autosomal dominant.
- Chronic liver disease.
- Protein wasting disorders.
- Heparin therapy.
- 3rd trimester of pregnancy.
- Acute leukaemia.
- Burns.
- Renal disease.
- Gram –ve sepsis.

Protein S

- Reduced levels predispose to VTE. Individuals with 30–60% normal level may suffer recurrent thrombosis.
- ↓ PS.
- Inherited (autosomal dominant).
- Pregnancy.
- Oral anticoagulants, e.g. warfarin.
- Nephrotic syndrome.
- Liver disease.

Protein C

- Similar to PS; autosomal dominant inheritance in genetic cases.
- ↓ PC.
- Hereditary.
- Liver disease.
- Malignancy.
- Warfarin therapy.
- Pregnancy.

Bone marrow examination

This is a key investigation in haematology. It may be diagnostic in the follow-up of abnormal peripheral blood findings and is an important staging procedure in defining the extent of disease, e.g. lymphomas. It is a helpful investigative procedure in unexplained anaemia, splenomegaly, or selected cases of pyrexia of unknown origin (PUO).

Preferred sites: Posterior iliac crest is the usual site (allows aspirate and biopsy to be obtained). The sternum is suitable only for marrow aspiration and is not a test for the squeamish.

The marrow aspirate provides
- Cytology of nucleated cells.
- Qualitative and semiqualitative analysis of haematopoiesis.
- Assessment of iron stores (if Perls' iron stain used).
- Smears for cytochemistry (helps in the diagnosis of leukaemias).

Marrow cells can also be used for
- Chromosomal (cytogenetic) analysis.
- Immunophenotype studies using monoclonal antibodies.

Marrow trephine biopsy provides information about
- Marrow cellularity.
- Identification and classification of abnormal cells.
- Immunohistochemistry on infiltrates.

Contraindications
None, other than physical limitations, e.g. pain or restricted mobility. Avoid sites of previous radiotherapy (inevitably grossly hypocellular and not representative).

See Table 3.13.

Procedure

1 BM aspiration may be performed under local anaesthetic (LAn) alone, but short acting IV sedative (e.g. midazolam) is preferred when trephine biopsy is performed. General anaesthetic used in children.

2 Place patient in (L) lateral position, or use right if s/he cannot lie on left side.

3 Infiltrate skin and periosteum over the posterior iliac spine with local anaesthetic.

4 Make a small cutaneous incision before introducing the aspirating needle, which should penetrate the marrow cortex 3–10mm before removal of the trocar.

5 Aspirate no more than 0.5–1mL marrow initially (to avoid dilution of sample with blood).

6 Make smears promptly (▶ the sample clots rapidly!).

7 If further samples are needed, e.g. for immunophenotyping, cytogenetics, etc., these can be aspirated after making initial slides.

8 For trephine biopsy use Islam or Jamshidi needle.

9 Advance the needle through the same puncture site to penetrate the cortex.

10 Remove the trocar and, using firm hand pressure, rotate the needle clockwise and advance as far as possible.

11 Remove the needle by gentle anticlockwise rotation.

12 Following the procedure apply simple pressure dressings.

13 Minor discomfort at the location may be dealt with by simple analgesia, such as paracetamol.

Table 3.13 Tests carried out on bone marrow

Test	Purpose
Chromosomes	Standard cytogenetic analysis, looking for rearrangements suggestive of acute or chronic leukaemias and myelodysplasia
	Fluorescence *in situ* hybridization (FISH) looking for additions or losses of chromosomes, as well as more subtle changes seen in leukaemias and lymphomas
DNA or RNA analysis	Using PCR to look for mutations or translocations that help classify leukaemias and lymphomas; also useful for monitoring disease levels in some disorders
Immunophenotype	Cell surface marker profile helps in the diagnosis of most leukaemias and lymphomas; may also be used to monitor disease levels post-treatment
Microbiology	E.g. TB culture (not routine, but occasionally useful in cases of PUO)
Cytochemical stains	To help define type of leukaemia

Cytochemistry tests (leukaemia diagnosis)

These staining methods have been around for many years (for decades they were all that was available), but remain extremely useful in the diagnosis and classification of leukaemias. Modern technologies, such as flow cytometry and nucleic acid analysis have refined leukaemia and lymphoma diagnosis, but the examination of well-stained cytochemistry bone marrow smears remains the cornerstone of good haematology practice.

After performing a bone marrow aspirate and spreading the material onto glass slides, the air-dried unfixed microscope slides are passed to the cytochemistry laboratory who will fix and stain the slides according to the likely diagnosis (stains for AML differ to those for acute lymphoblastic leukaemia (ALL), for example; Table 3.14). Positive results with particular stains will point to a specific diagnosis. This will then be augmented by flow cytometric or molecular assays (Fig. 3.16).

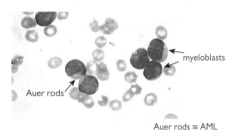

Auer rods ≡ AML

Fig. 3.16 AML marrow showing myeloblasts (leukaemic cells) and an Auer rod in one cell. Auer rods are pathognomonic of AML, since they do not occur in any other disorder.

Table 3.14 Cytochemical stains

Cytochemical stain	Substrate/cell
Myeloperoxidase (MPO)	Lysosomal enzyme found in neutrophils and monocytes
Sudan black (SB)	Phospholipids in neutrophil granules
Chloroacetate esterase	Stain specific esterase in granulocytes and mast cells. Makes it easier to diagnose AML M4 subtype
α-naphtholacetate esterase (ANAE)	Esterase stain, useful for diagnosis of AML subtypes
Acid phosphatase	Enzyme found in many different WBCs. Useful for T cell malignancies
Periodic acid-Schiff (PAS)	Detects glycogen in cells. Granulocytes have diffuse staining whereas lymphocytes staining is much coarser

Table 3.15 Cytochemical stains in acute leukaemia

	Acute lymphoblastic leukaemia		Acute myeloid leukaemia		
	B lineage	T lineage	M1–3	M4–5	M6–7
Myeloperoxidase	–	–	+/++	+	–
Sudan black	–	–	+/++	+	–
Chloroacetate esterase	–	–	–/++	–	–
α-Naphthol acetate esterase	–	–	–	++	–
Acid phosphatase	–	+ (focal)	–	+ (diffuse)	+ (focal)
Periodic acid–Schiff	+ (blocks)	–	–	+ (fine granular)	+

+, Positive; ++, strongly +ve; –, –ve.

From Hoffbrand et al. (2000).[1]

Further reading

🔗 http://www.rcpa.edu.au/pathman/cytochem.htm

1 Hoffbrand AV, Lewis SM, Tuddenham EGD. *Postgraduate Haematology*, 4th edn, Oxford: Butterworth-Heinemann, 2000.

Neutrophil alkaline phosphatase

Uses

This is a cytochemical stain used to demonstrate the presence and quantity of the neutrophil enzyme alkaline phosphatase. Historically, the NAP score was of value in differentiating 'reactive' states from myeloproliferative disorders, such as CML, polycythaemia rubra vera, etc.—now more often features in examination MCQs! (**Note**: sometimes termed leucocyte alkaline phosphatase, LAP.)

Procedure

Best performed on fresh blood films, made without the use of anticoagulant. EDTA samples may be used, but are less satisfactory. The film should be made, air-dried, fixed, and then stained—all within 30 min. Positive neutrophil alkaline phosphatase (NAP) activity is indicated by the presence of bright blue granules in the neutrophil cytoplasm (the nucleus is stained red; Fig. 3.17).

Scoring: films are scored from 0 to 4 on the basis of stain intensity:
0: Negative, no granules seen.
1: Weak positive, few granules.
2: Positive, few–moderate numbers of granules.
3: Strongly positive.
4: Very strong.

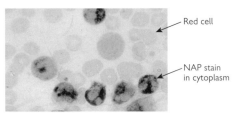

Red cell

NAP stain
in cytoplasm

Fig. 3.17 NAP-stained blood film: shows positively stained neutrophils. Red cells do not take up the stain.

Interpretation & significance (Table 3.16)

Table 3.16 NAP

High NAP score	Low NAP score
Polycythaemia rubra vera (PRV)	Chronic myeloid leukaemia
Leukaemoid reaction	Paroxysmal nocturnal haemoglobinuria
Neutrophilia—any cause	Acute myeloid leukaemia
Myelofibrosis	
Essential thrombocythaemia	
Hepatic cirrhosis	
Hodgkin's disease	
Aplastic anaemia	
Down's syndrome	
Cushing's disease	

The NAP score is affected by corticosteroids, oestrogens, and pregnancy (↑ NAP). In Hodgkin's disease, the NAP score offers no advantage over simpler tests, such as ESR, for assessment of disease activity. Occasionally of value in a patient with aplastic anaemia who is developing PNH—the NAP score is seen to fall (both of these are very rare disorders). NAP score has been replaced in most hospitals by flow cytometry and other methods.

Further reading

Lewis SM, Bain BJ, Bates I (eds). *Dacie & Lewis Practical Haematology*, 9th edn, Edinburgh: Churchill Livingstone, 2001

Blood transfusion

Due to space limitations it is inappropriate to go into major details about the investigations used in transfusion medicine. However, we have provided the more important tests in current use which include:
- Blood group & antibody screen.
- Cross-match (compatibility test).
- DAT.
- Antiplatelet and antineutrophil antibody testing.

Safe transfusion practice

Each year patients are transfused with the wrong blood. In 2007, 12 patients were given ABO incompatible blood, while 46 patients given wrong blood (not just ABO incompatible) in 2007.[1] Note that reporting is currently voluntary and very likely underestimates actual incidents. However, with nearly 3 million transfusions it is a small % overall.

The most common error is clerical and generally involves the cross-match sample being taken from the wrong patient and so the compatibility test is performed on the wrong sample. Occasionally, the staff carrying out the transfusion connect the blood up to the wrong patient. In any event, the result varies from no symptoms to shock and possible death.

How to minimize errors

- First, ask yourself *does this patient really need to be transfused* with blood or blood products (e.g. FFP, platelets, etc.)? For example, a post-operative patient who is asymptomatic with a Hb of 9g/dL probably does not require red cell transfusion. Use clinical judgement in helping decide whether or not to proceed with transfusion.
- Before taking the blood sample check that you are taking blood from the correct patient—ask for his/her name and check the identity bracelet.
- Label the patient's blood bottle at the bedside (i.e. no prelabelling of bottles). Many transfusion laboratories insist on 1, 2, 5, 6, & 7, and either 3 or 4 from:
  1 Surname & forename (correctly spelt)
  2 DoB
  3 Hospital/A&E/new NHS number
  4 First line of address
  5 Sex
  6 Time and date blood taken
  7 Signature of person taking blood
- Ensure details on form match those on the bottle.
- Complete the request form properly:
  - State what is required (e.g. 2 units of packed cells, etc.).
  - Detail any previous transfusions, reactions, antibodies (if known).
  - Let the laboratory know when you want the blood or blood product.

▶▶ Adhesive patient labels are fine for forms, but are not suitable for specimen bottles, and are usually not accepted by transfusion laboratoriess. Transfusion specimens should be labelled by hand—at the bedside.

If this sounds cumbersome and bureaucratic:

Remember many people die annually because they are transfused with the *wrong blood*. In most cases clerical error is to blame—people have filled out bottles in advance and failed to check patient identity.

Further reading

McClelland B. *Handbook of Transfusion Medicine*, 2nd edn. London: HMSO, 2001.
🖑 http://www.blood.co.uk/
🖑 http://www.transfusionguidelines.org.uk/
🖑 http://www.scotblood.co.uk/
🖑 http://www.bcshguidelines.com/pdf/tme203.pdf

1 http://www.shotuk.org/Summary%202007.pdf

▶▶ Transfusion reactions

See Table 3.17

Rapid temperature spike (> 40°C) at start of transfusion indicates transfusion should be stopped (suggests acute intravascular haemolysis).

If slow rising temperature (< 40°C), providing patient not acutely unwell, slow intravenous infusion (IVI). Fever often due to antibodies against WBCs (or to cytokines in platelet packs).

▶▶ Immediate transfusion reaction

Intravascular haemolysis (→ haemoglobinaemia & haemoglobinuria). Usually due to anti-A or anti-B antibodies (in ABO-mismatched transfusion). Symptoms occur in minutes/hours. *May be fatal.*

Table 3.17 Transfusion reactions

Symptoms	Signs
Patient restless/agitated	Fever
Flushing	Hypotension
Anxiety	Oozing from wounds or venepuncture sites
Chills	Haemoglobinaemia
Nausea & vomiting	Haemoglobinuria
Pain at venepuncture site	
Abdominal, flank or chest pain	
Diarrhoea	

Immediate transfusion reaction or bacterial contamination of blood

If predominantly extravascular may only suffer chills/fever 1 h after starting transfusion—commonly due to anti-D. Acute renal failure is not a feature.

Mechanism

Complement (C3a, C4a, C5a) release into recipient plasma → smooth muscle contraction. May develop DIC or oliguria (10% cases) due to profound hypotension.

Initial steps in management of acute transfusion reaction

- Stop blood transfusion immediately.
- Replace giving set, keep IV open with 0.9% saline.
- Check patient identity against donor unit.
- Insert urinary catheter and monitor urine output.
- Give fluids (IV colloids) to maintain urine output > 1.5mL/kg/h.
- If urine output < 1.5mL/kg/h insert CVP line and give fluid challenge.
- If urine output < 1.5mL/kg/h and CVP adequate give furosemide 80–120mg.
- If urine output still < 1.5mL/kg/h consult senior medical staff for advice.
- Contact blood transfusion laboratory before sending back blood pack and for advice on blood samples required for further investigation (*see below*).

Complications
Overall mortality ~10%.

Urgent investigations

Your local blood transfusion department will have specific guidelines to help you with the management of an acute reaction. The following guide lists the samples commonly required to establish the cause and severity of a transfusion reaction. If you are uncertain about the laboratory procedure or management of a patient who appears to have suffered a severe reaction you must notify your hospital's haematology medical staff who will provide advice.

▶▶ Delays may threaten the patient's life.

1 Check compatibility label of blood unit matches with patient's id band, forms and case notes.
2 If mistake found *tell the blood bank urgently*—the unit of blood intended for your patient may be transfused to another patient.
3 Take blood for:
    - **Haematology**:
        - FBC.
        - DAT.
        - Plasma Hb.
        - Repeat cross-match sample.
        - Coagulation screen.
    - **Chemistry**: U&E.
    - **Microbiology**: blood cultures.
4 Check urinalysis and monitor urine output.
5 Do ECG and check for evidence of $\uparrow[K^+]$.
6 Arrange repeat coagulation screens & biochemistry 2–4 hourly.

Febrile transfusion reactions

Seen in 0.5–1.0% of blood transfusions. Mainly due to anti-HLA antibodies in recipient serum or granulocyte-specific antibodies (e.g. sensitization during pregnancy or previous blood transfusion).

Delayed transfusion reaction

Occurs in patients immunized through previous pregnancies or transfusions. Antibody weak (so not detected at pre-transfusion stage). 2° immune response occurs—antibody titre ↑.

Symptoms and signs
- Occur 7–10 days after blood transfusion.
- Fever, anaemia, and jaundice.
- ± Haemoglobinuria.

Management
- Discuss with transfusion laboratory staff.
- Check DAT and repeat compatibility tests.
- Transfuse patient with freshly cross-matched blood.

Further reading

⚕ http://www.emedicine.com/emerg/topic603.htm

Bacterial contamination of blood products

Uncommon but *potentially fatal* adverse effect of blood transfusion (affects red cells and blood products, e.g. platelet concentrates). Implicated organisms include Gram −ve bacteria, including *Pseudomonas*, *Yersinia*, and *Flavobacterium*.

Features

Include fever, skin flushing, rigors, abdominal pain, DIC, ARF, shock, and possible cardiac arrest.

Management

As per ***Immediate transfusion reaction***
- Stop transfusion.
- Urgent resuscitation.
- IV broad-spectrum antibiotics if bacterial contamination suspected.

Antiglobulin test

The old term is Coombs' test. DAT detects antibodies or complement or both on the RBC surface and the indirect antiglobulin test (IAT) detects presence of antibodies in serum. A useful investigation when investigating haemolytic anaemia.

Sample: EDTA.

Interpretation

- Positive DAT in most AIHA.
- Lymphoproliferative disorders, e.g. CLL.
- Drug-induced haemolysis (e.g. α-methyl dopa, L-dopa).
- Haemolytic disease of the newborn, e.g. Rhesus haemolytic disease of the newborn (HDN).

Note: As with many tests in medicine, things are never entirely black or white—a +ve DAT does not necessarily imply that haemolysis is actively occurring and a −ve DAT does not exclude haemolysis.

Further reading

Coombs RRA. A new test for the detection of weak and 'incomplete' Rh agglutinins. *Br J Exp Pathol* 1945; **26**: 255.

Kelton JG. Impaired reticuloendothelial function in patients treated with methyldopa. *N Engl J Med* 1985; **313**: 596–600.

Kleihauer test

Uses

To determine whether fetal red cells have entered the maternal circulation and, if so, the volume of such fetal cells.

Background

If an Rh (D)-negative mother has a baby that is Rh (D) +ve she may develop antibodies (maternal anti-D) against fetal red cells. This may result in fetal red cell destruction termed *Rhesus haemolytic disease of the newborn*, a serious haemolytic disorder that is seen less today due to greater understanding of the underlying mechanism and our ability to prevent it. Sensitization to the fetal red cells occurs when fetal RBCs enter the maternal circulation, e.g. at birth or through obstetric manipulations, e.g. amniocentesis, previous pregnancies, etc.

Fetal RBCs in the mother's circulation can be detected and quantified (in mL) using the Kleihauer test, which exploits the resistance of fetal red cells to acid elution (acid washes adult Hb out of the mother's red cells, but the fetal RBCs contain HbF, which is not washed out). The Kleihauer test should be performed on all Rh (D) −ve women who deliver a Rh (D) +ve infant.

Fetal cells appear as darkly staining cells against a background of ghosts (these are the maternal red cells). An estimate of the required dose of anti-D can be made from the number of fetal cells in a low power field.

Sample: maternal peripheral blood EDTA.

Calculating the volume of fetal RBCs in maternal circulation

Basically, a calculation is made by the laboratory staff based on the number of fetal RBCs seen in the Kleihauer film. The actual calculation is:

$$1800^* \times \text{ratio of fetal/adult RBCs} \times {}^4/_3 \text{ (correction factor)}$$

For example, if there are 1% fetal RBCs in maternal circulation:

$$1800 \times {}^1/_{100} \times {}^4/_3 = 24\text{mL}.$$

where 1800 is the maternal red cell volume

A 4mL bleed (i.e. 4mL fetal RBCs) requires 500IU anti-D given IM to the mother with a further 250IU anti-D for each additional mL of fetal RBCs.

Don't panic!

The laboratory carrying out the Kleihauer test will tell you the volume of fetal RBCs detected since they will count the cells and do the calculation for you. After this you will need to calculate the dose of anti-D to give the mother, but *if you are unsure either discuss with the Haematology medical staff or contact your local transfusion centre.*

Further reading

Chanarin I (ed.) *Laboratory Haematology: an Account of Laboratory Techniques*, Edinburgh: Churchill Livingstone, 1989.

Erythropoietin assay

Erythropoietin (Epo) is the hormone produced largely by the kidney that drives red cell production. The typical anaemia found in renal disease is a result of failure of Epo production. Epo assays are of value in renal medicine and haematology. For example, in the assessment of polycythaemic states an ↑ Epo level may be appropriate (e.g. in hypoxia where the body is attempting to increase O_2 availability to tissues) or inappropriate (e.g. some tumours). The Epo assay is carried out using a radioimmunoassay method and is not available in all haematology laboratories (may need to be sent to another hospital or laboratory).

Normal range: 35–25mU/mL, steady state level, no anaemia. May rise to 10,000mU/mL in hypoxia or anaemia.

Causes of ↑ Epo (appropriate)
- Anaemias.
- High altitude.
- Hypoxia:
  - Lung disease.
  - Sleep apnoea syndromes.
- Cyanotic heart disease (e.g. R → L shunts).
- High affinity haemoglobins.
- Cigarette smoking.
- Methaemoglobinaemia.

Causes of ↑ Epo (inappropriate)
- Renal disease:
  - Hypernephroma.
  - Nephroblastoma.
  - Post-renal transplant.
  - Renal cysts.
  - Renal artery stenosis.
- Hepatoma.
- Uterine fibroids.
- Cerebellar haemangioblastoma.
- Phaeochromocytoma.

Other causes of ↑ Epo
- Androgen therapy.
- Cushing's disease.
- Hypertransfusion.
- Neonatal polycythaemia.

Causes of ↓ Epo
- Renal failure.
- Polycythaemia vera.
- Rheumatoid arthritis, and other chronic inflammatory diseases.
- Myeloma and other cancers.

Further reading
Cotes PM et al. The use of immunoreactive erythropoietin in the elucidation of polycythemia. N Engl J Med 1986; **315**: 283–7.

Immunohaematology

Immunohaematology is the study of the effects of the immune system on the blood and its components. This includes red cells, white cells, platelets, and coagulation proteins.

Tests for antiplatelet and antineutrophil antibodies

These tests are usually requested by the Haematology Department for patients with either thrombocytopenia or neutropenia, respectively. These assays are used to detect the presence of specific antibodies against platelet or neutrophil antigens on the cell surface.

Antibodies may be *alloantibodies* (e.g. antibody produced by the mother against fetal antigens) or *autoantibodies*, which are antibodies produced by the patient against his/her own antigens (Table 3.18).

Antiplatelet antibody tests

Generally platelet immunofluorescence tests (PIFT) or monoclonal antibody immobilization of platelet antigens (MAIPA) are used. These are useful for detecting even weak antibodies or where there are only a few antigenic sites per cell.

Table 3.18 Disorders with neutrophil-specific allo- and autoantibodies

Disorders with neutrophil-specific alloantibodies
- Neonatal alloimmune neutropenia.
- Febrile transfusion reactions (HLA antibodies).
- Transfusion-related acute lung injury (TRALI).

Disorders with neutrophil-specific autoantibodies
- Primary autoimmune neutropenia.
- Secondary:
  - SLE.
  - Evans' syndrome (AIHA + ↓ platelets).
  - Lymphoproliferative disorders (e.g. CLL).
  - Immune dysfunction (e.g. HIV, GvHD).

Elegant though these tests are, they are actually not useful in clinical practice for the diagnosis of neutropenia or thrombocytopenia where the cause is autoimmune, since these are largely clinical diagnoses. (Platelet-associated IgG or IgM may be high in autoimmune thrombocytopenia. However, it may also be high in non-immune causes of thrombocytopenia.) Where these tests are of value is in the neonatal setting where the neonate has low platelets or neutrophils.

Further reading

Roitt I *Essential Immunology*, 10th edn. Oxford: Blackwell Science, 2001.

Immunophenotyping

This describes the identification and counting of cell types using powerful monoclonal antibodies specific for cell surface proteins.

Uses (Table 3.19)

- Diagnosis and classification of leukaemias and lymphomas.
- Assessment of cellular DNA content and synthetic activity.
- Determination of lymphocyte subsets, e.g. CD4$^+$ T cells in HIV infection.
- Assessment of clonality.
- Allows identification of prognostic groups.
- Monitoring of minimal residual disease (MRD, the lowest level of malignancy that can be detected using standard techniques).

Terminology and methodology

Cell surface proteins are denoted according to their cluster differentiation (CD) number. Most cells will express many different proteins and the pattern of expression allows cellular characterization. Monoclonal antibodies recognize specific target antigens on cells. Using a panel of different antibodies an immunophenotypic *profile* of a sample is determined. Immunophenotyping is used in conjunction with standard morphological analysis of blood and marrow cells. The antibodies are labelled with fluorescent markers and binding to cell proteins is detected by laser. For each analysis thousands of cells are assessed individually and rapidly. Some antibodies can detect antigens inside cells.

Sample: heparin.

Monoclonal antibodies

These are so-called because they are derived from single B lymphocyte cell lines and have identical antigen binding domains (idiotypes). It is easy to generate large quantities of monoclonal antibodies (MoAbs) for diagnostic use.

- Cell populations from, e.g. PB or bone marrow (BM) samples are incubated with a panel of MoAbs, e.g. anti-CD4, anti-CD34, which are directly or indirectly bound to a fluorescent marker antibody.
- Sample is passed through a fluorescence-activated cell sorter (FACS) machine.
- FACS instruments assign cells to a graphical plot by virtue of cell size and granularity detected as forward and side light scatter by the laser.
- Allows subpopulations of cells, e.g. mononuclear cells, in blood sample to be selected.
- The reactivity of this cell subpopulation to the MoAb panel can then be determined by fluorescence for each MoAb.
- A typical result for a CD4 T lymphocyte population is shown:
  CD3, CD4 +ve; CD8, CD13, CD34, CD19 –ve.

Leukaemia diagnosis: common patterns (profiles)

- **AML**: CD13+, CD33+, ± CD34, ± CD14 +ve.
- **cALL**: CD10 and TdT +ve.
- **T-ALL**: cCD3, CD7, TdT +ve.
- **B-ALL**: CD10, CD19, surface Ig +ve.
- **CLL**: CD5, CD19, CD23, weak surface Ig +ve.

Table 3.19 Uses of immunophenotyping

Surface immunophenotyping	Leukaemias
	Lymphomas
	CD4:CD8 ratios in HIV infection
DNA content of tumours	Ploidy
	S phase analysis
	Proliferation markers
TdT measurement	In leukaemias & lymphomas
BMT/stem cell transplantation	
Antiplatelet antibody detection	
Reticulocyte counts & maturation	
Apoptosis	
Detection of small numbers of cells	E.g. fetal cells in mother's circulation, microorganisms in blood

Adapted from Provan et al. (2004).[1]

Clonality assessment

Particularly useful in determining whether there is a monoclonal B cell or plasma cell population.

► Monoclonal B cells from, e.g. non-Hodgkin's lymphoma (NHL) will have surface expression of κ or λ light chains, but not both.

► Polyclonal B cells from e.g. patient with infectious mononucleosis will have both κ *and* λ expression.

Further reading

🕮 http://pleiad.umdnj.edu/hemepath/immuno/immuno.html
🕮 http://www.bcshguidelines.com/pdf/CLH135.PDF
🕮 http://www.bcshguidelines.com/pdf/clh253.pdf
🕮 http://www.bcshguidelines.com/pdf/clh190.pdf

1 Provan D et al. Oxford Handbook of Clinical Haematology, 2nd edn, Oxford: Oxford University Press, 2004.

Cytogenetics

Uses

- The study of chromosomes.
- Looks at the number of chromosomes in each cell.
- Detects structural abnormalities between chromosome pairs.

Chromosome abnormalities may be constitutional (inherited) or acquired later in life. Cytogenetic analysis of chromosome structure and number has been used for many years for the study of disorders, such as Down's syndrome. Acquired chromosomal abnormalities are found in malignancies, especially haematological tumours. The analysis and detection of cytogenetic abnormalities is known as *karyotyping*. Because of the complexity of this subject area, we will concentrate on two main areas where chromosome analysis is of value.

- Prenatal diagnosis of inherited disorders:
  - Detection of common aneuploidies (gain or loss of chromosomes).
  - Detection/exclusion of known familial chromosome abnormalities.
- Detecting acquired chromosome abnormalities for:
  - Diagnosis of leukaemia subtypes, e.g. t(15;17) characteristic of AML M3 subtype.
  - Markers of prognostic information in a variety of diseases such as leukaemias, e.g. t(9;22) in acute leukaemias, N-myc amplification in neuroblastoma.
  - Monitoring response to treatment (in CML the Philadelphia chromosome, t(9;22), should disappear if the malignant cells are killed).

Principal indications for cytogenetic analysis are therefore

- Haematological malignancies at diagnosis (assuming the bone marrow is infiltrated).
- Infiltrated solid tumour tissue at diagnosis.
- Patients with equivocal morphology (e.g. type of leukaemia not clear using microscopy and other markers).
- FISH analysis when required in certain treatment protocols, e.g. MRC.
- Confirmation of disease relapse.
- Accelerated phase or blast crisis in CML.

Cytogenetic assays are expensive (around £250 for a leukaemia or lymphoma karyotype) and if there is any doubt as to whether the test is indicated we would suggest you discuss the case with one of your seniors or the cytogenetics staff. Arranging karyotyping before or during pregnancy is generally carried out by the obstetrician in charge of the woman's care.

See Table 3.20.

Table 3.20 Cytogenetic terminology

Constitutional	Present at conception or arising during embryonic life
Acquired	Arise later in fetal life or after birth
Translocation	Exchange of material between chromosomes
Deletion	Loss of part of a chromosome
Duplication	Part of a chromosome is gained
Inversion	Part of a chromosome is rotated through 180°
Diploid	46 chromosomes (somatic cell)
Haploid	23 chromosomes (germinal cell, e.g. egg or sperm)
Trisomy	Extra copy of a chromosome
Monosomy	Loss of a chromosome
Aneuploidy	Loss or gain of certain chromosomes, e.g. monosomy or trisomy

Cytogenetics: prenatal diagnosis

This allows both the detection of genetic diseases associated with specific chromosomal abnormalities, thereby offering the possible prevention of an affected child. With the advent of chorionic villus sampling (ChVS) in the first trimester, karyotyping can be done at an early stage of development (Figs 3.18 & 3.19). Pre-implantation genetic diagnosis allows abnormalities to be detected even before implantation has occurred.

Sample: amniotic fluid (15–16 weeks' gestation).

Tests available

- α-Fetoprotein level.
- Chromosome analysis.
- Biochemical tests, e.g. acetylcholinesterase.

Sample: ChVS (9–12 weeks' gestation).

Tests available

- DNA analysis.
- Chromosome analysis.
- Biochemistry tests.

Procedure (in brief)

1 Cells are obtained using amniocentesis, ChVS, or fetal blood sampling.
2 Cells are cultured in medium.
3 Cell division is arrested at metaphase using, e.g. colchicine.
4 Chromosomes are spread onto slides and stained.
5 Chromosomes are examined directly using light microscopy or with the aid of a computerized image analysis system.

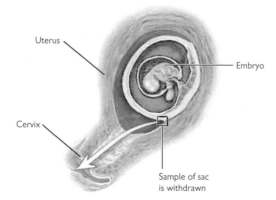

Fig. 3.18 Diagram showing method of chorionic villus sampling.

1	2	3			4	5

6	7	8	9	10	11	12

13	14	15	16	17	18

19	20	21	22	X	Y

Fig. 3.19 Normal karyotype showing metaphase chromosomes (22 autosomes, 1–22, and 2 sex chromosomes, XX or XY depending on sex of patient).

Chromosome anatomy

Note: the banding pattern which helps identify individual chromosomes, along with position of the centromeres (mitotic spindle attaches to these during cell division), short (*p*) and long (*q*) arms, and telomeres (chromosome ends). See Fig. 3.20.

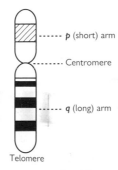

----- *p* (short) arm

------- Centromere

----- *q* (long) arm

Telomere

Fig. 3.20 Chromosome anatomy: note short (*p*) arms and long (*q*) arms.

Further reading

Rooney DE. *Human Cytogenetics*, Vol 2, 2nd edn, Oxford: Oxford University Press, 2001.
✍ http://www.pathology.washington.edu/galleries/Cytogallery/
✍ http://www.infobiogen.fr/services/chromcancer/Anomalies/Anomliste.html

Cytogenetics: haematological malignancies

Uses
- Aids the diagnosis and classification of haematological malignancy.
- Assessment of clonality.
- Identification of prognostic groups.
- Monitoring response to therapy.
- Determining engraftment and chimerism post-allogeneic transplant.

Terminology
- Normal somatic cell has 46 chromosomes; 22 pairs, and XX or XY.
- Numbered 1–22 in decreasing size order.
- 2 arms meet at centromere—short arm denoted *p*, long arm is *q*.
- Usually only visible during condensation at metaphase.
- Stimulants and cell culture used—colchicine disrupts the spindle apparatus thereby arresting cells in metaphase.
- Chromosomes are G-banded using Giemsa or Leishman's stain to create characteristic banding patterns along the chromosome. The regions and bands are numbered, e.g. p1, q3, etc.

Common abnormalities
- **Whole chromosome gain**: e.g. trisomy 8 (+8).
- **Whole chromosome loss**: e.g. monosomy 7 (−7).
- **Partial gain**: e.g. add9q+, or partial loss, e.g. del5q−.
- **Translocation**: material exchanged with another chromosome; usually reciprocal, e.g. t(9;22)—the Philadelphia translocation.
- **Inversion**: part of chromosome runs in opposite direction, e.g. inv(16) in M4Eo.
- Many translocations involve breakpoints around known oncogenes, e.g. bcr, ras, myc, bcl-2.

Molecular cytogenetics
- Molecular revolution is further refining the specific abnormalities in the genesis of haematological malignancies.
- Techniques such as fluorescence *in situ* hybridization (FISH) and PCR can detect cryptic abnormalities.
- Bcr-abl probes are now used in diagnosis and monitoring of treatment response in CML.
- IgH and T cell receptor (TCR) genes are useful in determining clonality of suspected B and T cell tumours, respectively.
- Specific probes may be used in diagnosis and monitoring of subtypes of acute leukaemia, e.g. AML, e.g. *PML-RARA* in AML M3, t(9;22), t(12;21), and 11q23 rearrangements in paediatric acute lymphoblastic leukaemias.

Table 3.21 Karyotypic abnormalities in leukaemia and lymphoma

CML	
t(9;22)	Philadelphia chromosome translocation creates bcr-abl chimeric gene.

AML	
t(8;21)	AML M2, involves AML-ETO gene—has better prognosis.
t(15;17)	AML M3 involves PML-RARA gene—has better prognosis.
inv(16)	AML M4Eo—has better prognosis.
−5, −7	Complex abnormalities have poor prognosis.

MDS	
−7, +8, +11	Poor prognosis.
5q− syndrome	Associated with refractory anaemia and better prognosis.

Myeloproliferative disease	
20q− and +8	Common associations.

ALL	
t(9;22)	Philadelphia translocation, poor prognosis.
t(4;11)	Poor prognosis.
Hyperdiploidy	Increase in total chromosome number—good prognosis.
Hypodiploidy	Decrease in total chromosome number—bad prognosis.

T-ALL	
t(1;14)	Involves tal-1 oncogene.

B-ALL and Burkitt's lymphoma	
t(8;14)	Involves myc and IgH genes, poor prognosis.

CLL	
+12, t(11;14)	

ATLL	
14q11	

NHL	
t(14;18)	Follicular lymphoma, involves bcl-2 oncogene.
t(11;14)	Small cell lymphocytic lymphoma, involves bcl-1 oncogene.
t(8;14)	Burkitt's lymphoma, involves myc and IgH genes.

Further reading

Heim S, Mitelman F. *Cancer Cytogenetics*, 2nd edn, New York: Wisley-Liss,1995.

Kingston HM. *ABC of Clinical Genetics*, 2nd edn, London: BMJ Books,1994.

Sandberg AA.*The Chromosomes in Human Cancer and Leukemia*, 2nd edn, New York: Elsevier Science, 1990.

Human leucocyte antigen (tissue) typing

The HLA (human leucocyte antigen) system or major histocompatibility complex (MHC) is the name given to the highly polymorphic gene cluster region on chromosome 6, which codes for cell surface proteins involved in immune recognition.

Uses

Tissue typing patients (to ensure compatibility between donor and recipient) who are undergoing transplantation to reduce the likelihood of rejection or graft-versus-host disease in the following types of transplant:

- Heart.
- Lung.
- Liver.
- Kidney.
- Bone marrow.
- Stem cells.

The gene complex is subdivided into 2 regions

Class 1
- The A, B, and C loci.
- These proteins are found on most nucleated cells and interact with CD8+ T lymphocytes.

Class 2
- Comprised of DR, DP, DQ loci present only on B lymphocytes, monocytes, macrophages, and activated T lymphocytes.
- Interact with CD4+ T lymphocytes.

- Class 1 and 2 genes are closely linked so one set of gene loci is usually inherited from each parent, although there is a small amount of cross-over.
- There is ~25% chance of 2 siblings being human leucocyte antigen (HLA) identical.
- There are other histocompatibility loci apart from the HLA system, but these appear less important generally except during HLA matched stem cell transplantation when even differences in these minor systems may cause graft versus host disease (GvHD).

Typing methods

Class 1 and 2 antigens were originally defined by serological reactivity with maternal antisera containing pregnancy-induced HLA antibodies. There are many problems with the technique and it is too insensitive to detect many polymorphisms. Molecular techniques are increasingly employed, such as SSP. Molecular characterization is detecting enormous class 2 polymorphism.

Importance of HLA typing

- Matching donor/recipient pairs for renal, cardiac, and marrow stem cell transplantation.
- Degree of matching more critical for stem cell than solid organ transplants.
- Sibling HLA-matched stem cell transplantation is now treatment of choice for many malignancies.
- Unrelated donor stem cell transplants are increasingly performed, but outcome is poorer due to HLA disparity. As molecular matching advances, improved accuracy will enable closer matches to be found and results should improve.

Functional tests of donor/recipient compatibility

- **Mixed lymphocyte culture (MLC)**: now rarely used.
- **Cytotoxic T lymphocyte precursor assays (CTLp)**: determine the frequency of cytotoxic T lymphocytes in the donor directed against the recipient. Provides an assessment of GvHD occurring.

HLA-related transfusion issues

- HLA on WBC and platelets may cause immunization in recipients of blood and platelet transfusions.
- May cause refractoriness and/or febrile reactions to platelet transfusions.
- Leucodepletion of products by filtration prevents this (the National Blood Service removes the WBCs at source routinely nowadays).
- Diagnosis of refractoriness confirmed by detection of HLA or platelet-specific antibodies in patient's serum.
- Platelet transfusions matched to recipient HLA type may improve increments.

Further reading

℘ http://www.ebmt.org/4Registry/Registry_docs/HLA%20MANUAL%2003_2004.pdf
℘ http://content.nejm.org/cgi/content/full/343/10/702?ijkey=oOilwRsUqacag
℘ http://medind.nic.in/jaa/t0J/i3/jaat03iJp79.pdf

Southern blotting

This technique has been around since the mid-1970s. It explained much about the physical structure of genes and was a major advance in the diagnosis of many single gene disorders. The method is simple and elegant, but time-consuming. Not used as much today with the advent of PCR technology. Southern blotting relies on the physical nature of DNA, whereby single strands are able to recognize and bind to their complementary sequences (Fig. 3.21).

Sample: EDTA sample (heparin can be used, but beware inhibitory effect on PCR amplification; if any chance PCR required, send EDTA).

Procedure

1 Genomic (i.e. total) DNA is extracted from WBC in EDTA blood sample.
2 DNA is digested with bacterial restriction endonucleases (enzymes cleave DNA at specific sequences—each enzyme recognizes a different DNA sequence).
3 After digestion of the DNA, the fragments are separated on the basis of size using agarose gel electrophoresis (smallest fragments travel the farthest).
4 The fragments are transferred to a nylon membrane and fixed permanently to the membrane using ultraviolet (UV) light.
5 Membranes are 'probed' using specific (known) gene probes that are radioactively labelled using ^{32}P.
6 The location of specific binding is detected by placing the membrane next to radiographic film (standard X-ray film).
7 The film is developed using standard techniques and the autoradiograph generated will show bands corresponding to the position of binding of the labelled probe.
8 Fragment sizes are calculated and the presence or absence of mutations is worked out by determining whether enzyme cutting sites have been lost through mutation.

Applications

• Historically, many diseases caused by single base changes (loss of restriction enzyme cutting site) have been diagnosed using Southern blotting.
• Globin gene disorders:
• Sickle cell anaemia (mutation in β-globin gene).
• Thalassaemia (mutations or deletions in α- or β-globin genes).
• Clotting disorders:
• Haemophilia.
• Analysis of immunoglobulin or TCR genes to detect clones of cells in suspected leukaemia or lymphoma.
• Detection of chromosomal translocations in leukaemia and lymphoma (e.g. t(9;22) in CML, t(14;18) in follicular lymphoma).

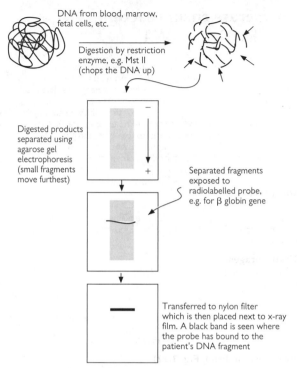

DNA from blood, marrow, fetal cells, etc.

Digestion by restriction enzyme, e.g. Mst II (chops the DNA up)

Digested products separated using agarose gel electrophoresis (small fragments move furthest)

Separated fragments exposed to radiolabelled probe, e.g. for β globin gene

Transferred to nylon filter which is then placed next to x-ray film. A black band is seen where the probe has bound to the patient's DNA fragment

Fig. 3.21 Southern blotting method.

Further reading

Southern EM. Detection of specific sequences among DNA fragments separated by gel electrophoresis. *J Mol Biol* 1975; **98**: 503–17 (▶▶ Southern's classic paper and probably *the* most cited molecular biology paper ever).

🔎 http://www.accessexcellence.org/RC/VL/GG/southBlotg.html

🔎 http://users.rcn.com/jkimball.ma.ultranet/BiologyPages/G/GelBlotting.html

Polymerase chain reaction amplification of DNA

The ability to use an enzyme to amplify specific DNA sequences has revolutionized modern diagnostic pathology. Whereas Southern blotting might take up to 1 week to produce a result, PCR can do the same thing in 2–3 h! PCR is now in routine use in the analysis of oncogenes, haematological malignancies, general medicine, infectious disease, and many other specialties. Because the system amplifies the starting DNA up to a million-fold there need only be one cell as starting material; in practice, much more DNA is required but because of the extreme sensitivity of the technique PCR has been used in forensic medicine where there may be only a few cells available for analysis (e.g. blood or semen stain).

See Fig 3.23.

Advantages
- Requires very little DNA.
- DNA quality does not matter (can be highly degraded, e.g. with age and still be amplified—DNA from Egyptian mummies has been amplified).
- Rapid results.

Disadvantages
- Expensive, but less so than it used to be.
- DNA sequence of the gene of interest must be known in order to design the short PCR primers (oligos). With the near completion of the Human Genome Project this is less of a problem now.
- Highly sensitive, and contamination of samples may occur (DNA fragments float through the air constantly; if these drop into the reaction tube a false +ve result may be obtained).

Procedure (in brief; Fig. 3.22)
- Two short DNA primers on either side of the gene of interest bind to the fragment of interest.
- The region between the primers is filled in using a heat-stable DNA polymerase (Taq polymerase).
- After a single round of amplification has been performed the whole process is repeated.
- This takes place 30 times (i.e. through 30 cycles of amplification) leading to a million-fold increase in the amount of specific sequence.
- After the 30 cycles are complete, a sample of the PCR reaction is run on agarose gel and bands are visualized.
- Information about the presence or absence of the region or mutation of interest is obtained by assessing the size and number of different PCR products obtained after 30 cycles of amplification.

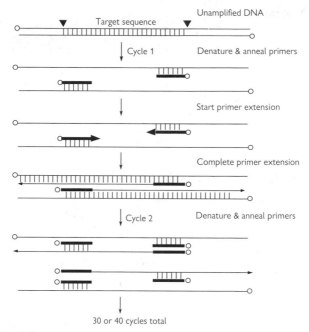

Fig. 3.22 PCR amplification method.

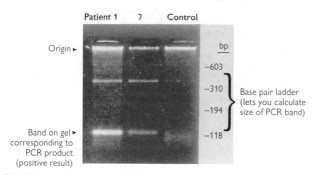

Fig. 3.23 Detection of residual leukaemia using PCR. Patients 1 and 2 have undergone chemotherapy, but as can be seen (arrow) there is still some leukaemia-specific DNA sequence present, i.e. they have minimal residual disease.

Applications

- PCR is currently used to amplify immunoglobulin genes, HIV loci, tuberculosis genes, and many other targets that are of use in molecular medicine (cystic fibrosis, haemophilia, thalassaemia, sickle cell disease, and many others).
- PCR can be used to quantitate mRNA species in blood samples and tissue samples. Allows gene 'activity' to be measured.

Further reading

Saiki RK. Primer-directed enzymatic amplification of DNA with a thermostable DNA polymerase. *Science* 1988; **239**: 487–91 (classic PCR method paper).

♪ http://nobelprize.org/chemistry/educational/pcr/

♪ http://allserv.rug.ac.be/~avierstr/principles/pcr.html

In situ hybridization & fluorescence *in situ* hybridization

Like PCR and other techniques, *in situ* hybridization and FISH are conceptually simple techniques that rely on the ability of a DNA probe to 'find' its counterpart on a chromosome, bind, and if a fluorescent tag is present it will light up the region of binding (this modification is termed fluorescence *in situ* hybridization, or FISH). These techniques have evolved from standard cytogenetic analysis of metaphase chromosomes in which metaphase chromosomes were prepared on glass slides to which specific labelled probes were applied.

Sample: Discuss with your local Cytogenetics or Haematology laboratory (they will have specialized medium for maintaining cells from blood or marrow, so that they will divide and be suitable for hybridization studies).

In situ hybridization

The location of binding of the probe is detected by visualizing the signal produced after coating microscope slides with photographic emulsion, which generate a black area around the probe which is labelled with ^{32}P.

FISH

A further modification based on the original principles, whereby specific gene probes are hybridized to chromosomes without the need for metaphase preparations (interphase cells can be used). Instead of ^{32}P the probes are labelled with fluorescent dye and hybridization may be detected as red, blue, or other coloured dots over the cells (Fig. 3.24).

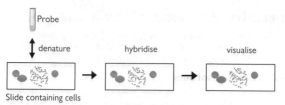

Fig. 3.24 FISH analysis. Metaphase chromosomes are placed on microscope slide, and the probe (e.g. for the gene of interest) is applied. The chromosome region to which the probe binds will fluoresce—highlighting its exact location in the genome.

Applications of FISH

- Used in the analysis of trisomies (chromosome gains) and monosomies (chromosome losses) associated with leukaemias and lymphomas. The presence of trisomy is detected as three fluorescent dots within the cell, whilst monosomy is seen as a single fluorescent dot within the cell.
- FISH has been used widely within paediatric leukaemias, such as ALL, where abnormalities of chromosome number are common.

Further reading

Mathew P *et al*. Detection of the t(2;5)(p23;q35) and NPM-ALK fusion in non-Hodgkin's lymphoma by two-color fluorescence *in situ* hybridization. *Blood* 1997; **89**, 1678–1685.
Sinclair PB *et al*. Improved sensitivity of BCR-ABL detection: a triple-probe three-color fluorescence in situ hybridization system. *Blood* 1997; **90**: 1395–402.
Vaandrager JW. Direct visualization of dispersed 11q13 chromosomal translocations in mantle cell lymphoma by multicolor DNA fiber fluorescence *in situ* hybridization. *Blood* 1996; **88**: 1177–82.
℘ http://www.slh.wisc.edu/cytogenetics/procedures/fish/fish-method.php

Specialized haematology assays

The following laboratories provide specialized molecular, biochemical and cellular investigations for rare haematological disorders. Please contact the laboratory before tests are requested to confirm the specimen(s) required.

Thalassaemia disorders

Dr John Old
National Haemoglobinopathy Reference Laboratory, Institute of Molecular Medicine, John Radcliffe Hospital, Headington, Oxford OX3 8DU

Tel: 01865-222449; Fax: 01865-222500

E-mail: jold@hammer.imm.ox.ac.uk

Professor Swee Lay Thein
Haematological Medicine, King's College Hospital, Denmark Hill, London SE5 9RS

Tel: 020-7346-1682; Fax: 020-7346-6168

E-mail: sl.thein@kcl.ac.uk

Dr Mary Petrou
Perinatal Centre, University College Hospital, 84–86 Chenies Mews, London WC1E 6HX

Tel: 020-7388-9246; Fax: 020-7380-9864

E-mail: m.petrou@ucl.ac.uk

Dr Tom Vulliamy
Haematology, ICSTM, Hammersmith Hospital, London W12 0HS

Tel: 020-8383-1136; Fax: 020-8742-9335

E-mail: t.vulliamy@ic.ac.uk

Haemoglobin variants, unstable, and altered affinity haemoglobins

Dr John Old
National Haemoglobinopathy Reference Laboratory, Institute of Molecular Medicine, John Radcliffe Hospital, Headington, Oxford OX3 8DU

Tel: 01865-222449; Fax: 01865-222500

E-mail: jold@hammer.imm.ox.ac.uk

Professor Sally Davies & Joan Henthorn[2]
Department of Haematology, Central Middlesex Hospital, Acton Lane, London NW10 7NS

Tel: 020-8453-2112; Fax: 020-8965-1115

E-mail: sally.davies@dol.gso.gov.uk

Professor Joan Henthorn
Department of Haematology, Central Middlesex Hospital, Acton Lane, London NW10 7NS

Tel: 020-8453-2323

Dr Barbara Wild
Haematological Medicine, King's College Hospital, Denmark Hill, London SE5 9RS

Tel: 020-7737-4000 Ext 2283; Fax: 020-7346-3514

E-mail: *barbara.wild@kcl.ac.uk*

Glycolytic defects, G6PD deficiency other erythroenzymopathies

Dr Mark Layton
Haematology, ICSTM, Hammersmith Hospital, London W12 0HS

Tel: 020-8383-2173; Fax: 020-8742-9335

E-mail: m.layton@ic.ac.uk

Dr Barbara Wild
Haematological Medicine, King's College Hospital, Denmark Hill, London SE5 9RS
Tel: 020-7737-4000 Extn 2283; Fax: 020-7346-3514
E-mail: barbara.wild@kcl.ac.uk

Porphyrias

Dr Allan Deacon
Clinical Biochemistry, King's College Hospital, Denmark Hill, London SE5 9RS
Tel: 020-7346-3856; Fax: 020-737-7434

Dr Michael Badminton
Porphyria Service, Medical Biochemistry, University Hospital of Wales, Cardiff CF14 4XW

Tel: 02920-748349; Fax: 02920-748383

E-mail: badminton.mn@cardiff.ac.uk

Ms J Woolf/Dr S Whatley
Porphyria Service, Medical Biochemistry, University Hospital of Wales,

Cardiff CF14 4XW

Tel: 02920-743565

Red cell membrane defects

Dr May-Jean King
International Blood Group Reference Laboratory, Southmead Road, Bristol BS10 5ND

Tel: 0117-991-2111; Fax: 0117-959-1660

E-mail: may-jean.king@nbs.nhs.uk

Immunology & allergy

Serum immunoglobulins

Units: g/L.

Normal range (adults):
- **IgG**: 5.8–15.4g/L
- **IgA**: 0.64–2.97g/L
- **IgM (♂)**: 0.24–1.90g/L
- **IgM (♀)**: 0.75–2.30g/L

Principles of assay

The 3 main classes of immunoglobulins (Igs) are measured by either rate nephelometry or turbidimetry on automated analysers. Principles are similar, dependent on immune complex formation, using antisera specific for the class of antibody. Rarely radial immunodiffusion may be used—this is slow and less accurate. For automated analysers, coefficients of variation should be in the 5–10% range. Results are standardized against international standards. In the UK, an EQA scheme operates. Laboratories should provide normal ranges, which vary according to age and sex. Unfortunately, many laboratories do not adjust ranges for age and sex, which may lead to confusion.

Indications for testing

Measurement of serum immunoglobulin is indicated in the following:
- Suspected immunodeficiency (1° or 2°), diagnosis and monitoring.
- Suspected myeloma, plasmacytoma, diagnosis and monitoring.
- Lymphoma.
- Liver disease (1° biliary cirrhosis, hepatitis, cirrhosis).
- Sarcoidosis (diagnosis).
- Post-bone marrow/stem cell transplantation; monitoring.

Interpretation

Measurement of serum immunoglobulins does not provide categorical diagnosis in any disease. Normal serum immunoglobulins do not exclude immunodeficiency. In all cases, measurement of immunoglobulins must be accompanied by serum electrophoresis, and immunofixation to look for paraproteins (see ☐ Electrophoresis and immunofixation, p315).

Causes of hypogammaglobulinaemia

- X-linked agammaglobulinaemia (absent B cells; all immunoglobulins low/absent).
- Common variable immunodeficiency (reduced T/B cells; low immunoglobulins).
- Hyper-IgM syndrome (normal/raised IgM, low/absent IgG, IgA).
- Selective IgA deficiency (absent IgA, normal IgG, IgM).
- Severe combined Immunodeficiency (mainly children; all immunoglobulins low; absent T cells).
- Lymphoma (reduced IgM, IgA normal; IgG normal or low; disease, chemotherapy, or radiotherapy).
- SLE (rare).

- **Infections**:
  - HIV (rare).
  - Herpes viruses (rare, Epstein–Barr virus in X-linked lympho-proliferative disease).
  - Acute bacterial infections.
  - Measles/rubella.
- Drugs (immunosuppressives, e.g. cyclophosphamide, azathioprine, chemotherapy).
- Plasmapheresis.
- Renal loss (IgM normal, IgG, and IgA reduced).
- Gastrointestinal loss (IgM normal, IgG, and IgA reduced).

Causes of hypergammaglobulinaemia

- **Chronic infection**: all immunoglobulins ↑.
  - Osteomyelitis.
  - Bacterial endocarditis.
  - Tuberculosis.
  - Chronic inflammation.
- **SLE, rheumatoid arthritis**: all immunoglobulins ↑.
- **Sjögren's syndrome**: ↑ IgG (all IgG$_1$).
- **Sarcoidosis**: ↑ IgG and IgA, IgM usually ↔.
- **Liver disease**:
  - Primary biliary cirrhosis (IgM, may be very high e.g. > 30g/L) with small monoclonal bands on a polyclonally raised background.
  - Alcohol-related (↑ IgA, polyclonal, β–γ bridging on electrophoresis).
  - Autoimmune hepatitis (↑ IgG, IgA; IgM ↔).
- **Hodgkin's disease**: IgE ↑ (also eosinophilia).
- **Viral infections**:
  - Acute common viral infections: ↑ IgM, ↔ IgG and IgA.
  - Human immunodeficiency virus (HIV)—all immunoglobulins ↑ (IgG very high but *polyclonal*).
  - Epstein–Barr virus (EBV)—all ↑.

Critical action

All patients with recurrent infections* should be reviewed by an immunologist or paediatric immunologist. Any patient with recurrent infections and ↓ serum immunoglobulins has an immunological problem until proven otherwise.

Patients with unusual infections, or with illness caused by opportunist or normally non-pathogenic organisms infections, and patients with infections in unusual sites (without good reason) should all be referred for further investigation.

---

*Recurrent infections can be pragmatically defined as 2 or more major microbiologically/virologically proven infections, requiring hospitalization, within 1 year. One major and recurrent minor infections should also be referred, where minor are documented infections requiring treatment in the community.

Immunoglobulin G subclasses

Units: g/L.

Normal range (adults):
- **IgG₁**: 2.2–10.8g/L
- **IgG₂**: 0.5–8.0g/L
- **IgG₃**: 0.05–0.9g/L
- **IgG₄**: 0.0–2.4g/L

Principles of test

As for serum immunoglobulins, IgG subclasses are normally measured by nephelometry or turbidimetry. Radial immunodiffusion is still occasionally used.

Indications for testing

There are no absolute indications for testing, as significant immunodeficiency can occur in the presence of normal subclasses and, conversely, complete genetic absence of a subclass may be completely asymptomatic. Measurement is usually performed as part of the work-up of patients with recurrent infections.

Interpretation

Low levels may be significant in the context of presentation with recurrent infections. Deficiency of IgG3, which is involved in immunity against viruses, associated with asthma, and intractable epilepsy. IgG2 deficiency may be seen in patients with IgA deficiency and may be associated with poor responses to polysaccharide antigens, such as the capsular polysaccharides of bacteria.

Raised IgG1 with normal or reduced IgG2, IgG3, and IgG4 is seen in Sjögren's syndrome and is a specific pattern, which may occasionally be helpful in diagnosis.

Evaluation of specific antibody production (anti-bacterial and anti-viral antibodies)

Units: Variable: u/L, IU/mL, μg/mL.

Ranges: Variable, check with reporting laboratory.
- **Pneumococcal antibodies**: >20u/L (asplenics >35)
- **Tetanus antibodies**: >0.1IU/mL (minimum protective level)
- **Haemophilus influenzae type B**: >1.0μg/mL (full protection; asplenics >1.5)

Principles of test

Measurement of antibody production against defined pathogens or antigens purified from pathogens plays an important role in the investigation of suspected immunodeficiency. Most assays carried out by enzyme-linked immunoassay, but some viral antibodies are still measured by haemagglutination or complement fixation. Pre- and post-immunization samples should be run on the same run for direct comparison as the coefficients of variation for the assays tend to be high: 15–25%! An EQA scheme exists. Assays have tended to focus on agents for which there are safe and effective vaccines. **Live vaccines should never be given to any patient in whom immunodeficiency is suspected**.

Antibodies normally assayed in immunology laboratories include: pneumococcal polysaccharides (which may be further differentiated as IgG1 and IgG2), *Haemophilus influenzae* type B (Hib), and tetanus. Diphtheria antibodies are not run by many laboratories as the assays' performance has been so poor. Meningococcal C polysaccharide antibodies are run by a few specialized laboratories, but correlation with known clinical status has been poor. ASOT may be helpful.

Viral antibodies may be valuable, to natural exposure and immunization antigens such as polio, measles, mumps, rubella, chickenpox, EBV, and hepatitis B (if immunized).

Indications for testing

These assays should be used in the work-up of patients with suspected immunodeficiency, or in monitoring change in such patients. Responsiveness to immunization is a helpful marker of immunological recovery post-bone marrow transplant. Annual monitoring of levels may be valuable in asplenic patients, as such patients lose immunity more rapidly than a eusplenic population.

Interpretation

The interpretation is entirely dependent on the context. Assays for pneumococcal polysaccharides measure a composite of responses to the 23-strains in the Pneumovax® vaccine. This can be misleading as not all strains represented in the vaccine are equipotent as immunostimulators. This means that a 'normal' response, may actually mean a good response to the immunogenic strains masking failure of response to the less immunogenic strains. For this reason evaluation of such patients should be carried out by an immunologist with an interest in immunodeficiency. More weight should be placed on changes in response to immunization than on actual values.

A 'normal' response to immunization has never been standardized, publications frequently using different criteria, rendering comparison impossible. The following is a useful working definition:

A 4-fold rise in titre, which rises to well within the normal range.

Antibody deficiency in adults

This usually presents with upper and lower respiratory tract infections (*Streptococcus pneumoniae*, *Haemophilus*, *Staphylococcus*, *Klebsiella*), leading to chronic bronchiectasis and sinusitis. Gastrointestinal infections (*Salmonella*, *Giardia*, *Campylobacter*). Skin infections (recurrent boils); autoimmune features (idiopathic thrombocytopenic purpura (ITP), haemolytic anaemia, diabetes, thyroid disease) only in CVID not XLA. Increased incidence of lymphoma.

Normal serum immunoglobulins do not exclude antibody deficiency (IgG subclass deficiency, specific failure of antibody production against polysaccharides). Use test immunization with killed or purified component vaccines to test humoral responses.

Asplenia

Patients are at increased risk of overwhelming sepsis: *Streptococcus pneumoniae*, *Haemophilus influenzae*, *Staphylococcus aureus*, Meningococcus, *Klebsiella* species, *Capnocytophaga canimorsus* (from dog-bites), fulminant malaria, and babesiosis. Risk is lifelong. Asplenia may result from trauma, involvement in malignancy, removal for diagnosis (rarely performed for this indication today), coeliac disease and sickle disease, and rarely due to congenital absence. Serum immunoglobulins and IgG subclasses are normal, but responses to polysaccharide antigens are often poor, especially in patients with lymphoma. Blood film will show Howell–Jolly bodies. Absence of the spleen (if not known from records) will be shown by ultrasound.

Immunoglobulin D

IgD is rarely measured in clinical practice, as its main function is as a membrane receptor. Elevated levels may be seen in the periodic fever syndrome, hyper-IgD syndrome, due to deficiency of mevalonate kinase, and in IgD-secreting myeloma (very rare). Measurement is usually by radial immunodiffusion.

Electrophoresis & immunofixation

Units: Not applicable to electrophoresis (qualitative). Paraprotein quantitated by scanning densitometry reported in g/L.

Normal range: N/A.

Principles of testing

In serum or urinary electrophoresis, the relevant body fluid is applied to an electrolyte-containing agarose gel. A current is applied across the gel and causes the proteins to migrate through the gel on the basis of their charge, and to a lesser extent size, until they reach a neutral point in the electric field. The proteins are then visualized with a protein-binding stain. If the total protein is known, then the electrophoretic strip can be scanned and the absorption by the stain measured, which will be proportional to the amount of protein in the particular region in the gel. Thus, any monoclonal bands can be measured directly. This is useful for patients with myeloma, as immunochemical methods for measurement of immunoglobulins may be inaccurate in patients with myeloma.

Immunofixation is the technique by which monoclonal immunoglobulins are identified by overlaying the electrophoresed strips with anti-sera against heavy and light chains. These precipitate with the monoclonal proteins in the gel and unbound anti-sera can be washed free prior to staining.

The same techniques can be carried out with urine, although this may require concentration to provide the clearest results.

Indications for testing

Electrophoresis and, if necessary, immunofixation of serum is an integral part of measurement of serum immunoglobulins. All requests for serum immunoglobulins must have electrophoresis carried out—failure to do so will lead to important abnormalities being missed. There is no place for carrying out electrophoresis as a stand-alone test.

Interpretation

Serum electrophoresis gives valuable information, not only of immunological status, but also of other organ systems. Reports are poorly understood by clinicians and not explained by laboratories. The reports shown in Table 4.1 may be seen:

Table 4.1 Interpretation

Report	Interpretation
Reduced albumin	Chronic inflammation, nephritic syndrome
Absent α1 band	Absent/reduced α-1-antitrypsin
Increased α2 band	Chronic inflammation/infection; also seen in nephrotic syndrome, due to selective retention of α 2 macroglobulin
Increased β	Seen in pregnancy (raised β-lipoprotein) and iron deficiency (transferrin)
β–γ bridging	Caused by raised polyclonal IgA, e.g. cirrhosis of liver
Increased	Caused by polyclonal increase in IgG: infection/inflammation
Faint band(s) on polyclonal background	Caused by monoclonal escape during polyclonal response to infection/inflammation (does NOT indicate myeloma)
Monoclonal band in γ	Due to myeloma, lymphoma, and MGUS*
Absent/reduced γ	Due to inherited or acquired immunoglobulin deficiency (further investigation *essential*)

*MGUS = monoclonal gammopathy of uncertain significance—most evolve to myeloma given time (years).

Monoclonal proteins may polymerize to give more than one band. Some patients will have more than one clone present producing different immunoglobulins.

Densitometry cannot be used where the monoclonal protein overlies the beta-region, as the figures include non-immunoglobulin proteins.

Serum free light chains

Modifications in the techniques for measurement of free, as opposed to bound, light chains have been proposed as a valuable adjunct to monitoring light-chain only myelomas, which had previously been monitored by measurement of 24 h urinary light chain excretion. The urinary measurement can be problematic where there is renal impairment, and as light chains are nephrotoxic, as the disease advances, urinary measurements become less accurate.

'Bence Jones proteins'; urine electrophoresis and immunofixation

Bence Jones proteins are urinary free light chains, i.e. unbound to heavy chains. During normal antibody synthesis a small excess of light chains are produced, which are excreted. Hypergammaglobulinaemic states, such as rheumatoid arthritis and chronic infection, may therefore be accompanied by excretion of polyclonal free light chains. Monoclonal free light chains are seen in myeloma, and may be the only marker in light-chain only myelomas, which do not produce any heavy chains at all. Testing is carried out as for serum.

Cryoglobulins

Units: Usually reported qualitatively, but a 'cryocrit' can be measured in a similar way to a manual haematocrit using capillary tubes.

Normal range: Tiny amounts of cryoglobulins may be found in normal individuals.

Principle of test

Cryoglobulins are immunoglobulins that precipitate when serum is cooled. The temperature at which this occurs determines whether disease will result. If the blood circulates through a part of the body where the temperature is below the critical temperature, then the protein will precipitate in the capillaries, causing obstruction, vascular damage, and eventually necrosis. The temperature of the hand is approximately 28°C at ambient room temperature. To check for the presence of cryoglobulins, take blood using a warmed syringe into a warmed bottle and transport to laboratory at 37°C, using a thermos flask with either pre-warmed sand or water at 37°C. The laboratory will allow the blood to clot at 37°C and then cool the serum. Cryoglobulins will form a precipitate as the temperature drops. The precipitate is then washed and redissolved for analysis by electrophoresis and immunofixation. Cryoglobulins are not the same as cold agglutinins (a feature of *Mycoplasma pneumoniae* infection; see 📖 Haematology, Chapter 3).

Indications for testing

All patients with Raynaud's phenomenon of new onset, or with winter onset of purpuric or vasculitic lesions on the extremities should be tested. Chronic hepatitis C infection is often accompanied by type II cryoglobulinaemia and a characteristic syndrome: 'mixed essential cryoglobulinaemia' = autoimmune phenomena, arthritis, ulceration, glomerulonephritis, neuropathy. C3 normal, C4 ↓. Patients with myeloma, SLE, Sjögren's syndrome, and rheumatoid arthritis also at risk.

Interpretation (Table 4.2)

Table 4.2 Interpretation

Type	Nature of cryoprecipitate
Type I	All monoclonal immunoglobulin; myeloma, lymphoma
Type II	Monoclonal immunoglobulin with rheumatoid factor activity; myeloma, lymphoma, connective tissue diseases, infections (esp. HCV, SBE)
Type III	Polyclonal rheumatoid factor: connective tissue diseases, infections

Cryofibrinogen

This is found less commonly than cryoglobulins. It will not be detected unless both ethylenediamine tetra-acetic acid (EDTA) and heparinized blood samples are sent warm to the laboratory. The main association is with occult malignancy (and thrombophlebitis migrans). Also associated with: connective tissue disease, pregnancy, oral contraceptive pill (OCP) use, diabetes mellitus, and cold urticaria.

β_2-microglobulin

Units: mg/L.

Normal range: 1–3mg/L.

Principles of test

The test measures free β_2-microglobulin, which normally forms the light chain of human leucocyte antigen (HLA) class I molecules, but is shed when there is increased lymphocyte turnover. It is usually rapidly cleared by the kidneys. Measurement is usually by automated analyser, nephelometry or turbidimetry. Radial immunodiffusion (RID) is still used.

Indications for testing

The main indication is as part of the routine monitoring of patients with myeloma and HIV.

Interpretation

Levels ↑ in:
- HIV infection (surrogate marker of progression).
- Myeloma (marker of tumour mass).
- Lymphoma.
- Common variable immunodeficiency (correlation with severity).
- Renal dialysis (depending on type of membrane).

Acute phase proteins (C-reactive protein, erythrocyte sedimentation rate, serum amyloid A)

Units:
- **C-reactive protein (CRP)**: mg/L
- **Erythrocyte sedimentation rate (ESR)**: mm/hour
- **Serum amyloid A (SAA)**: mg/L

Normal ranges:
- **CRP**: 0–6mg/L
- **ESR**: see 📖 Erythrocyte sedimentation rate, p233.
- **SAA**: not measured routinely

Principles of test

As serum proteins CRP and SAA are amendable to measurement by nephelometry or turbidimetry. Measurement of the ESR is covered in Chapter 3 (📖 Haematology, Chapter 3).

Indications for testing

Acute and chronic infections, vasculitis, connective tissue disease, arthritis.

Interpretation

Clinicians are usually confused by ESR and CRP—they do not give the same information and should be used together. CRP is like blood glucose while ESR is like HbA_{1c}. CRP rises within hours of onset of inflammation/infection and falls quickly once treatment is instituted. It is therefore useful for rapid diagnosis and for monitoring response. The ESR rises slowly, being dependent, in part, on fibrinogen—a long-lived protein—and falls equally slowly (see Fig. 4.1). In active SLE, the ESR is high, but the CRP is not elevated. CRP is driven by IL-6 and may be in myeloma.

See Table 4.3 for interpretation.

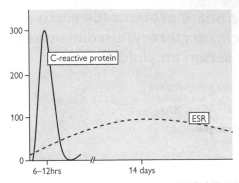

Fig. 4.1 Time course of acute phase response proteins. ESR in acute phase response parallels fibrinogen level.

Table 4.3 Causes of elevated CRP

Level of CRP	Common associations
Little or no change: (< 4–100mg/L)	Most viral infections
	Active SLE
	Systemic sclerosis & CREST
	Inactive RA
	Myeloma
	Most tumours
Moderate elevation (100–200mg/L)	EBV/CMV infection
	Bacterial infection
	Active rheumatoid arthritis
	Polymyalgia rheumatica
	Temporal arteritis
	Lymphoma
	Hypernephroma
Large elevation: (> 200mg/L)	Severe bacterial sepsis
	Legionella
	Active vasculitis (Wegener's, rheumatoid)
Huge elevation (> 400mg/L)	Overwhelming sepsis (deep tissue abscess)
	Fulminant Legionella
	At this level, death usually ensues!

Levels in very young children may be much lower for a given stimulus. A very small number of patients do not make inflammatory responses that exceed the normal range, but seem to run on a lower 'normal' range (10-fold less): ultra-sensitive assays for low level CRP are available.

Amyloidosis

Amyloid refers to the deposition of altered proteins in tissues in an insoluble form. The precursor protein varies according to the cause and can often be measured specifically. Amyloid is usually confirmed by special stains on histological examination of biopsies. Measurement of serum immunoglobulins and electrophoresis, β_2-microglobulin, and CRP is essential if amyloid is suspected (see Table 4.4).

Table 4.4 Types of amyloid

Amyloid protein	Protein precursor	Clinical syndrome
AL, AH	Light or heavy chain of immunoglobulin	Idiopathic, multiple myeloma, gamma-heavy chain disease
AA	Serum amyloid A	Secondary, reactive: inflammatory arthritis, familial Mediterranean fever, hyper-IgD syndrome, TRAPS, CINCA (periodic fever), Behçet's, Crohn's disease
Aβ_2M	β_2-microglobulin	Dialysis amyloid
ACys	Cystatin C	Hereditary cerebral angiopathy with bleeding (Iceland)
ALys, AFibA	Lysozyme, fibrinogen Aa	Non-neuropathic hereditary amyloid with renal disease
AIAPP	Islet amyloid polypeptide	Diabetes mellitus type II; insulinoma
AANF	Atrial natriuretic peptide	Senile cardiac amyloid
ACal	Procalcitonin	Medullary carcinoma of the thyroid
AIns	Porcine insulin	Iatrogenic
ATTR	Transthyretin	Familial amyloid polyneuropathy, senile cardiac amyloid
A	Aβ-protein precursor	Alzheimer's disease
AprP	Prion protein	Spongiform encephalopathies

Serum complement components

Units: g/L.

Normal ranges:
- **Complement C3**: 0.68–1.80g/L
- **Complement C4**: 0.18–0.60g/L
- Factor B (rarely measured routinely)
- Other components usually reported as percentage of normal human plasma

Principles of test

C3, C4, and factor B are usually measured by rate nephelometry or turbidimetry. Other components are measured by RID or simply by double diffusion, where presence or absence is the only result of interest. Complement breakdown products are measured by RID or enzyme-linked assay (EIA).

Indications

Valuable in suspected
- SLE (C3, C4, C3d).
- Complement deficiency (C3, C4, haemolytic complement).
- Anaphylaxis (anaphylatoxins C4a, C5a).
- Hereditary angioedema (C3, C4, C1q, C1 esterase inhibitor, immunochemical, *and* functional).

Complement deficiency is common (esp. C4 and C2 deficiency); predisposes to recurrent neisserial disease, bacterial infections (C3 deficiency) and immune complex disease (lupus-like). Anyone with more than one episode of systemic neisserial disease has a complement deficiency until proven otherwise.

C1 esterase inhibitor

Units:
- **Immunochemical**: g/L
- **Functional**: reported as percentage activity compared with normal fresh plasma

Normal range:
- **Immunochemical**: 0.18–0.54g/L (paediatric ranges not well defined, but lower than adults)
- **Functional**: 80–120% normal plasma

Principles of tests

Immunochemical measurement carried out by RID; functional assay is usually a colorimetric assay.

Indications for testing

Key indication is angioedema occurring *without* urticaria at any age. If urticaria is present, diagnosis is *never* C1-esterase inhibitor deficiency. C4 is a useful screen—normal C4 during an attack excludes C1-esterase inhibitor deficiency.

Interpretation

C1-esterase inhibitor deficiency causes hereditary angioedema.

Three types
- **Type I (common, 80%)**: absence of immunochemical C1-esterase inhibitor (C1-inh).
- **Type II (rare 20%)**: presence of non-functional C1-inh; immunochemical levels normal or high.
- **Type III**: very rare: due to gain of function mutation in Factor XII (not linked to C1-inh)

Both are inherited as autosomal dominants. Presents with angioedema, NO urticaria; may involve larynx and gut, usual onset at puberty. C4 absent during acute attacks. Treat with purified C1-inh (FFP may be a substitute, but can make attacks worse) or bradykinin antagonist icatibant; maintenance therapy with danazol, stanozolol, or tranexamic acid to decrease frequency of attacks. Pregnancy/oral contraceptive exacerbate.

Rare acquired form due to autoantibody to C1-inh (systemic lupus erythematosus (SLE), lymphoma); C1q levels are reduced and paraproteins may be present.

Haemolytic complement (lytic complement function tests)

Units: Can be reported in arbitrary units or percentage of normal plasma, but better reported as normal, reduced, or absent.

Normal range: Present (80–120% of reference plasma).

Principles of test

Haemolytic complement assays screen for the integrity of the classical, alternate pathways, and the terminal lytic sequence, and use either antibody-coated sheep cells (CH100, classical pathway) or guinea-pig red cells (CAPCH100, alternate pathway). Either a gel or liquid assay can be used, but the gel is easier! Both tests must be performed in parallel.

Indications for testing

Any patient in whom deficiency of a complement component is suspected.

Interpretation

Reduced levels of haemolytic activity will be seen during infections and during immune complex diseases, such as serum sickness and SLE. Testing for absence of a component needs to be undertaken a minimum of 4–6 weeks after recovery from infection. Absence of both CH100 and APCH100 indicates a deficiency in the terminal lytic sequence C5–C9 (C9 deficiency will give slow lysis). Absence of CH100 indicates a missing component in the classical pathway C1–C4. Absence of APCH100 indicates deficiency in alternate pathway (factor D, factor B, C3).

Follow-up testing to identify missing component will be performed by laboratory automatically (if they are doing their job!).

Critical action

Anyone who has a single episode of neisserial meningitis with an unusual strain or a second episode *must* be assumed to have a complement deficiency until proven otherwise. *Refer* after recovery to immunologist for investigation.

Immune complexes

Used in the past to monitor connective tissue disease activity, but the many different assays have given different results and have proven impossible to standardize. Therefore no longer recommended for routine clinical use.

Complement breakdown products

Measurement of specific complement breakdown products, such as C3bi and C3d are more valuable as markers of complement turnover. A number of different assays are available—your laboratory will advise. Special samples are usually required.

Factor H and factor I

Deficiency of either of these factors may lead to haemolytic-uraemic syndrome (HUS). Measurement is possible in specialized centres, with follow-up genetic testing.

Anti-C1q autoantibodies

These may be found in the hypocomplementaemic urticarial vasculitis syndrome (HUVS) and in patients with SLE, especially with proliferative nephritis.

Autoimmunity

Autoantibodies are usually divided into organ specific and organ non-specific, but clinical testing rarely follows this pattern. They are therefore covered in convenient groups, associated with types of testing.

Rheumatoid factor

Units:
- Titre (particle agglutination assay)
- IU/mL (nephelometry, EIA)

Normal range:
- **Titre <1/20**: < 16 yrs
- **Titre <1/40**: 16–65 yrs
- **Titre <1/80**: > 65 yrs
- **<30IU/mL**

Principles of test

Tests detect autoantibodies binding to human immunoglobulin: these can be of any class, but assays commonly recognize IgG and IgM auto-antibodies. Suggestions that IgA RF may be helpful have not been widely accepted. Assays use either agglutination of immunoglobulin-coated particles (visual assay) or latex particle enhanced nephelometry.

Indications for testing

Difficult to think of any indications where this test is essential. Widely abused by clinicians.

Interpretation

Not a diagnostic test for rheumatoid arthritis! Only +ve in 70–80%. High titre in patient with known rheumatoid arthritis is risk factor for extra-articular manifestations.

RF also found in:
- Healthy elderly (asymptomatic).
- Chronic bacterial (SBE) & viral infections (HIV, hepatitis C virus (HCV)).
- Acute viral infections (transient, esp. Adenovirus).
- Myeloma (often type II cryoglobulins).
- Lymphoma.
- Connective tissue diseases (SLE, Sjögren's, systemic sclerosis, polymyositis, undifferentiated connective tissue disease (UCTD)).

Antibodies to cyclic citrullinated peptides (anti-CCP, anti- mutated citrulli-nated vimentin (MCVm)) may be more valuable in identifying and monitoring RhA and are now available routinely.

Autoantibody screen

Another abused test! Usually used as an immunological fishing expedition. Multiple tissues (rodent), often with human Hep-2 cell line; gives rapid and semi-quantitative results for the following autoantibodies:
- Anti-nuclear antibodies (see Table 4.5).
- Anti-ribosomal antibodies.
- Anti-mitochondrial antibodies.
- Anti-smooth muscle antibodies.
- Anti-liver-kidney microsomal antibodies.
- Anti-gastric parietal cell antibody.

Where Hep-2 cells are used other patterns of nuclear and cytoplasmic fluorescence may be seen. See Fig. 4.2 for examples.

Principles of test

The traditional method is to overlay suitably diluted serum into frozen sections of rodent liver kidney and stomach, and human Hep-2 cells. Bound antibody in the serum is then identified using a fluoresceinated anti-human IgG (or IgM, IgA) as second stage. Slides are then read manually. Enzyme-based immunoassays are being introduced for screening, including multiplex bead-laser array systems. These can be very specific when purified or recombinant antigens are used, but lose out because of their inability to pick up unexpected patterns.

Enzyme-linked assays are used for confirming antigens, such histone antibodies and ds-DNA antibodies.

Indications

The correct use of testing is to identify which specific autoantibody is being sought as part of the differential diagnosis.

Interpretation

Because of the multiple patterns detected in this system, the interpretation for each is covered separately.

Table 4.5 Patterns of anti-nuclear antibodies (ANA)

Homogeneous	SLE, drug-induced SLE (ds-DNA or histones)
Coarse speckled	UCTD*, SLE (U1-RNP)
Fine speckled	SLE, Sjögren's (Ro and La)
Nucleolar	Systemic sclerosis, polymyositis, SLE
Centriole	Commonest in mycoplasma pneumonia; also scleroderma
Proliferating cell nuclear antigen (PCNA)	SLE—highly specific, but rare
Centromere	'CREST' syndrome, limited scleroderma, Raynaud's, never diffuse scleroderma; may be confused with multi-nuclear dot pattern, which is seen in mitochondrial antibody –ve primary1° biliary cirrhosis
Nuclear matrix Nuclear mitotic spindle	SLE and UCTD Non-specific: SLE, RhA, CREST, UCTD, and Sjögren's syndrome
Histones	SLE, drug-induced SLE (>90% of patients); other connective tissue diseases (low frequency)

*UCTD = undifferentiated connective tissue disease (previously mixed connective tissue disease).

Note: ribosomal antibodies associated with SLE especially neuro-lupus (cytoplasmic pattern not nuclear).

Titre of antibodies does NOT correlate with disease activity.

Anti-nuclear antibodies may be seen transiently after viral infections, especially in children. Therefore, observe low titre antibodies occurring in the absence of clinical symptoms compatible with a juvenile arthritis.

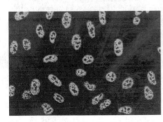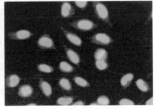

Fig. 4.2 ANA on Hep-2 cells with a speckled pattern (L) and homogeneous pattern (R).

Double-stranded DNA antibodies

Units: IU/mL.

Normal range: Varies according to assay.
- **<30IU/mL**: –ve
- **30–50IU/mL**: borderline
- **>50IU/mL**: +ve

Principles of assay

Original and still best assay is Farr assay—a radioisotope based assay. EIA tends to be widely used, but is less specific, due to frequent contamination with single-stranded DNA. Crithidia assay used only rarely as quick fluorescent screen (kinetoplast is pure ds-DNA).

Indications

Suspected SLE or autoimmune hepatitis. Used to monitor SLE, in conjunction with complement studies.

Interpretation

Sensitive and specific for SLE and AIH: +ve result is significant (in correct clinical context).

Antibodies to extractable nuclear antigens

Units: reported qualitatively.

Normal range: dependent on antibody, normally –ve.

Principles of test

Usually carried out by enzyme-linked immunoassay or immunoblot. However, counter-current immunoelectrophoresis and Western blotting are still widely used, especially for rare antibodies. EIA is much more sensitive than other methods and has led to clinical confusion.

Indications

Should always be carried out in patients with suspected connective tissue disease. Monitoring at yearly intervals should be carried out in diagnosed patients as the antibody pattern may change with time and this may correlate with changes in the clinical profile.

Interpretation

Reported qualitatively; normally laboratories will carry out a six-antigen screen: Ro, La, ribonucleoprotein (RNP), Sm, Jo-1, and Scl-70. See Table 4.6.

Table 4.6 Antibodies to extractable nuclear antigens (ENA)

Ro/SS-A	SLE, Sjögren's, neonatal lupus, neonatal congenital complete heart block (cause of ANA-negative lupus, as not picked up by standard ANA screen, which does not include Hep-2 cells)
La/SS-B	SLE, Sjögren's, neonatal lupus, neonatal congenital complete heart block (rare)
(U1)-RNP	Mixed (undifferentiated) connective tissue disease (if present alone); SLE (if present with ds-DNA)
Sm	Highly specific marker for SLE (mainly West Indians; rare in Caucasians)
Jo-1	Polymyositis, dermatomyositis; transferase syndrome (fibrosing lung disease; 65% +ve); many other specificities are known (all recognizing tRNA-transferases)
Scl-70	Systemic sclerosis (diffuse scleroderma); only 30% of patients are +ve
Pm-Scl (PM1)	Scleroderma–myositis overlap
Ku, Ki	Rare: SLE, UCTD, Sjögren's syndrome, polymyositis
Mi-2	Rare: steroid-responsive polymyositis

Monitor with CRP (differential between infection and flare of disease), C3, C4, C3d and ds-DNA antibodies (no value from serial ANA); rising titre DNA antibodies often heralds relapse (actual titre not related to disease activity; see Table 4.7).

Table 4.7 Diagnosis and monitoring of SLE

Antinuclear antibodies double-stranded DNA antibodies	Both +ve
C3 & C4	Both ↓
Complement breakdown products	↑ in active disease (C3d)
CRP	Normal
Anti-Ro	Often +ve in ANA-negative lupus
Anti-Sm	+ve in West Indian lupus
Cardiolipin antibodies & lupus anticoagulant (dRVVT)	These should usually be checked (📖 Antiphospholipid antibodies, p332)
Ribosomal P antibodies	May be a marker for neuropsychiatric lupus
C1q autoantibodies	Lupus nephritis

Antiphospholipid antibodies

Principles of testing

Many types of antibodies to phospholipids are recognized. However, routinely available tests are IgG and IgM anti-cardiolipin antibodies, detected by EIA, and the presence of a 'lupus anti-coagulant', detected using the dilute Russell viper venom test (dRVVT). *Both* tests must be carried out together as either may be positive without the other but the clinical significance is the same. Antibodies to β_2-glycoprotein I are also important as the protein is key co-factor for pathogenic antibodies. Other specificities are available only as research tools.

Indications

Patients with unexplained venous or arterial thrombosis; recurrent miscarriage (> 3), connective tissue disease, early transient ischaemic attack (TIAs) or stroke (< 60 years). Livedo reticularis is a cutaneous marker.

Interpretation

- Prolonged APTT and reduced platelet count ($80-120 \times 10^9$/L) are typical features. May get false +ve VDRL.
- Persistent +ve IgM anti-cardiolipin antibodies as only marker of syndrome unusual, but clinically significant.
- Hughes' syndrome = anti-phospholipid antibodies without evidence of other connective tissue disease or vasculitis. Presents with recurrent miscarriage, thrombosis, or strokes. Fulminant disease causes multiorgan failure.
- Antibodies also found in SLE, but NOT cerebral lupus, Behçet's, and Sneddon's syndrome. Also seen after EBV infection (asymptomatic and disappear).
- Treatment is lifelong warfarinization if symptomatic (heparin in pregnancy) if symptomatic; aspirin may be acceptable if asymptomatic (but no controlled studies). No indication for intensive immunosuppression.

Other patterns of autoantibodies identified on 'autoantibody screen'

Anti-mitochondrial antibodies (AMA) and anti-M2 antibodies

Units: Reported as titre (AMA). Anti-M2 reported as +ve or –ve.

Normal range: Not usually detectable in health.

Principles of testing

AMA are identified on fluorescent screen and previously unknown +ves should be followed up with EIA or blot-based test for anti-M2 antibodies.

Indications

Suspected liver disease, especially with ↑ alkaline phosphatase (and in females); investigation of unexplained pruritus (early feature of 1° biliary cirrhosis).

Interpretation

95% of PBC patients +ve for anti-mitochondrial antibodies (anti-M2, against dihydrolipoamide acyltransferase, E2). Remainder may have antibodies against S100 antigen of nuclear membrane (Nsp-II pattern; multinuclear dots) or gp210, another nuclear antigen. Type of antibody present has no influence on prognosis or response to therapy. Marked elevation in IgM.

Autoantibodies in autoimmune hepatitis

Units: Reported as titres (anti-smooth muscle antibodies (ASMA), anti-liver–kidney microsomal (LKM) antibodies). Anti-liver cytosol (LC-1) and soluble liver antigen (SLA) reported as +ve or −ve.

Normal range: Not usually detectable in health.

Principles of testing

ASMA and LKM are identified on fluorescent screen, and previously unknown +ves should be followed up with EIA or blot-based test for anti-LC and anti-SLA antibodies. Also do ANCA (see 📖 Vasculitic Syndromes, ANCA, p342).

Indications

Suspected autoimmune liver disease (abnormal liver function tests (LFTs), alcohol and viral infections excluded).

Interpretation

Antibodies to HCV or HCV polymerase chain reaction (PCR) +ve = exclusion criteria for auto-immune hepatitis.

Autoimmune hepatitis

- Type 1 (AIH-1) is ANA+, smooth muscle Ab (SMA)+, P-ANCA+, and soluble liver antigen (SLA) Ab+. Typically occurs in adults and has a better prognosis and responds well to therapy.
- Type 2 (AIH-2) is typically liver–kidney microsomal (LKM-1, LKM-3) Ab+ and liver cytosol (LC-1) Ab+. AIH-2 is seen in children and has a worse prognosis with poor response to therapy.
- In serological studies AIH-1 50% are ANA+/SMA+, 15% are ANA+ only and 35% are SMA+ only; however there are biopsy proven serologically −ve hepatitis. 8% of AIH-1 are SLA+ only. 43% of AIH-2 are LC-1+ only. Therefore necessary to do SLA and LC-1 tests. Prognosis is dependent on type and early diagnosis.
- Liver–kidney microsomal antibodies are also associated with drug-induced hepatitis (esp. halothane) and chronic hepatitis C or D.
- Non-actin smooth muscle antibodies may be seen in SLE and after viral infections (especially adenovirus).
- Sclerosing cholangitis may be associated with atypical P-ANCA.

Gastric parietal cell and intrinsic factor antibodies

Units: GPC may be reported as titre or simply +ve/–ve (as titre of no clinical value); IF antibodies reported +ve/–ve.

Normal range: GPC antibodies found in healthy normals without evidence of B_{12} deficiency or gastritis—may be at risk of later pernicious anaemia (PA). IF antibodies only found in PA.

Principles of testing

GPC antibodies are detected as part of the 'autoantibody screen'; IF antibodies usually detected by either radioimmunoassay or EIA, but assays are inconsistent. There is a robust EQA scheme for GPC antibodies, but none currently for IF antibodies.

Indications for testing

GPC antibodies should be checked in all patients with thyroid disease, as there is a close association ('thyrogastric disease'). Also check in patients with unexplained macrocytosis ± low B_{12}. Positive antibodies identified incidentally should be followed up with a blood count and if the MCVm is high, a B_{12} level. Intrinsic factor antibodies may help in patients with high MCVm and low B_{12} to confirm pernicious anaemia (but Schilling test is gold standard).

Interpretation

Gastric parietal cell antibodies found in 90% of patient with pernicious anaemia and in 40% of patients with other organ-specific autoimmune diseases; antigen is b-subunit of gastric H^+/K^+ ATPase. Anti-intrinsic factor antibodies are of two types: those that block B_{12} binding to IF (70% of patients with PA) and those that block uptake of the B_{12}–IF complex (35% of patients with PA).

Thyroid disease

Thyroid microsomal antibodies; thyroid peroxidase antibodies

Units: Variable—check with laboratory.

Normal range: Low levels of antibodies may be found in asymptomatic individuals, although higher levels may indicate predisposition to later development of thyroid disease.

Principles of testing

Previously, particle agglutination assays for thyroid microsomal antibodies were the mainstay; now being replaced by thyroid peroxidase (EIA). Thyroglobulin antibodies not monitored now except as part of monitoring for thyroid carcinoma (interfere with assays for thyroglobulin, which is used as a tumour marker). Antibodies to thyroid stimulating hormone (TSH)-receptor may be stimulating or blocking, but these can only be identified by bioassay or radioimmunoassay in specialized laboratories.

Indications for testing

Suspected thyroid disease and as reflex testing when thyroid function is abnormal; often now combined with thyroid testing on same analyser. Also check in patients with pernicious anaemia. Use thyroid peroxidase (or microsomal) antibodies. Other antibodies are for specialist use only.

Interpretation (Table 4.8)

Table 4.8 Interpretation	
Thyroid peroxidase (thyroid microsomal)	95–100% Hashimoto's thyroiditis 70% Graves' disease
	Highest titres seen in Hashimoto's
Thyroglobulin antibodies	Add little to diagnosis (also found in other endocrinopathies and thyroid carcinoma).
Antibodies to TSH-R (stimulating or blocking)	95% Graves' patients

Islet cell antibodies, anti-glutamic acid decarboxylase antibodies, insulin-receptor, & insulin antibodies

Units: Qualitative (previously measured in JDF units).

Normal range: 0.4% of normal population +ve for islet cell antibodies (ICA).

Principles of testing

Islet cell antibodies can be detected by immunofluorescence on pancreatic sections; other antibodies detected by EIA.

Indications for testing

All newly diagnosed early onset diabetics should be tested; they should also be tested for coeliac disease using endomysial or tissue transglutaminase antibodies. May be used to screen normoglycaemic first degree relatives for likelihood of developing diabetes.

Interpretation

Islet cell antibodies found in 75–86% of type I diabetics, but only 10% type II diabetics and 2–5% first-degree relatives. Levels decline with time and may disappear completely in longstanding type I patients. Antigen is glutamic acid decarboxylase, glutamic acid decarboxylase (GAD; similar antibodies cause stiff man (person!) syndrome although a different epitope on the molecule is recognized). Other target antigens for autoantibodies, with high specificity for diabetes, are:

- Insulin/proinsulin (seen at diagnosis in 40% type I diabetics).
- Insulin receptor (associated with acanthosis nigricans and insulin resistance).
- Pancreatic decarboxylase.
- β-cell granule protein.

Monitoring is of no value.

Note: IgE antibodies to porcine or bovine insulin may occur in insulin allergy, due to exogenous 'foreign' insulin. These may be useful in the investigation of local allergic reactions to insulin injection. Specialist advice is required on the management of this problem.

Adrenal antibodies & other endocrine autoantibodies

Units: Qualitative.

Normal range: Not detectable.

Principles of testing

Usually detected by immunofluorescence on appropriate tissue (adrenal, ovary, testis, parathyroid, pituitary). EIA for 21-hydroxylase, 17-hydroxylase, and P450 side-chain cleavage enzymes (targets of adrenal antibodies) in research centres.

Indications for testing

Suspected autoimmune endocrinopathy (adrenal insufficiency, premature ovarian failure, hypoparathyroidism).

Interpretation

Positives indicate autoimmune disease of relevant organ.

Classification of autoimmune polyglandular syndromes

Table 4.9 Classification of autoimmune polyglandular syndromes

Syndrome	Major criteria	Minor criteria
Type I	Candidiasis Adrenal failure Hypoparathyroidism	Gonadal failure Alopecia Malabsorption Chronic hepatitis
Type II (Schmidt's syndrome)	Adrenal failure Thyroid disease IDDM	Gonadal failure Vitiligo Non-endocrine autoimmunity (myasthenia)
Type III	Thyroid disease	*either* IDDM *or* Pernicious anaemia *or* Non-endocrine autoimmunity (myasthenia)

Autoantibodies & neurological disease

Principles of testing

Most neurological autoantibodies of interest are rare and are available from the Neuroimmunology Research Laboratory in Oxford. A variety of methods are used; some assays are reported with numeric values.

Indications for testing

These are restricted to very specific neurological syndromes.

Interpretation

- **Acetylcholine receptor antibodies** (ACRAb): associated with myasthenia gravis (90%). Reported numerically as high and low +ves distinguish different clinical phenotypes. May also be found in asymptomatic relatives. Striated muscle antibodies (immunofluorescence on striated muscle section) strongly associated with underlying thymoma.
- **Anti-muscle specific kinase (MUSK) antibodies**: associated mainly with bulbar and ocular myasthenia. Patients often suffer from respiratory crises.
- **Lambert–Eaton myasthenic syndrome**: occurring with small cell carcinoma of the lung, associated with autoantibodies to voltage-gated calcium channels, α & β subunits. Same tumour also associated with retinal autoantibodies (cancer-associated retinopathy, anti-recoverin antibodies). Antibodies to voltage-gated potassium channels are associated with neuromyotonia.
- **Anti-ganglioside antibodies** associated with Guillain–Barré syndrome (GM-1, GD1a) and variants (Miller–Fischer—GQ1b, GT1a), chronic variants (chronic inflammatory demyelinating polyneuropathy), and neuropathy associated with paraproteins.
- **Myelin associated glycoprotein associated antibodies (MAG)**: associated with paraproteinaemic neuropathy especially with Waldenström's macroglobulinaemia.
- **Antibodies to myelin basic protein**: found in multiple sclerosis, but not useful diagnostically.
- **Anti-Yo (Purkinje cell antibodies)**: found in paraneoplastic cerebellar degeneration (gynaecological or breast tumours associated); anti-Hu (anti-neuronal nuclear antibodies, ANNA) associated with paraneoplastic neuropathies and myelopathies (small cell carcinoma). Anti-Ri (anti-neuronal nuclei) associated with cerebellar ataxia and opsiclonus (small cell carcinoma, gynaecological or breast tumours associated).
- **Anti-neuronal antibodies**: in CSF of 74% of patients with cerebral lupus; also associated with anti-ribosomal P antibodies.
- **Anti-GAD antibodies**: found in stiff-person syndrome; same antigen to that found in pancreatic islets; diabetes usually occurs in stiff person syndrome. Antibodies appear to inhibit the production of γ-aminobutyric acid (GABA), an inhibitory neurotransmitter. Rasmussen's encephalitis associated with autoantibodies to GluR3 receptor, which cause hyperexcitability of neurones.

Vasculitic syndromes

ANCA

Units: Usually expressed as titre (qualitative EIAs are used in some centres).

Normal range: In adults, normally undetectable.

Principles of testing

Screening is usually carried out by immunofluorescence on ethanol-fixed human neutrophils. Rapid EIA screening tests exist for positive–negative testing in emergencies. EIA to specific antigens is an essential follow-up. Distinction between anti-nuclear and perinuclear staining may require the use of Hep-2 cells.

Indications for testing

Suspected vasculitis; acute glomerulonephritis.

Interpretation

- **Two main patterns recognized**: cANCA (mostly Wegener's; 90% of Wegener's ANCA +ve) and pANCA (some Wegener's, microscopic polyarteritis, Churg–Strauss syndrome, glomerulonephritis, sclerosing cholangitis, autoimmune hepatitis ulcerative colitis).
- **cANCA pattern due to antibodies against proteinase-3**: pANCA pattern due to antibodies against myeloperoxidase, lactoferrin, cathepsin, elastase. Follow-up EIA required to identify antigenic specificity: minimum PR3 and MPO enzyme-linked immunosorbant assay (ELISA); other antigens available through supra-regional referral laboratories.
- In Wegener's, monitoring titre of ANCA is useful: rising titre in a patient in clinical remission heralds relapse.
- ANCA may be seen as epiphenomenon in states of chronic neutrophil activation and turnover, e.g. cystic fibrosis.

Anti-glomerular basement membrane (GBM) disease (Goodpasture's syndrome)

Units: Qualitative (quantitation available through reference centres—used only to follow patients post-plasmapheresis or transplant).

Normal range: Not detectable in health.

Principles of testing

Usually carried out by EIA; screening by immunofluorescence is not sensitive. Biopsies will show linear IgG deposition in glomeruli (and alveoli). Antibodies recognize the NC1 region in the α3 chain of type IV collagen.

Indications for testing

Acute glomerulonephritis, particularly if associated with pulmonary haemorrhage.

Interpretation

Positive antibodies confirm Goodpasture's syndrome. Urgent plasmapheresis is required and monitoring reduction of antibody with treatment is advisable. Disease may recur in transplanted kidneys, so monitoring of antibody is advised. Some patients may be both ANCA and anti-GBM antibody +ve.

Allergic disease

Total IgE
Units: kU/L.

Normal range: <100kU/L (>14 yrs old).

Principles of testing
Previously carried out by radioimmunoassay (RIA), now by enzyme immunoassay.

Indications for testing
There are FEW indications for testing. Screening for atopic disease; investigation of suspected hyper-IgE syndrome (Job's syndrome, a rare immunodeficiency), Churg–Strauss vasculitis. Gating requests for RAST tests on the basis of IgE is scientifically unsound (see below).

Interpretation
Significant allergic disease is possible with low levels of total IgE (including anaphylaxis). Only patients with undetectable IgE (<7kU/L) are unlikely to have allergic disease. Conversely, levels above the normal range are compatible with no clinical allergic disease. IgE >1000kU/L associated with atopic eczema; IgE >50,000kU/L confirms hyper-IgE syndrome (although patients may have lower levels—diagnosis is clinical). Raised levels are also seen in parasitic infections of the bowel, filariasis, lymphoma (especially Hodgkin's disease), and Churg–Strauss vasculitis.

Further reading
🖉 http://www.worldallergy.org
🖉 http://www.aaaai.org/professionals.stm
🖉 http://www.medscape.com/allergy-immunologyhome

Skin prick tests

Units: mm wheal size, compared with histamine and saline controls.

Normal range: No wheal.

Principles of testing

This remains the gold standard for allergy diagnosis. It identifies IgE-mediated reactions (type I), such as inhalant allergy, anaphylaxis, food allergy. It is dependent on triggering release of histamine from cutaneous mast cells. Solution of allergen or controls (histamine or saline) placed on skin and pierced through by lancet. After 15 min wheal will be visible. Positive is at least 2 mm greater than −ve control. Histamine control must be +ve. Not interpretable if patient is dermographic (−ve = +ve). Can use factory prepared allergens; also use double-prick technique with fresh foods (prick food then patient)—useful where allergens are labile, e.g. fruits.

Indications for testing

Mainstay for diagnosis of all types of allergic disease. Contraindicated when there is significant skin disease, previous severe allergic reactions (use RASTs first), patients on anti-histamines (need to be off drug for a week). Other drugs will interfere, e.g. calcium channel blockers, tricyclic anti-depressants.

Interpretation

Results can only be interpreted in the context of the clinical history. Testing should be tailored to individual patients to answer specific questions. May need to be followed up by open or blinded challenges, where −ve results are obtained in patients with good histories.

Good specificity for inhalant allergens and some foods (nuts, fish); results comparable with RAST testing.

Many known families of cross-reactivity between biological families

- Latex allergy associated with food reactions: banana, avocado, kiwi fruit, chestnut, potato, tomato, cannabis, lettuce. Also birch pollen allergy commoner.
- Birch pollen allergy (asthma, rhinitis) with food-related reactions to nuts, apples, plums, cherries, carrots, and potatoes ('oral allergy' syndrome).
- Mugwort pollen and celery.
- Ragweed pollen with melon and banana.

Specific immunoglobulin E: 'RAST tests'

Units: Reported as Grades 1–6. Also as continuous numeric scale in IU/mL.

Normal range: Grades 0 & 1 indicate insignificant specific IgE (Table 4.10).

Table 4.10 Grades

Grade	IU/mL
0	<0.35
1	0.35–0.70
2	0.70–3.50
3	3.50–17.50
4	17.5–50.0
5	50–100
6	>100

Principles of testing

Previously tested by radioimmunoassay (hence, acronym RAST = radio-allergosorbent test); now identified by enzyme-linked or fluorimetric assays.

Indications for testing

'RAST' tests are expensive and should be reserved for cases where skin prick testing is not possible. Extensive skin disease, patient on anti-histamines, severe reactions, small children, dermographic patients. Testing *must* be guided by history—do not request 'allergen screen'.

Interpretation

Presence of specific IgE does *not* equate to allergic disease—indicates sensitization only. Must be interpreted in the context of the clinical history. Numerical value does *not* correlate with severity of clinical reactions.

RAST tests of little value for identifying allergy to fruits and vegetables as the allergens are labile and drugs (unreliable). False +ves possible when total IgE is very high due to non-specific binding (less of a problem with newer assays).

Mast cell tryptase

Units: mg/L.

Normal range: 2–14mg/L.

Principles of testing

Measured by EIA. Analyte is stable in clotted blood.

Indications for testing

Valuable test for the investigation of acute ?allergic reactions. Released when mast cells degranulate and stable in serum for up to 24 h. Also useful for monitoring patients with mastocytosis.

Interpretation

Raised levels indicate mast cell degranulation and will help distinguish anaphylactic and anaphylactoid reactions from other causes of reactions (vasovagal, hyperventilation, carcinoid, phaeochromocytoma, etc.).

Drug allergy testing

Investigation of severe drug allergy is a specialized field and all patients should be referred to an appropriate expert for an opinion, usually a consultant in allergy or clinical immunology in a regional centre. Testing will usually involve skin prick testing followed by intradermal testing and patch testing, and if necessary blind challenge.

Patch tests

Units: Scored qualitatively.

Normal range: –ve.

Principles of testing

This test identifies cell-mediated reactions = delayed type hypersensitivity (type IV reactions). It should not be confused with skin prick testing. Allergens in petrolatum jelly are placed in contact with the skin for 48 h under occlusion with aluminium cups. Test result is read at 96 h, looking for eczematous change and blistering. Usually carried out by Dermatology departments.

Indications for testing

Investigation of contact reactions, e.g. eczema.

Interpretation

Positive results are invariably significant. Common allergens include metals such as nickel and chromium, dyes and chemical in leather, rubber chemicals (accelerators), cosmetic chemicals. Panels of allergens used depending on clinical history.

Cellular function assays

Investigation of cellular function of lymphocytes, neutrophils, macrophages, and NK cells are restricted to specialized regional immunology laboratories. The tests are labour-intensive and difficult to standardize, with the exception of basic lymphocyte markers. EQA schemes are available only for basic lymphocyte markers.

All tests, other than basic lymphocyte markers, should only be requested after discussion with a consultant immunologist. Their role is in the investigation of suspected cellular immunodeficiency, particularly severe combined immunodeficiency (SCID) and 1° disorders of neutrophils. In such cases urgent referral of the patient to an appropriate paediatric or adult immunologist is more appropriate than fiddling around trying to get tests done, as the immunologist will have direct and immediate access to the appropriate tests. Lives have been lost due to delay in transfer while inexperienced clinicians have tried to make diagnoses.

Lymphocyte surface markers
Units: cells/mL.

Normal range (Table 4.11)

Table 4.11 Normal range	
CD3+ (total T cells)	690–2540
CD19+ (total B cells; CD20 is equivalent)	90–660
CD3+CD4+ (T helper cells)	410–1590
CD3+CD8+ (cytotoxic T cells)	190–1140
CD16+CD56+ (NK cells)	90–590

Principles of testing
Lymphocyte surface markers should be carried out on a single platform flow cytometer, which will give a direct absolute count, not requiring a total lymphocyte count from a haematology analyser. Absolute counts are the preferred value; percentages are not useful. Fresh samples are required for optimum results. Many other surface markers are available to answer more specific immunological questions, but these will usually be of interest only to clinical immunologists. An EQA scheme operates.

Indications for testing
There are no absolute indications. Investigation of lymphocyte subsets is an important part of the work-up of any patients with suspected 1° or 2° immunodeficiency and of patients with unexpected lymphopenia. Serial measurements are valuable in patients undergoing bone marrow or stem cell transplantation, with 1° immunodeficiencies, in patients on any immunosuppressive therapy and with HIV on therapy with HAART.

Interpretation

Results can only be interpreted in the context of the clinical question. Lymphocyte surface marker analysis *cannot* be used as a surrogate for HIV testing, as many acute viral and bacterial infections, as well as other medical problems, will give rise to a reduction in CD4+ T cells.

Critical action

Baby <6 months with lymphocyte count <2 × 10^9/L = SCID until proven otherwise: *immediate* referral to SCID Bone Marrow Transplant (BMT) Unit (In UK, Newcastle General Hospital, Newcastle upon Tyne and Great Ormond Street Hospital for Sick Children, London). Look at the differential white count not just the total white count!

Lymphocyte function tests

These are highly specialized and should only be carried out on the recommendation of a clinical immunologist.

Indications for testing

There are no absolute indications for testing, but it is usually carried out as part of the specialized work-up of patients with known or suspected severe combined immunodeficiency, and in the monitoring of immunological reconstitution post bone marrow transplant.

Interpretation

Is complex and dependent on the precise clinical circumstances.

Neutrophil & macrophage function

This is a specialized test. Samples do not transport well and results are often abnormal if the patient has active infection or is on antibiotics. It is preferable to refer patients to a clinical immunologist who will organize testing if appropriate.

Indications for testing

Patients with deep-seated abscesses, recurrent major abscesses (exclude diabetes, staphylococcal carriage, and hidradenitis suppurativa first), major oral ulceration, unusual fungal, or bacterial infections (*Pseudomonas*, serratia, staphylococci, *Aspergillus*). Atypical granulomatous disease, including atypical Crohn's disease. Genetic defects of neutrophil function may present at any age.

Interpretation

Interpretation is complex; defects of oxidative metabolism may indicate chronic granulomatous disease; defects of phagocytosis are recognized. Also myeloperoxidase deficiency. Neutropenia may be chronic or cyclical. Genetic testing to follow-up may be required.

NK cell function

Is rarely required. Main indication is in recurrent severe infection with herpes viruses. Assays are complex and need specialist interpretation. Always discuss cases with a clinical immunologist.

Immunology websites

Immunology and general medicine

ℳ http://www.specialtylabs.com/books/default.asp
ℳ http://www.emedicine.com/

European Federation of Immunological Societies

ℳ http://www.efis.org/

American Academy of Allergy, Asthma, & Immunology

ℳ http://www.aaaai.org/professionals.stm

Infectious & tropical diseases

Introduction to infectious diseases

Everything about microscopic life is terribly upsetting…how can things so small be so important? (Isaac Asimov—1920–92).

An old enemy

Infectious diseases have had a huge impact on the human species. Throughout history mighty armies have been humbled by microbiology. After the introduction of effective antibiotics during the Second World War, there was great optimism that the fight against infectious diseases had been won. In recent years this hope has been dramatically dashed. Almost all new diseases are infections, and some of the 21st century's most pressing problems are pathogens that have only appeared in the 30 yrs prior to this book being written. Globally, the most important of the newer organisms are human immunodeficiency virus (HIV) and hepatitis C, though old enemies such as tuberculosis (TB), pneumococcus, and malaria are still killing millions throughout the world.

New challenges

As we enter the 21st century several factors are serving to increase the relative importance of infection over other areas of medicine. New infections such as SARS and avian/swine influenza are continually emerging. Anti-microbial resistance is increasing, methicillin-resistant *Staphylococcus aureus* (MRSA) being the most infamous example. There are more immunosuppressed patients as a result of increased use of chemotherapy agents and organ transplantation. Tourists and other travellers are making their way to ever more remote parts of the world. Migration of populations has always spread disease and this continues today. Most alarmingly, there are concerns of bioterrorism. All of these factors mean that the infectious differential diagnosis—even in the developed world—grows ever longer.

It is always worth bearing in mind that the infectious diseases in a differential diagnosis are often treatable. Accordingly, it is always better to consider treatable options over incurable ones. Furthermore, some infectious diseases like MDR-TB and avian/swine influenza have major public health consequences.

A challenge to the clinician

The same infectious disease is often capable of causing a wide variety of clinical pictures. HIV, for example, is a great mimicker. This is not so surprising given the genetic variety of mankind; hence, individually-tailored responses to a bewildering variety of infecting agents. Some clinical syndromes can be caused by many quite different pathogens. Good examples include pneumonia, hepatitis, and endocarditis.

Furthermore, some infectious diseases can resemble non-infectious diseases. For example, amoebic colitis can resemble ulcerative colitis, syphilis can present with serious psychiatric symptomatology, a brain abscess or a tuberculoma can resemble a brain tumour, and tuberculosis of the vertebral column can resemble metastatic malignancy. Getting it wrong can be catastrophic for the patient.

Other diseases can mimic infections

Non-infectious diseases can resemble infection. Examples include gout of the first metatarso-phalangeal joint, rather than cellulitis; cervical lymphade-nopathy due to lymphoma, rather than tuberculosis; familial Mediterranean fever as a cause of PUO; SLE leading to Libman–Sachs endocarditis; adult Still's disease as a cause of fever and neutrophilia; inflammatory carcinoma of the female breast resembling a pyogenic breast abscess.

The importance of epidemiological factors

Epidemiology is fundamental to determining which, if any, infecting agents, and therefore investigations, are relevant in a given patient.

Geography: This is very important.

Some infections are common the world over and include
- *Salmonella* infections.
- Pneumococcal pneumonia.
- Gonorrhoea.
- Thrush (candidiasis).
- Tuberculosis.
- Influenza.
- Epstein–Barr virus (EBV).
- HIV (although sub-Saharan Africa is the worst affected area).
- Hepatitis C.
- Herpes simplex.
- Threadworm (*Enterobius*).

Some infectious diseases are only common in the developing world, e.g.
- Malaria.
- Syphilis.
- Diphtheria (although still common in Eastern Europe).
- Rheumatic fever.
- Enteric fever (typhoid and paratyphoid).
- Hepatitis E.
- Poliomyelitis.
- Rabies (although Eastern Europe has significant disease).
- Viral haemorrhagic fever.
- Onchocerciasis (river blindness).
- Schistosomiasis.
- Leishmaniasis (although commonly found around the Mediterranean sea).
- Ascariasis.
- Cutaneous myiasis (e.g. tumbu fly).

Some infectious diseases are common in some parts of the developed world, but not in others including
- Lyme disease.
- Babesiosis.
- Ehrlichiosis.
- Histoplasmosis.
- Hydatid disease.
- Anisakiasis.

In the USA, only certain areas are endemic for
- Lyme disease.
- Coccidioidomycosis.
- Babesiosis.
- Histoplasmosis.

Travel history: This is important for many reasons. Travel exposes patients to new infectious agents to which they have no immunity. The clinician must therefore be aware of the distribution of common infections. Great variation in antibiotic resistance patterns can be observed in different parts of the world; this clearly has in impact on choice of empirical treatment. Finally, travel often has an impact on patterns of sexual and risk-taking behaviour (Fig. 5.1).

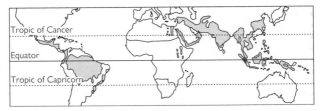

Fig. 5.1 The importance of taking a geographic history. Malaria, which can be life-threatening, is a very common disease in many parts of the world, but is not indigenous to most parts of the developed world. Making a diagnosis depends heavily upon the clinician eliciting the clues in the patient's history. Even if s/he has been taking antimalarial drugs, a patient who has been on holiday to Kenya, Thailand, or Brazil may die if the disease is not diagnosed. Clinical suspicion should lead to blood films (on 3 consecutive days) and a platelet count. Bear in mind that the patient may not have been taking adequate prophylaxis, may have been missing tablets, or may not have been absorbing them.

Sexual and drug-taking activity: Searching and personal questions may need to be asked. This is always difficult to do, even with great experience. Patients will rarely admit to high risk sexual activity or the use of illegal substances and may need to be pressed. The clinician must maintain a high clinical suspicion at all times, even and especially when the patient does not fit a social stereotype. Bear in mind that any patient may have a 'double life' that even his/her spouse is unaware of. It is dangerous for the clinician to assume that being married equates to sexual fidelity or even heterosexuality.

It may not be immediately obvious that the fever, rash, and hypotension in a woman may be related to her tampon usage (toxic shock syndrome), yet menstruation can be a difficult subject to discuss in some cultural settings. TB of the female genital tract may present as infertility or menorrhagia. 'Lumpy semen' may be indicative of *Schistosoma haematobium* infection, and a 'urinary tract infection' in a 19-yr-old man may be gonorrhoea.

Social and professional: Pets, hobbies, and jobs may well be important. The patient with pneumonia and a budgerigar could have psittacosis. The tropical fish salesman with a chronic rash on his hand could have *Mycobacterium marinum* infection (aka 'fish tank granuloma'). The jaundiced volunteer cleaning out canals at weekends could have leptospirosis related to contact with rats. The cat owned by the middle-aged lady with recurrent axillary lymphadenopathy may be the key to her problem.

Sexual history
e.g. HIV, syphilis, PID, herpes simplex, etc.

Contact with animals (job, hobbies, pets, etc.)
e.g. tuberculosis, brucella, psittacosis, leptospirosis, etc.

Travel history
(holidays, business, military, etc.)
e.g. malaria, VHF, Legionnaire's disease, gastroenteritis, etc.

Drug-injecting history
e.g. HIV, HCV, HBV, endocarditis, deep sepsis

Menstrual history
Toxic shock syndrome

Fig. 5.2 Infection and history taking.

Assessing the patient
The recognition of an infectious disease in a patient (or the absence of one) goes far beyond the Petri dish, the microbiology bench and polymerase chain reaction (PCR) testing technology. The Andromeda Strain phenomenon (with all due credit to Michael Crichton MD) should be borne in mind. The disease in front of you might be the first ever presentation! Almost the only significant new human diseases that will appear in the future will be infectious diseases and they will keep appearing till the end of the human species (Fig. 5.2).

Assessment should include
- A detailed history.
- Full physical examination (including temperature).
- The generation of a differential diagnosis.
- Laboratory tests.
- Non-invasive procedures (including radiological tests where appropriate).
- Invasive procedures.
- The making of a definitive diagnosis (wherever possible).

When considering the possibility of an infective process, one should always consider the basic infection groups
- Bacteria (including primitive forms).
- Mycobacteria.
- Fungi.
- Viruses.
- Protozoa.
- Helminths.
- Prions.
- Myiasis.

Investigations available to the ID or general physician

Many tests will be performed with a view to making a diagnosis. Investigation of a patient should be rational and evidence-based wherever possible. Although the interrogative armamentarium of the infectious diseases and tropical medicine physician is enormous—as with any other branch of medicine, the history, and examination will point the way. Results will emerge which, while not producing a diagnosis as such, will nevertheless require following up. For example, low C5 levels in recurrent meningococcal septicaemia may need immunological assessment. IgG deficiency leading to recurrent pneumonia may require regular infusions of gamma globulins. A low CD4+ cell count, which is not due to HIV infection, could be a feature of sarcoidosis.

Making a diagnosis alone is not the only issue at stake. Some tests must be done if a patient is going to be treated safely. Examples might include: glucose-6-phosphate dehydrogenase (G6PD) levels before administering primaquine for hypnozoite eradication in malaria; TB cultures for antibiotic sensitivity prior to starting empirical therapy; exclusion of pregnancy before using certain antibiotics such as doxycycline and ciprofloxacin. Other tests relate to the fact that some infectious diseases are dangerous to others: prime examples of this would be multi-drug-resistant tuberculosis (MDR and XDR-TB) and SARS, both of which are potentially dangerous for the population at large and need to be identified (or at least suspected wherever appropriate) and treated in an isolation unit.

Investigating the infectious diseases/ tropical medicine case

Available diagnostic techniques

Direct detection
- **Microscopy**:
  - *Direct*—e.g. faecal parasites (± iodine) or malarial and trypanosomal blood films.
  - *Special stains*—these include Gram and Ziehl–Nielsen stains.
  - *Electron microscopy*—for viruses and other pathogens.
- **Presence of toxin**: e.g. *Clostridium difficile*.
- **Antigen detection**: see ☐ Serology, p364.
- **Molecular assays**: see ☐ Molecular diagnostics, p373. These include gene probes, amplification assays, e.g. PCR.

Culture
- Almost all body fluid and tissues can be cultured. As a general principle, the larger the sample sent, the greater the yield. It is good practice to forewarn the laboratory before sending any unusual samples. Laboratory preparation and specialist containers may be required. Adequate clinical details should be written on any request forms. The choice of culture technique can vary dramatically depending on the organism that is being sought. There may be only one chance to culture the correct bacteria so it should not be wasted.
- Identification through special growth media, culture temperature or atmosphere.[1]
- Identification of individual colonies by biochemical reactions (e.g. catalase or coagulase).
- Identification with specific antisera (i.e. latex agglutination).
- Identification using molecular-based methods (e.g. specific probes, restriction enzyme patterns, DNA sequencing).
- Antimicrobial susceptibility testing, if indicated.

Serology (☐ Serology, p364).

Other tests as appropriate (see appropriate sections)
- Biochemistry.
- Haematology.
- Immunology.
- Molecular tests.
- Radiology.
- Stool & bowel contents.
- Tissue biopsy and deep aspiration specimens.
- Other tests.

Culture techniques

Micro-organisms exist in nature as mixed populations. Diagnosis of an infection means identifying the relevant pathogen in the face of this plethora of 'pretenders to the crown'. Furthermore, different organisms can cause the same disease (e.g. pneumonia), and require very different treatment and management and have different prognoses. While some specimens (e.g. stool, sputum) contain extremely large numbers of varied organisms, some specimens (e.g. blood, cerebrospinal fluid (CSF), urine) should be sterile unless infected or contaminated during their collection.

Microbiological culture assists with the aetiological diagnosis of bacterial, fungal, protozoal, or viral illness by enabling identification and susceptibility testing of the isolated organism(s). Bacterial culture was the first to evolve, but useful data on other pathogenic groups can also be obtained through the use of culture-based methodologies (although options for treatment are currently more limited for viruses and fungi than for bacteria). Furthermore, culture of viruses and fungi usually takes longer than most bacterial culture; therefore, the data obtained is most valuable for the late confirmation of the diagnosis or for epidemiological purposes (e.g. for predicting the appropriate constituents for a polyvalent influenza vaccine).

Bacteria

3 major steps are involved in extracting pure cultures from a diverse population of micro-organisms and identifying a pathogen. Many of these processes can now be automated (Fig. 5.3).

1. **An isolation plate is created**: To do this, the mixture must be diluted until the various individual micro-organisms have been dispersed far enough apart on an agar surface so that, after incubation, they will form visible colonies isolated from the colonies of their neighbours. Specialized culture media (such as selective media, differential media, enrichment media, and combination selective and differential media—a great many exist) may be used to supplement mechanical techniques of isolation. Culture can be aerobic or anaerobic. (**Note**: specimens for the isolation of anaerobic pathogens require special care as anaerobic bacteria die in the presence of oxygen. Such specimens should therefore be transported in a reduced container.) Lastly temperature can be used to further select for pathogenic organisms, for example *Campylobacter jejuni* is unusual as it will grow at 41°C.

2. **A pure culture is created**: To achieve this, an isolated colony will be selected out and carefully 'picked off' the isolation plate for transferring to a new sterile medium. Following incubation all the organisms in the new culture will be descendants of the same organism.

3. The organism can then be identified through various manoeuvres:

- The colony appearance and susceptibility to specific antibiotic discs.
- The microscopic appearance.
- The staining responses (e.g. Gram +ve vs. Gram –ve).
- The use of a range of biochemical tests designed to uncover characteristics typical of a particular organism, e.g. catalase reaction, sugar fermentation. The presence of the enzyme coagulase is useful for distinguishing *Staphylococcus aureus* from less pathogenic coagulase-negative staphylocci (normal skin commensals).
- The use of antisera (direct serology) for culture confirmation:
  - Agglutination and latex agglutination tests are used on colonies to identify *Escherichia coli* 0157, *Streptococcus pneumoniae*, serogroups of *Neisseria meningitidis*, *Shigella*, and *Salmonella*, Lancefield groups of β-haemolytic streptococci and serotypes of *Haemophilus influenzae*.
  - Detection of specific antigens by DFA (direct fluorescent antibody) staining can be used to identify colonies of *Streptococcus pyogenes*, *Bordetella pertussis*, and the species and serotypes of *Legionella*.
  - The Quellung reaction, which employs specific antisera to interact with capsular polysaccharides of *Streptococcus pneumoniae*, can be used to confirm the identification of the pneumococcus as well as to determine the serotype of the cultured organism.

Ideally, specimens for bacterial culture should be taken before antibiotics are administered. This may not always be feasible, but the information yielded may well be less than ideal.

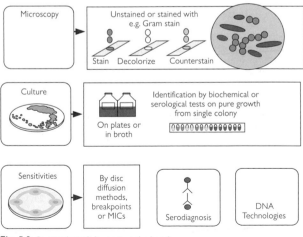

Fig. 5.3 Bacteriological diagnosis at the bench.
🔊 htttp://www.medmicro.mds.qmw.ac.uk/underground/diagnose/diagnose.html

Antibiotic sensitivity

Once a bacterium is isolated, it can be cultured in the presence of antibiotic(s) to assess if it is susceptible to that agent or not (i.e. resistant). The minimum inhibitory concentration (MIC) is the lowest antibiotic concentration at which the micro-organism under assessment shows no visible growth in vitro. The MIC can provide the clinician with precise information about the infecting bacterium's degree of antibiotic susceptibility and enable him/her to avoid antibiotics to which the organism shows resistance.

For organisms exhibiting unusual resistance patterns, susceptibility panels using methodologies such as broth microdilution, gradient diffusion, and/or disc diffusion have been created to assist clinicians.

On occasions, these data will need to be linked to testing of blood levels for some antibiotics (e.g. gentamicin, vancomycin, cycloserine). Serum bactericidal test (sbt) can be used to determine whether concentrations of the antibiotic in a patient's serum are capable of killing the infecting micro-organism.

Viruses

Viral culture differs from bacterial culture, i.e. viruses require a very different type of medium to grow in. They grow in cell cultures and are detected through the cytopathic effects that appear in cell culture (Figure 5.4). New techniques appear regularly. Indeed, viral culture is being used less commonly as molecular techniques, such as PCR become more effective and can quantitate the amount of virus present.

The appropriate type of specimen to collect, the best means of transport and the most appropriate cell culture to use will vary with the particular virus suspected, the specimen site, and the time of the year.

- The choice of specimen is very important: numerous viruses enter via the mucosa of the upper respiratory tract, yet that virus may compromise multiple or distant tissues and organs.
- Swabs can be used to collect a variety of specimens from the body surfaces for viral detection, e.g. nose, throat, eye, skin, and rectum. A naso-pharyngeal aspirate may be the more appropriate specimen if influenza is suspected. Deeper specimens, such as blood and CSF, will be appropriate for some viruses. Different viruses will need different collection approaches—for example, heparin, citrate, and ethylenediamine tetra-acetic acid (EDTA) are all acceptable for the detection of cytomegalovirus (CMV) by culture or by antigenaemia testing, but for some other viruses only citrate should be used if they are to be cultured.
- Unlike many bacterial or fungal pathogens, the time of year is important to keep in mind when making a diagnosis of certain viral diseases. For example, enteroviruses (e.g. poliomyelitis) circulate almost exclusively in the summer months and influenza likewise circulates during the winter months.

- Timing is important when collecting specimens for viral detection. They should be collected as early as possible after the onset of symptoms as once viral shedding ceases, culture will be impossible and serological and molecular techniques may be the only way of diagnosing the viral pathogen.
- Some viruses cannot be cultured—e.g. viral agents of diarrhoea (caliciviruses, astroviruses, and coronaviruses), hepatitis C virus (HCV), and hepatitis B virus (HBV).

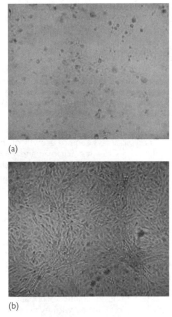

(a)

(b)

Fig. 5.4 Diagnosing viral infections using cell culture. (a) Enterovirus cytopathogenic effect from a sample of stool in monkey kidney tissue culture, and (b) normal monkey kidney tissue culture. From Grist et al. (1987).[1]

1 Grist NR et al. Diseases of Infection—an Illustrated Textbook. Oxford: Oxford University Press, 1987.

Cell culture techniques enable detection of a wide range of viral pathogens, and can allow for dual or mixed viral infections to be diagnosed. Once specimens arrive at the laboratory, they are processed and inoculated into a variety of cell cultures that support the growth of common viral isolates. The inoculated cell cultures are then examined daily for the development of a viral cytopathic effect. Viruses vary in their cell culture requirements, and laboratories must use more than one cell line for culture. For example, the respiratory viral pathogens, influenza, and para-influenza viruses favour replication in 1° cell lines, such as 1° Rhesus monkey kidney (RhMK) cells. However, respiratory syncytial virus (RSV) and adenoviruses prefer heteroploid cell lines such as human epidermoid larynx carcinoma (Hep-2) cells.

Among the newer viral culture techniques are shell vial spin amplification cultures. These offer a more rapid turnaround time than traditional viral cultures for detection of the more common respiratory viruses and some other agents. Rather than having to examine for a cytopathic effect, fluorescein-labelled monoclonal antibodies are employed to detect antigens of replicating viruses. This system can be utilized for detecting CMV, HSV, influenza A and B, parainfluenza 1, 2, and 3, adenovirus and RSV, and can detect, for example, HSV in as little as 1 or 2 days.

Laboratory assays for antiviral susceptibility testing include phenotypic and genotypic assays. Phenotypic assays require growth of the virus in vitro, and are useful for HSV and CMV for aciclovir and ganciclovir, respectively. These assays cannot be used in the viruses for which in vitro culture systems are not available such as HBV. In these circumstances genotypic assays (📖 Molecular diagnostics, p373) may be available and useful.

Fungi

Unlike bacterial and viral diseases, direct microscopy can often be used to diagnose fungal infections (based on distinctive morphological characteristics of the invading fungi, e.g. tinea, and/or the judicious use of special stains such as methylene blue). However, histopathological diagnoses should be confirmed by culture wherever possible. Conversely, although diagnoses are usually made by isolating the causative fungus from bodily samples, the presence of a fungus in a culture from a non-sterile site does not mean that it is pathological (e.g. *Candida* isolation from sputum). Fungal infection can only be definitively established with evidence of tissue invasion. There are also a range of serological tests available for systemic mycoses (📖 Serology, p364), but few provide definitive diagnoses by themselves. A recent innovation that may prove useful is galacotomannan. This is an antigen released in blood by invasive aspergillosis, and when taken serially it can be used for both diagnosis and treatment response.

Fungal culture techniques are similar to the bacterial scenario. They are most useful for detecting the dimorphic fungi, which manifest both mycelial and yeast forms. This group includes *Candida* spp., *Cryptococcus neoformans*, *Blastomyces dermatidis*, *Histoplasma capsulatum*, and *Coccidioides immitis*.

Protozoa

Protozoa of the genera *Acanthamoeba* and *Naegleria* may cause fatal CNS disease. *Acanthamoeba* spp. are free-living amoebae associated with keratitis; they may also cause a granulomatous encephalitis. Another free-living amoeba, *Naegleria fowleri*, is able to cause an acute fulminant meningoencephalitis, and is usually associated with a history of swimming in freshwater lakes or brackish water. In suspected cases, CSF and other suspicious clinical material may be cultured on a non-nutrient agar plate seeded with a 'lawn' of a Gram −ve bacteria (such as *E. coli*). Pathogenic amoebae can be identified microscopically.

Worldwide the most important protozoan infection are plasmodia causing malaria. This can be cultured but this is rarely of use clinically. The mainstay of malarial identification is direct microscopy, although antigen detection tests are now available.

Serology

Immunological methods are in wide usage to detect pathogens present in clinical samples. Serology refers to the laboratory usage of antigen–antibody reactions for such diagnostic purposes. Diagnosis is made by detecting antibody or antigen in blood and/or other bodily fluids, or by the identification of pathogens in culture.

Both *direct* and *indirect* serological tests exist

Indirect serological techniques: Employ antigen–antibody reactions to detect specific antibodies manufactured in response to an antigen or antigens on an infecting pathogen's surface. These antibodies are found circulating in the patient's blood or present in other body fluids.

Direct serological techniques: Employ antibodies to detect specific antigens. Because this technique can be used to identify and type cultured organisms ($\square$ Culture techniques, p358), it not only has individual clinical value, but also has important epidemiological applications.

HBV is a good example of an infection where both antigen and antibody profiles are diagnostically, therapeutically, prognostically, and epidemiologically important:

- Antibody detection of specific antibody, e.g. antihepatitis B$_e$ antigen (anti-HB$_e$ antibody), anti-Hepatitis B surface antigen (anti-HB$_s$ antibody).
- Antigen detection, e.g. hepatitis B 'e' antigen (HB$_e$Ag), hepatitis B surface antigen (HB$_s$Ag).
- More recently, pre-core mutants of HBV have emerged that are not picked up by the common antigen tests.

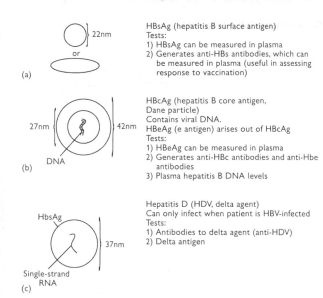

(a) HBsAg (hepatitis B surface antigen)
22nm
Tests:
1) HBsAg can be measured in plasma
2) Generates anti-HBs antibodies, which can be measured in plasma (useful in assessing response to vaccination)

(b) HBcAg (hepatitis B core antigen, Dane particle)
27nm 42nm
Contains viral DNA.
DNA
HBeAg (e antigen) arises out of HBcAg
Tests:
1) HBeAg can be measured in plasma
2) Generates anti-HBc antibodies and anti-Hbe antibodies
3) Plasma hepatitis B DNA levels

(c) Hepatitis D (HDV, delta agent)
HbsAg
37nm
Can only infect when patient is HBV-infected
Single-strand RNA
Tests:
1) Antibodies to delta agent (anti-HDV)
2) Delta antigen

Fig. 5.5 Antibody tests in Hepatitis B and D.

Antibody tests

A wide variety of methodologies for assessing antibody response are available, such as immunofluorescence, agglutination, enzyme-linked immunosorbant assay (ELISA), and complement fixation. This is complex and beyond the range of this book.[1]

Sub-classification of organisms, through serogrouping, is very valuable epidemiologically, e.g. while investigating an outbreak of meningococcal (*Neisseria meningitides*) disease; if the culprit is determined to be type C, vaccination can be utilized to control the outbreak.

In the 'direct fluorescent antibody' (DFA) technique, a fluorescent mono-clonal antibody is used to react with an antigen specific for a given organism (e.g. Herpes simplex virus) and a positive result will be detected micro-scopically. If the fluorescent antibody does not react with the antigen, the antibodies will be washed off the slide and the antigen will not fluoresce.

1 ☞ www.eawag.ch/publications_e/proceedings/oecd/proceedings/Torrance.pdf

General principles (Fig. 5.6)

1 ↑ Specific IgM levels indicates a 'new' infection.
2 ↑ Specific IgG levels indicates a 'new' or a 'previous' infection, or, in some cases, immunity generated by vaccination.
3 Increasing IgG ('rising titre') when two samples ('paired sera') are taken with an appropriate intervening interval between them indicates a 'new' infection or re-infection. Diagnosis (as indicated by seroconversion) necessitates a diagnostic antibody titre or a four-fold increase in antibody titre.
4 *Seroconversion* is said to have occurred in situations 1 and 3.

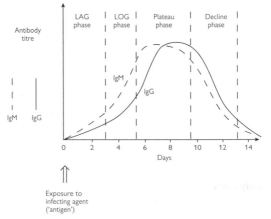

Fig. 5.6 Relative rate of appearance and disappearance of IgM and IgG.

Viral antibody tests

These can be very useful because, once viral shedding has ceased, viral culture is of no further value. They include tests for HIV-1, HIV-2, HTLV-1, HTLV-2, hepatitis A, hepatitis B, hepatitis C, delta agent (hepatitis D), hepatitis E, EBV, CMV, dengue, Ebola fever, Lassa fever, RSV, mumps, measles, rubella, influenza, parainfluenza, St Louis encephalitis, West Nile virus, yellow fever, SARS and many more (Fig. 5.7).[1]

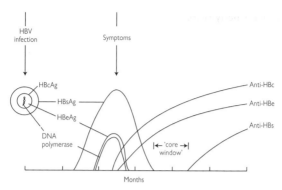

Fig. 5.7 Hepatitis B antigens and antibodies.

Bacterial antibody tests

These include ASO (anti-streptolysin) and anti-DNAse B for strepto-coccal infection.

Can also be useful for non-culturable or difficult to grow organisms, e.g. cat scratch fever (*Bartonella henselae*), *Bordetella pertussis*, Lyme disease (*Borrelia burgdorferii*), *Brucella abortus*, *Burkholderia pseudomallei* (melioidosis), *Campylobacter jejuni*, *Chlamydia* spp., Q fever (*Coxiella burnetti*), *E. coli* 0157, *Francisella tularensis*, *Helicobacter pylori*, *Legionella pneumophila*, *Leptospira interrogans*, *Listeria monocytogenes*, *Mycoplasma pneumoniae*, *Neisseria meningitidis*, *Neisseria gonorrhoeae*, *Rickettsia prowazekii*, *Salmonella* spp., *Treponema pallidum* (including TPHA, VDRL, FTA-ABS, IgM-FTA, IgM-ELISA), *Yersinia enterocolitica/,Y. pseudotuberculosis*, (Widal test).[1]

Protozoal antibody tests

Include tests for malaria (*Plasmodium* spp.), amoebiasis, toxoplasmosis, leishmaniasis (kala azar), African trypanosomiasis (sleeping sickness), American trypanosomiasis (Chagas' disease), babesiosis, *Toxoplasma gondii*.[1]

Helminthic antibody tests

Include tests for *Echinococcus granulosus* (hydatid disease), *Echinococcus multilocularis* (alveolar echinococcosis), *Microsporidium* spp., *Pneumocystis jiroveci* (formerly *Pneumocystis carinii*), schistosomiasis (bilharzia), strongyloidiasis, filariasis, onchocerciasis, *Trichinella spiralis*, *Toxocara* canis, *Taenia solium* (cysticercosis, or pork tapeworm), paragonimiasis (Chinese lung fluke), gnathostomiasis.[1]

1 ♘ http://www.mic.ki.se/Diseases

Fungal antibody tests

Include tests for *Aspergillus fumigatus*, *Aspergillus niger*, *Aspergillus nidulans*, *Aspergillus versicolor*, *Blastomyces dermatitidis*, *Candida albicans*, *Coccidioides immitis*, *Cryptococcus neoformans*, *Histoplasma capsulatum*, *Mukorazeen*.[1]

Note: In the case of complement fixation (CF) antibody assays for antibodies to coccidiomycosis, these are specific and do not require proof of rising levels. They can provide indispensable confirmatory evidence for a diagnosis of coccidiomycosis as well as an indication of the relative risk of extrapulmonary dissemination. In a case of chronic meningitis, a positive CF for anti-coccidioidal antibodies in the CSF often provides the only definite diagnostic indication of the need for aggressive antifungal therapy.

Antigen tests

Antigen measurement is achieved through techniques such as complement fixation and immunodiffusion. A variety of bodily fluids can yield diagnostically useful antigens, including serum, urine, CSF, and fresh stool. The choice depends upon the clinical context.

Viral antigen tests

Include mumps, cytomegalovirus, influenza, HIV, hepatitis B and C, respiratory syncytial virus, parainfluenza viruses, adenovirus, rota virus, and varicella-zoster virus.

Bacterial antigen tests

Include *Legionella pneumophila* (serotype 1) and *Borrelia burgdorferii* (in urine), β-haemolytic *Streptococci*, *pneumococcus*, *Clostridium difficile*, *Haemophilus influenzae*, *Neisseria meningitidis*, *Helicobacter pylori*, *Campylobacter jejuni*.

Helminthic antigen tests

Filariasis.[1]

Protozoal antigen tests

Include malaria, giardiasis, *Trypanosoma cruzi* (Chagas' disease).

Fungal antigen tests

Include *Cryptococcus neoformans* (CrAg), *Histoplasma capsulatum*, mannoprotein antigen in *Candida albicans*.[2]

℘ http://www.clinical-mycology.com/

---

1 ℘ http://www.who.int/mediacentre/facs102/en/
2 Sendid B *et al.* New enzyme immunoassays for sensitive detection of circulating *Candida albicans* mannan and antimannan antibodies: useful combined test for diagnosis of systemic candidiasis. *J Clin Microbiol* 1999; **37**: 1510–17.

Collection of specimens

Principles of good specimen collection

- Good-quality specimen and clinical information produce the most valuable data.
- Optimal time of collection, e.g. take bacterial specimens before administering antibiotics.
- Collect the optimal type of specimen wherever possible, e.g. pus is preferable to a 'pus swab'.
- Acquire expertise in specimen collection: ensure minimal contamination by normal flora (e.g. mid-stream specimen of urine (MSU), use of a tongue depressor for throat swab collection).
- Freshness of specimens—rapid transport to the laboratory is essential (especially for anaerobic organisms, and for 'hot stools' for parasite diagnosis).
- Collect the appropriate number of specimens at the appropriate intervals, e.g. paired antisera should be taken at least 1–6 weeks apart if a diagnostic rising titre is to be demonstrated.
- Be aware of biological hazards: category 3 organisms (e.g. tuberculosis, *Burkholderia pseudomallei*, hepatitis C, HIV) and category 4 organisms (e.g. viral haemorrhagic fever, possible bioterrorism cases such as smallpox).

Surface specimens include

- **Anal/anorectal**: e.g. gonococcus (*Neisseria gonorrhoeae*).
- **Cervical swab**: e.g. HSV, gonococcus, HPV.
- **Ear swab**: e.g. otitis externa, otitis media, bacterial and fungal infections.
- **Foreign bodies**: almost always infected if causing trouble! (includes iatrogenic foreign bodies, such as arthroplasties, cardiac valves, pacemakers, ventriculo-peritoneal shunts, etc.). Foreign bodies in the ear, nose or vagina can lead to prolonged (and often unpleasant) discharges.
- **Genital ulcers**: dark ground microscopy for syphilis organisms. Also chancroid, *Entamoeba histolytica*.
- **In-dwelling catheters**: include urinary catheters, IV cannulae, Portacaths, etc. If a catheter is thought to be the source of an infection, cultures should performed, and if the catheter or cannula is removed, this should be sent for culture. Urinary catheters are always colonized by bacteria. Intravascular foreign bodies such as central venous catheters and prosthetic heart valves are often affected by bacteria which are normally non-virulent such as coagulase –ve staphylococci.
- **Laryngeal swab**: can be useful for tuberculosis.
- **Nasal, pharyngeal, gingival and throat**: e.g. meningococcus, *Staphylococcus aureus* carriage, streptococcal infections, pertussis, adenovirus. Naso-pharyngeal aspirates are useful diagnosing for influenza and RSV through direct immunofluorescence (DIF) tests and culture. In lepromatous leprosy, a swab from the anterior nares may reveal acid-fast bacilli indicative of this infection.

- **Ophthalmic**: e.g. bacterial conjunctivitis, adenovirus, rabies (from corneal impressions.[1] For trachoma, direct fluorescein-labelled monoclonal antibody (DFa) and enzyme immunoassay (EIA) of conjunctival smears is useful.[2]
- **Skin**:
  - *Abscess*—culture for bacteria and other, unusual, organisms.
  - *Dermal scrapings, nail clippings*—fungal infections (tinea—includes pedis, capitis, cruris, versicolor forms).
  - *Petechial rash scrapings*—meningococcus (occasionally gonococcus).
- **Throat**: e.g. *Candida albicans*, diphtheria, gonococcus, croup organisms.
- **Urethral**: e.g. *Chlamydia*, gonococcus.
- **Vagina (high vaginal swab)**: e.g. *Staphylococcus aureus* in toxic shock syndrome (including toxin testing), *Gardnerella*, gonococcus.

Normally sterile fluids include

- **Amniotic fluid**: bacterial infection can cause premature delivery, and rDNA was detected by PCR (🕮 Molecular diagnostics, p373) in samples from 15 (94%) of 16 patients with positive amniotic fluid cultures.[3] Hydrops fetalis can be caused by congenital infections (e.g. CMV, parvovirus B19, toxoplasmosis, syphilis and Chagas' disease), and making a diagnosis may involve analysis of amniotic fluid with cultures, PCR, etc.
- **Ascites**: consider TB (consider laparoscopy for biopsying peritoneal lesions for culture as well as histology, 🕮 Gastrointestinal tract investigations, p379).
- **Blood**: multiple samplings at separate times from separate body sites may need to be taken, e.g. in endocarditis. For some organisms and pathologies, an extended period of culture may be needed.
- **CSF**: possibilities include, e.g. meningococcus, pneumococcus, *Listeria monocytogenes*, TB, fungi (e.g. *Cryptococcus neoformans*), viruses (🕮 Tissue biopsy & deep aspiration specimens, p384).
- **Ejaculate (semen)**: if the semen contains a high number of leucocytes, this may be an indication of either infection or inflammation. WBCs are considered significant if >1 million found in each mL of ejaculate. Sexually transmitted diseases (STDs), e.g. gonorrhoea, or urea, plasma, and prostate infections come into the differential diagnosis. *Schistosoma haematobium* (bilharzia) may cause haemospermia, and be found in ejaculate.[4] Acute mumps orchitis can be associated with loss of spermatozoa.
- **Ocular fluids (intra-)**: include aqueous humor, vitreous humor. Bacterial, fungal, and parasitic problems can affect the interior of the eye.

1 Zaidman GW, Billingsley A. Corneal impression test for the diagnosis of acute rabies encephalitis. *Ophthalmology* 1998; **105**: 249–51.
2 🕭 http://www.emedicine.com/OPH/topic118.htm
3 Hitti J et al. Broad-spectrum bacterial rDNA polymerase chain reaction assay for detecting amniotic fluid infection among women in premature labor. *CID* 1997; **24**: 1228.
4 Torresi J, Yung A. Usefulness of semen microscopy in the diagnosis of a difficult case of Schistosoma haematobium infection in a returned traveler. *J Travel Med* 1997; **4**: 46–7.

- **Pericardial fluid**: the most common organisms will include staphylococci, streptococci, pneumococci, *Haemophilus influenzae*, meningococci, and tuberculosis.
- **Pleural fluid**: numerous pathologies, including underlying bacterial pneumonia, tuberculous pleurisy, parasitic infections (such as strongyloidiasis), and fungal diseases (such as histoplasmosis).
- **Synovial fluid (joint aspirate)**: bacterial infections can be very destructive and the options are legion. TB must always be borne in mind. Viral arthritides are usually self-limiting and treatment is supportive.
- **Urine**: standard culture and sensitivity, e.g. midstream specimen (MSU), catheter specimen (CSU)—useful for diagnosing cystitis, pyelonephritis, prostatitis, etc. (prostatic massage may be helpful for improving diagnosis of prostatic infections); EMU ('early morning urines') for tuberculosis and a terminal specimen for *Schistosoma haematobium* (bilharzia) best collected around midday.

Normally infected fluids include

- **Pus**: e.g. abscess contents, wound swab/aspirates, drainage swabs. Usually bacterial (consider both aerobic and anaerobic), but amoebic and hydatid options need to be considered when the lesion is in the liver.
- **Saliva**: normally contains a wide range of commensal flora. Cannulation of a parotid gland duct may yield a specific pathogen that is causing a problem in that gland.
- **Sputum**: includes tracheal aspirate, induced sputum (obtained with physiotherapy assistance) and bronchoalveolar lavage (BAL), which may be needed in sicker patients unable to produce sputum or in conditions where copious sputum production may not be a feature (such as *Pneumocystis jirovecii* pneumonia (PCP) in HIV infection). Culture and sensitivity assists with identifying a vast range of organisms, including and especially tuberculosis (always ally sputum culture to direct microscopy).
- **Stool**: vast range of uses (📖 Gastrointestinal tract investigations, p379). Includes direct microscopy for parasites, ova and cysts, i.e. giardia and ascariasis, culture for *Salmonella*, *Campylobacter*, *Shigella*, *E. coli* 0157, typhoid and paratyphoid, *Plesiomonas shigelloides*, enteroviruses, and antigen detection of rotavirus. 'Hot stools' (from patient to the microbiology bench in less than 1 h) may be helpful for amoebae, strongyloides larvae, etc.

Molecular diagnostics

These tests are expensive and are often only available in larger or specialist laboratories, but their potential power is considerable. While a full understanding of these complex technologies can present some conceptual difficulties to the average clinician, they are destined to become an increasingly important part of mainstream clinical practice. HIV viral load and anti-retroviral drug resistance are considered mainstream tests, while examination of the CSF for JC virus DNA by PCR is the method of choice for the diagnosis of progressive multifocal leucoencephalopathy.

The areas of greatest value include

- Detection and quantification of viruses to monitor therapy, e.g. HCV, HIV, HBV, CMV.
- Detection of slow-growing organisms, e.g. TB, atypical mycobacteria.
- Diagnosis of pathogens, which are potentially too dangerous for the laboratory staff to handle, e.g. viral haemorrhagic fever, smallpox, avian/swine flu.
- Detection of organisms killed by antibiotics prior to culture samples being taken, e.g. meningococcal sepsis.
- Detection of organisms that cannot be cultured, e.g. hepatitis C virus (HCV).
- Detection of unusual diseases, e.g. helminthic diseases, fungi.
- Detection of toxins elaborated in small quantities by bacteria, e.g. toxic shock syndrome toxins.
- To quantify the level of an infection (e.g. viral load in HIV disease).
- Detection of mutations manifesting resistance to antimicrobial agents (genotypic resistance testing), e.g. HIV, CMV, TB.
- Elucidation of pathogens that are as yet 'undiscovered'.

Available molecular techniques include

PCR (polymerase chain reaction): This test uses probes to look for the presence of the genes of infecting organisms (💷 Polymerase chain reaction amplification of DNA, p302).

There are numerous PCR tests available, and it is particularly valuable for hepatitis C (including for genotyping), HIV and TB. A universal eubacterial PCR (for genus and species identification of prokaryotes) and universal fungal PCR (genus and species identification of fungi) are available. HBV DNA quantification is accomplished through PCR.

Choosing the appropriate sample for the application of PCR testing is important (e.g. biopsy of possible Kaposi's sarcoma lesion and KSHV (HHV-8); BAL fluid and PCP; small bowel biopsy and Whipple's disease; CSF and meningococcal disease, herpes simplex virus or *Mycobacterium tuberculosis*). **Note**: Fluid samples for PCR usually have a higher yield when not spun in a centrifuge.

LCR (ligase chain reaction): Works through specific probe amplification through the use of DNA-ligase. Greatest value in *Chlamydia* infection.

TMA (transcription-mediated amplification): Uses an isothermal amplification system. Amplified telomerase products are rna, detected using a non-isotopic hybridization protection (HPA) system. Identification of HCV, tuberculosis, gonococcus, and *Chlamydia* are among its potential uses.

Branched chain DNA (bDNA): A signal amplification methodology able to quantify HIV RNA levels.

Nucleic acid sequence-based amplification (NASBA): A quantitative test for HIV RNA, also of value with CMV.

Hybridization with nucleic acid probes: Detects specific ribosomal RNA, and is most widely used for culture confirmation of an organism (e.g. fungi, mycobacteria).

Sequencing: Organisms are identified by direct sequencing of amplified gene fragments. Has been applied to tuberculosis, *H. pylori*, enteroviruses, and HIV (for assessing drug resistance).

Restriction fragment length polymorphisms (RFLP): Restriction enzymes are used to cut up DNA into pieces, and the fragments are then subjected to gel electrophoresis (such as Southern blotting, 📖 Southern blotting, p300). The patterns produced can be used to identify organisms.

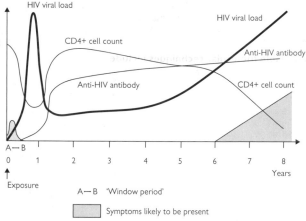

Fig. 5.8 The immunological profile of HIV disease.

Further reading
Shanson DC. *Microbiology and Clinical Practice*, 3rd edn. Oxford: Butterworth-Heinemann, 1999.

Haematology

Many infectious diseases manifest haematological changes that are diagnostically valuable.

Blood film: The blood smear examination provides general data on the size and appearance of cells, as well as data on particular cell segments, while pathogens may be seen, e.g. malaria, African trypanosomiasis, Chagas' disease, babesiosis, borreliosis, bartonellosis, ehrlichiosis, filaria (time of day the blood is taken may be significant in this condition), haemolysis, and evidence of hyposplenism. Thick and thin blood films should be considered, especially where malaria is concerned; at least 3 blood films each taken 24 h apart should be performed. Blood films are also useful in assessing if a patient has disseminated intravascular coagulation (DIC).

Bone marrow examination: Culture (for e.g. TB, brucellosis, *Mycobacterium avium intracellulare*, typhoid/paratyphoid, CMV), microscopy (for e.g. leishmaniasis), and establishing cell line integrity (e.g. white blood cell (WBC) abnormalities). An aspirate is generally useful for culture purposes and for establishing what cells are present in the marrow, but a trephine is needed if structural information is needed (e.g. to establish if granulomata suggestive of tuberculosis are present).

Coagulation studies, fibrin degradation products, D-dimers: Useful where DIC is suspected. DIC is a common association of severe sepsis (especially meningococcal disease). Coagulation abnormalities are also present in conditions such as viral haemorrhagic fevers, *Plasmodium falciparum* malaria, rickettsial diseases, etc. D-dimers may assist with the diagnosis of deep venous thrombosis, although this is not universally accepted.

Cold agglutinins: A haemagglutination-based test. Can be caused by *Mycoplasma pneumoniae* (most commonly), influenza A, influenza B, parainfluenza, and adenoviruses.

Differential white cell count in peripheral blood: Useful associations include:
- Eosinophilia and parasite infection.
- Neutrophilia and bacterial sepsis.
- Neutropenia and atypical pneumonias.
- Atypical lymphocytes and EBV.
- Neutropenia and pyrexia.

ESR: Together with the CRP (🕮 Biochemical tests, p382), the rate of erythrocyte sedimentation is sensitive to the extent of a body's response to a lesion or disease. The ESR is important for pointing to the possible existence of an organic disease, but a normal result does not exclude the presence of disease. An ↑ ESR points to the need for additional investigations and, if ↓, is very useful in monitoring the course of a disease. Procalcitonin (PCT) may eventually prove to have even greater value in a similar role.[1]

Ferritin levels: ↓ In iron deficiency, e.g. associated with hookworm infestation of the bowel (*Ancyclostoma duodenale*, *Necator americanus*) or *Helicobacter pylori*-associated gastritis. Ferritin levels are often extremely high in Still's disease, an important non-infective cause of pyrexia and neutrophilia. Serum iron and TIBC may be helpful in a fuller evaluation (🕮 Biochemical tests, p382).

G6PD: Useful in therapy of benign malarias, e.g. *Plasmodium vivax* and *P. ovale* (a deficiency will cause severe haemolysis when primaquine is used to kill the hypnozoite phase to prevent relapse).

Hb concentration and red cell parameters (especially mean cell volume (MCV)): Useful in, e.g. anaemia of chronic infection, haemolysis, iron deficiency (microcytosis) associated with hookworm infestation of the bowel or *H. pylori*-associated gastritis, macrocytosis due to vitamin B_{12} deficiency with *Diphyllobothrium latum* (fish tapeworm) infestation.

Hb electrophoresis: Can detect haematological conditions, such as thalassaemia, sickle cell disease, etc.

Haemolysis screen (including reticulocyte count): May be abnormal in, e.g. DIC, EBV, viral haemorrhagic fever, *E. coli* 0157 gastroenteritis due to haemolytic uraemic syndrome, rickettsial infections, dengue, gas gangrene. Haptoglobin levels can be useful (🕮 Biochemical tests, p382) since they are generally ↓/absent in haemolysis.

Monospot test (Paul Bunnell test): Diagnostic of EBV infection.

Sickling test: Uncovers sickle cell disease, known to be associated with *Salmonella* osteomyelitis, chronic leg ulcers, etc.

Thrombocytopenia: Characteristic in some conditions, e.g. HIV disease, *Plasmodium falciparum* malaria, and dengue.

Vitamin B12 levels: ↓ In *Diphyllobothrium latum* infestation, tuberculosis of the terminal ileum, etc.

---

1 🕭 http://www.pubmedcentral.nih.gov/articlerender.fcgi?artid=29013

Radiology

Plain X-rays

- **Chest**: the potential diagnoses are legion, including pneumonia, TB, pleural effusion/empyema, bronchiectasis, PCP, tropical eosinophilia, and other parasite-related diseases (e.g. paragonimiasis), occupational risks for infections (e.g. silicosis and TB), post-varicella calcification. Also useful to exclude non-infectious causes of fever such as cancer or sarcoidosis
- **Plain abdominal X-ray**: e.g. bowel dilatation, perforation, calcification of adrenal glands and lymph nodes (e.g. TB, histoplasmosis), 'babies head' sign of schistosomal bladder calcification.
- **Dental radiography (orthopantomogram)**: occult dental sepsis.
- **Elsewhere**: e.g. limbs for osteomyelitis, skeletal muscles for calcified cysticercosis lesions, joints for Charcot changes (such as in syphilis).

More sophisticated imaging

ERCP

Using contrast medium and radiographs to define the anatomy of the biliary tree and pancreatic duct. Useful for HIV-associated biliary tree disease (including porta hepatis nodal lymphoma), parasites (e.g. *Clonorchis sinensis*, *Ascaris lumbricoides*), and pancreatic disease such as tuberculosis.

Jugular venous pressure (IVP, intravenous urogram (IVU))

Defines renal anatomy. Renal infection such as pyelonephritis, renal calculi, malignancy or anatomical abnormalities (including congenital) leading to recurrent infections. CT-IVP is generally considered superior now.

MRI

Including with contrast enhancement

- **Cranial**: variant Creutzfeldt–Jakob disease (vCJD; exhibits bilateral pulvinar high signal), encephalitis, rabies, sagittal sinus thrombosis, PMLE. Magnetic resonance imaging (MRI) is also more sensitive than CT when looking for infective space occupying lesions such as tuberculoma, especially in and around the cerebellum.
- **Elsewhere in the body**: defining solid lesions, fluid-filled lesions, etc.
- **Magnetic resonance cholangiopancreatography (MRCP)**: non-invasively defines the hepatopancreatic-biliary tree anatomy.
- **New techniques**: e.g as cardiac MRI imaging, show great promise in the diagnosis of valvular disease.

Computed tomography (CT)

Including with contrast enhancement

- **Cranial**: e.g. brain abscess, paranasal sinus disease, middle ear disease, orbital sepsis, cysticercosis, mastoid air cells.
- **Chest**: e.g. cardiac lesions (possibly with associated endocarditis risk), mediastinum (e.g. lymphadenopathy, including retrosternal), lung lesions such as bronchiectasis, lung abscess, other non-infectious pathologies.
- **Abdomen**: delineates intra-abdominal abscesses and abnormalities in retroperitoneal and mesenteric lymph nodes, defects in the spleen, liver, kidneys, adrenals, pancreas and pelvis.

- **CT-IVP (CT-IV pyelography)**: powerful tool for defining the anatomy of the urinary tract.
- *Spiral CT pulmonary angiography scan (CTPA)*: e.g. for defining pulmonary emboli as a cause of pyrexia of unknown origin (PUO).
- **CT guided biopsy**: to specifically pick out an area for sampling, e.g. liver lesion, lymph node, mediastinal mass.
- **New techniques**: such as 'CT colonoscopy' and cardiac CT scanning have value in diagnosing colonic and cardiac disease (including valvular disease), respectively, especially in older patients unable to undergo invasive testing (e.g. when looking for an associated colonic tumour in a patient with *Streptococcus bovis* endocarditis.)

Ultrasound
- **Abdomen**: evidence of pancreatic, liver, renal, and biliary tree/gallbladder abnormalities (e.g. abscess, hepatic cyst, presence or absence of spleen, ascites, gallstones, etc.).
- **Thoracic**: pleural effusion, empyema (can assist with drainage).
- **Echocardiography**: to help exclude the cardiac vegetations of endocarditis, TB pericarditis (with effusion), myocarditis. *Note*: both transthoracic and transoesophageal echocardiogram (TOE) approaches are available, each yielding data of differing value in different situations.
- **Doppler studies of blood vessels**: to exclude deep vein thrombosis (DVT), such as in the legs.
- **Guided biopsy**: to specifically pick out an area for sampling, e.g. liver lesion, lymph node.
- **Drainage**: to specifically pick out an area for draining, e.g. liver abscess, pleural effusion.

Radionuclide scanning
- Has limited value.
- **Indium (^{111}In)-labelled granulocyte scan**: may help localize many infectious or inflammatory processes (i.e. deep sepsis).
- **^{99m}Technetium bone scan**: bone and joint sepsis.
- **V/Q scan**: to exclude pulmonary embolus as cause of PUO, to delineate consolidation, abscess, bronchiectasis, etc.

Positron emission tomography (PET)
Enormous potential for locating localized infective processes, especially in the brain. Limited availability at time of writing.

These techniques are all described in detail in 📖 Radiology, Chapter 13.

Gastrointestinal tract investigations

Biopsy-based

- **Duodenal biopsy (Crosby capsule and endoscopic methods, ± electron microscopy)**: e.g. Whipple's disease, giardiasis, cryptosporidium, strongyloidiasis.
- **Gastric biopsy**: *H. pylori*.
- **Laparoscopy**: useful to exclude TB and other infections in the presence of ascites (biopsies should be sent for histology, culture and sensitivity).
- **Liver biopsy**: 📖 Tissue biopsy and deep aspiration specimens, p384.
- **Oesophageal biopsy**: e.g. candidiasis, cytomegalovirus (e.g. in advanced HIV disease).
- **Sigmoidoscopy and bowel biopsy**: e.g. amoebiasis, pseudomembranous colitis (*Clostridium difficile* infections), exclusion of idiopathic colitis and Crohn's disease.

Gastrointestinal contents-based

- **Baermann concentration technique**: the method of choice for the detection of *Strongyloides stercoralis*.
- **Capsule endoscopy**: involving the swallowing of a pill-sized capsule containing digital video recording equipment, which broadcasts to a receiver outside of the body. Enormous potential for diagnosing pathology within the gastrointestinal tract, including small bowel infective processes such as tuberculosis.[1]
- **Duodenal aspirate**: e.g. giardiasis, cryptosporidium, strongyloidiasis.
- **Enterotest (string test)**: e.g. giardiasis, cryptosporidium, strongyloidiasis.
- **Hot stools**: 📖 Culture techniques, p358.
- **Salivary amylase**: mumps.
- **Stool culture and sensitivity**: 📖 Culture techniques, p358.
- **Stool microscopy**: for ova, cysts, parasites (e.g. amoebae, helminths such as *Ascaris lumbricoides*).
- **Stool electron microscopy**: good for viruses, e.g. rotavirus and norovirus.
- **Stool chromatography**: *Clostridium difficile* toxin, though microscopy of cell cultures in the presence and absence of a specific *Clostridium difficile* antibody is also used.
- **Sellotape® (adhesive) strip test**: for the threadworm, *Enterobius verminformis*. To perform this test, roll some clear adhesive tape around 4 fingers of a hand, sticky side out, while an assistant spreads the buttocks. In good lighting, identify the involved perianal area, and apply the tape 1–2 times to the affected perianal area. Place the tape on a slide with the clean side downwards, trim the tape, label the slide and send to the laboratory.
- **Toxin tests**: most widely used for *Clostridium difficile* toxins A and/or B, the definite diagnosis of botulism food poisoning is the examination of faeces for *Clostridium botulinus* and toxin (EMG is also helpful). In wound botulism (common in drug injectors), the organism may grow in material taken directly from the wound(s); also used for *E. coli* 0157.

Gastrointestinal tract function

- **D-xylose absorption test**: for malabsorption syndromes, such as Whipple's disease and tropical sprue.
- **^{13}C breath test**: for detection of *H. pylori*.[2]
- **Faecal elastase**: for diagnosis of pancreatic exocrine insufficiency in conditions such as HIV
- **Vitamin levels**: diagnosis of fat soluble vitamin malabsorption in pancreatic or small bowel disease or of B12 levels in terminal ileal problems such as with TB.

1 ॐ http://www.nzma.org.nz/journal/116-1183/633/).
2 ॐ http://www.infai.de/scripten/iquery.cgi?res=ae1

Immunology

Cutaneous hypersensitivity tests are discussed elsewhere (Ω Other tests, p388).

Complement (especially 'terminal' complements C5–C9): Deficiencies can lead to recurrent meningococcal sepsis, pneumococcal disease, etc.

Cytokine studies: Currently experimental.

Differential white cell count (Ω Haematology, p375): Neutropenia and lymphopaenia are associated with bacterial sepsis.

Immunoglobulins: Deficiencies lead to recurrent infections (some cases may be hereditary, and family history is important). Levels may also be higher—IgM tends to be ↑ in brucellosis, malaria, trypanosomiasis, and toxoplasmosis.

Splenic dysfunction: Indicated by a history of surgical removal (not always clear!) or a condition associated with hyposplenism (e.g. coeliac disease/dermatitis herpetiformis), an abnormal blood film, and absent spleen on abdominal imaging. This state may be associated with recurrent meningococcal infection and life-threatening pneumococcal sepsis. Once diagnosed, the patient will need appropriate vaccinations and advised to always carry a warning card and/or wear a MedicAlert® bracelet or similar.

T cell subsets: The absolute CD4+ (T4) cell count and the CD4+/CD8+ (T4/T8) cell ratio is of value. HIV disease, tuberculosis, and sarcoidosis are associated with reduced CD4+ cell levels, HIV with a reversed CD4+/CD8+ cell ratio.

Biochemical tests

A number of biochemical tests are useful in the diagnosis and assessment of a range of infectious illnesses.

α-fetoprotein (AFP): ↑ In hepatocellular carcinoma (associated with HCV and HBV). Note: much higher AFP than in other causes of hepatocellular damage.

Arterial blood gases: Assessment of sepsis, assessment of pneumonia.

CA-125: ↑ False positive in peritoneal tuberculosis.

C-reactive protein (CRP): Together with the ESR, a valuable method for monitoring infections. CRP is an acute phase reactant, ↑ in bacterial infections and ↓ in viral infections. PCT may be of value.

Creatinine phosphokinase (CPK) level: ↑ In *Legionella pneumophila* infection[1]. Also ↑ with zidovudine (AZT) usage in HIV disease.

Glucose metabolism: Diabetes mellitus is a common association of infection, particularly TB. Consider performing a fasting glucose level, an oral glucose tolerance test (OGTT) or checking haemoglobin A_{1c} levels.

Haptoglobin levels: Part of haemolysis screen (📖 Haematology, p375). Iron levels (serum iron), total iron binding capacity (TIBC): iron ↓ (TIBC ↑) in iron deficiency, e.g. associated with hookworm infestation of the bowel (*Ancyclostoma duodenale*, *Necator americanus*) or *H. pylori*-associated gastritis. Serum ferritin may be helpful.

Lactate levels: May be ↑ in HIV-associated mitochondrial toxicity syndrome. Also high in severe sepsis syndrome.

Lipid abnormalities (cholesterol, triglycerides): HIV drug toxicity.

Liver function tests: Abnormalities are present in many conditions, e.g. hepatitis, leptospirosis, yellow fever, antimicrobial drug toxicity (e.g. in TB).
- **Alkaline phosphatase (ALP)**: in the serum of healthy adults, ALP mostly originates from the liver. Biliary obstruction, often associated with sepsis, leads to an ↑ in serum concentration of ALP.
- **Bilirubin**: determination of the bilirubin levels (conjugated and unconjugated) is important in the differential diagnosis of jaundice.
- **γGT**: ↑ in serum concentration of γGT is most sensitive indicator of liver damage.

Pancreatic amylase level: ↑ With pancreatitis in, e.g. mumps (consider also salivary amylase), toxicity with antiretroviral drugs (e.g. didaonosine or DDI).

Pleural fluid analysis: Analysis for lactate dehydrogenase (LDH) levels is useful (as well as albumin, total protein and amylase). An exudate, which implies infection in the differential diagnosis, is defined by at least one of the following criteria: pleural fluid/serum total protein ratio >0.5, pleural fluid/serum LDH ratio >0.6 or pleural fluid LDH >$^2/_3$ upper limits of normal of serum LDH.

Pregnancy test: Some infections, e.g. varicella, genital herpes (simplex) and TB, are often more serious in pregnancy. The use of some antibiotics, e.g. ciprofloxacin and tetracyclines, is relatively contra-indicated in pregnancy. There is the potential to prevent vertical transmission of HIV if diagnosed prior to delivery.

Procalcitonin: Shows promise for detecting and following 'inflammation induced by microbial infections'.[1]

Serum Na+ levels: Hyponatraemia associated with Legionnaire's disease[2], but may also be related to intracranial sepsis or hypocortisolaemia

Synacthen test: TB and histoplasmosis can damage the adrenal glands, leading to an Addisonian state (hypocortisolaemia).

Vitamin D levels: If deficient, may predispose to TB and may lead to difficulties with treating TB infections due to hypocalcaemia (consider checking levels in patients with darkly pigmented skins, especially those with a culture of wearing clothing over most of their body surface).

1 ♒ http://www.pubmedcentral.nih.gov/articlerender.fcgi?artid=29013.
2 Kociuba KR et al. Legionnaires' disease outbreak in south western Sydney, 1992. Clinical aspects. Med J Aust 1994; **160**: 274–7.

Tissue biopsy & deep aspiration specimens

Whatever part of the anatomy they are taken from, biopsy specimens should be evaluated both histopathologically (with specialized stains used wherever appropriate) and by culture for bacteria, mycobacteria, fungi, viruses, and prions (using specialized culture techniques where appropriate).

Bone marrow biopsy: 📖 Haematology, p375. Important for TB, brucellosis, MAI, typhoid/paratyphoid, leishmaniasis.

Cerebrospinal fluid (CSF): While the main objective of a lumbar puncture is usually to obtain fluid for microscopy, culture, and sensitivity, there are other useful tests that can be performed. The opening pressure should be between 10–20cm H_2O—infective and other processes may alter this. While the usual approach to obtaining CSF is through a lumbar puncture, if the pressure is high a cisternal puncture can be performed instead (normally the advice and help of a neurosurgeon would need to be sought). In neonates, foramenal puncture is a possibility. A CT scan is usually performed beforehand to assess the risk of 'coning', although it is by no means a guarantee.

Along with the Gram-staining process and microscopy, other tests to consider include a complete blood cell count, and differential measurement of glucose and protein levels, Ziehl–Nielsen staining for TB, and bacterial, mycobacterial, viral and fungal cultures. On occasions, other tests that might be considered include:

- Wet mount (for amoebae such as *Acathamoeba*; 📖 Culture techniques, p358).
- PCR for herpes simplex virus, herpes varicella-zoster, enteroviruses tuberculosis, JC virus, cryptococcosis (📖 Molecular diagnostics, p302, p373).
- Antibodies to specific pathogens (e.g. arboviruses; 📖 Serology, p364).
- India ink capsule stain (for cryptococcosis).
- Cryptococcal antigen (CrAg) (📖 Serology, p364).
- VDRL, etc., for syphilis (📖 Serology, p364).
- 14-3-3 protein—specific protein marker present in CSF of patients with vCJD.
- Xanthochromia to help exclude subarachnoid haemorrhage also seen in leptospirosis.
- Cytology to help exclude carcinomatous meningitis.
- Assessing comparative CSF protein-cellular levels if Guillain–Barré syndrome (recognized association of infections, such as *Campylobacter gastroenteritis*) is being considered.

Liver biopsy

Indications are numerous and include assessment of viral hepatitis (especially HBV and HCV, including possible cirrhosis and/or hepatocellular carcinoma), assessment of PUO (including TB and lymphoma) and determining if a patient has a medication-induced liver disease. Only on <1% of occasions does the liver biopsy overestimate the amount of hepatic damage (Fig. 5.9).

The biopsy is commonly preceded by an USS examination of the liver to determine the best and safest biopsy site. Usually, the biopsy is conducted under ultrasonic guidance to avoid major blood vessels. Coagulation status should be optimized at the time of biopsying including by the administration of clotting factors.

The risks of the traditional liver biopsy (not performed under ultrasound guidance) include
- Pain (1 in 5 patients).
- Haemorrhage (1 in 500 patients).
- Bleeding requiring transfusion or surgery (1 in 1000 patients).
- Pneumothorax and/or puncture of the gallbladder, kidney, or bowel (1 in 1000 patients).
- Death (1 in 5000 patients).[1]

Equivalent figures are not available for USS-guided liver biopsy, but the technique is well established. Liver biopsy material should be subjected to microbiological culture, as well as to histological assessment.

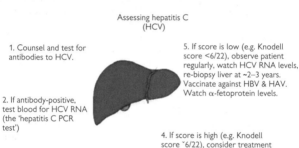

Assessing hepatitis C
(HCV)

1. Counsel and test for antibodies to HCV.

2. If antibody-positive, test blood for HCV RNA (the 'hepatitis C PCR test')

3. If PCR-positive, organize liver ultrasound and biopsy, and check hepatic enzymes and coagulation profile. Histology looks at inflammation, focal necrosis, bridging necrosis and fibrosis, and the histological appearance is scored, e.g. Knodell score (X/22).

4. If score is high (e.g. Knodell score ˘6/22), consider treatment for HCV. Vaccinate against HBV & HAV.

5. If score is low (e.g. Knodell score <6/22), observe patient regularly, watch HCV RNA levels, re-biopsy liver at ~2–3 years. Vaccinate against HBV & HAV. Watch α-fetoprotein levels.

Fig. 5.9 Assessing hepatitis C.

Lymph node sampling
The likely pathologies depend upon whether or not the lymphadenopathy is regional or generalized, and upon the site.

Biopsy: For histology and culture, especially for TB, for tropical infections such as chancroid, and for other relevant infections, such as the cat scratch fever (*Bartonella henselae*). If regional, the differential diagnosis varies with the site; if intra-abdominal, for example, TB, *Yersinia enterocolitica*, and adenovirus should be considered.

1 ℘http://pages.prodigy.com/hepc/hepc6.htm.

Fine needle aspirate (FNA): Useful as full biopsy for culture purposes, but no structural information available (similar to the aspirate vs. trephine issue in bone marrow sampling).

Respiratory samples

Sputum tests
- **Microscopy**: can perform direct microscopy (e.g. for *Aspergillus* spp., eggs of paragonimiasis), Gram stain, Ziehl–Neelsen (ZN), PCP (silver staining needed).
- **Induced sputum**: e.g. for TB, PCP, *Aspergillus*.
- **Tracheal aspirate**: used in ill individuals. May produce similar material.

Bronchoscopy
- **Bronchoalveolar lavage (BAL)**: Useful for TB and other mycobacteria, PCP, fungi, melioidosis, resistant bacteria (e.g. *Pseudomonas*), RSV, paragonimiasis.
- **Lung biopsy**: useful for TB and other mycobacteria, PCP (needs silver staining, IFT or PCR), fungi, melioidosis, resistant bacteria (e.g. *Pseudomonas*), RSV, paragonimiasis. Also for exclusion of non-infective causes of non-resolving pneumonia.

Open lung biopsy
When not feasible to obtain intrathoracic tissue by less invasive means.

Pleural disease: effusion, empyema, biopsy
Consider, e.g. TB, pneumococcal sepsis, underlying neoplasm (and rarer conditions, like strongyloidiasis). Biochemical analysis of pleural fluid can help (📖 Biochemical tests, p382). An empyema will have white cell count, protein, pH, LDH changes compatible with an exudate, and, possibly, organisms visible and/or culturable within the fluid. A pleural biopsy can be obtained blindly with an Abraham's needle, but in recent times pleuroscopy has developed into a better option.[1]

Skin biopsy

Biopsy and hair sampling
- Useful for, e.g. TB, Kaposi's sarcoma (caused by HHV-8 and associated with HIV), onchocerciasis, the aetiology of warts (common viral warts versus molluscum contagiosum—the distinction can be important in view of the therapeutic options and the potential for malignant change in some sites, such as the female cervix).
- The identification of pathogenic arthropod parasites, e.g. myiasis (the invasion and feeding on living tissues of humans or animals by dipterous larvae, such as that of the tumbu fly), scabies, lice, ticks, and chigger fleas, depends on the offending agent being seen and correctly recognized or the appropriate specimen (e.g. excision biopsy) being taken and examined histologically.

Skin snips
- **Filarial infestations**: examination of skin snips will identify microfilariae of *Onchocerca volvulus* and *Mansonella streptocerca*. Skin snips can be obtained using a corneal-scleral punch, or more simply a scalpel and needle. The sample must be allowed to incubate for 30 min to 2 h in saline or culture medium, and then examined microscopically

for microfilariae that would have migrated from the tissue to the liquid phase of the specimen. In onchocerciasis, nodulectomy is also of value, as is examination of the eye with a slit lamp.
- **Leprosy**: acid-fast bacilli are present in the skin.
- **Ebola virus**: these have diagnostic value.[2]

Other tissues and collections are numerous and include
- **Bone infection/abscess/osteomyelitis**: consider e.g. pyogenic sepsis, TB, atypical mycobacteria, sickle cell disease, ectopic ova of schistosomiasis. History is important, e.g. with a history of fight trauma to a hand, anaerobic bony infection may be more likely.[3]
- **Brain lesions and abscesses**: biopsy and drainage useful for, e.g. TB, herpes simplex, rabies, cysticercosis, encephalitis, vCJD, JC virus, and toxoplasmosis (in HIV infection).
- **Cervix**: HPV, HSV, *Neisseria gonorrhoeae*.
- **Joint infections**: aspirate synovial fluid and consider, e.g. pyogenic sepsis, TB. An acute attack of gout (diagnosed through identifying the birefringent crystals of sodium urate) can mimic an acute infective arthritis (including a systemic inflammatory response with neutrophilia) and should be excluded.[4]
- **Liver abscess**: consider *Streptococcus milleri*, hydatid disease, amoebic dysentery, necrotic hepatocellular carcinoma in hepatitis C or hepatitis B, obstruction of biliary tree by *Ascaris lumbricoides* or liver flukes, such as *Clonorchis sinensis*.
- **Muscle biopsy**:
  - *Cardiac*—may point towards a myocarditis or Chagas' disease.
  - *Skeletal*—may be used to identify parasites, including, e.g. trichinosis, cysticercosis.
- **Nerve biopsy**: peripheral nerve biopsy (e.g. posterior auricular nerve) may reveal tuberculoid leprosy.
- **Ocular**:
  - *Vitreous humor*—e.g. intraocular infections, including fungal, HSV, HVZ, pyogenic bacterial.
  - *Cornea*—e.g. rabies, CJD.
  - *Retina*—e.g. herpes varicella-zoster, toxocariasis, CMV.
- **Paranasal sinus aspirates**: e.g. bacteria, fungal (such as mucomycosis).
- **Pericardial biopsy**: particularly important for establishing a diagnosis in a chronic pericarditis, e.g. tuberculosis, fungal.
- **Peritoneal infection**: via laparoscopic tissue sampling and ascites sampling (☐ Gastrointestinal tract investigations, p379).
- **Splenic aspiration**: useful in the diagnosis of visceral leishmaniasis (kala-azar) by microscopic examination and culture and demonstration of the organism.[5]
- **Tonsillar biopsy**: of particular value for diagnosing vCJD: also consider MRI scanning (☐ Radiology, p377), EEG, and 14-3-3 protein in CSF.[6]

1 ✍ http://blue.temple.edu/~pathphys/pulmonary/pleural_disease.html
2 ✍ http://www.uct.ac.za/microbiology/promed21.htm
3 ✍ http://www.worldortho.com/database/etext/infection2.html
4 ✍ http://www.rheumatology.org/publications/primarycare/number6/hrh0033698.html
5 ✍ http://www.who.sci.eg/Publications/RegionalPublications/Specimen_Collection/
6 ✍ http://www.mad-cow.org/~tonsil_human.html

Other tests

Antibiotic plasma concentration monitoring

Some drugs are toxic if the plasma levels rise too high and their use is futile if the levels are too low. Monitoring serum drug levels ensures that plasma drug levels remain within the therapeutic range. Anti-microbial drugs that may require this approach include gentamicin, vancomycin, kanamycin, amikacin, tobramycin, chloramphenicol, streptomycin, cycloserine, amphotericin B, 5-fluorocytosine, and itraconazole.

Cardiac

- **ECG**: serial ECGs can be of value in Lyme disease, rheumatic fever, pericarditis, myocarditis, and toxic shock syndrome. Also of value in conditions where cardiac conduction mechanism has been damaged, e.g. Chagas' disease (American trypanosomiasis) and with a valve root abscess in severe infective endocarditis. In cholera and enteric fever (typhoid and paratyphoid), the cardiac rate will often be slower than one might anticipate for the degree of fever.
- **Echocardiography**.

Dermatological tests

- **Tuberculosis skin tests**: measure delayed hypersensitivity. The Mantoux test usually involves the intradermal injection of 10 tuberculin units of purified protein derivative (ppd), and the response is quantified. The reaction is read at 48–72 h. Most useful epidemiologically, their individual clinical value being relatively limited. Multiple puncture techniques (the Heaf and Tine tests) are likely to be more convenient for large group study. Interpretation of these tests is more difficult in patients inoculated with the BCG vaccine and interferon gamma release assays (e.g. Quartit FERON®) are generally more helpful as they distinguish between T cell responses to BCG and TB.
- **Casoni test**: immediate hypersensitivity skin test employed to detect sensitization to hydatid antigen (*Echinococcus granulosus*). No longer used.
- **Histoplasmin test**: a +ve intradermal skin reaction to histoplasmin (the histoplasmin test) may be only sign of past infection with *Histoplasma capsulatum*. Main value is epidemiological. A similar skin test exists for *Coccidioides immitis*.
- **Mazzotti (DEC) test**: for filariasis. This test relied on the intense pruritic response induced by microfilariae after treatment with the antifilarial agent diethylcarbamazine* (DEC). Used in a minute quantity, it can nevertheless be associated with side effects, ranging from mild discomfort, fever, headaches and intolerable pruritus to tachypnoea, tachycardia, and even pulmonary oedema.

---

* Diethylcarbamazine is not licensed for use as a filaricide.

- **Schick test**: for assessing susceptibility to diphtheria. A small amount of diphtheria toxin is injected into the skin; in individuals with low levels of specific antibody the injection will produce an area of redness and swelling, indicating that vaccination is needed. When the patient is immune to diphtheria, serum antibody to diphtheria toxin will neutralize the injected toxin, and no skin reaction will develop. Seldom used.
- **Skin testing for antibiotic allergy**: this can be performed in the same way as for other allergens.

Narcotics and anabolic steroids screen

If positive, these may point towards occult drug use, and a concomitant risk of blood-borne viruses (e.g. HIV, hepatitis C, hepatitis B). vCJD has been transmitted through anabolic steroid injecting.

Neurological

- **EEG**: may help with making a diagnosis of encephalitis (e.g. in patients with HSV encephalitis, the EEG may exhibit focal unilateral or bilateral periodic discharges localized in the temporal lobes), of brain abscess, or of cerebral cysticercosis. It may also be of value in vCJD.
- **Lumbar puncture**: material for culture and sensitivity can be obtained, but much additional information is also gathered, for example, the opening pressure is usually elevated in infections (Tissue biopsy & deep aspiration specimens, p384).
- **EMG**: offers rapid bedside confirmation of the clinical diagnosis of botulism. It shows a pattern of brief, small, abundant motor unit potentials. In Guillain–Barré syndrome (associated with *Campylobacter* gastroenteritis) EMG may be helpful in excluding 1° muscle disease.
- **Nerve conduction studies**: helpful with diagnosing neuropathies (e.g. HIV, leprosy, Guillain–Barré syndrome).

Ophthalmology

- **Slit lamp examination**: can help with the diagnosis of infective and parasitic ocular problems, e.g. uveitis (syphilis, Reiter's syndrome), *Onchocerca volvulus* larvae, toxocariasis, toxoplasmosis, candidiasis.
- **Colour vision testing (Ishihara)**: used to assess toxicity associated with ethambutol in treatment of TB.
- **Direct and indirect opthalmoscopy**: essential for the diagnosis of CMV retinitis in all HIV positive patients with a CD4 cell count less than 100.

Pulmonary

Pulmonary function tests: Bronchial hyperreactivity can be assessed for (often provoked by infection, e.g. allergic bronchopulmonary aspergillosis) and interstitial lung disease checked for (which can include, for example, tuberculosis, fungal infections, etc.).

Clinical investigation in action: pyrexia of uncertain origin

Common problem in hospital medicine, with huge potential differential diagnosis.

PUO is best defined as a body temperature $\geq 38.3°C$ centrally (rectally) for 3 weeks or longer without the cause being discovered, despite extensive investigation for at least 1 week.

Assessment should include

Observation of the fever pattern

Some conditions, such as typhoid and malaria, may exhibit characteristic fever patterns.

Complete and repeated detailed history, with emphasis on the recognized differential diagnosis including

- Travel history.
- Antimalarial usage.
- Vaccination history.
- Past use of medical services in foreign parts may be especially important (e.g. blood transfusions, splenectomy post-trauma, needlestick assaults).
- Drug-using history (including illicit drugs and especially injecting).
- Exposure to certain agents and/or animals (e.g. pet ownership, occupational risk of animal contact, such as veterinary medicine, nursing, farming, meat packing).
- Hobbies (e.g. caving is linked to histoplasmosis and canal fishing to leptospirosis).
- Sexual history (and risk taking).
- Menstrual history.

Complete and repeated physical examination, including re-evaluation of previous findings, e.g.

- Check the skin, eyes, nail beds, lymph nodes, heart, and abdomen.
- A new sign, e.g. cardiac murmur, may have developed over time.
- The judicious use of repeated tests also critical, depending upon context
- Laboratory and radiological tests, taking into account new data, e.g. blood cultures, blood films, autoantibody screen, radiological findings.
- Non-invasive procedures, taking into account new data, e.g. genitourinary assessment, such as high vaginal swab.
- Invasive procedures, e.g. liver biopsy, bone marrow biopsy, laparoscopy, Waldeyer's ring assessment by otolaryngologist.

Common groups of causes of a PUO in an adult are

- Infections.
- Connective tissue diseases.
- Occult neoplasms (esp. leukaemia, lymphoma, and renal carcinoma).

A list of relevant pathologies might include

HIV, tuberculosis, endocarditis, osteomyelitis, malaria, syphilis, zoonoses (e.g. brucellosis, Lyme disease, tularaemia), viral hepatitis (especially hepatitis C and B), typhoid/paratyphoid, pelvic inflammatory disease, chronic meningo-coccaemia, dental sepsis, tumours, such as lymphoma, renal carcinoma, liver metastases, familial Mediterranean fever, multiple pulmonary emboli, drugs, rheumatological (Still's disease, temporal arteritis, SLE, Wegener's granulo-matosis, vasculitis), atrial myxoma, factitious fever, Munchausen's syndrome, Munchausen's syndrome by proxy.

With improved non-invasive and microbiological techniques, most cases of PUO are found not to be caused by infections, but rather by other systemic diseases, such as sarcoidosis, SLE and temporal arteritis. However, there are also infectious diseases capable of causing prolonged fever that should always be considered and factored into the assessment because they are often treatable and/or transmissible to others and will have serious con-sequences if missed. A definitive diagnosis is not made in around 25% of patients, however, they tend not to come to any harm when observed over a long period.

Endocarditis

Endocarditis is a deep-seated infection that behaves like a deep-seated abscess. Indeed, an abscess can form adjacent to an infected cardiac valve or shunt. The diagnosis involves thoughtful clinical assessment, including whether or not there is a history of injecting drug use, and requires mul-tiple blood cultures and cardiac assessment. The Duke criteria form the basis of the diagnosis.[1] Assess clinically for likelihood, e.g. background of injecting drug use, congenital heart disease, prosthetic valves, rheumatic fever, scarlet fever. Endocarditis may manifest changing cardiac murmurs over a period of time, as well as a number of additional signs.

- **Establish diagnosis**: echocardiography (especially TOE)—to look at valves, cardiac chambers, shunts, etc.
- **Establish aetiology**:
  - *Blood cultures (multiple)*—consider culturing for unusual organisms such as fungi, HACEK organisms (*Haemophilus* sp., e.g. *H. parainfluenzae*, *H. aphrophilus*, and *H. paraphrophilus*, *Actinobacillus actinomycetemcomitans*, *Cardiobacterium hominis*, *Eikenella corrodens*, and *Kingella* spp.), *Listeria monocytogenes*, etc.
  - *Serology*—Q fever (*Coxiella burnetti*) phase I and II, *Candida albicans*.
- **Assess clinical status**:
  - *ECG*—tachycardia, conduction abnormalities.
  - *CXR*—cardiac size, pulmonary emboli with right-sided endocarditis.
  - *U&E*—to assess renal compromise, if any.
  - *Haematology*—WBC.
  - *Inflammatory markers*—ESR, CRP.
  - *Proteinuria*—to assess renal compromise, if any.
  - *Blood-borne virus status*—HIV, hepatitis C, hepatitis B if there is a history of drug injecting.

---

1 ℘ http://www.medcalc.com/endocarditis.html

- **Assistance with therapy**:
  - Antibiotic sensitivity testing.
  - Serum antibiotic levels (e.g. gentamicin, vancomycin).
- **Prevention: dental assessment**: for prevention in the future.
  Endocarditis warning card. MedicAlert® bracelet.

Tuberculosis

Consider pulmonary vs. extrapulmonary disease and other epidemiological parameters.

- **Establish diagnosis/aetiology**:
  - Radiological evidence.
  - Bodily fluids (e.g. sputum, early morning urines, gastric washings, CSF) and biopsies—always consider performing induced sputum even with a normal CXR; histology may show caseating granulomata (Fig. 5.10).
  - PCR testing.
  - Mantoux test.
  - Interferon gamma release assays such as Quantiferon.
  - CA-125 levels—abdominal TB in women.
- **Assess clinical status**:
  - Inflammatory markers—ESR, CRP.
  - T cell subsets—low CD4+ cell count characteristic.
  - Body weight.
  - HIV testing—now essential in all patients.
  - Glucose metabolism—may be an association (fasting glucose, OGTT, HbA_{1c}).
- **Assistance with therapy**:
  - Antibiotic sensitivity testing.
  - Serum antibiotic levels (e.g. cycloserine).
  - Liver function tests.
  - Skin testing.
  - Calcium and vitamin D levels.
  - Gene probes (for rifampicin resistance).
- **Prevention**: notify cases to public health authorities. Contact tracing.

CASEOUS GRANULOMA

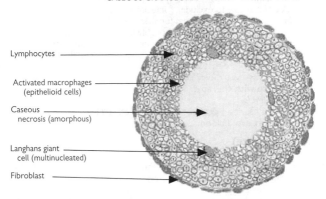

Lymphocytes

Activated macrophages
(epithelioid cells)

Caseous
necrosis (amorphous)

Langhans giant
cell (multinucleated)

Fibroblast

Fig. 5.10 Caseating granulomata are the principal histological feature of tuberculosis together with acid-fast bacilli (detected using the ZN stain). In any tissue affected by tuberculosis, caseating granulomata may be present and are accordingly of immense assistance diagnostically.

Tuberculosis and biopsies: when a biopsy is being obtained of any organ or tissue, the possibility of extrapulmonary TB should be borne in mind. If histology is performed, caseating granulomata may be seen, and appropriate staining for acid-fast bacilli (such as the ZN stain) may reveal the presence of TB organisms. However, because of the increasing risk of MDR and XDR-TB material should always be sent to the microbiology laboratory and appropriate cultures for TB should be set up, both for diagnostic and for drug sensitivity purposes. Molecular techniques, including gene probes and PCR, are now essential parts of the diagnostic armoury for TB. In many instances, having a biopsy taken is an unpleasant experience for a patient and remembering to perform a TB culture at the outset may prevent the patient from having to undergo an unpleasant procedure more than once.

Malaria (fever in the returning traveller)

Always consider malaria in the febrile individual returning from overseas. A detailed geographical history and malaria prophylaxis history is essential. Always consider the possibility of a coexistent second diagnosis (especially in *P. falciparum* infestation), such as *Salmonella* septicaemia (so-called 'algid malaria').

- **Establish diagnosis/aetiology**:
  - *Thick and thin blood films*—perform 3 (each 24h apart).
  - *Antigen tests*—such as ParaSightF® and OptiMAL®.
  - *Blood sugar*—hypoglycaemia is common and needs immediate treatment.
  - *Platelet count*—thrombocytopenia suggestive of *P. falciparum*.
  - *Haematology*—WBC.
  - *Inflammatory markers*—ESR, CRP.

- **Assess clinical status**:
  - *Blood cultures*—to exclude 2° infection.
  - *Haemoglobinopathy*—assess for sickle cell disease.
  - Assess the very ill patient thoroughly for markers of severity (includes LFTs, blood film for haemolysis, coagulation status, CXR, ECG, arterial blood gases, glucose levels, lactate levels, conscious level etc.). Note that severe *Plasmodium falciparum* malaria can present as a diarrhoeal illness.
- **Assistance with therapy**:
  - *G6PD levels.*
  - *Tests of hearing*—deafness can occur with quinine.
- **Prevention**: avoid blood donation for 18 months.

Jaundice (acute)

Jaundice can be pre- or post-hepatic, or a combination of both. Epidemiological factors are important (drug injecting, travel, unsafe food, unsafe sex, job, hobbies, vaccination history, alcohol, prescribed medications, herbal remedies, etc.). The patient may have an acute exacerbation of a chronic disease e.g. hepatitis C. Always remember Courvoisier's law (distended gall bladder in a patient with obstructive jaundice means cancer) and Charcot's triad (the characteristic presentation of acute cholangitis, with biliary colic, jaundice, and spiking fevers with rigors). Haemolysis may lead to jaundice without liver disease being present.

- **Establish diagnosis**:
  - *LFTs*—conjugated and unconjugated bilirubin levels.
  - *Urinalysis.*
  - *Stool examination*—colour, flushability.
  - *Haemolysis screen*—blood film, coagulation studies, antiglobulin test, etc.
  - *Hepatobiliary ultrasound*—serial scans can assess hepatobiliary status sequentially.
  - *α-fetoprotein levels*—may suggest hepatocellular carcinoma associated with hepatitis C and hepatitis B infection.
- **Establish aetiology**:
  - *Serology*—e.g. hepatitis A through to E, EBV, CMV, toxoplasmosis, leptospirosis, hantavirus, yellow fever.
  - *Blood culture.*
  - *Stools for ova, cysts and parasites*—e.g. *Clonorchis sinensis*, ascariasis).
  - *Monospot for EBV.*
  - *Hepatobiliary ultrasound*—obstruction by malignancy or parasites, liver parenchyma status, gallstones.
  - *ERCP/MRCP*—may diagnose parasitic invasion of biliary tree, CMV/crypotosporidial disease, porta hepatis lymphadenopathy associated with HIV, etc.
  - *Paracetamol levels.*

- **Assistance with therapy**:
  - *HIV testing*—if appropriate; co-infection with HIV, HCV, and HBV an increasing problem world-wide.
  - *Ethanol assessment*—γGT levels, ↑ MCV.
  - *Molecular tests*—PCR testing for HCV, circulating DNA levels in HBV.
  - *Antigens*—hepatitis B.
- **Prevention**:
  - Notify cases to public health authorities; safe sex education; safe drug-injecting education possible once viral diagnosis of HCV, HBV and/or HIV established.
  - Assess family, sexual partners, etc. for possible infection (HIV, HBV, HCV) and/or need to vaccinate (HBV).
  - Vaccination strategies: HBV, hepatitis A virus (HAV) as appropriate.

Diarrhoea

Diarrhoea can be acute *vs.* chronic, or acute on chronic. For example, a gastroenteritis illness may uncover pre-existing inflammatory bowel disease, such as Crohn's disease, or malabsorption (such as coeliac disease or pancreatic insufficiency). Drugs such as opiates can lead to 'overflow' diarrhoea. Also bear in mind that where there is one bowel pathogen, another one might be present. Antibiotic resistance is common among some bowel pathogens. Diarrhoea can appear infective, but for example, might be endocrine in origin (e.g. carcinoid syndrome, Zollinger–Ellison syndrome, medullary carcinoma of thyroid), while the possibility of bowel cancer must always be borne in mind. Note that the presence of *Streptococcus bovis* in blood cultures is always highly indicative of the presence of a bowel cancer until proven otherwise. Irritable bowel disease is being increasingly diagnosed. Malaria can present as diarrhoea.

- **Establish diagnosis**:
  - Examine stools.
  - Keep stool chart on ward.
- **Establish aetiology**:
  - Stool culture and sensitivity.
  - Stool microscopy for ova, cysts, and parasites.
  - Faecal fat and elastase for pancreatic insufficiency.

Pneumonic illness

Pneumonia is multi-aetiological. If recurrent, this throws up certain diagnostic possibilities that must be considered. Many epidemiological considerations are important, such as travel history, occupation, pet keeping, hobbies, sexual activity, etc. Osler's triad of rigors, pleuritis, and rust-coloured sputum is said to be characteristic of pneumococcal pneumonia.

- **Establish diagnosis/aetiology**:
  - *CXR* (or CT chest).
  - *Serology*—atypical pneumonia organisms (*Legionella pneumophila*, *Mycoplasma pneumoniae*, *Coxiella burnetti*, *Chlamydia psittaci*), hantavirus, RSV, influenza.
  - *Sputum*—including induced sputum, bronchoscopy and BAL: microscopy and culture.
  - *Blood cultures*.
  - *Serum Na$^+$ level*— ↓ in *Legionella*.

- *Antigen*—pneumococcal (blood), *Legionella* (urine).
- *Nasopharyngeal aspirate (NPA) for viral culture*—RSV, influenza.
- *Cryoglobulins*—e.g. *Mycoplasma pneumoniae*.
- *Molecular*—various PCR tests.
- *HIV test*—if appropriate.
- **Assess clinical status**.
- **(CURB65 score)**:[1]
  - *Arterial blood gases.*
  - *Ultrasound of chest*—if effusion developing (drain if necessary).
  - *Pulmonary function tests* if appropriate.
- **Assistance with therapy**:
  - Antibiotic sensitivity testing.
  - If recurrent: consider tuberculosis testing (*see earlier*), HIV testing, immunoglobulin levels (to check for deficiency), assessing for hyposplenism, checking terminal complement levels (C5–C9).
- **Prevention**:
  - Notify appropriate cases to public health authorities (e.g. *Legionella*, tuberculosis); isolate as necessary.
  - Vaccination strategies: influenza, *Pneumococcus*, *Haemophilus influenzae* B (Hib).
  - Stop smoking, if relevant.

Meningitic illness (headache and photophobia)

Meningitis can be extremely serious, particularly bacterial, mycobacterial, fungal, and protozoal forms, but viral meningitis is generally less serious. Meningitic infection is often mimicked by much less serious infections, such as urinary tract infection (UTI, especially in women), throat infections (ASO, monospot), atypical pneumonias and sinusitis (especially ethmoidal, sphenoidal). A similar picture can also be generated by a subarachnoid haemorrhage. Meningococcal infection can be life-threatening without ever causing meningitis. If a bacterial meningitis is recurrent, certain diagnostic possibilities must be considered. Brain abscess (consider injecting drug use, congenital heart disease, immunodeficiency, etc.) and, under certain circumstances, encephalitis can present in a similar fashion to meningitic illnesses. Where the patient has a marked petechial rash and a history of travel to Africa, Ukraine or South America, even viral haemorrhagic fever (particularly the Congo-Crimean variety) comes into the picture (Fig. 5.11).

1. A detailed travel history and a high index of suspicion are essential in making the diagnosis of VHF. A recent travel history to an area where one of these viruses are known to be particularly prevalent is suggestive, particularly Africa (e.g. Uganda and Ebola, Nigeria and Lassa) and South America — the incubation period ranges from 3 to 21 days, depending upon the variety. Many VHF cases presenting together may suggest a bioterrorism attack.

Biohazard

5. Almost always, the true diagnosis will not be a VHF, but they must be considered where appropriate. Strict adherence to isolation and infection control precautions has prevented secondary transmission in almost all cases.

2. VHFs are severe febrile illnesses that can be complicated by a haemorrhagic tendency, petechiae, hypotension (and even shock), flushing of the face and chest, and oedema. Constitutional symptoms such as headaches, myalgia, vomiting and diarrhoea may occur. Some VHFs manifest particular features not shared by the others.

3. Once suspected, VHFs are category 4 pathogens, so precautions for healthcare workers must be instituted and the case notified to the proper authorities. Isolation measures and barrier nursing procedures are indicated (Marburg, Ebola, Lassa and Congo-Crimean HF viruses may be particularly prone to aerosol nosocomial spread), usually in a special infectious diseases/tropical medicine unit staffed with clinicians with expertise in the field. Intensive supportive care may be required.

4. Diagnosis requires clinical expertise in infectious diseases/tropical medicine. The differential diagnosis includes malaria, yellow fever, dengue, typhoid/paratyphoid fever, non-typhoidal salmonellae, typhus and other rickettsial diseases, leptospirosis, shigella dysentery, relapsing fever (borreliosis), fulminant hepatitis and meningo coccal disease. Antigen tests, antibody detection and viral culture are all available for most of the VHFs. The patient should be fully investigated and treated accordingly.

Fig. 5.11 Investigating a possible case of viral haemorrhagic fever (VHF) case.

- **Establish diagnosis/aetiology**:
  - *LP/cisternal puncture/foramenal puncture (in neonates)*—for CSF pressure, microscopy, bacterial, and mycobacterial culture (including special cultures, e.g. for *Listeria*), viral culture, biochemistry (e.g. protein, glucose), differential cell count, viral PCR, xanthochromia, India ink stain, cryptococcal antigen testing.
  - *CT scan of head*—sometimes necessary to exclude a space-occupying lesion prior to performing LP, CT is little better than a clinical assessment in the exclusion of raised intracranial pressure. When ↑ ICP is found, cisternal puncture and foramenal puncture is possible in skilled hands.
  - CXR and assessment for atypical pneumonia if appropriate.
  - NPA (see earlier).
  - *Petechial rash sampling*—aspirate material from a fresh purpuric lesion using a small-needle insulin syringe, Gram stain and culture.

- *Molecular*—meningococcal PCR (blood and CSF), pneumococcal PCR (blood and CSF).
- *Serology*—urine and blood for cryptococcal antigen; blood for pneumococcal antigen; urine and saliva for mumps antigen; ASO, antibodies to mumps, EBV, *Cryptococcus*, *Neisseria meningitidis*.
- Nasopharyngeal swab for meningococcus.
- Stool for enteroviral culture.
- Monospot test for EBV.
- **Assess clinical status**:
  - *CT scan/MRI scan of head*—assess for raised intracranial pressure, exclude subarachnoid haemorrhage (SAH; xanthochromia), sagittal vein thrombosis; exclude skull fracture, especially of cribriform plate or middle ear (this can lead to recurrent pneumococcal meningitis—if there is a nasal drip, test fluid for glucose to exclude presence of CSF as CSF contains glucose).
  - Differential WBC in blood.
  - *Inflammatory markers*—ESR, CRP.
  - Coagulation screen and platelet count: for meningococcal sepsis.
  - *Arterial blood gases*—to assess acid-base balance in severe cases.
  - *Synacthen® test* (□ Short synacthen test, p209)—adrenal failure in severe meningococcal sepsis (Waterhouse–Friederichsen syndrome).
  - *HIV test*—suggested by some pathologies, and may be the overall underlying problem.
  - *TB assessment*—may be the underlying pathology.
- **Assistance with therapy**:
  - Antibiotic sensitivity testing.
  - Serum antimicrobial levels, e.g. amphotericin, flucytosine.
- **Prevention**:
  - Notify relevant cases to public health authorities; isolate as necessary.
  - *Vaccination strategies*—meningococcus A and C, pneumococcus, influenza, Hib.
  - *History of skull fracture*—may need neurosurgery, etc.

Urethritis (with or without haematuria)

Pain on micturition can simply represent a urinary tract infection or there may be a sexually transmitted disease, such as gonorrhoea present. The patient's sexual and travel history is important. Renal calculi can produce clinical pictures resembling infection, as can dermatological condition such as Stevens–Johnson syndrome. Urinary tract infections are more common during pregnancy. Prostatitis can be a problem in older men.

- **Establish diagnosis/aetiology**:
  - *Urine collection (MSU)*—culture (bacterial infections), microscopy (parasites, etc., such as schistosomiasis—use terminal specimen), molecular techniques (LCR for *Chlamydia*).
  - *Sexually transmitted diseases and pelvic inflammatory disease*—perform HVS and urethral swabs, screen for gonococcus (includes throat and anal swabs).
  - *Calcular disease*—exclude with urine microscopy, radiology, etc.

- *Prostatitis*—prostatic massage, cryptococcal antigen.
- *Tuberculosis*—can present like any other UTI.
- *Reiter's syndrome*—slit lamp examination of the eye, urine and stool culture/LCR for *Chlamydia*.
- **Assess clinical status**:
  - *Biochemistry*—exclude renal failure (urea, creatinine, etc.).
  - *Markers of inflammation*—CRP, ESR.
  - *White cell count.*
  - Check all other mucosal surfaces of the body (mouth, conjunctivae, nose, etc.) to help exclude Stevens–Johnson syndrome.
- **Assistance with therapy**:
  - Pregnancy test.
  - PSA to exclude prostatic carcinoma (recurrent UTIs in older men).
  - Radiology of renal tract—ultrasound, IVP (to exclude underlying renal tract anatomical problems, TB involvement, calculi, etc.).
- **Prevention**:
  - *History of unsafe sex, recent new sexual partner, drug injecting*—consider VDRL, HIV, viral hepatitis testing.
  - *Tuberculosis*—notify, contact trace, etc.
  - *Calculi*—exclude hypercalcaemia, hyperuricaemia, etc.

Red painful swollen lower leg

One of the most difficult things in medicine is to distinguish effectively between a distal deep venous thrombosis, and cellulitis—and a combination of both! Less commonly a ruptured Baker's cyst of the knee can present in almost the same way, the key is in the history. Sometimes the problem is in the tissues, and sometimes in the joints (even gout and pseudogout can look like cellulitis) or the bone (osteomyelitis). Ulceration may be present on the legs. Venous and arterial insufficiency may complicate the picture—infected legs in older people can be very difficult to treat with antibiotics alone. Recent long-haul air travel may point more towards thrombosis, but swollen legs with compromised veins can easily get infected. Although rare, syphilis, yaws, and *Mycobacterium ulcerans* can cause leg ulcers that are potentially amenable to treatment. Pyoderma gangrenosum can resemble infection of the leg, but is associated with non-infectious systemic diseases.

- **Establish diagnosis/aetiology**:
  - Exclude DVT with Doppler ultrasound (and possible embolic disease on occasions).
  - Swabs: from ulcers, between the toes usually not helpful.
  - Blood cultures.
  - ASO titre, antistaphylococcal titres (on occasions), VDRL.
  - Joint assessment: urate levels for gout, assess (if relevant) for pseudogout, rheumatological screen, synovial fluid analysis (if relevant), Lyme disease titres (depends on the travel history, etc.).
  - Leg ulcers in the young: consider sickle cell disease, hereditary spherocytosis.
- **Assess clinical status**:
  - *White cell count.*
  - *Inflammatory markers*—ESR, CRP.
  - *Assess blood vessel integrity*—e.g. compression ultrasound for venous problems, lower limb arteriography.

- **Assistance with therapy**:
  - *Exclude diabetes.*
  - *X-ray, bone scanning*—is osteomyelitis present?
- **Prevention**:
  - Treat diabetes if present.
  - Treat other underlying conditions if present.
  - Patient advised to take care in future (e.g. DVT avoidance while travelling).

Vesicular rash

Many vesicular rashes are infective, many are not. In particular, the distribution of the rash should be carefully assessed and joint assessment and management with a dermatologist is often valuable. If atopic, eczema herpeticum comes into the picture. Staphylococcal impetigo can cause vesiculation. If there is a relevant travel history, rickettsial pox, and monkey pox, come into the picture. Erythema multiforme, which often has an infective basis, but can also be produced by medications, can produce a vesiculating rash (so check the mouth, eyes and genitalia, and determine the medication history). Non-infective blistering conditions include dermatitis herpetiformis (coeliac disease), pompholyx, and pemphigus.

- **Establish diagnosis/aetiology**:
  - *Vesicular fluid*—PCR, EM, IFT, culture, etc.
  - *Serology*—HSV, HVZ, rickettsial pox, coxsackievirus, ASO titre.
- **Assess clinical status**:
  - *CXR*—chickenpox (if compromised, ABGs will be needed).
  - *EEG* if cerebral symptoms present (e.g. cerebellar encephalitis can occur with HVZ).
  - *Monkey pox, small-pox, rickettsial pox*—the patient will be ill and will require full assessment, even possibly intensive care.
- **Assistance with therapy**: **pregnancy test**: HVZ a bigger problem in pregnancy.
- **Prevention**:
  - Avoid precipitants with erythema multiforme.
  - Manage atopy optimally.

Further reading

Chin J (ed.) *Control of Communicable Diseases Manual*, 18th edn. Washington DC: American Public Health Association, 2004.

Cohen J, Powderly WG (eds) *Infectious Diseases*, 2nd edn. St Louis: Mosby, 2003.

Cook GC, Zumla AI (eds) *Manson's Tropical Diseases*, 22nd edn. Philadelphia: WB Saunders, 2008.

Mandell GL, Douglas JE, Dolin R, Bennett RE (eds) *Principles and Practice of Infectious Diseases*, 7th edn. London: Churchill Livingstone, 2009.

Peters W, Pasvol G. *Color Atlas of Tropical Medicine and Parasitology*, 5th edn. St Louis: Mosby-Year Book, 2001.

Shanson DC. *Microbiology and Clinical Practice*, 3rd edn. Oxford: Butterworth-Heinemann, 1999.

Steffen R, Dupont HL, Wilder-Smith A. *Manual of Travel Medicine and Health*, 3rd edn. Ontario: BC Decker, 2007.

Chapter 6

Cardiology

Cardiac catheterization

Principle

Cardiac catheterization is an invasive procedure during which catheters are placed within the cardiac chambers, coronary arteries and great vessels to provide information on cardiac anatomy, pressures, disease states, function, and oxygen saturations.

Indications

- Diagnosis of suspected coronary artery disease (after appropriate non-invasive assessment or if results are equivocal).
- Assessment of coronary artery disease burden and suitability for intervention, e.g. percutaneous coronary intervention (PCI), coronary artery bypass surgery or cardiac transplantation.
- Measurement of intracardiac pressures in patients with valvular heart disease (largely superseded by non-invasive imaging).
- Detailed measurement of left and right ventricular cardiac output and pulmonary hypertension in patients considered for cardiac transplantation or with suspected congenital heart disease (CHD).
- Evaluation of O_2 saturations in cardiac chambers to identify cardiac shunting.
- Myocardial biopsy in patients with cardiomyopathy of unknown cause.
- Monitoring of cardiac transplantation success/rejection.

Contraindications

- Pregnancy is an absolute contraindication to coronary angiography.
- Relative contraindications include:
  - Severe peripheral vascular disease.
  - Aortic aneurysm.
  - Renal failure.
  - Unstable cardiac failure or arrhythmias.
  - Haemodynamic instability.
  - Sensitivity to contrast agents.

Patient preparation

The patient is fasted for 4 h prior to the procedure. Intravenous access is required, together with haemodynamic and electrocardiographic monitoring. Sedation may be used according to patient request or operator direction. It is important that the patient understands the risks of the procedure and gives informed, written consent. The contrast agents used can provoke renal failure in susceptible patients. Metformin should be withdrawn for 48 h prior to the procedure. In patients with renal impairment, pre-treatment with acetyl-cysteine is advised and a less nephrotoxic contrast agent may be considered. Contrast agent volume should be minimized.

Procedure

1. The patient lies flat on a couch and appropriate monitoring is applied.
2. Local anaesthetic is used and an aseptic technique employed. For a left heart procedure, arterial access is required. The proximal femoral artery is the most commonly employed, but the radial or brachial arteries provide alternative routes, especially if peripheral vascular disease is present.
3. The chosen artery is cannulated using the Seldinger technique and an access sheath inserted.
4. Fluoroscopic screening is used to monitor the passage of a guide wire and catheter to the heart.
5. Catheters are pre-shaped according to the structure being examined. Typically, a Judkin's left 4 catheter is used for the left coronary artery, Judkin's right 4 catheter for the right coronary artery, and an angled pigtail catheter is placed in the left ventricle (LV) and/or aorta for examination of these structures.
6. A contrast agent is injected for image acquisition. Images of the coronary arteries are acquired in multiple planes in order to optimally identify coronary artery stenoses. Continuous pressure transducers can be used for dynamic left heart pressure monitoring, e.g. left atrium, LV, and aorta.
7. Evaluation of the right heart necessitates venous access. The most common access point is the femoral vein, but the central veins, e.g. subclavian or internal jugular vein, can also be used.
8. A right heart or Swan–Ganz catheter is passed towards the right heart. Right-sided pressures, e.g. vena cavae, right atrium, right ventricle (RV), pulmonary artery (PmA) and pulmonary capillary wedge pressure (indirect left atrial (LA) pressure), can be measured.
9. Blood samples obtained from these sites can be analysed for oxygen saturation and used to identify the presence and site of cardiac shunts, e.g. atrial or ventricular septal defects. Cardiac output studies can also be performed.

Risks

Cardiac catheterization is an invasive technique and so there are inherent risks to the procedure (1:200 patients). Full cardiopulmonary resuscitation facilities should be immediately available.

These risks include

- Trauma to arterial/venous access site, including haematoma, occlusion, aneurysm, pseudo-aneurysm, nerve damage.
- Aortic/coronary artery dissection.
- Cerebrovascular accident (embolus).
- Myocardial infarction (MI; embolus/dissection).
- Arrhythmias.
- Pulmonary oedema (left main stem stenosis).
- Renal failure.
- Vasovagal response to arterial access/sheath removal.

Additionally the patient is exposed to ionizing radiation and so screening/image acquisition times should be reduced as much as possible. Serial studies should be avoided.

Possible results

Results from a left heart study can provide information on
- Coronary artery anatomy and distribution of disease, to aid decisions regarding the need for revascularization (Fig. 6.1).
- Left ventricular size and function.
- Left heart pressures.
- Aortic and mitral valve integrity.
- Aortic size and disease.
- Congenital abnormalities.

A right-sided study can provide information on
- Right ventricular size and function.
- Tricuspid and pulmonary valve integrity.
- PmA anatomy.
- Right heart pressures.
- Congenital abnormalities, e.g. shunts.
- Myocardial histopathology, where biopsy is taken.

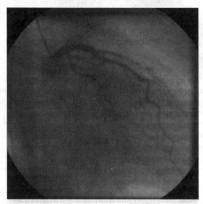

Fig. 6.1 Coronary angiogram showing a normal left coronary artery.

Advantages over other tests

Invasive coronary angiography has high resolution for the evaluation of coronary artery disease and is the current gold standard imaging technique for this application. However cardiac CT is rapidly becoming an accurate alternative means of depicting coronary artery atheroma, particularly in the proximal vessels. Advances in echocardiography and cardiac magnetic resonance have reduced the need for right heart catheterization, but the latter is still the only means with which to obtain direct histopathological information from myocardial structures.

Pitfalls

The procedure is invasive and the risks involved are not insignificant. Whilst coronary angiography is the gold standard for the demonstration of anatomical coronary arterial lesions, it provides little information regarding their physiological significance on the myocardium. The information should therefore be used in conjunction with imaging techniques that can assess the adequacy of myocardial perfusion, e.g. stress nuclear imaging, stress echocardiography or cardiac magnetic resonance.

Further reading

Scanlon PJ Faxon DP, Audet Am *et al*. ACC/AHA Guidelines for Coronary Angiography: Executive Summary and Recommendations. *Circulation* 1999; **99**: 2345–57.

Cardiac markers of myocardial necrosis

Principle

When cardiac muscle is damaged, certain substances, e.g. myoglobin, creatine kinase, troponins I and T, are released into the bloodstream and can be measured by biochemical assays. Such assays can be helpful in making the diagnosis of acute coronary syndromes or myocardial contusion. Myoglobin and creatine kinase (CK and CK-MB) are relatively non-specific cardiac markers of myocardial necrosis (CK is also released by skeletal muscle) that are elevated within 2–4 h of myocyte damage. Troponins (cTnT and cTnI) are cardiac muscle proteins that are released into the peripheral circulation more slowly and are highly specific for myocardial injury. Circulating levels may be undetectable within the initial 12 h after MI (Fig. 6.2).

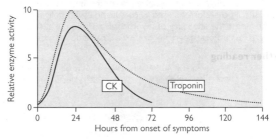

Fig. 6.2 Changes in levels of cardiac markers following acute MI.

Patients presenting with unstable ischaemic cardiac pain are initially labelled as having an acute coronary syndrome (ACS) and are categorized on the basis of their initial 12-lead electrocardiogram (ECG) into ST segment elevation ACS (which requires urgent reperfusion via 1° PCI or thrombolysis) or non-ST segment elevation ACS (which requires appropriate antiplatelet, and antithrombotic therapy). MI is confirmed later if there is a rise in markers of myocardial necrosis, most commonly troponins. When these markers are raised, those presenting with an ST-segment elevation ACS are classified as ST-elevation myocardial infarction (STEMI) and those with non-ST elevation ACS are classified as non-ST elevation MI (NSTEMI).

Indications

Cardiac markers of myocardial necrosis are useful

- In conjunction with the clinical history and 12-lead ECG to diagnose and to categorize suspected acute coronary syndromes.
- To stratify risk in acute coronary syndromes.
- To ascertain the extent of any myocardial injury following coronary revascularization procedures.
- To identify myocardial contusion following thoracic trauma.

Procedure

A 10mL venous blood sample is sufficient, ideally taken 12 h after the patient's most severe symptoms. Repeat sampling may be necessary, especially if a sample has been taken too soon after symptom onset.

Risks

In patients who have had thrombolysis for acute MI, bleeding, or haematoma formation may occur spontaneously at venepuncture sites.

Possible results

In the appropriate clinical setting of chest pain typical of acute MI ± ECG changes:
- An elevated troponin is diagnostic of STEMI or NSTEMI.
- Acute MI (STEMI and NSTEMI) can be confidently excluded if troponin is within normal limits 18 h after the onset of symptoms.

Pitfalls

Creatine kinase may be elevated in skeletal muscle injury, as well as with MI. Direct estimation of CK-MB, the isoenzyme that is more specific for cardiac muscle, may be helpful. Troponins are much more specific for cardiac injury, but may also be elevated in cardiac failure, arrhythmias, renal failure, or pulmonary embolus, and so the clinical context should always be taken into account. Timing of blood samples is critical since values may be normal if blood is taken too soon after symptom onset. Troponins may remain elevated for 7–10 days following a cardiac event and so the diagnosis of re-infarction using troponins alone may be unreliable. Troponin assays vary between hospitals so always check local laboratory normal ranges.

Further reading

Ammann P Pfisterer M, Fehr T. *et al.* Raised cardiac troponins. *BMJ* 2004; **328**: 1028–9.
ESC/ACC. Myocardial infarction redefined. *J Am Coll Cardiol* 2000; **36**: 959–69.
Timmis A. Acute coronary syndromes: risk stratification. *Heart* 2000; **83**: 241–6.

Cardiac volumetric imaging: magnetic resonance & computed tomography

Principle

Cardiac volumetric imaging is now established as a powerful tool to visualize anatomy, size, and function of cardiac structures, i.e. valves, chambers, myocardium, pericardium, and great vessels. Advanced technology magnetic resonance imagers and multislice computed tomography (CT) scanners are increasingly available to clinicians. These techniques provide information regarding aetiology and severity of most congenital and acquired cardiac abnormalities.

Indications

The indications for cardiac magnetic resonance (CMR) and CT are shown in Table 6.1. CMR is especially useful in patients with ischaemic heart disease, where a comprehensive assessment of left ventricular function, reversible myocardial ischaemia and myocardial viability can be made. Cardiac CT is of particular value in screening for coronary artery disease, and for assessment of the great vessels and coronary arteries.

Table 6.1 Indications for CMR and CT

Condition	MRI	CT
Congenital heart disease	+++	++
Anatomy, size or mass of the cardiac chambers (left atrium, LV, right atrium, RV)	++++	+++
Global and regional left ventricular function	++++	+++
Screening (cardiomyopathy, including arrhythmogenic right heart)	++++	+
Valvular heart disease (aortic, mitral, tricuspid, and pulmonary)	+++	+
Prosthetic heart valves	+++	+
Cardiac masses	+++	++
Pericardial disease	+++	++
Aortic disease	+++	++++
Coronary artery anatomy and patency	++	++++
Screening for coronary artery disease	+	++++
Myocardial perfusion	+++	−
Stress study in ischaemic heart disease	++++	−
Myocardial viability	++++	+

Contraindications

- Presence of any ferrous metal, e.g. intracranial clips, intra-ocular foreign bodies, shrapnel (magnetic resonance imaging (MRI)).
- Temporary or permanent pacing systems (MRI).
- Internal cardioverter–defibrillator (ICD) systems (MRI).
- Clinically dehiscing Starr–Edwards valve prostheses manufactured between 1960 and 1964 (MRI).
- Severe claustrophobia (more of an issue with MRI).
- Allergy to non-ionic contrast agents (CT).
- Haemodynamic instability.
- Pregnancy is a relative contraindication to MRI, but an *absolute* contraindication to CT.

Patient preparation

A patient questionnaire is performed to exclude contraindications. Patients should be relaxed and have the procedure explained so that they are able to co-operate effectively. Breath-holding techniques should be practiced prior to the scan to achieve optimal image quality. Height and weight are required for indexing cardiac measurements. Where stressors are to be used, a 12-lead ECG should be obtained. Intravenous access is required for contrast agent administration.

Procedure

The patient is positioned on the imaging couch. Electrodes are attached to allow image acquisition to be gated to the electrocardiogram. For CMR a cardiac coil is selected and earplugs supplied. Images are then acquired in order to evaluate the clinical problem.

The following MRI sequences are commonly performed

T1-weighted images

These are used for anatomical assessment and contribute, with optional contrast agent enhancement, towards tissue characterization.

Cine sequences

Cine sequences are used for anatomical assessment and particularly for cardiac function. Repetitive short axis slices from cardiac base to apex are summated to calculate left ventricular function. This is an extremely accurate method, since it avoids geometrical assumptions created by regional wall abnormalities. It is, therefore, a gold standard method for the calculation of left ventricular ejection fraction (EF), mass, and other cardiac volumes. The technique can be used in conjunction with pharmaceutical stress (e.g. dobutamine) in a manner analogous to stress echocardiography to identify regional reversible myocardial ischaemia.

First pass contrast agent imaging

Myocardial perfusion is assessed by imaging the first pass of a T1 shortening contrast agent, e.g. gadodiamide. The contrast agent passes through the right heart and lungs to the left heart. It is carried into the myocardium by the coronary circulation, giving rise to a rapid increase in myocardial signal intensity. Myocardial areas with reduced blood flow have slower and reduced signal change. The effect is enhanced by use of pharmaceutical volumetric imaging stressors, e.g. adenosine, and can be used for the identification of MI and reversible ischaemia. In contrast to nuclear perfusion imaging, high spatial resolution allows detection of subendocardial, as well as transmural ischaemia.

Delayed contrast agent imaging

Gadodiamide is an interstitial contrast agent and it accumulates in tissue where extracellular membranes are damaged within 10–15 min after administration. This is a powerful tool to delineate between myocardial scar tissue (increased signal intensity), and viable or hibernating myocardium (no change in signal intensity on delayed imaging).

Velocity encoded imaging

Velocities can be encoded into grey scale to measure motion of cardiac structures and flow within great vessels. This has similar applications to echocardiographic Doppler imaging and can be used to quantify valvular disease, e.g. stenosis or regurgitant volumes, and CHD, e.g. cardiac shunts.

Magnetic resonance angiography

A volume (3-dimensional) image acquisition is performed after a bolus of gadodiamide reaches an area of interest within the great vessels. This technique is useful for evaluating aortic disease, CHD, and the presence of renal artery stenosis.

Cardiac computed tomography

An infusion of iodinated contrast agent is given and a volumed image acquisition is attained during a 15–20 s breath-hold. Where coronary arteries are the area of interest, a coronary artery calcification score is performed initially, and this data can then be used to guide further imaging. A β-blocker may be required to lower heart rate to optimize image resolution. Images are then post-processed to reconstruct them to attain clinical information according to scan indication.

Risks

If appropriate screening is carried out to exclude patients with contra-indications then MRI carries minimal risk. Patients who are haemodynamically unstable, e.g. acute aortic dissection, should undergo an alternative form of imaging. CT exposes the patient to ionizing radiation and so this should limit its application.

Possible results

Fig. 6.3 shows the types of images that can be acquired by CMR imaging.

Advantages over other tests

Volumetric imaging is non-invasive, and facilitates excellent temporal and spatial definition of soft tissues. It overcomes difficulties of echocardiography where acoustic window availability limits the scan. CMR uses no ionizing radiation and so is ideal for serial imaging. A very comprehensive examination can be performed, and allows dynamic assessment of the heart and great vessels at a single visit. Multislice CT provides very accurate information regarding coronary artery disease and is a non-invasive alternative to traditional coronary angiography.

Pitfalls

CMR image quality may be impaired by artefact in some patients, especially if metal is present, e.g. non-ferrous surgical clips, spinal rods, or prosthetic valves. Rapid heart rates degrade image quality in multi-slice CT.

Further reading

Higgins CB, De Roos A. *Cardiovascular MRI and MRA*. Baltimore: Lippincott, Williams and Wilkins, 2003.

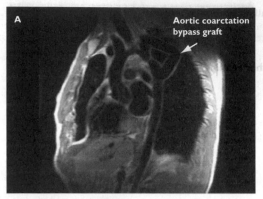

Fig. 6.3 (A) Examples of volumetric imaging techniques: (A) MRI Black blood sequence illustrating aortic coarctation bypass.

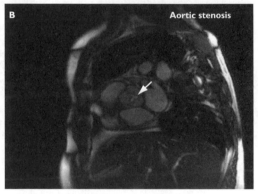

Fig. 6.3 (B) MRI cine sequence of aortic stenosis.

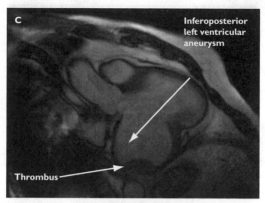

Fig. 6.3 (C) MRI cine sequence demonstrating huge inferoposterior left ventricular aneurysm containing thrombus.

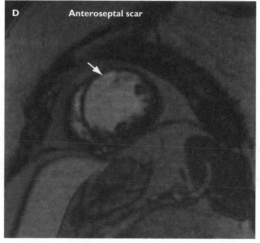

Fig. 6.3 (D) MRI delayed enhancement study delineating subendocardial scar tissue in the anteroseptal wall following MI.

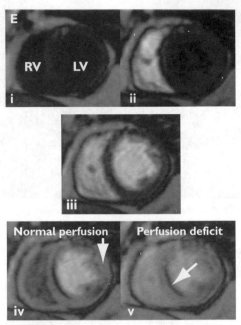

Fig. 6.3 (E) MRI first pass perfusion: (i) prior to contrast injection, (ii) contrast agent appears in the RV, (iii) LV, (iv, arrow) opacifies normally-perfused myocardium, (v, arrow), but identifies an inferoseptal subendocardial perfusion deficit.

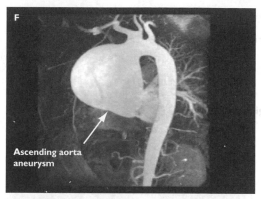

Fig. 6.3 (F) MRA of a severe ascending aortic aneurysm.

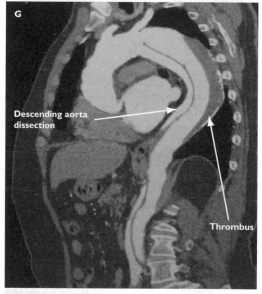

Fig. 6.3 (G) CT of type II aortic dissection and associated thrombus.

Echocardiography

Principle

Echocardiography is the use of ultrasound to visualize anatomy, size, and function of cardiac structures, i.e. valves, chambers, myocardium, pericardium, and great vessels. The technique provides information regarding aetiology and severity of most congenital and acquired cardiac abnormalities.

Imaging modalities

Several imaging modalities are available including 2-dimensional (2D), motion-mode (M-mode), Doppler, and contrast agent enhancement (Fig. 6.4).

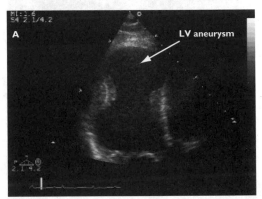

Fig. 6.4 (A) 2D transthoracic echocardiogram (TTE) image of LV demonstrating an apical aneurysm.

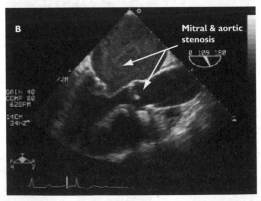

Fig. 6.4 (B) 2D transoesophageal echocardiogram (TOE) image of rheumatic heart disease (mitral and aortic stenosis).

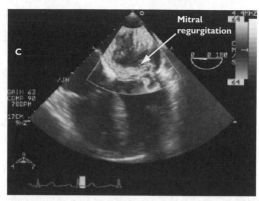

Fig. 6.4 (C) Colour Doppler of eccentric jet of severe mitral regurgitation secondary to mitral valve prolapse. (📖 Colour plate 1.)

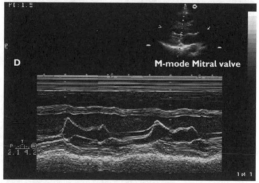

Fig. 6.4 (D) Normal M-mode through mitral valve leaflets.

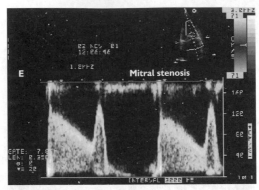

Fig. 6.4 (E) Laminar pulse wave Doppler flow in a patient with mitral stenosis. (📖 Colour plate 2.).

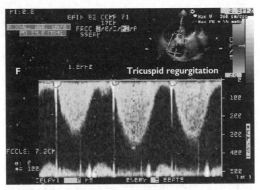

Fig. 6.4 (F) Continuous wave Doppler of tricuspid regurgitation, with PmA systolic pressure calculated as 54mmHg (plus right atrial pressure). (📖 Colour plate 3.)

2D imaging

2D echocardiography allows real time visualization of cardiac anatomy, abnormalities of cardiac structures, and their motion. Image quality is enhanced by use of harmonic imaging and contrast opacification. With some systems, 3-dimensional imaging is also possible.

M-mode imaging

M-mode imaging samples movement of cardiac structures along a single scan line, creating a graph of the motion of sampled structures against time. It is useful for accurate timing of cardiac events and measurement of cardiac dimensions.

Doppler

Doppler is the comparison of transmitted ultrasound beam frequency with received ultrasound frequency reflected from moving structures, e.g. soft tissues (Doppler tissue imaging) or blood cells. The direction of motion and its velocity can be assessed. When blood cells reflect ultrasound as they move towards the transducer, they compress ultrasound wavelength, whereas if they are moving away, ultrasound wavelength lengthens. The change in frequency between the transmitted and reflected wavelengths is the Doppler shift frequency.

Continuous wave Doppler

Continuous wave (CW) Doppler acquires velocity data along the ultrasound beam's entire path. Blood flow of varying strengths and velocities is demonstrated in blood vessels, and through the cardiac valves. The signal is represented graphically on a spectral display. Flow away from the transducer is reflected below the zero line, flow towards the transducer is positive in deflection. Signal density and shape give an indication of severity of any abnormalities.

CW Doppler velocity data can be used to measure the pressure gradients between the cardiac chambers according to the Bernoulli equation. The data thus obtained can be used to calculate the severity of valvular stenosis, expressed in terms of mean and peak pressure gradients, and effective orifice area. The pressure half-time can be used to estimate severity of diastolic valvular lesions, i.e. mitral stenosis and aortic regurgitation. It is defined as the time taken for the peak gradient to fall to half its original value. It is inversely related to effective orifice area.

Pulse wave Doppler

The velocity of blood is sampled within a small area. Since this involves only a small sample volume, it localizes blood flow. It is particularly useful for evaluating low velocity flow such as cardiac inflow and outflow tract velocities. At higher velocities it is limited by the problem of aliasing.

Colour Doppler

Colour Doppler colour codes direction and velocity of blood flow through cardiac structures. Blood flow in the direction away from the ultrasound probe is depicted as blue, whereas blood flowing towards the probe is red. Increased blood flow velocity is reflected by colour mixing, or turbulence. This is a useful screening tool for abnormal jets of blood and can be used to estimate the severity of some abnormalities.

Contrast echocardiography

Microbubbles, consisting of a gas core encapsulated by a protein shell, can be used as contrast agents to improve image quality. Typically, they are used in conjunction with harmonic imaging to allow opacification of left ventricular volume and thereby assess wall motion. Research is continuing into their use to assess myocardial perfusion.

Transthoracic and transoesophageal echocardiography

TTE, where the ultrasound beam is directed to the heart from outside the chest wall, is the most commonly performed examination. In certain clinical situations, more information is obtained by directing the ultrasound beam towards the heart from the oesophagus, and this is termed TOE.

This allows image acquisition without interference of the chest wall, i.e. ribs, soft tissues and lungs. Ultrasound beam attenuation is small and a high frequency transducer can be used, giving rise to higher spatial resolution than with TTE. This facilitates improved definition of the posterior cardiac structures, i.e. valves, atria, and aorta. Relatively small structures, such as cardiac vegetations may be visualized with greater accuracy.

Indications

Indications for TTE and TOE are shown in Table 6.2.

Table 6.2 Indications for TTE and TOE

Condition	TTE	TOE
Congenital heart disease	++	+++
Suitability for percutaneous closure of atrial septal defect	–	++++
Anatomy, size and function of the cardiac chambers (left atrium, LV, right atrium, RV)	+++	++++
Global and regional left ventricular function	+++	+++
Valvular heart disease (aortic, mitral, tricuspid and pulmonary)	+++	++++
Assessment for mitral valvuloplasty	+	++++
Prosthetic heart valves	++	++++
Infective endocarditis (and its complications)	++	++++
Guide to safe cardioversion (atrial fibrillation)	–	+++
Intra-operative assessment of valve disease/repair/replacement	–	+++
Pulmonary hypertension	++	+++
Unexplained pulmonary hypertension/right sided dilatation	+	++++
Cardiac source of embolus in TIA/CVA/peripheral embolism	+	+++
Cardiac masses	++	+++
Pericardial disease	+++	++
Aortic disease	+	+++
Screening (cardiomyopathy)	+++	++

Contraindications

TTE is a very safe imaging technique with no known side effects. Contraindications to TOE include:

- Cervical spine instability, e.g. rheumatoid arthritis, ankylosing spondylitis.
- Oesophageal disease, e.g. stricture, carcinoma, oesophageal varices.
- Haemodynamically unstable patients, including significant hypoxia.

Patient preparation

For both procedures, the patient is made comfortable on an imaging couch in the left lateral position with the head end raised to at least 60°. Cardiac electrodes should be applied to obtain an electrocardiographic trace. Aqueous gel is used on the probe to aid ultrasound beam conduction. For TOE, the patient should be nil by mouth for at least 4 h prior to the procedure and intravenous access sited. Any loose teeth or dentures should be removed. The throat should be sprayed with a local anaesthetic, e.g. xylocaine, and a bite guard inserted prior to intubation. The patient may be sedated according to the clinical situation, patient preference or operator recommendation. Antibiotic prophylaxis is not required.

Procedure

For TTE, the probe is applied to the chest in standard imaging positions (parasternal, apical, subcostal, and suprasternal) and the following imaging planes (Fig. 6.5) are acquired with use of all available modalities:

- Parasternal (long axis and short axis).
- Apical (2, 3, 4, 5 chamber).
- Subcostal and suprasternal.

For TOE, the probe is passed gently over the tongue towards the cricopharyngeal muscles. Gentle continuous pressure is applied and the patient is encouraged to swallow until the probe lies within the oesophagus. Views of the cardiac structures are acquired from varying levels within the oesophagus, gastro-oesophageal junction, and stomach.

Risks

TTE is extremely safe. TOE is a semi-invasive procedure and so informed written consent should be obtained. Intubation of the oesophagus carries a risk of approximately 1 per 2000 of oesophageal trauma. There is a small risk of laryngospasm and cardiac arrhythmia (usually supraventricular). This usually resolves spontaneously on probe withdrawal. Neither technique should be performed on a haemodynamically compromised patient where an interventional procedure is delayed by inappropriate image acquisition, e.g. aortic dissection, cardiac tamponade.

Advantages over other tests

TTE is cheap, non-invasive, and requires no ionizing radiation ensuring that serial examinations are without risk. It is portable and can easily be used at the bedside. The technique provides a comprehensive assessment of cardiac anatomy, function, and blood flow. In the future, additional information on myocardial perfusion may be available. TOE has similar advantages to transthoracic echocardiography, with the difference that it is a semi-invasive technique. Its superior imaging abilities compared with TTE are discussed above. It is a powerful tool for intra-operative use and in patients with limited transthoracic windows.

Pitfalls

Transthoracic image quality may be limited by inadequate acoustic windows in patients with obesity, lung disease, chest wall deformities, and those undergoing artificial ventilation. Structures at the posterior aspect of the heart are not well visualized. Optimal transoesophageal image quality is obtained at the posterior aspect of the heart and so the apex of the heart is less well seen. Image quality may be compromised in patients with hiatus hernia. Not all patients tolerate the procedure and so images relating to the suspected pathology should be acquired first in case the procedure has to be abandoned prematurely.

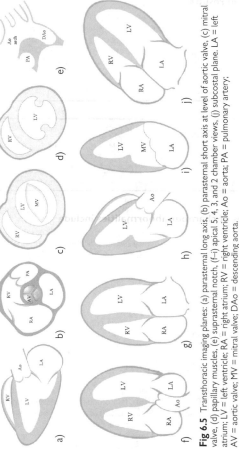

Fig 6.5 Transthoracic imaging planes: (a) parasternal long axis, (b) parasternal short axis at level of aortic valve, (c) mitral valve, (d) papillary muscles, (e) suprasternal notch, (f–i) apical 5, 4, 3, and 2 chamber views, (j) subcostal plane. LA = left atrium; LV = left ventricle; RA = right atrium; RV = right ventricle; Ao = aorta; PA = pulmonary artery; AV = aortic valve; MV = mitral valve; DAo = descending aorta.

Possible results

Anatomy and size of the cardiac chambers

Normal anatomy is demonstrated to exclude congenital heart disease. Each cardiac chamber and its connections are systematically identified and the presence of any shunts excluded. The size of the cardiac chambers and walls are assessed. Normal values are shown in Table 6.3.

Table 6.3 Normal values for cardiac dimensions (M-mode)

Parameter	Normal range
Left atrium	Male 30–40mm, Female 27–38mm
LV diastolic diameter	Male 42–59mm, Female 39–53mm
Septum diastolic diameter	6–12mm
Posterior wall diastolic diameter	6–12mm

Causes of chamber abnormalities include

- **LAt dilatation**: mitral valve disease, aortic valve disease, systemic hypertension, coronary artery disease, dilated cardiomyopathy, restrictive cardiomyopathy, hypertrophic cardiomyopathy, constrictive pericarditis.
- **Left ventricular dilatation**: mitral regurgitation, aortic regurgitation, severe aortic stenosis, systemic hypertension, ischaemic heart disease, dilated cardiomyopathy.
- **Left ventricular hypertrophy**: systemic hypertension, left ventricular outflow obstruction (aortic stenosis, supra-aortic membrane, sub-aortic membrane), hypertrophic cardiomyopathy (asymmetric), aortic coarctation, infiltrative cardiomyopathy (amyloidosis), restrictive cardiomyopathy.
- **Aortic root dilatation**: systemic hypertension, collagen disorders, e.g. Marfan syndrome, syphilitic aortitis, aortic coarctation, aortic valve disease, aortic aneurysm, aortic dissection.
- **Right atrial (RAt) dilatation**: tricuspid valve disease, pulmonary valve disease, pulmonary hypertension, dilated cardiomyopathy, restrictive cardiomyopathy, constrictive pericarditis.
- **Right ventricular dilatation**: 1° pulmonary hypertension, 2° pulmonary hypertension, e.g. mitral stenosis, pulmonary emboli, lung disease, left to right shunts, tricuspid regurgitation, pulmonary regurgitation, right ventricular cardiomyopathy (including arrhythmogenic), right ventricular infarction.
- **Right ventricular hypertrophy**: 1° pulmonary hypertension, 2° pulmonary hypertension, e.g. mitral stenosis, pulmonary emboli, lung disease, left to right shunts, pulmonary stenosis, right ventricular outflow tract obstruction.
- **Pulmonary trunk dilatation**: pulmonary hypertension, collagen disorders, e.g. Marfan syndrome, pulmonary atresia, pulmonary valve disease, idiopathic PmA dilatation.

Global and regional left ventricular systolic function

The size, shape, and function of the LV are evaluated with 2D imaging ± contrast opacification. Commonly measured echocardiographic parameters of LV function include ejection fraction, fractional shortening, stroke volume, and cardiac output. It should be remembered that, when calculated from the M-mode image, only the function of the base of the heart is assessed. This should not be extrapolated to global LV function unless the entire ventricle is normal. Ejection fraction can also be calculated from apical diastolic and systolic views (using the modified Simpson's rule). This is more reflective of global LV function, but is still limited since it is a 2D measurement and requires geometric assumptions. A more subjective assessment can be made by visually estimating LV function as normal or as having mild, moderate or severe impairment. Causes of impaired left ventricular systolic function are:

- Ischaemic cardiomyopathy.
- Hypertensive cardiomyopathy.
- Dilated cardiomyopathy.
- Valvular heart disease.

Regional wall motion abnormalities are confined to specific walls or segments of the LV. Systolic wall thickening is defined in Table 6.4.

Table 6.4 Categorization of regional wall motion

Severity	Description
Normal	>50% increase in systolic wall thickness compared with diastole
Hypokinetic	<50% increase in systolic wall thickness compared with diastole
Akinetic	Absent systolic wall thickening
Dyskinetic	Outward systolic wall motion

Causes of regional wall motion abnormalities are almost exclusively related to coronary artery disease

- MI.
- Left ventricular aneurysm.
- Myocardial hibernation.
- Myocardial ischaemia.
- Post-cardiac surgery.
- Cardiac tumour.

Stress echocardiography

Dobutamine stress may be used in conjunction with left ventricular global and regional wall functional assessment. As well as allowing distinction between normal, ischaemic and infarcted myocardium, it also permits the assessment of myocardial viability (regional dysfunction that will improve with revascularization) versus scar tissue (no effect on function from revascularization). It should be noted that cardiac magnetic resonance is now proven to be a superior technique for identification of myocardial scar/viability. Resulting interpretation with respect to regional wall motion responses to low dose and peak dose dobutamine stress is shown in Table 6.5.

Table 6.5 Interpretation of contractile responses to dobutamine stress

Interpretation	Rest	Low dose	Peak dose
Normal	Normal	Increased	Hyperdynamic
Inducible ischaemia	Normal or reduced	No change or reduced from baseline	Reduced from baseline
Scar tissue	Absent	Absent	Absent
Viability	Absent	Improved	Improved or reduced compared with low dose (biphasic response)

Left ventricular diastolic function

Left ventricular filling during diastole is an important component of left ventricular functional assessment. Normal LAt filling is passive throughout systole (S wave) and diastole (D wave), and is assessed from pulse wave Doppler sampling of pulmonary venous flow. Left ventricular filling is assessed from diastolic mitral valve flow. It is predominantly passive and early in diastole (E wave), with a small, later contribution from atrial systole (A wave). Diastolic dysfunction results in elevated left ventricular end diastolic pressure (LVEDP) and ultimately left atrial pressure (LAP) and so alters measured flow characteristics. There are three types of diastolic dysfunction (Table 6.6), depending on the degree of raised LAP that occurs in order to drive flow across the mitral valve.

Right heart function

Right heart failure is depicted by a dilated, poorly functioning RV. Raised right-sided pressures are indicated by a dilated right atrium and inferior vena cava (seen on subcostal view).

Pulmonary hypertension

Systolic PmA pressure, assuming there is no pulmonary valve stenosis, can be estimated from the pressure gradient between right atrium and ventricle. This is measured from any tricuspid regurgitant jet (Bernoulli equation) summated with estimated RAt pressure. Diastolic PmA pressure is measured by substituting end-diastolic velocity of pulmonary regurgitation into the Bernoulli equation, again summated with estimated RAt pressure. If systolic PmA pressure is raised but diastolic pressure is normal, this represents increased flow volume rather than pulmonary hypertension. Right atrial pressure is assessed by inferior vena cava diameter evaluation and its calibre reduction with inspiration (Table 6.7).

Table 6.6 Echo assessment of left ventricular diastolic dysfunction

Characteristics	Abnormal relaxation	Pseudonormalization	Restrictive
Haemodynamics	↑LVEDP Normal LAP Loss of passive filling gradient LA:LV filling from atrial systole	↑LVEDP ↑LAP LA:LV passive filling gradient restored Pulmonary vein: LA gradient lost	↑LVEDP ↑↑↑LAP LA:LV passive filling gradient ↑↑ Pulmonary vein: LA gradient lost
Mitral valve	(E:A reversal E↓ A↑)	Normal	(E↑↑, sharp descent, A↓)
Pulmonary venous flow	Normal	Diminished S wave, deeper broader A wave	Diminished S wave, deeper broader A wave
Doppler pattern (mitral valve above pulmonary vein below)			
LV impairment	Mild	Moderate	Severe
Significance	Slow early LV relaxation	Slow early relaxation, reduced compliance	Slow early LV relaxation, severely reduced compliance
Symptoms	Well at rest but SOB if heart rate increases	SOB on exercise and limited exercise tolerance	SOB on minimal exertion

Table 6.7 Estimation of RAt pressure

IVC size (cm)	IVC change with inspiration	Estimated RA pressure (mmHg)
<1.5	Collapse	0–5
1.5–2.5	Decreased >50%	5–10
1.5–2.5	Decreased <50%	10–15
>2.5	Decreased <50%	15–20
>2.5	No change	>20

Valvular heart disease
Echocardiography can identify and quantify valve abnormalities to decide whether long-term follow-up or referral for valve surgery is necessary.

Valves may be
- Stenosed (narrowed).
- Regurgitant (leaky).
- Infected (endocarditis).
- Affected by other cardiac pathological processes, e.g. cardiomyopathy, carcinoid.

Aortic stenosis
Aortic stenosis leads to left ventricular hypertrophy, increased left ventricular pressures and, if untreated, left ventricular failure and risk of sudden death (Table 6.8).
- **Aetiology**: congenital abnormality (bicuspid, unicuspid, or quadricuspid valve), calcific degenerative disease, rheumatic heart disease.
- **Differential diagnosis**: hypertrophic obstructive cardiomyopathy, sub-aortic membrane, supra-aortic membrane.
- **2D findings**: thickened, calcified and/or fused aortic cusps with reduced excursion, left ventricular outflow tract dimension (to calculate aortic valve area), effects on LV (hypertrophy/impaired systolic/diastolic function), post-stenotic dilatation of the ascending aorta/aortic coarctation.
- **Colour Doppler findings**: turbulent bright colour is seen through the valve.
- **CW/pulse wave (PW) Doppler findings**: peak and mean valvular gradients; aortic valve area; dimensionless severity index (DSI) is a useful parameter particularly where left ventricular function is impaired.

Table 6.8 Parameters of aortic stenosis severity

	Mild	Moderate	Severe
Mean gradient (mmHg)	<25	25–40	>40
Peak gradient (mmHg)	<36	36–64	>64
Effective orifice area (cm²)	1.5–2.0	1.0–1.4	<1.0

Aortic regurgitation

Aortic regurgitation leads to mild left ventricular hypertrophy, left ventricular dilatation, and failure.

- **Aetiology**: congenital abnormality (bicuspid, unicuspid, or quadricuspid valve), rheumatic heart disease, aortic leaflet prolapse, calcific or idiopathic degeneration, sub-aortic ventricular septal defect (VSD), infective endocarditis (presence of vegetations), aortic dissection (aortic root dissection flap), ascending aortic dilatation (hypertension, aortic stenosis, age), aortitis (syphilis, ankylosing spondylitis, giant cell arteritis, rheumatoid arthritis, Reiter's syndrome), degenerative disease, including collagen disease, e.g. Marfan syndrome.
- **2D findings**: aortic valve anatomy (including calcification, prolapse, vegetations, presence of sub-aortic VSD), size of aortic root/aortic dissection flap/aortic coarctation, effects on LV (hypertrophy/impaired systolic/diastolic function).
- **Colour Doppler findings**: a diastolic regurgitant jet is seen. The width of the jet (colour M-mode) comparative with left ventricular outflow tract diameter and its extent into the left ventricular cavity is measured.
- **CW/PW Doppler findings**: the density of the diastolic signal is assessed together with the pressure half time. Diastolic flow reversal in the aortic arch or descending aorta is indicative of significant aortic regurgitation, unless left ventricular diastolic pressure is high from a separate aetiology, e.g. MI. It can be difficult to differentiate between mild and moderate aortic regurgitation, especially with transthoracic imaging (Table 6.9).

Table 6.9 Parameters of aortic regurgitation severity

	Mild	Moderate	Severe
Jet width (as % of left ventricular outflow tract)	<25		≥65
Pressure half-time (ms)	>500		<250
Vena contracta width (cm)	<0.3		>0.6
Diastolic flow reversal	None	Aortic arch	Descending aorta

Mitral stenosis

Mitral stenosis causes LAt dilatation, increased pulmonary venous pressures, pulmonary oedema, pulmonary hypertension, right heart failure and functional tricuspid regurgitation. TOE should be used to assess the suitability of the patient for percutaneous mitral valvuloplasty (Table 6.10).

- **Aetiology**: rheumatic heart disease/calcification (valve leaflets, chordae or papillary apparatus), congenital abnormality (very rare), systemic lupus erythematosus (rare).
- **Differential diagnosis**: LAt myxoma, obstruction of the valve by thrombus or vegetations.
- **2D findings**: anatomy and degree of any calcification/fusion of the mitral valve leaflets and apparatus for suitability for valvuloplasty, effective orifice area (evaluated with planimetry), LAt size (dilated), presence of LAt thrombus, right heart size (hypertrophy) and function.
- **Colour Doppler findings**: turbulent flow is seen through the valve.
- **CW/PW Doppler findings**: peak and mean valvular gradients are calculated, pressure half time is measured and effective orifice area calculated. Pulmonary hypertension is estimated.

Table 6.10 Parameters of mitral stenosis severity

	Mild	Moderate	Severe
Mean gradient (mmHg)	<5	5–10	>10
Pressure half-time (ms)	71-139	140-219	>219
Mitral orifice area (cm²)	1.6-2.0	1.0–1.5	<1.0

Mitral regurgitation

Mitral regurgitation causes LAt dilatation, increased pulmonary venous pressures, pulmonary oedema, left ventricular failure, pulmonary hypertension, right heart failure, and functional tricuspid regurgitation. TOE gives an optimal assessment of severity (Table 6.11).

- **Aetiology**: rheumatic heart disease, mitral valve prolapse/redundant tissue, ischaemic heart disease (papillary muscle rupture/infarction/restriction of posterior leaflet), dilated/ischaemic cardiomyopathy (annular dilatation), hypertrophic obstructive cardiomyopathy (systolic anterior motion), infective endocarditis (presence of vegetations), congenital abnormality (very rare: note association of cleft mitral valve and primum atrial septal defect), systemic lupus erythematosus (rare).
- **2D findings**: mitral valve anatomy (calcification, prolapse, redundant tissue, leaflet excursion, vegetations, annular size, apparatus integrity), left ventricular size and function (hypertrophy, dilatation), LAt size (dilatation), right heart function (hypertrophy, dilatation) and PmA pressures.
- **Colour Doppler findings**: an abnormal systolic jet is seen through mitral valve into left atrium. The size of this is assessed. This can be deceptive with very eccentric jets associated with mitral valve prolapse.

- **CW/PW Doppler findings**: signal density and shape are characterized. Analysis of pulmonary venous flow with PW Doppler can be helpful.

Table 6.11 Parameters of mitral regurgitation severity

	Mild	Moderate	Severe
Jet area (cm²)	<4		>10
Signal density on CW Doppler	+	++	+++
Vena contracta width (cm)	<0.3		≥0.7
Pulmonary venous flow	Normal	Absent systolic component	Reversed systolic component

Tricuspid stenosis

Tricuspid stenosis causes RAt dilatation and increased systemic venous pressures.

- **Aetiology**: rheumatic heart disease (occurs in 10% patients with mitral stenosis), carcinoid disease, endomyocardial fibrosis, systemic lupus erythematosus.
- **2D findings**: tricuspid valve anatomy and degree of any doming, calcification, fusion of tricuspid valve leaflets and apparatus, size of right atrium, and inferior vena cava (dilated).
- **Colour Doppler findings**: turbulent flow is seen through the valve.
- **CW/PW Doppler findings**: peak and mean valvular gradients are calculated, pressure half time is estimated and effective orifice area calculated. Pulmonary hypertension is calculated from the velocity of any tricuspid regurgitant jet. Peak E wave velocity is elevated (normal peak is $<0.7\text{ms}^{-1}$) and there is a slow deceleration time. A mean gradient of 2–3mmHg may be clinically significant.

Tricuspid regurgitation

Tricuspid regurgitation leads to RAt dilatation, right ventricular hypertrophy, and failure (Table 6.12).

- **Aetiology**: rheumatic heart disease, infective endocarditis (intravenous drug abuse), functional (secondary to right ventricular dilatation, e.g. cardiac left to right shunts, right ventricular cardiomyopathy, pulmonary hypertension, permanent pacing system), carcinoid disease, Ebstein's anomaly, systemic lupus erythematosus, myxomatous degeneration, cardiac amyloidosis.
- **2D findings**: tricuspid valve anatomy (site, calcification, prolapse, redundant tissue, leaflet excursion, vegetations, annular size, apparatus integrity), right ventricular size (dilated) and function, size of right atrium, inferior vena cava (dilated), presence of pacing wires.
- **Colour Doppler findings**: abnormal systolic jet is seen through tricuspid valve into right atrium. The size of this is assessed compared with the right atrium.

- **CW/PW Doppler findings**: the density of the signal and shape is assessed. Analysis of hepatic flow with PW Doppler can be helpful. Pulmonary arterial pressure can be measured, but may be underestimated if there is severe tricuspid regurgitation.

Table 6.12 Parameters of tricuspid regurgitation severity

	Mild	Moderate	Severe
Jet area (cm^2)	<5	5-10	>10
Vena contracta width (cm)		<0.7	>0.7
Signal density on CW Doppler	+	++	+++
Shape of CW Doppler signal	Pansystolic	Pansystolic	Triangular
Hepatic venous flow reversal	None	Absent systolic component	Pansystolic flow reversal

Pulmonary stenosis

Pulmonary stenosis causes right ventricular hypertrophy and, if left untreated, right heart failure (Table 6.13).
- **Aetiology**: congenital, rheumatic heart disease, carcinoid.
- **Differential diagnosis**: right ventricular outflow obstruction (infundibular stenosis).
- **2D findings**: pulmonary valve anatomy (calcification, leaflet thickening, doming), size of pulmonary trunk (post-stenotic dilatation), effects on RV (hypertrophy/impaired function).
- **Colour Doppler findings**: turbulent systolic flow through pulmonary valve.
- **CW/PW Doppler findings**: The maximum gradient and pulmonary valve area are calculated.

Table 6.13 Parameters of pulmonary stenosis severity

	Mild	Moderate	Severe
Peak gradient (mmHg)	<40	40–75	>75

Pulmonary regurgitation

- **Aetiology**: congenital, infective endocarditis (intravenous drug abuse), pulmonary hypertension, PmA dilatation, carcinoid disease, post-pulmonary valvotomy.
- **2D findings**: pulmonary valve anatomy (calcification, prolapse, vegetations), size of pulmonary trunk, effects on RV (hypertrophy/impaired function).
- **Colour Doppler findings**: A diastolic regurgitant jet is seen. The width of the jet and its extent into the right ventricular outflow tract and cavity is measured.
- **CW/PW Doppler findings**: The density of the diastolic signal and its duration are estimated. Pulmonary regurgitation is haemodynamically significant if the jet is broad relative to the width of the pulmonary artery, extends >2cm into the right ventricular outflow tract and persists throughout diastole.

Prosthetic heart valves

Echocardiography is used for follow-up of prosthetic heart valves and potential dysfunction. It is important to consult tables of normal flow pattern values for each valve type according to its make and size. TOE is superior to TTE. The following parameters are assessed:

- Direct 2D imaging of the valve ring and leaflets.
- Presence of any rocking motion suggestive of valvular dehiscence.
- Forward blood flow through the valve.
- Valvular regurgitation (typical regurgitation on valve closure is normal).
- Infective endocarditis.
- Thrombus/pannus.
- Infective endocarditis
- The following features are characteristic of infective endocarditis
- Predisposing abnormal structure (valve lesion/congenital abnormality).
- Regurgitant lesion.
- Mobile echogenic masses (vegetations, usually in the path of regurgitant jets).
- Spread of infection to other valves (usually along the path of a regurgitant jet).
- Abscess (particularly around aortic root, prosthetic valves).
- Embolic potential (large, mobile vegetations, especially aortic valve).
- Valve destruction (degree of regurgitation and effect on cardiac chamber size and function).
- Chamber perforation and shunting.
- Prosthetic valve dehiscence.

Pericardial disease

The normal pericardium is poorly visualized with echocardiography, since it is a very thin structure. Pericardial abnormalities that may be identified are:

- Pericardial effusion (fluid between the pericardial layers).
- Pericardial thickening or calcification (constrictive pericarditis).
- Pericardial masses, e.g. cysts or tumour.

Pericardial effusion

A pericardial effusion gives rise to echo-free space around the heart. The anatomical relationship of pericardial fluid with the descending aorta distinguishes pericardial (anterior) and pleural (posterior) effusions. If the effusion is organizing or contains thrombus or tumour, then echodense structures may be identified within it. The width of this space is measured to give a rough guide as to the size of the effusion:

- Small   <1cm
- Moderate   1–2cm
- Large   >2cm

The most important assessment is whether fluid is causing any haemodynamic compromise, i.e. cardiac tamponade. This may occur regardless of the size of the effusion, particularly if it has accumulated rapidly. Features suggestive of tamponade include:

- Dilatation of inferior vena cava (>2.5cm), poor collapse with inspiration (<50%).
- Exaggerated reduction in transmitral velocities on inspiration (>40%).
- Right ventricular diastolic collapse.
- Low volume, poorly filled LV.

Constrictive pericarditis

This is typically caused by tuberculosis and constrains left and right ventricular filling. On 2D imaging the pericardium is thickened and appears bright when calcification is present. The period of left ventricular diastolic function is shortened. Systolic function is normal. Doppler shows:

- Exaggerated reduction of transmitral E wave velocity with inspiration.
- Shortened transmitral E wave deceleration time.
- Exaggerated flow reversal in the superior vena cava on expiration.

Cardiac masses

The most common intra-cardiac masses are thrombi and vegetations (infective endocarditis). Thrombus formation is increased in conditions causing slow blood flow, such as mitral or tricuspid valve stenosis, or cardiomyopathy. The most common cardiac tumours are atrial myxomas and metastatic deposits. An atrial myxoma is typically a pedunculated, frond-like mass that arises from the interatrial septum. Metastatic deposits can be found anywhere within the heart, including the pericardium. Extrinsic masses may cause compression of cardiac structures. Atrial pectinate muscles, Eustachian valve, Chiari network, papillary muscles, fibrin strands, sutures on prosthetic valves, large vascular structures, such as the aorta, coronary sinus, or left ventricular aneurysms may be incorrectly interpreted as cardiac masses.

- **Atrial masses**: thrombus, myxoma, lipomatous hypertrophy of the interatrial septum, ruptured mitral valve apparatus, 1° benign tumour, 1° malignant tumour, 2° tumour.
- **Ventricular masses**: thrombus, ruptured mitral valve apparatus, 1° benign tumour (fibroma, lipoma, rhabdomyoma, haemangioma), 1° malignant tumour (rhabdomyosarcoma, fibrosarcoma, angiosarcoma), 2° tumour.
- **Valvular masses**: vegetations, thrombus/pannus, fibroelastoma.

Aortic disease

The aorta is a predominantly posterior structure, and so the arch and descending aorta is best visualized by TOE.

- **2D findings**: integrity of the walls is assessed for atheroma (irregular wall thickening), intramural haematoma or dissection flap. The latter may be indirectly suspected from the presence of pericardial effusion or aortic regurgitation. Its anatomy and extent is noted to allow classification. Presence of regional left ventricular wall motion abnormalities may indicate coronary artery involvement. The size of the aorta is measured at several sites to assess dilatation or coarctation (Table 6.14). The normal aortic wall thickness is ≤4mm.

Table 6.14 Normal aortic dimensions

Site	Normal range (mm)
Annulus	17–25
Sinus of Valsalva	22–36
Sinotubular junction	18–26
Arch	14–29
Descending	11–23

- **Doppler findings**: colour, CW, and PW Doppler can all be used to distinguish between true (normal systolic velocity flow) and false (low or absent systolic flow) lumens in aortic dissection, to identify and determine severity of aortic regurgitation and aortic coarctation.

Congenital heart disease

It is important to recognize situs, and connections of cardiac chambers and great vessels.

- **The right ventricle is recognized by the following features**:
  - It is associated with the tricuspid valve.
  - The tricuspid valve is sited more towards the apex than the mitral valve.
  - The tricuspid and pulmonary valves are not continuous (compare aortic and mitral valves).
  - It is trabeculated and contains a moderator band.

- **The ventricles should be connected to the correct outflow tract**:
  - The aorta is a single vessel.
  - The PmA bifurcates soon after its origin unless hypoplasia/atresia is present.
- **The atria should be connected to the correct inflow**: the pulmonary veins normally drain into the left atrium. Drainage into alternative structures, e.g. superior or inferior vena cavae, hepatic veins, is referred to as anomalous pulmonary venous drainage and is associated with a left to right shunt.

There should be no shunts between systemic and pulmonary systems; such shunts include atrial septal defect (abnormal connection between left and right atria—Table 6.15), ventricular septal defect (abnormal connection between LVs and RVs—Table 6.16) or patent ductus arteriosus (abnormal connection between aorta and PmA).

Table 6.15 Types of atrial septal defect

Atrial septal defects	Site	Associations
Ostium secundum	Fossa ovalis	Mitral valve prolapse
Ostium primum	Low septum	Atrioventricular valve abnormalities
Sinus venosus	Upper septum	Anomalous pulmonary venous drainage

Table 6.16 Types of ventricular septal defect

Ventricular septal defects	Site	Associations
Membranous	Infundibular septum	
Sub-aortic	Below aortic valve	Aortic regurgitation Fallot's tetralogy
Muscular	Muscular septum	
Atrioventricular	Posterior septum near atrioventricular valves	Atrioventricular valve abnormalities

If shunts are identified, they are quantified. Pulmonary artery pressure is assessed together with evidence of shunt reversal (right to left) indicating Eisenmenger's syndrome. Fallot's tetralogy is a relatively common congenital condition, composed of a subaortic ventricular septal defect, overriding aorta, right ventricular outflow tract or pulmonary valve stenosis and right ventricular hypertrophy.

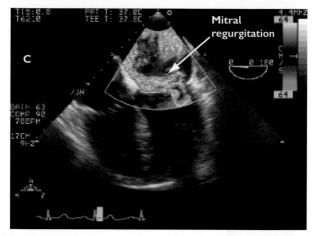

Plate 1 Colour Doppler of eccentric jet of severe mitral regurgitation secondary to mitral valve prolapse. (📖 See Fig. 6.4(c), p417)

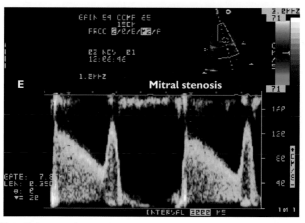

Plate 2 Laminar pulse wave Doppler flow in a patient with mitral stenosis. (See 📖 Fig. 6.4(e), p418)

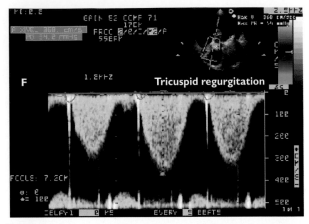

Plate 3 Continuous wave Doppler of tricuspid regurgitation, with PmA systolic pressure calculated as 54mmHg (plus right atrial pressure). (See 📖 Fig. 6.4(f), p418.)

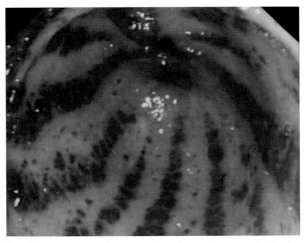

Plate 4 Endoscopic view of gastric antral vascular ectasia, one cause for blood transfusion-dependent iron deficiency anaemia, which may be treated using argon plasma coagulation. (See 📖 Fig. 7.1(a), p467.)

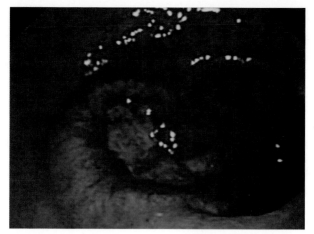

Plate 5 Endoscopic image of a rectal carcinoid tumour. (See 📖 Fig. 7.6, p485.)

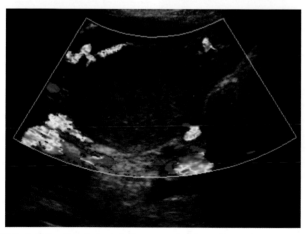

Plate 6 Colour Doppler image in the same patient shows abnormal vascularity in the wall of the gallbladder. (See 📖 Fig. 13.29, p753.)

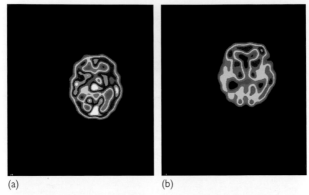

(a) (b)

Plate 7 ^{99m}Tc-HMPAO brain imaging. Transaxial tomographic slices: (a) normal and (b) dementia. (See 📖 Fig. 14.4, p801.)

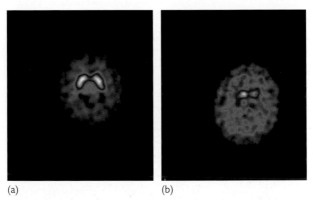

(a) (b)

Plate 8 ^{123}I-ioflupane brain transporter imaging: (a) normal dopamine transporters and (b) in Parkinson's disease. (See 📖 Fig. 14.5, p803.)

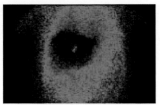

Anterior

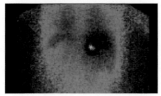

Posterior

(a)

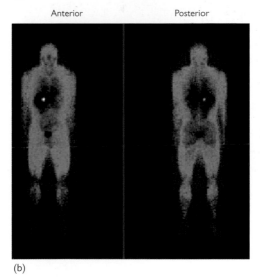

(b)

Plate 9 ^{123}I-MIBG scan: (a) right intra-adrenal phaeochromocytoma; (b) whole body scan—right intra-adrenal phaeochromocytoma. Excludes multifocal, ectopic and malignant tumour. (See 🕮 Fig. 14.9, p811.)

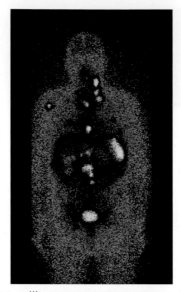

Plate 10 Whole body ^{111}In-octreotide scan showing neuroectodermal tumour with hepatic metastases. (See Fig. 14.10, p813.)

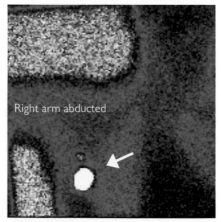

Right arm abducted

Plate 11 ^{99m}Tc-nanocolloid sentinel node study—anterior thorax, right arm abducted. Peri-tumoural, subcutaneous injection right breast and sentinel node (arrow). (See Fig. 14.12, p817.)

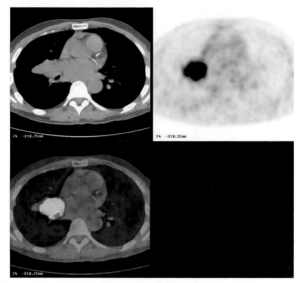

Plate 12 ^{18}F-FDG PET scan—transaxial views showing CT (top left) correlation with PET (top right). The image fusion is shown bottom left. (See 📖 Fig. 14.15, p822.)

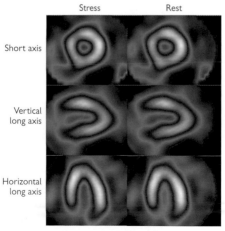

Plate 13 Normal myocardial perfusion scan. (See 📖 Fig. 14.18, p826.)

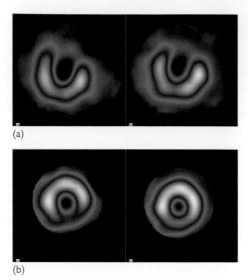

Plate 14 Myocardial perfusion scan: (a) in fixed perfusion loss (anterolateral infarction) and (b) in inferior stress-induced (reversible) ischaemia. (See 📖 Fig. 14.19, p826.)

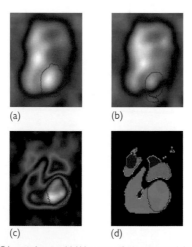

Plate 15 MUGA scan showing (a) LV regions of interest at end diastole and (b) end systole for ejection fraction calculation; (c) amplitude image showing relative anteroseptal hypokinesis, but (d) synchronous LV contraction. (See 📖 Fig. 14.21, p828.)

Valves and outflow tracts should be morphologically normal
- **Aortic valve**: may be unicuspid, bicuspid, quadricuspid, or associated with a sub-aortic or supra-aortic membrane.
- **Pulmonary valve/right ventricular outflow tract**: may be obstructed.
- **Mitral valve**: cleft leaflet associated with primum atrial septal defect, mitral stenosis, parachute valve.
- **Tricuspid valve**: ventricularization of site = Ebstein's anomaly.
- **Aortic and pulmonary arteries** should be normal situs, size, anatomy and unobstructed:
- Left sided aortic arch, aortic coarctation.
- Pulmonary hypoplasia, atresia, affecting either of the pulmonary arteries after trunk bifurcation.

Further reading

ACC/AHA/ASE. Guidelines for the Clinical Application of Echocardiography. 2003. ℘ http://www.acc.org/clinical/guidelines/echo/index_clean.pdf

British Society of Echocardiography. ℘ http://www.bsecho.org

Houghton AR. Making sense of echocardiology. London: Hodder Arnold, 2009.

Leeson P, Mitchell ARJ, Becher H. *Echocardiography*. Oxford: Oxford University Press, 2007.

Otto CM. *Textbook of Clinical Echocardiography*, 3rd edn. Philadelphia: Elsevier Saunders, 2004.

Electrocardiogram

Principle

The ECG records the heart's electrical activity. It can provide valuable information about not just arrhythmias, but also a host of other disorders that affect the electrical activity of the myocardium, such as ischaemia, cardiomyopathy and electrolyte disturbances.

Indications

- Investigation of suspected arrhythmias, both to 'capture' the cardiac rhythm, whilst the patient is experiencing symptoms and also to look for predisposing abnormalities, e.g. short P–R interval, pre-excitation (delta waves), conduction abnormalities, long QT interval.
- Investigation of chest pain, e.g. myocardial ischaemia or infarction, pericarditis, pulmonary embolism.
- Assessment of suspected cardiomyopathy and/or left ventricular failure (a normal ECG is unusual in the presence of left ventricular systolic dysfunction).
- Assessment of electrolyte disturbances, particular where these might have pro-arrhythmic potential, e.g. hyperkalaemia.
- Assessment of drug effects on the heart, e.g. digoxin, tricyclic antidepressants.

Contraindications

None. However, always check if the patient has a known allergy to the self-adhesive pads used to attach the electrodes to the skin.

Patient preparation

- Explain what the procedure involves.
- Ask the patient to lie supine on a bed or examination couch.
- Prepare the skin by shaving, where necessary, and cleaning with alcohol wipes.
- Ask the patient to relax and lie still whilst the recording is in progress.

Procedure

- Having prepared the patient for the test, attach the chest and limb electrodes in the appropriate positions.
- Before recording the ECG, check that the calibration settings of the ECG machine are appropriate. Standard settings are an amplitude of 10mm/1mV and a paper speed of 25mm/s. Ensure that these settings are noted on the ECG.
- After recording the ECG, ensure that the patient's identification details and the time and date of the recording are noted on it.
- It is good practice to make a record on the ECG of any symptoms, e.g. chest pain, palpitations, that the patient was experiencing at the time of the recording, or to write 'asymptomatic' where appropriate.
- Ensure that the ECG is seen and reported by an appropriate staff member as soon as practicable.

Reporting the findings

Always use a systematic approach to ECG reporting to ensure nothing is overlooked.

Report the ECG in the following order

- **Heart rate**: bradycardia vs. tachycardia.
- **Rhythm**: regular vs. irregular, supraventricular vs. ventricular, broad complex vs. narrow complex.
- **QRS axis**: left or right axis deviation.
- **P wave**: presence or absence, inverted, tall (peaked), or wide (bifid).
- **P–R interval**: long, short, or variable.
- **Q waves**: are pathological Q waves present?
- **QRS complex**: large, small, broad, or abnormally shaped.
- **ST segment**: elevated or depressed.
- **T wave**: tall, small or inverted.
- **QT interval**: short or long.
- **U wave**: are prominent U waves present?
- **Additional waves**: are delta or J waves present?

Possible results

The range of possible ECG results is almost endless. Some of the more significant findings and their possible significance, are listed below:

Heart rate

Heart rate can be calculated in one of two ways

- By counting the number of large squares between two successive QRS complexes and dividing this number into 300, e.g. 4 large squares = 300/4 = 75 beats/min. This method is preferred when the heart rhythm is regular.
- By counting the number of QRS complexes along a 15cm rhythm strip (30 large squares), and multiplying this number by 10, e.g. 8 complexes in 15cm = 8 × 10 = 80 beats/min. This method is preferred when the heart rhythm is irregular.

Bradycardia is arbitrarily defined as a heart rate <60 beats/min, **tachycardia** as a heart rate >100 beats/min.

If the patient is bradycardic, consider

- Sinus bradycardia.
- Sick sinus syndrome.
- Second- and third-degree AV block.
- Escape rhythms, e.g. AV junctional escape rhythms, ventricular escape rhythms, asystole and drug-induced conditions.

If the patient is tachycardic, consider

- **Narrow complex tachycardia**: e.g. sinus tachycardia, atrial tachycardia, atrial flutter, atrial fibrillation, AV re-entry tachycardias.
- **Broad complex tachycardia**: e.g. narrow complex tachycardia with aberrant conduction, ventricular tachycardia, accelerated idioventricular rhythm, torsades de pointes.

Cardiac rhythm

To identify the cardiac rhythm ask the following questions
- How is the patient?
- Is ventricular activity (QRS complexes) present?
- What is the ventricular rate?
- Is the ventricular rhythm regular or irregular?
- Are the QRS complexes narrow or broad?
- Are there P waves (atrial activity)?
- What is the correlation between P waves and QRS complexes?

Being able to describe the cardiac rhythm in these terms will narrow down the range of possible diagnoses in most cases and you will, at least, be able to describe the key features of the rhythm clearly over the telephone to an expert.

Rhythms to consider include
- **Sinoatrial nodal rhythms**:
  - Sinus rhythm.
  - Sinus bradycardia.
  - Sinus tachycardia.
  - Sinus arrhythmia.
  - Sick sinus syndrome.
- **Atrial rhythms**:
  - Atrial tachycardia.
  - Atrial flutter (Fig. 6.6).
  - Atrial fibrillation (Fig. 6.7).
  - AV junctional rhythms.
  - AV re-entry tachycardias (Fig. 6.8).
- **Ventricular rhythms**:
  - Accelerated idioventricular rhythm.
  - Ventricular tachycardia (Fig. 6.9).
  - Polymorphic ventricular tachycardia (torsades de pointes, Fig. 6.10).
  - Ventricular fibrillation (Fig. 6.11).
- **Conduction disturbances**.
- **Escape rhythms**.
- **Ectopic beats**.

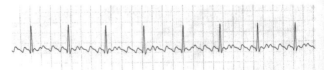

Fig. 6.6 Atrial flutter with 4:1 atrioventricular block.

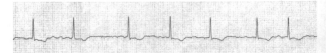

Fig. 6.7 Atrial fibrillation.

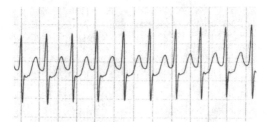

Fig. 6.8 AV re-entry tachycardia.

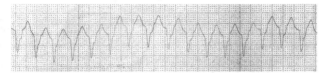

Fig. 6.9 Ventricular tachycardia.

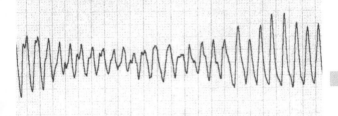

Fig. 6.10 Polymorphic ventricular tachycardia.

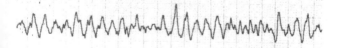

Fig. 6.11 Ventricular fibrillation.

QRS axis
- **Left axis deviation**: left anterior hemiblock, Wolff–Parkinson–White syndrome, inferior MI, ventricular tachycardia (with left ventricular apical focus).
- **Right axis deviation**: left posterior hemiblock, right ventricular hypertrophy, Wolff–Parkinson–White syndrome, anterolateral MI, dextrocardia.

P wave
- **P waves absent**: atrial fibrillation, sinus arrest, or sinoatrial block (persistent or intermittent), hyperkalaemia.
- **P waves inverted**: dextrocardia, retrograde atrial depolarization, electrode misplacement.
- **Tall or peaked P waves**: RAt enlargement.
- **Wide, often bifid P waves**: LAt enlargement.

P–R interval
- **Short P–R interval (<0.12s)**: AV junctional rhythm, Wolff–Parkinson–White syndrome (Fig. 6.12), Lown–Ganong–Levine syndrome.
- Long P–R interval (>0.2s): first degree AV block (Fig. 6.13), e.g. ischaemic heart disease, hypokalaemia, acute rheumatic myocarditis, Lyme disease, digoxin, beta-blockers, certain calcium channel blockers.
- Variable P–R interval: second degree AV block (Mobitz type I (Fig. 6.14), Mobitz type II, 2:1 AV block), third degree AV block (Fig. 6.15).

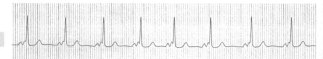

Fig. 6.12 Wolff-Parkinson-White syndrome.

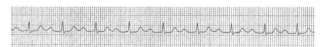

Fig. 6.13 First degree AV block.

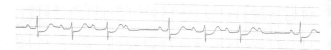

Fig. 6.14 Second degree AV block (Mobitz type I).

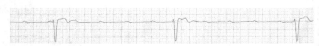

Fig. 6.15 Third degree AV block.

Q waves

Pathological Q waves: MI, left ventricular hypertrophy, bundle branch block.

QRS complex

- **Large R or S waves**: incorrect ECG calibration, left ventricular hypertrophy, right ventricular hypertrophy, posterior myocardial infarction, Wolff–Parkinson–White syndrome (left-sided accessory pathway), dextrocardia, bundle branch block.
- **Small QRS complexes**: incorrect ECG calibration, obesity, emphysema, pericardial effusion.
- **Broad QRS complexes (>0.12s)**: bundle branch block, ventricular rhythms, hyperkalaemia.
- **Abnormally-shaped QRS complexes**: incomplete bundle branch block, fascicular block, Wolff–Parkinson–White syndrome.

ST segment

- **Elevated ST segments**: acute MI (Fig. 6.16), left ventricular aneurysm, Prinzmetal's (vasospastic) angina, pericarditis (concave appearance), high take-off.
- **Depressed ST segments**: myocardial ischaemia, acute posterior MI, drugs e.g. digoxin (reverse tick), ventricular hypertrophy with 'strain'.

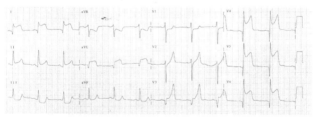

Fig. 6.16 Anterolateral ST-elevation MI.

T wave

- **Tall T waves**: hyperkalaemia, acute MI.
- **Small T waves**: hypokalaemia, pericardial effusion, hypothyroidism.
- **Inverted T waves**: normal (aVR, V1, sometimes V2–V3 and III), myocardial ischaemia, MI, ventricular hypertrophy with 'strain', digoxin toxicity.

QT interval

- **Short QT interval**: hypercalcaemia, digoxin effect, hyperthermia.
- **Long QT interval**: hypocalcaemia, drug effects, acute myocarditis, hereditary syndromes (Jervell and Lange–Nielsen syndrome, Romano–Ward syndrome).

U wave

Prominent U waves: hypokalaemia, hypercalcaemia, hyperthyroidism.

J wave

Present: hypothermia.

Pitfalls

- A common error is to interpret an ECG in isolation. To avoid this error, always consider the clinical context in which it was recorded. Begin your assessment of the ECG by asking, 'How is the patient?' before rushing to conclusions about the clinical relevance of any abnormalities that may be present.
- A normal ECG does not necessarily exclude a significant cardiac problem, particularly when recorded whilst the patient is asymptomatic. This is particularly the case when investigating palpitations and chest pain.
- Technical artefacts are often mistaken for significant abnormalities. Follow the advice given above regarding patient preparation and how to perform the procedure to minimize the risk of artefact.

Further reading

Houghton AR, Gray D. *Making Sense of the ECG*, 3rd edn. London: Hodder Arnold, 2008.

Electrocardiographic monitoring

Principle

Electrocardiographic monitoring allows continuous observation of a patient's ECG in an ambulatory setting over an extended period of time. This is typically from 24 h all the way up to a year or more, depending upon the technique used. There are three types of device available for ambulatory ECG monitoring:

• 24 h ambulatory ECG (Holter) monitor.
• External loop recorder.
• Implantable loop recorder (Reveal™).

The choice of device is largely determined by how frequently the patient experiences symptoms, as the key to successful ECG monitoring is to maximize the chances of capturing a typical symptomatic event during the monitoring period. A Holter monitor is typically worn for 24–48 h, but becomes somewhat impractical over longer periods. It is therefore ideally suited to patients with frequent (daily) symptoms. An external loop recorder (often called an event monitor) is carried for around 7 days and is, therefore, used for patients with less frequent symptoms. Instead of recording a continuous ECG they capture brief periods of the ECG, usually when activated by the patient. Transtelephonic monitors allow captured loops to be relayed to a cardiac centre by telephone, allowing an immediate analysis of the recorded ECG.

An implantable loop recorder (ILR) is used to detect infrequent events. It is used to monitor a patient's cardiac rhythm over an extended period (up to its battery life, usually at least 12 months). An ILR is implanted subcutaneously and contains a battery, a digital memory and diagnostic software to analyse the ECG recording. It records the ECG on a digital 'loop', continuously overwriting older ECG data with the most current data. It can store up to 42 min of ECG recording in its memory, either as one single block or a number of shorter blocks, e.g. 3 blocks of 14 min each. Should a symptomatic event occur, the patient can 'freeze' the loop using an external hand-held device that is held over the ILR ('patient activated mode'). Alternatively or additionally, the device can be programmed to detect and store abnormal cardiac rhythms automatically ('auto activated mode'). The device will usually store the ECG leading up to an event and also a short segment of ECG following the event. Stored ECG loops can subsequently be downloaded for further analysis via a telemetry device at the hospital clinic.

Indications

Where patients have symptoms suggestive of a paroxysmal arrhythmia (palpitation and/or dizziness/syncope), ECG monitoring can provide a diagnosis by capturing the cardiac rhythm during a typical event. This allows the underlying arrhythmia to be identified or, where the rhythm proves to be normal, an arrhythmic aetiology to be ruled out. The choice of method depends upon the frequency of the symptoms (📖 Principle, p446).

Contraindications

None. However, always check if the patient has a known allergy to the self-adhesive pads used to attach the electrodes to the skin.

Patient preparation

For external monitoring no specific preparation is required apart from ensuring that the electrodes make good contact with the patient's skin, so that an ECG of diagnostic quality can be recorded. For the implantation of an ILR:

- Explain what the procedure involves.
- Obtain written informed consent.
- Check FBC (and clotting profile if bleeding risk).
- Local anaesthesia.
- Sedation if the patient is anxious.

The best site for the device is established by optimal ECG signal measurement prior to insertion.

Procedure

External monitors are attached to the patient's skin via electrodes, ensuring good contact is maintained. The recorder itself is carried on a belt or in a pouch. The patient should be given a diary with clear instructions on how to operate the monitor, and how to note the timing and nature of any symptoms that occur. Some event monitors are carried by the patient and only applied to the skin during symptomatic episodes. The patient should be given clear instructions on how to operate such a monitor and a 'test run' should be conducted.

An ILR is implanted subcutaneously under aseptic technique and using local anaesthetic. The implantation takes around 15 min and can be done as a day case procedure. The device is self-contained since, unlike a pacemaker, there are no associated leads. The ILR is commonly implanted near the left deltopectoral groove or below the left breast. This requires an incision approximately 2cm in length. Once implanted, the device is interrogated using an external programmer to ensure that a high-quality ECG is being recorded. If not, the orientation of the device relative to the heart is adjusted until the ECG signal is optimized. The device is then secured in position using sutures and the incision is closed.

Risks

External monitoring carries no significant risks. Implantation of an ILR carries a risk of:

- Infection.
- Erosion through the skin (if patient is thin).

Possible results

Depending upon the underlying cause of the patient's symptoms, almost any cardiac rhythm disturbance (or, indeed, no rhythm disturbance whatsoever) may be revealed by ECG monitoring. The most important aspect of interpreting the results is to correlate recordings with symptoms. Patient activated recordings are, as one might expect, usually made in relation to a symptomatic episode. In this case, it's essential to find out precisely what symptoms were experienced at the time (including a witness account where appropriate). Auto-activated recordings may be asymptomatic and made by the device without the patient being aware of a problem. The most useful outcome is to assess the ECG recorded during a typical symptomatic event. It is then usually straightforward to make a diagnosis and plan further treatment as appropriate.

Advantages over other tests

Ambulatory ECG monitoring allows the chance of capturing paroxysmal arrhythmias, an opportunity that is unlikely to arise with a 12-lead ECG recording unless the patient happens to be symptomatic at the time. Each of the methods of ECG monitoring has advantages over the others. External monitoring is non-invasive, but can only be performed for relatively short periods. An ILR allows continuous ECG monitoring over a much longer period, making it extremely useful for investigating patients with infrequent, but nonetheless troublesome symptoms. It does, however, involve an invasive procedure (with the attendant risks) and is more expensive than other forms of ambulatory monitoring. It can, however, prove very cost-effective if it avoids the need for multiple short-term ambulatory recordings.

Pitfalls

As with any other form of ambulatory monitoring, a failure to correlate symptoms with recorded events can lead to inappropriate diagnoses.

Further reading

ACC/AHA. *Guidelines on Ambulatory Electrocardiography*, 1999. ℘ http://circ.ahajournals.org/cgi/reprint/100/8/886

ESC Task Force on Syncope. Guidelines on management (diagnosis and treatment) of syncope. *Eur Heart J* 2004; **25**: 2054–72.

Exercise testing

Principle

Exercise testing permits the dynamic assessment of cardiac function. There are many different indications for exercise testing, but the commonest is the investigation of suspected or known coronary heart disease.

Indications

- Assessment of likelihood of coronary heart disease (CHD) in patients with chest pain.
- Risk stratification of patients with known CHD and hypertrophic cardiomyopathy.
- Evaluation of response to treatment or revascularization in CHD.
- Assessment of exercise-induced arrhythmias.
- Assessment of symptoms in valvular heart disease.
- Objective assessment of exercise capacity.

Contraindications

The absolute and relative contraindications to exercise testing are listed in Table 6.17.

Table 6.17 Absolute and relative contraindications to exercise testing

Absolute contraindications
- Recent myocardial infarction (within 2 days)
- Unstable angina (rest pain within previous 48 hours)
- Uncontrolled cardiac arrhythmias (causing symptoms or haemodynamic compromise)
- Symptomatic severe aortic stenosis
- Uncontrolled symptomatic heart failure
- Acute pulmonary embolus or pulmonary infarction
- Acute myocarditis or pericarditis
- Acute aortic dissection

Relative contraindications
- Left main stem coronary stenosis
- Moderate valvular stenosis
- Electrolyte abnormalities
- Uncontrolled hypertension (systolic >200mmHg, diastolic >110mmHg)
- Tachyarrhythmias or bradyarrhythmias
- Outflow obstruction, e.g. hypertrophic cardiomyopathy
- Inability to exercise adequately
- High-degree atrioventricular block

Patient preparation

Unless the exercise test is being performed to assess response to treatment, patients should be advised to discontinue anti-anginal drugs, e.g. β-blockers, calcium channel blockers, long-acting nitrates, nicorandil and also digoxin 48 h prior to the test. Patients should attend for the test wearing suitable clothing and footwear.

Procedure

The test should be carefully explained to the patient so that they are familiar with the exercise protocol being used. A resting ECG is recorded and the patient's blood pressure measured. An appropriately trained team comprising at least two personnel, trained in advanced life support, should supervise the test. Full resuscitation and defibrillation facilities must be readily available. Exercise can be performed using either an exercise treadmill or an exercise bicycle. A variety of protocols are available, of which the most common are the Bruce protocol and the Modified Bruce protocol (see Table 6.18). The workload during exercise normally increases at 3-min intervals, with the blood pressure and ECG being recorded at each stage. The patient should be asked to report any symptoms during the test.

Table 6.18 Modified Bruce and Bruce protocols

Protocol	Modified Bruce			Standard Bruce				
Stage	01	02	03	1	2	3	4	5
Speed (kph)	2.7	2.7	2.7	2.7	4.0	5.5	6.8	8.0
Slope (°)	0	1.3	2.6	4.3	5.4	6.3	7.2	8.1

Exercise should be stopped if there is
- A fall of >10mmHg in systolic blood pressure from baseline associated with ischaemia.
- Moderate–severe angina.
- Increasing ataxia, dizziness, or near syncope.
- Evidence of poor perfusion.
- Difficulty in monitoring the ECG or blood pressure.
- Sustained ventricular tachycardia.
- 1.0mm or more ST elevation (in leads without Q waves, other than V_1 or aVR).

One should also consider stopping exercise if there is
- A fall of >10mmHg in systolic blood pressure from baseline even in the absence of ischaemia.
- >2mm of ST segment depression or marked axis shift.
- Arrhythmias (other than sustained ventricular tachycardia, see Table 6.17).
- Fatigue, breathlessness or wheezing, leg cramps, claudication.
- Development of bundle branch block that cannot be distinguished from ventricular tachycardia.
- Increasing chest pain.
- Rise in blood pressure above 250/115.

At the end of exercise the patient may be permitted to sit. Monitoring of the ECG and blood pressure must continue until heart rate and blood pressure have returned to baseline and any ECG changes have resolved.

Risks

Exercise testing is generally well tolerated with a morbidity of 2.4 in 10,000 and a mortality of 1 in 10,000 (within 1 week of testing). Risks include arrhythmias and cardiac arrest, MI and cardiac rupture, and are more likely in those with a recent history of acute coronary syndrome. Facilities for resuscitation and defibrillation must be immediately available.

Possible results

Myocardial ischaemia is indicated by ≥1mm horizontal or down-sloping ST segment depression 80ms after the J point. Some cardiologists use ≥2mm of ST segment depression as the diagnostic criterion—this increases the specificity of the test, but reduces the sensitivity. Up-sloping ST segment depression and T wave changes are not reliable indicators of ischaemia. A fall in blood pressure (or a failure of blood pressure to rise) during exercise can also indicate ischaemia, particularly if accompanied by ST segment depression and chest pain.

Generally speaking, the earlier and the more marked the ST segment changes, the more severe the underlying coronary artery disease. The prognostic value of exercise testing is well established. Patients can be risk stratified using the Duke Treadmill Score, calculated as follows:

Duke Treadmill Score = Exercise time (Bruce protocol) − [5 × ST depression (mm)] − (4 × exercise angina index)

where: 0 = no exercise angina; 1 = exercise angina; 2 = exercise angina that led to termination of test

The Duke Treadmill Score defines a high risk group with a score of equal to or greater than −11, with an annual cardiovascular mortality of ≥5%. Low risk patients have a score of equal to or greater than +5, with an annual cardiovascular mortality of 0.5%.

Almost any arrhythmia or conduction disturbance can occur during exercise testing. If the exercise test is being performed to investigate arrhythmias this can indicate a diagnostic result.

Advantages over other tests

Exercise testing is a relatively simple and inexpensive investigation with a strong evidence base that is useful in a large number of clinical situations. Alternative tests for myocardial ischaemia include stress echocardiography, cardiac magnetic resonance (MR) and myocardial perfusion imaging.

Pitfalls

Exercise test results are commonly reported as 'positive' or 'negative', giving the erroneous impression that the results are 'black or white'. The sensitivity and specificity of exercise testing varies widely between different patient populations, but in a 'typical' population has a modest sensitivity of 50%, but a reasonably good specificity of 90%. False negative and false positive results are therefore not uncommon. If the pretest probability of CHD is low, e.g. an asymptomatic young woman, exercise testing is of little value as even a 'positive' result is unlikely to be true. Similarly, if the pretest probability of CHD is high, e.g. a male in his 60s with typical anginal symptoms, a 'negative' result is also unlikely to be true. The test is therefore of most use in diagnostic decision-making when the pretest likelihood of CHD is intermediate.

Further reading

ACC/AHA 2002 Guideline for Exercise Testing. ℘ http://www.acc.org/clinical/guidelines/exercise/exercise_clean.pdf

Myocardial perfusion imaging

Principle

Since myocardial perfusion abnormalities occur early following the onset of ischaemia, evaluation of regional myocardial perfusion heterogeneity is a sensitive marker for the presence of coronary artery disease. Myocardial perfusion imaging is most commonly performed with radionuclide imaging. Optional, but less readily available modalities include contrast echocardiography and contrast magnetic resonance imaging.

The radioisotopes thallium-201 or technetium-99m are taken up by the myocardium in proportion to blood flow. Images are then acquired by a gamma camera. The images are processed to provide colour mapping of myocardial perfusion. Information is obtained regarding the presence of reversible or fixed myocardial ischaemia. Late repetition of image acquisition allows redistribution of the isotope in areas of slow blood flow for assessment of myocardial viability.

As with all investigational methods for evaluation of ischaemia, perfusion imaging is enhanced by the addition of cardiac stress. This may be in the form of physical exercise, e.g. treadmill or bicycle, or with use of pharmacological stressors. The latter are particularly useful if the patient is physically unable to exercise sufficiently or has electrocardiographic abnormalities that prohibit accurate interpretation, e.g. left bundle branch block or ventricular pacing. The two most commonly used pharmacological stressors are the vasodilators, dipyridamole, and adenosine. Adenosine is preferred as it has a very short half-life. Dobutamine can also be used in patients with contraindications to adenosine, but it is a less effective vasodilator. Adenosine gives rise to a 4- or 5-fold hyperaemia, whereas dobutamine only has a 2-fold vasodilatory effect. During adenosine stress, there is a four- to 5-fold increase in blood flow to normal myocardial territories compared with the basal state. In the presence of coronary artery stenosis, there is impaired vasodilatation and a reduction in the stress:rest ratio, precipitating myocardial ischaemia.

Indications

- To assess the presence and degree of coronary artery stenoses in patients with suspected coronary artery disease.
- To assist in the management of patients with known coronary artery disease:
  - To determine likely prognosis and probability of future cardiac events, e.g. following MI or during proposed non-cardiac surgery.
  - To guide proposed revascularization procedures by determining the physiological significance of known coronary artery lesions, including the effects of anomalous coronary arteries, muscle bridging, and coronary artery ectasia in Kawasaki's disease.
  - To assess the success of performed revascularization strategies.
- To differentiate between areas of myocardial scar tissue and viable myocardium prior to proposed revascularization.

Contraindications and risk

Pregnancy is a contraindication to nuclear imaging. Contraindications to physical exercise testing are listed in Table 6.17

Contraindications to adenosine are

- Known hypersensitivity to adenosine.
- Untreated 2nd or 3rd degree heart block, sick sinus syndrome, long QT syndrome.
- Asthma, chronic obstructive airways disease with known bronchospasm.
- Hypotension (systolic blood pressure <90mmHg).
- Acute coronary syndrome not successfully stabilized with medical therapy.
- Decompensated heart failure.
- Concomitant use of dipyridamole (within last 24 h) or xanthines (within last 12 h).

Contraindications to dobutamine include those for physical exercise testing and

- Known hypersensitivity to dobutamine.
- Glaucoma.
- Hypokalaemia.
- Concomitant use of β-blockade.

Patient preparation

β-blockers and rate-limiting calcium antagonists should be withdrawn for 48 h prior to the test if physical exercise or dobutamine stress is planned. Xanthines and dipyridamole should be withdrawn for 24 h prior to adenosine stress, and any foods or drugs containing caffeine should be avoided. Peripheral intravenous access should be sited.

Procedure

The stress study is generally performed first, since if this is normal there may be no need to acquire resting images. The radioisotope is injected at peak stress so that myocardial uptake of the tracer reflects maximal blood flow and optimizes visualization of any perfusion deficit. The protocols for the varying forms of stress are given in Table 6.19.

Table 6.19 Radionuclear exercise and imaging protocols

Stress	Protocol	Injection time of radioisotope
Physical exercise	As directed by physician, e.g. Bruce, Sheffield, to ≥85% max predicted heart rate (MPHR)	1–2 min prior to cessation of peak exercise
Adenosine	140μg/kg/min for 6 min	3–4 min after start of infusion
Dipyridamole*	140μg/kg/min for 4 min	4 min after infusion completion
Dobutamine	In 3 min stages: 5–10, 20, 30, 40μg/kg/min	When ≥85% MPHR and/or maximal dose dobutamine

* See Pellika PA, Nagueh SF, Elhendy AA, et al. American Society of Echocardiography recommendations for performance, interpretation, and application of stress echocardiography. Journ Amer Soc Echo, 20: 1021–41.

Heart rate and blood pressure should be measured throughout physical or pharmaceutical stress. A 12-lead ECG should be observed continuously for evidence of ST segment or T wave changes suggestive of ischaemia and arrhythmias.

Redistribution imaging for assessment of myocardial viability can be performed 3–4 h after stress imaging. To enhance redistribution imaging, particularly if any perfusion deficits seen with stress are severe, sublingual nitrate can be given, followed by a further resting injection of the radio-isotope and image acquisition an hour later. This is known as a stress-redistribution-reinjection protocol.

A single or dual head gamma camera is used for image acquisition. This rotates 180° round the patient from 45° in the right anterior oblique position to 45° in the left posterior oblique position. The tomographic data are reconstructed into double oblique imaging planes. Stress and rest images are aligned carefully with accurate image registration for comparison. Image quality is assessed, and then the long and short axis images are evaluated for myocardial perfusion deficits.

Risks

It should be remembered that the patient is exposed to ionizing radiation, especially if sequential studies are planned. Physical or pharmaceutical stress may induce severe myocardial ischaemia, infarction, and potentially life-threatening arrhythmias (0.01–0.05%).

The test should be stopped if the patient is physically unable to complete the test or if s/he develops
- Severe angina.
- ST segment elevation of >0.1mV in leads without Q waves.
- A fall in systolic blood pressure >10mmHg below baseline.
- A severe hypertensive response (blood pressure >250/115).
- Clinical loss of peripheral perfusion, i.e. pallor or cyanosis.
- Dizziness or near syncope.

Possible results

Perfusion deficits are identified as areas of reduced tracer uptake. These may be assessed qualitatively or semiquantitatively. Semi-quantitative classification expresses regional myocardial uptake as a percentage of the maximal uptake seen according to the following scale:
- **Absent**:10–9%
- **Severely reduced**: 10–29%
- **Moderately reduced**: 30–49%
- **Mildly reduced**: 50–69%
- **Normal**: 70–100%

Perfusion deficits may be categorized as either reversible (present on stress imaging alone) or fixed (present on stress and rest imaging). When the redistribution protocol is followed, areas of reduced perfusion can be examined for the presence of viability (revascularization will improve regional function) or scar tissue (revascularization is futile). The size of the left and RVs can also be determined (Table 6.20).

Table 6.20 Possible results for myocardial perfusion imaging

	Stress	Rest	Clinical conclusion
Myocardial perfusion	Normal/increased	Normal	Normal
	Reduced	Normal	Myocardial ischaemia (reversible defect)
	Reduced/absent	Reduced/absent	MI (fixed defect)
Late redistribution	Reduced	↑ from baseline	Viable myocardium
	Reduced	Reduced	MI (scar)

Advantages over other tests

Radionuclide imaging is readily available and non-invasive. It is inexpensive compared with coronary angiography. In contrast to magnetic resonance imaging, where the number of imaging planes that can be acquired may be limited, radionuclide imaging provides full myocardial coverage. There are many studies supporting the ability of the technique to give accurate diagnostic information and prognostic data.

Pitfalls

Qualitative or semiquantitative analytical techniques, whereby signal intensity is compared with the area of maximal myocardial uptake, may limit accuracy in the presence of triple vessel disease where there is globally reduced myocardial perfusion. Additionally, the study may be suboptimal if peak stress is not achieved. Radionuclide imaging has poor spatial resolution in comparison with other techniques. Perfusion defects limited to the subendocardium may not be visualized. Image quality can be degraded by patient movement and by artefacts. Such artefacts include attenuation from breast tissue in the anterior wall and inferior signal loss.

Further reading

Anagnostopoulos C. et al. (2004) Procedure guidelines for radionuclide myocardial perfusion imaging. Heart **90**, Suppl 1.

Radionuclide ventriculography

Principle

Radionuclide ventriculography (RNV) is a technique to provide accurate assessment of cardiac chamber size, morphology, and function. The patient's red blood cells are radiolabelled with ^{99m}Tc pertechnate *in vitro* or *in vivo*. The labelled blood pool within the cardiac chambers is then imaged with a gamma camera, gated to the electrocardiogram. Multiple image acquisitions are acquired throughout the cardiac cycle, typically over at least 16 systolic and 32 diastolic frames. These images can be assessed based on either the radioactive count or by geometric analysis.

Indications

- Prognostic estimation in patients with heart failure or coronary artery disease.
- Estimation of operative coronary risk for non-cardiac surgery.
- Diagnosis of coronary artery disease where conventional exercise testing is inadequately performed or result equivocal.
- Evaluation of the efficacy of revascularization or medical management strategies in patients with coronary artery disease.
- Monitoring of cardiac function in patients undergoing chemotherapy.

Contraindications

The technique is contraindicated in pregnant or lactating women.

Patient preparation

No special preparation is required for a resting study. If an exercise study is to be performed, the patient should fast for 3–4 h prior to the procedure. If pharmacological stress agents are used, the same preparation as for myocardial perfusion imaging should be followed. A resting ECG is helpful to exclude arrhythmias.

Procedure

For a resting study, the patient lies supine whilst anterior and left anterior oblique images are acquired. Stress studies may be performed with either physical exercise, e.g. bicycle ergometry, or with pharmacological stressors, e.g. dobutamine. Images are acquired at intervals once the heart rate has stabilized at each new level of exercise or stress. The patient should have haemodynamic and ECG monitoring throughout. Cardiopulmonary resuscitation facilities should be available. Images are then analysed to obtain the required morphological and functional parameters. High activity areas, such as spleen or aorta, may be filtered out for optimal assessment of cardiac parameters.

Risks

Technetium has a 6-h half life. Although the heart receives the largest dose, 5% of the total radiation dose is sequestered by bone marrow, the most radiosensitive body tissue. Radiation dose is up to 1100 MBq and so a typical examination carries a fatal cancer risk of 1 in 3300. Serial studies should be avoided where alternative forms of imaging suffice.

Possible results

- Dilatation or hypertrophy of the cardiac chambers and great vessels may be identified.
- Left and right ventricular ejection fractions can be measured. Normal left ventricular ejection fraction is 60–80% at rest and slightly more during exercise. Right ventricular ejection fraction is 46–70%. Both values decline with age. The extent of any global left ventricular dysfunction can therefore be identified.
- Regional wall dysfunction at rest, low and peak dose stress, and during recovery may be described in a manner analogous to stress echocardiography in order to identify areas of reversible myocardial ischaemia, myocardial hibernation or scar.

Advantages over other tests

RNV is non-invasive and repeatable, and provides serial measurements especially in patients who are difficult to scan echocardiographically or cannot tolerate MRI. It can be used in critically-ill patients soon after acute MI.

Pitfalls

Patients receive a significant radiation dose. Echocardiography is safer and cardiac MRI is likely to replace this technique as the gold standard. Red cell labelling may be inefficient in chronic renal failure. Technical factors are important; in particular, radioactivity in the left atrium must be separated from that in the LV to obtain an accurate ejection fraction. A poor ECG signal and inappropriate gating may render data uninterpretable, heart rate variability may compromise diastolic filling indices and inadequate frame counts decrease statistical reliability.

Further reading

ACC/AHA/ASNC Guidelines for the Clinical Use of Cardiac Radionuclide Imaging, 2003. ℘ http://www.acc.org/clinical/guidelines/radio/index.pdf

Schwaiger M, Melin J. et al. Cardiological applications of nuclear medicine. *Lancet* 1999; **354**: 661–6.

Swan–Ganz catheterization

Principle

A Swan–Ganz catheter is a multi-lumen catheter that is passed percutaneously from a central vein, e.g. femoral, subclavian, or jugular to the right heart structures. It can be used to measure venous, RAt, right ventricular, PmA and LAt (indirect) pressures, to obtain blood samples for oxygen saturation estimation, to measure cardiac output and systemic vascular resistance and additionally to act as a central venous infusion port.

Indications

- Aid in the diagnosis of cardiovascular shock and pulmonary oedema.
- Management of complicated acute MI, especially right ventricular infarction, cardiogenic shock.
- Management of patients with cardiac failure.
- Fluid therapy/inotropic delivery in severely ill patients, e.g. sepsis, burns, multi-organ failure, cardiac surgery, trauma.
- Diagnostic right heart catheterization, including congenital heart disease, pulmonary hypertension, intracardiac shunts.

Contraindications

- Right-sided endocarditis.
- Prosthetic tricuspid or pulmonary valve.
- Right heart tumour or thrombus.
- Unstable ventricular arrhythmia.

Patient preparation

Local anaesthetic is injected into the skin at the site of venous access. The patient is positioned flat on a couch, generally with a head-down orientation if cephalad access is to be used. Pressure transducers are made ready and zeroed for accurate measurements. Fluoroscopic screening should be available if required.

Procedure

An access sheath is placed in the vein using a Seldinger technique. The Swan–Ganz triple lumen catheter is flushed with saline and the integrity of the flotation balloon assessed by inflation with air. Under fluoroscopic guidance or by observation of intracardiac pressure traces, the catheter is passed through the venous system towards the right heart and into a branch of the PmA. At each stage, pressure and oxygen samples can be measured. The balloon can be inflated to assist passage through the right heart. The balloon is wedged briefly into a PmA branch to obtain an assessment of indirect LAt pressure (PmA wedge pressure). Cardiac output can be calculated using a thermodilution method. Iced saline at a known temperature is injected through the proximal lumen and a thermistor at the catheter tip measures the temperature rise in the blood-warmed saline as it passes through the tricuspid valve, RV, and pulmonary valve. Systemic peripheral resistance can also be estimated.

Risks
- Arterial puncture, pneumothorax, haemothorax.
- Sepsis.
- Pulmonary embolus or infarction (if right heart contains masses or if balloon remains inflated in wedge pressure position).
- Pulmonary artery rupture (balloon over-inflation).
- Arrhythmia.

Possible results
Swan–Ganz catheterization can be used to assess pulmonary and systemic venous filling pressures and fluid status, right and left cardiac function, and also where indicated to provide information on valve dysfunction, intracardiac shunts, tamponade, and pulmonary hypertension.

Advantages over other tests
This technique has traditionally been a useful adjunct to patient monitoring in the intensive care setting, in particularly for accurate pressure evaluation of the right heart and left atrium, and for continuous cardiac output assessment. However, recently several less invasive devices have been designed for cardiac output monitoring, e.g. oesophageal Doppler.

Pitfalls
The procedure is generally well-tolerated, but it is an invasive procedure not without risk. It is essential that the Swan–Ganz catheter is inserted only by suitably-trained individuals to assist diagnosis and to monitor treatment in carefully selected patients. If a non-invasive alternative is available then this should be preferentially employed. Care must be taken in data interpretation as misleading results may be obtained if the system is not systematically and accurately zeroed for serial measurements. Indirect LAt pressure measurements may be inaccurate in patients with pulmonary disease.

Tilt table testing

Principle
On standing, gravity redistributes up to 800mL of blood to the legs. The normal compensatory response is increased sympathetic and decreased parasympathetic stimulation, which maintains blood pressure with a small increase in heart rate. Head-up tilt table testing uses gravity-induced venous pooling to assess autonomic control and to attempt to reproduce symptoms of autonomic dysfunction of dizziness or collapse, i.e. neuro-cardiogenic (vasovagal) syncope.

Indications
Testing is appropriate in the investigation of sudden, unpredictable loss of consciousness thought to be neurally-mediated (vasovagal syncope, carotid sinus syncope or situational syncope) in the absence of structural heart disease.

Contraindications

Testing is not appropriate for frail patients who cannot weight-bear for up to an hour or those with a suspected psychogenic cause of syncope.

Patient preparation

The patient should be asked to omit all cardioactive drugs for 24 h, if possible, and to fast overnight.

Procedure

The patient is laid supine and lightly strapped to a table with a weight-bearing footboard. Blood pressure, pulse and ECG are measured every 5 min for 15–20 min, and then the table is mechanically tilted to about 70°. Recordings are made for a further 30 min. If responses are normal and symptoms not reproduced, an infusion of isoprenaline adjusted to achieve a heart rate 20% higher than resting for 20 min or carotid massage may provoke a response.

Risks

Syncopal symptoms (or in extreme cases loss of consciousness), hypotension and bradycardia may be induced, albeit transiently, so full cardiopulmonary resuscitation facilities should be available. Intravenous access is necessary.

Possible results

A normal response is a <20% decrease in blood pressure associated with a modest rise in pulse rate. The test is negative in the absence of a fall in blood pressure, fall in heart rate and lack of syncopal symptoms, and positive if syncopal symptoms are induced by hypotension and/or bradycardia. A cardio-inhibitory response is characterized by a fall in heart rate (asystole in extreme cases), a vasodepressor response by a fall in blood pressure with no pulse change and a mixed response by a fall in both pulse and blood pressure.

Advantages over other tests

Monitoring of ECG and blood pressure during a 24 h ambulatory period or during a Valsalva manoeuvre: measurement of plasma catecholamines, mineralocorticoids and glucose have a role in the investigation of autonomic dysfunction and syncope, but only tilt table testing provides a dynamic objective, witnessed assessment.

Pitfalls

The test is time-consuming, and requires technical and medical personnel trained in the conduct and interpretation of the procedure and in resuscitation.

Further reading

ESC Task Force on Syncope. Guidelines on management (diagnosis and treatment) of syncope. *Eur Heart J* 2004; **25**: 2054–72.

Gastroenterology

Endoscopy

This allows direct visualization of the gastrointestinal tract mucosa and offers further diagnostic investigations to obtain tissue for histology, cytology, or microbiology, as well as therapeutic possibilities.

Consent (general)

Consent is a vital component of the endoscopy process. Patients should receive written information before attending for the procedure. This should describe pre-test preparation, the procedure itself, risks and possible complications, after-care advice (particularly for those patients requiring sedation), and contact details in the event of problems and include the consent form that the patient will be asked to sign.

Sedation

While the majority of oesophagogastroduodenoscopy (OGD) procedures can be performed using local anaesthetic spray to the oropharynx, sedation will be required for more complex or prolonged procedures. An IV combination of a sedative with amnesic effects such as midazolam or diazepam is usually combined with an analgesic such as pethidine or fentanyl. Finally, hyoscine butylbromide (Buscopan®) may act to reduce intestinal motility, which is useful for colonoscopy, endoscopic retrograde cholangiopancreatography (ERCP), or enteroscopy. An alternative to hyoscine butylbromide (Buscopan®) is glucagon which may be used for patients with glaucoma or ischaemic heart disease where hyoscine butylbromide (Buscopan®) is contraindicated.

Antibiotic prophylaxis

Guidelines have recently changed with prophylaxis indicated for percutaneous endoscopic gastrostomy or jejunostomy palcement, those patients undergoing ERCP where biliary drainage is unlikely to be achieved at the first procedure or finally for those with severe neutropenia (<0.5 10^9/L) and/or severe immunocompromise undergoing procedures with a high risk of bacteraemia such as oesophageal dilatation or variceal sclerotherapy.

Anticoagulation guidelines

For diagnostic OGD, colonoscopy, flexible sigmoidoscopy and enteroscopy, including simple biopsies and thermocoagulation techniques, it is possible to continue anticoagulation as long as the international normalized ratio (INR) is within the therapeutic range. However, therapeutic procedures such as PEG placement, ERCP, polypectomy, or dilatation require normal coagulation and specialist advice should be sought.

Risks and points for consent

Table 7.1 shows the common complications of endoscopic procedures with morbidity and mortality figures for each.

Table 7.1 Risks and complications of most commonly performed endoscopic procedures

Procedure	Risks	Morbidity for each complication	Overall mortality	Other issues
OGD	Perforation Haemorrhage	0.03% 0.002%	0.0001%	Greatest risk for therapeutic procedures Cardiorespiratory sedation-related complications 0.005%
Flexible sigmoidoscopy/ colonoscopy	Perforation Haemorrhage	0.005% 0.001%	0.001%	Cardiorespiratory complications related to sedation—0.01%
Colonic polypectomy	Perforation Haemorrhage	0.06%, 0.26%	0.007%	As above
PEG placement	Perforation Haemorrhage Infection	Overall risk 5–10%	1–2%	30-day mortality of approximately 10% (often resulting from underlying condition)
ERCP	Perforation Haemorrhage Cholangitis Pancreatitis	1.1%, 0.9% 5%, 3.8% Cardiorespiratory complications related to sedation—2.3%	1.0%	Greatest risks overall with dilated bile duct, placement of stent and high dose buscopan Risk of pancreatitis greatest with age <40 yrs, placement of stent and dilated bile duct

Further reading

Allison M. BSG Antibiotic prophylaxis in gastrointestinal endoscopy. 2009. ℘ www.bsg.org.uk. (British Society of Gastroenterology).

Christensen M, Matzen P, Schulze S, Rosenberg J. Complications of ERCP: A prospective study. *Gastrointest Endosc* 2004; **60**: 721–31.

Green J (ed). Complications of gastrointestinal endoscopy. 2006. ℘ www.bsg.org.uk (British Society of Gastroenterology guidelines)

Veitch AM, Baglin TP, Gershlick AH, et al. Guidelines for the management of anticoagulant and antiplatelet therapy in patients undergoing endoscopic procedures. *Gut* 2008. **57**: 1322–9.

Oesophagogastroduodenoscopy

- Endoluminal visualization of oropharynx to second part of duodenum.
- Allows direct testing for *Helicobacter pylori*.
- In preparation for OGD, patients should not eat for 4–6 h beforehand with clear fluids allowed up to 2 h before the procedure.
- They should remain nil-by-mouth for at least 30 min afterwards to allow local anaesthetic spray or sedation to wear off.
- Stop proton pump inhibitors 2 weeks before elective diagnostic OGD to prevent masking of appearances (risk of partial healing and thus misdiagnosing malignant oesophageal or gastric ulcers).

Alternative investigations

As an alternative procedure to OGD or enteroscopy, barium swallow, meal, or follow through may be performed depending upon symptoms (for oesophageal, gastric, or duodenal, and jejunal pathology, respectively). Investigations are limited by their lower sensitivity for mucosal pathology and inability to obtain tissue for histology or *H. pylori* testing.

Indications

Symptoms/signs

- Dysphagia.
- Haematemesis and melaena.
- Dyspepsia despite appropriate therapy.
- Iron deficiency anaemia (Fig. 7.1a).
- Weight loss.
- Vomiting or nausea.
- Investigation of suspected giardia to obtain duodenal aspirates.
- Investigation of suspected coeliac disease to obtain duodenal/jejunal biopsies.
- Investigation to obtain histology and cultures of *H. pylori*.
- Abnormal barium swallow, meal, or early follow through.

Surveillance/screening

- Ensures healing of oesophageal and gastric ulceration.
- Barrett's oesophagus.
- Establishes response to a gluten-free diet in coeliac disease.
- Diagnosis of polyps in familial polyposis syndromes.

Therapeutic

- Treatment of bleeding lesions (peptic ulceration, angiodysplasia, varices, vascular malformations).
- Palliation of oesophageal cancers using stent placement, argon plasma coagulation or Nd:Yag laser therapy.
- Placement of PEG or jejunostomy tubes (Fig. 7.1b).
- Direct placement of nasogastric or nasojejunal feeding tubes.

- Dilatation of strictures of the oesophagus or pylorus.
- Polypectomy.
- Endoscopic mucosal resection of tumours (Fig. 7.1c,d).
- Placement of luminal stents

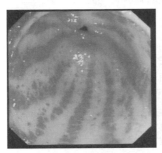

Fig. 7.1 (a) Endoscopic view of gastric antral vascular ectasia, one cause for blood transfusion-dependent iron deficiency anaemia, which may be treated using argon plasma coagulation. (📖 Colour plate 4).

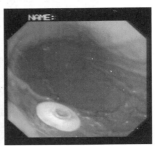

Fig. 7.1 (b) Endoscopic view of internal bumper of percutaneous endoscopic gastrostomy (PEG) holding this *in situ* in the stomach to allow feeding. PEG placement is a therapeutic possibility by using OGD to allow direct visualization.

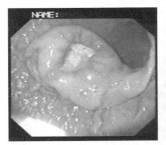

Fig. 7.1. (c) Endoscopic view of a gastric carcinoma (note rolled and heaped edges).

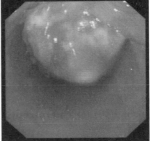

Fig. 7.1 (d) Endoscopic view of oesophageal carcinoma (note active oozing of blood).

Conventional enteroscopy

- Similar to OGD, but allows views of distal duodenum and jejunum using a 2.4m instrument.
- An overtube allows less looping, but increases complications.
- Preparation as for OGD; usually requires sedation, analgesia, and hyoscine butylbromide (Buscopan®).

Double-balloon enteroscopy

- Allows views of entire small bowel from oral or rectal approach.
- Preparation is as for OGD or colonoscopy, and requires sedation, analgesia, and buscopan.
- Consists of two balloons, one attached to distal endoscope and one to a transparent overtube sliding over the endoscope allowing movement forward by telescoping the small bowel by gripping and pleating it over the endoscope.

Alternative investigations

Diagnosis

Barium investigations are limited by a lower sensitivity for mucosal pathology. Wireless capsule endoscopy is a more effective (but less frequently available) alternative. Sonde enteroscopy uses a thinner endoscope with a balloon at its tip passing through the entire small bowel over 6–8 h, with examination occurring on withdrawal of the instrument after deflation of the balloon. However, each of these is limited by an inability to obtain tissue or provide therapeutic interventions.

Treatment (and diagnosis)

Double-balloon enteroscopy allows visualization and treatment of any lesions within the full length of the small bowel, and may replace conventional enteroscopy. Conventional enteroscopy will diagnose and treat lesions within the upper small bowel (to jejunum), but is limited by patient tolerance. Intra-operative enteroscopy allows complete examination of the entire small bowel and therapeutic possibilities via an enterotomy.

Indications for enteroscopy

Symptoms/signs

- Investigation of obscure gastrointestinal bleeding (following non-diagnostic OGD and colonoscopy).
- Investigation of lesions found on barium follow-through/computed tomography (CT) scan abdomen.
- Investigation of severe iron deficiency anaemia (following non-diagnostic OGD and colonoscopy).
- Therapeutic.
- Treatment of bleeding lesions found at enteroscopy or by wireless capsule endoscopy (WCE).
- Polypectomy.

Wireless capsule endoscopy

- Allows imaging of the entire small bowel by using an 11 × 27mm capsule ('M2A') with up to 7.5 h of battery life.
- When swallowed, the capsule transmits images to aerials attached by adhesive pads to the abdominal wall and stored on a recorder attached round the waist.
- Propelled by the patient's own peristalsis so symptom-free.
- Views of the distal small bowel are improved by using one sachet of sodium picosulfate 1 day beforehand to remove residue.
- Specialist procedure, but with a higher diagnostic yield than other small bowel investigations.
- Prior barium small bowel imaging may be advisable to rule out stricturing, where WCE could precipitate obstruction.

Indications

- WCE has a role in visual diagnosis, but is unable to obtain samples for subsequent analysis or allow therapeutic management.
- Occult gastrointestinal bleeding with non-diagnostic OGD and colonoscopy.
- Possible small bowel polyposis (e.g. Peutz–Jegher syndrome).
- Unexplained diarrhoea and malabsorption not diagnosed by other methods.

Points for consent

- 1–2% risk of obstruction reported especially if stricturing (e.g. small bowel Crohn's disease) or previous small bowel surgery.
- Contraindicated in patients with a pacemaker.

Table 7.2 Diagnostic yield of small bowel investigations for occult bleeding lesions

	Sensitivity	Specificity	Diagnostic yield
Enteroscopy	37%	97%	30–32%
Wireless capsule endoscopy	64%	92%	55–68%

Further reading

Mylonaki M, Fritscher-Raven A, Swain CP. Wireless capsule endoscopy: a comparison with push enteroscopy in patients with gastroscopy and colonoscopy negative gastrointestinal bleeding. *Gut* 2003; **52**: 1122–6.

Swain P. Wireless capsule endoscopy. *Gut* 2003; **52**: 48–50.

Flexible sigmoidoscopy & colonoscopy

- Allows examination from anus to splenic flexure (flexible sigmoidoscopy) or from anus to caecum/terminal ileum (colonoscopy).
- Flexible sigmoidoscopy may be performed without sedation.
- Colonoscopy usually requires a sedation and analgesia together with smooth muscle relaxant (buscopan).
- Preparation for flexible sigmoidoscopy: phosphate enema 30–60 min prior to the procedure.
- Preparation for colonoscopy: oral preparation using 2 sachets of sodium picosulfate on the day before the procedure with a low residue diet for the 3 days pre-procedure.

Alternative investigations

Alternative procedures are radiological: barium enema or CT colonography. Neither allows tissue to be taken, for histotopy nor polypectomy, nor other therapeutic procedure to be performed. Sensitivity is lower for detecting adenomas using CT colonography than colonoscopy; for lesions ≤10mm, sensitivity is 55% against 99% for colonoscopy. Colonoscopy is 'gold standard' for investigating likely colon cancer, diarrhoea, anaemia, and rectal bleeding.

Indications

Symptoms and signs
- Rectal bleeding (bright red = flexible sigmoidoscopy and dark red = colonoscopy), but beware as some right-sided colonic lesions do present with bright red bleeding.
- Positive faecal occult bloods (colonoscopy).
- Abnormal barium enema (depends upon site of pathology found).
- Iron deficiency anaemia (colonoscopy).
- Diarrhoea (colonoscopy with biopsies).

Surveillance/screening
- Extensive ulcerative colitis or colonic Crohn's disease for more than 8 yrs.
- High risk of adenomatous colonic polyps, or carcinoma, or previous history of adenomatous polyps or carcinoma.
- Familial polyposis syndrome (FAP), hereditary non-polyposis colorectal carcinoma (HNPCC), or other family cancer syndromes.

Therapeutic
- Treatment of bleeding lesions (angiodysplasia, vascular abnormalities, haemorrhoids).
- Dilatation of benign strictures.
- Palliation of malignant strictures (placement of stents, argon plasma coagulation, or Nd:Yag laser therapy).
- Decompression of sigmoid volvulus and non-malignant toxic megacolon.
- Endoscopic mucosal resection of tumours.

Further reading

Cairns S, Scholefield JH. (2002) Guidelines for colorectal cancer screening in high risk groups. *Gut* 2002; **51** (suppl V): V1–21.

Endoscopic retrograde cholangiopancreatography

- Side-viewing endoscope used to find the ampulla of Vater, and guide cannulation of the biliary and pancreatic ducts by injecting radio-opaque contrast medium to allow visualization of the ducts using fluoroscopy.
- Magnetic resonance cholangiopancreatography (MRCP) has replaced ERCP in 1° diagnosis. ERCP is used for interventional procedures and to obtain biopsy and cytology specimens.
- ERCP requires sedation, an analgesic and buscopan.

Alternative investigations

MRCP allows imaging of the biliary and pancreatic systems and is the best (and safest) option for diagnosis, although no therapeutic procedures are possible. A percutaneous transhepatic cholangiogram (PTC) allows imaging, stent placement and drainage of a dilated biliary tree using a trans-abdominal approach. PTC is indicated if therapeutic ERCP fails.

Indications

Symptoms and signs

- Endoscopic diagnosis of periampullary polyps, and tumours.
- Obtaining bile/brushings for cytology in suspected cholangiocarcinoma.
- Investigation of dilated ducts found on ultrasound scan with contraindications to MRCP.
- Assessment of sphincter of Oddi pressures in suspected sphincter of Oddi dysfunction syndromes (SOD).

Therapeutic

- Biliary stenting:
  - Palliation of pancreatic, ampullary and cholangiocarcinomas.
  - Treatment of biliary leak following surgery.
  - Benign biliary stricture.
- Biliary sphincterotomy:
  - Gaining access to perform diagnostic or therapeutic procedures.
  - Choledocholithiasis.
  - Ampullary carcinoma.
  - Treatment of a biliary leak following surgery.
  - Treatment of SOD.
  - Treatment of acute severe pancreatitis secondary to gallstones.
- Pancreatic stenting:
  - Drainage of pseudocysts (via stomach).
  - Following sphincterotomy for SOD (as this increases risk of pancreatitis in short-term).
- Pancreatic sphincterotomy:
  - Pancreatic stone disease.
  - Gaining access prior to stent placement.
  - Minor duct papillotomy in pancreatic divisum to prevent pancreatitis.

Endoscopic ultrasound

- Combines endoscopy with ultrasound imaging to allow visualization of organs such as the pancreas and accurate assessment of degree of invasion of luminal tumours.
- Higher frequency ultrasound probe allowed by proximity of probe to organ results in increased spatial resolution compared with transabdominal ultrasound, CT or magnetic resonance (MR) scanning.
- Two different modes of imaging are possible: radial—which allows a 360° view around the shaft of the instrument—or linear—which is in line with the endoscope and allows 90° up to 270° views.
- Specialist technique provided in few centres.
- Pre-procedure preparation is as for OGD or ERCP.
- Consent procedures differ, depending upon indications and potential pathology.

Alternative investigations

Transabdominal ultrasound, CT and MRI scanning allow views of the pancreas and liver, but do not allow such fine detail for diagnosis or therapy.

Indications

- Staging of oesophageal, gastric, pancreatic, and distal biliary tumours.
- Diagnosis and staging for gastrointestinal stromal tumours.
- Fine needle aspiration of 'Trucut' biopsy of mediastinal or coeliac axis lymph nodes, pancreatic lesions, or submucosal lesions.
- Defining mucosal abnormalities, such as Barrett's oesophagus.
- Coeliac axis nerve block to treat pancreatic pain (chronic pancreatitis or pancreatic carcinoma).
- Evaluation and treatment of pancreatic pseudocysts.
- Detection of common bile duct stones.

Further reading

Allum WH, Griffin SM, Watson A, *et al*. Guidelines for the management of oesophageal and gastric cancer. *Gut* 2002; **50** (suppl V): v1–23.

Soriano A, Castells A, Ayuso C, *et al*. Preoperative staging and tumor resectability assessment of pancreatic cancer: prospective study comparing endoscopic ultrasonography, helical computed tomography, magnetic resonance imaging, and angiography. *Am J Gastroenterol* 2004; **99**: 492–501.

Tests for *Helicobacter pylori*

Indications for testing

- 'Test and treat': patients <55 yrs of age with a low probability of significant pathology and dyspeptic symptoms do not require OGD. Non-invasive testing for *H. pylori* allows treatment of those found to be positive to assess effect on symptoms. Although it is essential that all patients with alarm symptoms (weight loss, anaemia, or dysphagia) should undergo urgent OGD.
- Ensure effective eradication in patients with confirmed peptic ulceration or MALT-lymphoma.

Non-invasive tests

Serology

Serum IgG antibodies to *H. pylori* may be detected by ELISA with sensitivity of 90% and a specificity of 70–90%. IgG levels take up to 1 year to fall so are not useful to confirm response to eradication. Other organisms may cause cross-reactivity. False negatives occur in elderly or immuno-compromised patients.

Urea breath test

Expired air is collected after ingestion of ^{13}C-labelled urea. If *H. pylori* present, bacterial urease breaks down urea → ammonium and bicarbonate then → carbon dioxide and ammonia. Expired $^{13}CO_2$ is collected into a tube 30 min after ingestion, measured by mass spectrophotometer, and compared with one collected prior to ingestion. This test is almost 100% sensitive and specific, and remains the gold standard to confirm eradication.

Faecal antigen test

H. pylori antigens in faeces are measured using an immunochromatographic test. Sensitivity exceeds 91% and specificity exceeds 92%. Commercially available kits allow testing for initial diagnosis or to confirm eradication.

Invasive tests (performed at OGD)

Investigations are based on biopsy samples. *H. pylori* density is usually greatest in the antrum, but during acid suppression the greatest concentration is found in the corpus. Colonization is patchy so may yield sampling errors.

Histology

H. pylori can be detected on routine histology using the modified Giemsa stain. Sensitivity is 85% with a specificity of almost 100%.

Culture

This is useful in those few patients who have failed eradication to establish antibiotic sensitivities. Sensitivity is over 95% with specificity of almost 100%.

Rapid urease test

A biopsy is placed into a urea solution containing phenol red. *H. pylori* contains urease, releasing ammonia from urea thus changing pH, detected as a colour change with phenol red dye turning from straw to pink/purple. Commercial kits such as the *Campylobacter*-like organism (CLO) test are available. Specificity is 97%, and sensitivity between 70 and 95%.

Further reading

Calam J. *Clinicians guide to* Helicobacter pylori. Chapman and Hall Medical, London, 1996.

Gatta L, Perna F, Ricci C *et al.* A rapid immunochromatographic assay for *Helicobacter pylori* in stool before and after treatment. *Aliment Pharmacol Ther* 2004; **15**: 469–74.

Faecal occult blood

Indications

- Population screening for colorectal neoplasms in UK started 2006–2008 with a planned screening programme from Department of Health for 60–69-yr-olds every 2 yrs. Full colonoscopy is performed for those with positive results. Mortality from colorectal carcinoma is decreased by 15–18%.
- Pre-menopausal women to establish whether iron-deficiency anaemia is related to gastrointestinal blood loss (in all other groups, the gastrointestinal (GI) tract should be investigated in iron-deficiency anaemia using OGD and colonoscopy).

Investigation

- Simple and inexpensive, performed by the patient in their own home.
- Samples taken onto test card from 3 consecutive bowel motions and card sent to screening centre.
- Test card uses the 'guaiac' reaction with pseudoperoxidase in haemoglobin causing a colour change in an indicator dye.
- Dietary changes advised (avoid red meat, horseradish, broccoli, and turnips as these have high perioxidase activity, which may cause false positive results) and vitamin C tablets (high ascorbic acid activity).

Results

- Sensitivity of the non-hydrated test is 70%; this increases to 90% with rehydration, but at the loss of specificity. Sensitivity improves with the number of samples taken.
- Individuals who are positive require full colonoscopy.
- Multicentre UK trial invited 486,355 for screening using FOB (take up 56%), finding 2% FOB positive and of these, 10.9% have carcinoma, 35% adenoma, and 54.1% to be normal

Limitations

Polyps and carcinomas may bleed intermittently, but FOB are more likely to be positive with early-stage cancers than polyps.

False positives

Rehydration of the sample, non-colorectal blood source (upper GI tract or nosebleed), red meat, broccoli, or turnips (peroxidase activity).

False negatives

'Old' sample with bacterial degradation of haemoglobin, presence of ascorbic acid, reduced, or absent bleeding.

Further reading

Hardcastle JD, Chamberlain JO, Robinson MHE, et al. Randomised controlled trial of faecal-occult-blood screening for colorectal cancer. Lancet 1996; **348**: 1472–7.

Tappenden P et al. Option appraisal of population-based colorectal cancer screening programme in England. Gut 2007; **56**: 677–84.

Valori, R. Bowel cancer screening. 2007. ✍ www.18weeks.nhs.uk

Serological & faecal testing in inflammatory bowel disease

At present, there are no tests that are sufficiently sensitive or specific to confidently diagnose either ulcerative colitis or Crohn's disease, but antibodies to *Saccharomyces cerevisiae* (ASCA) and perinuclear antineutrophil cytoplasmic antibodies (pANCA) cannot be measured in isolation as the sensitivity and specificity of each increases if the other serological marker is negative.

Perinuclear antineutrophil cytoplasmic antibodies

Occur in the serum of 50–80% of patients with histologically confirmed ulcerative colitis, but only 10% of those with Crohn's disease. This is likely to be genetically determined. These antibodies are particularly associated with 1° sclerosing cholangitis in association with ulcerative colitis. Overall sensitivity is 55.3% with a specificity of 88.5%. In a paediatric cohort with negative ASCA, sensitivity increased to 70.3% with 93.4% sensitivity.

Antibodies to *Saccharomyces cerevisiae*

Found in 60% of patients with Crohn's disease, but only 5% of those with ulcerative colitis. In Crohn's disease, the presence of high titres of ASCA appears to be associated with early age of onset, and both fibrostenosing and fistulating disease types. Here, sensitivity is 54.6% with specificity of 92.8% if pANCA is negative.

Faecal calprotectin

This is a neutrophil granulocyte cytosol protein which acts as a marker of intestinal inflammation. It is positively correlated with inflammation scores in Crohn's disease and ulcerative colitis. However, it is non-specifically elevated in neoplasia and radiation proctitis. At present it is available in few centres and it identifies a group of patients who require further investigation from those with probable irritable bowel syndrome who do not. Sensitivity for diagnosing pathology is 93% with specificity of 100%. This is likely to become more widely available with easier assays and a reduction in price compared with the cost implications of avoiding tests such as colonoscopy for those patients who do not require them.

Faecal lactoferrin

This is a neutrophil-derived protein, which acts as a marker of intestinal inflammation. As for calprotectin, it aims to use non-invasive testing to differentiate those who require intestinal imaging, such as colonoscopy, from those more likely to have functional disease, such as irritable bowel syndrome. It is not as effective as calprotectin in this regard as sensitivity for diagnosing pathology is 82% and specificity is 84%.

Further reading

Reese GE. *et al.* Diagnostic precision of anti-*Saccharomyces cervisiae* antibodies and perinuclear antineutrophil cytoplasmic antibodies in inflammatory bowel disease. *Am J Gastroenterol.* 2006; **101**: 2410–22.

Schröder O, et al. Prospective evaluation of faecal neutrophil-derived proteins in identifying intestinal inflammation: combination of parameters does not improve diagnostic accuracy of calprotectin. *Aliment Pharmacol Ther.* 2007; **26**: 1035–42.

Tumour markers

- As a result of generally low sensitivities and specificities, these should not be first-line investigations.
- They are best used for tracking patients following diagnosis of carcinoma through subsequent surgery, and chemo-radiotherapy when levels should fall to normal unless disease recurrence.

Carcinoembryonic antigen

- ↑ in 60% of those with localized colorectal carcinoma and 80–100% of those with metastatic disease.
- Non-specific and non-diagnostic—also ↑ in bronchial carcinoma, heavy smokers, inflammatory bowel disease.
- Levels do not relate to tumour load, but a rising level, which was previously low or normal, may imply recurrence of colorectal carcinoma.

α-fetoprotein

- Normally produced by fetal liver.
- High levels in non-pregnant adults imply hepatocellular carcinoma (raised in over 90% cases).
- ↑ Serological concentrations in pregnancy suggest neural tube defect.
- Blood levels may be ↑ in hepatocyte regeneration, acute viral hepatitis, cirrhosis, choriocarcinoma, and teratoma.
- May be used 6 monthly (with liver ultrasound scan) to screen cirrhotic patients for development of hepatocellular carcinoma

Carbohydrate antigen 19-9 (CA 19-9)

- ↑ in pancreaticobiliary obstruction with the highest levels in pancreatic carcinoma.
- Levels >40IU/L have 75–90% sensitivity and 80–95% specificity for ductal pancreatic carcinoma.
- Serum levels may be elevated in jaundice, cholangitis, choledocholithiasis, and chronic pancreatitis.

Cancer antigen 125 (Ca 125)

- Glycoprotein antigen to an epidermal growth factor receptor (p110 sEGFR).
- Blood levels ↑ with menstruation, endometriosis, pelvic inflammatory disease, pregnancy, and ascites.
- Highest levels with ovarian malignancy, but also ↑ with ovarian, pancreas, breast, lung, and colon cancers.
- 20% ovarian cancers have little/no expression of Ca 125.
- Useful in monitoring response of ovarian carcinoma to treatment (if initially positive) as rising level Ca 125 precedes clinical recurrence by up to 3 months (>90% cases).
- As isolated values lack sensitivity and specificity, serial Ca 125 readings may be used to achieve specificity of 99.6%, but with a sensitivity of only 80%.

Further reading

Sakamoto K, Haga Y, Yoshimura R, Egami H, Yokoyama Y, Akagi M. Comparative effectiveness of the tumour diagnostics, CA 19-9, CA 125 and carcinoembryonic antigen in patients with diseases of the digestive system. *Gut* 1987; **28**: 323–9.

Investigations for small bowel pathology

General investigations

Presenting features of small bowel pathology include diarrhoea (or steator-rhoea), abdominal pain, weight loss, and nutritional deficiencies. Investigation of diarrhoea is shown in Fig. 7.4. Occasionally, occult GI bleeding may originate in the small bowel and an algorithm for investigation of anaemia is shown in Fig. 7.5.

Serology

Anti-endomysial antibodies (almost 100% sensitivity for coeliac disease, but may be false −ve in presence of a low IgA)—this can be confirmed using duodenal or jejunal biopsies, which would reveal partial villous atrophy. Now largely replaced by anti-tissue transglutaminase (see 📖 Endomysial & tissue transglutaminase antibodies, p339).

Endoscopy

OGD and enteroscopy allow views of the proximal small intestine to obtain tissue and allow therapeutic possibilities. Wireless capsule endoscopy permits diagnosis from the whole small intestine, but does not allow therapeutic options.

Radiology

Barium follow-through involves ingestion of dilute barium with images taken every 10–30 min until barium reaches the caecum. Small bowel enema (enteroclysis) uses insertion of a nasoduodenal tube to infuse barium slowly, with this column followed continuously using fluoroscopy. Both studies define structural abnormalities. Small bowel enema allows more focused views of areas of interest, such as the terminal ileum (Fig. 7.2).

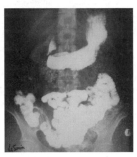

Fig. 7.2 Barium follow-through image showing a terminal ileal stricture.

Nuclear medicine

Radiolabelled white cell scintigraphy for inflammation/infection

This uses ^{99m}-technetium-hexamethylpropyleneamine oxide (^{99m}Tc-HMPAO) to show intensity and extent of inflammation or infection 1 & 3 h after injection of autologous, radiolabelled leucocytes, and is used in Crohn's disease and ulcerative colitis to delineate disease extent (Fig. 7.3). False negative results occur, particularly with small bowel Crohn's disease. There is a sensitivity of 96% and specificity of 97% for inflammatory bowel disease, and a sensitivity of 85–100% and specificity of 100% for detecting abscesses.

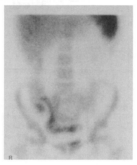

Fig. 7.3 Radiolabelled white cell scintigraphy using ^{99m}-Tc-HMPAO to show inflammation of the terminal ileum consistent with Crohn's disease (taken at 3 h).

Radionuclide studies to detect Meckel's diverticulum

Intravenous ^{99m}Tc pertechnate accumulates in gastric mucosa with a time course of 5–60 min. Uptake in ectopic mucosa (e.g. Meckel's diverticulum) occurs simultaneously. Imaging at 5–10 min intervals up to 2 h after injection allows localization of the site of ectopic mucosa. False positives are caused by early gastric emptying and duplication cysts. Sensitivities vary from 90% in children to 60% in adults. (See 📖 Meckel's scan: ectopic gastric mucosa localization, p844.)

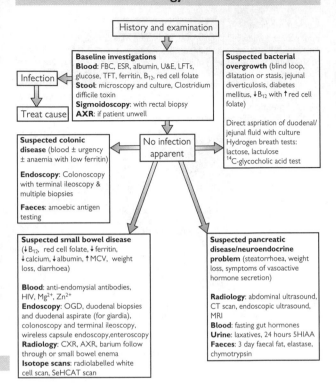

Fig. 7.4 Investigation of diarrhoea.

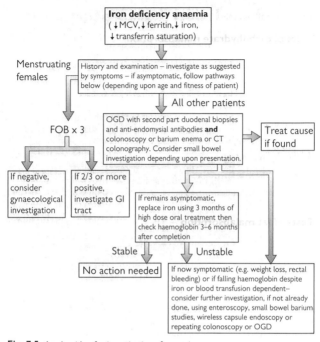

Fig. 7.5 An algorithm for investigation of anaemia.

Further reading

Cooney DR, Duszynski DO, Gamboa E *et al.* The abnormal technetium scan (a decade of experience). *J Paediatr Surg* 1982; **17**: 611–19.

Tests of small bowel absorption

Tests of carbohydrate malabsorption

D-xylose tolerance test

Xylose is absorbed from the proximal small bowel, and urinary excretion and blood levels reflect absorption. It is used mainly in paediatric practice and has a low sensitivity.

Lactose tolerance test

Oral administration of 50g lactose is followed by blood sampling every 30 min for 2 h. A rise in blood glucose <1.1mmol/L suggests deficiency of disaccharidases, especially with colicky abdominal pain and diarrhoea.

Lactose-hydrogen test

This is similar to the hydrogen breath test for bacterial overgrowth. Lactase-deficient individuals fail to metabolize lactose, which then undergoes luminal metabolism by lactase-producing colonic bacteria to yield hydrogen.

Tests of fat malabsorption

Patients with fat malabsorption secondary to small bowel diseases, such as coeliac disease or tropical sprue, may malabsorb between 10 and 20g/day of fat, while patients with pancreatic insufficiency may malabsorb 30–50g/24 h. A normal faecal fat excretion is less than 6g/day (17mmol/day).

3-day faecal fat

- Unpleasant test, fallen into disuse, but remains gold standard.
- Fat content measured in a 3-day faecal collection.
- Patient takes standard diet of 100g fat/day.
- Does not differentiate small bowel and pancreatic malabsorption.

Radiolabelled ^{14}C fat breath test

- [14]C triolein is ingested and [14]CO2 measured in breath.
- Small bowel malabsorption shows delayed $^{14}CO_2$ excretion.
- Pancreatic malabsorption shows low $^{14}CO_2$ excretion, which is corrected using oral pancreatic enzyme supplements such as Creon.

Fat microscopy

- Examines faeces for neutral fat, fatty acid crystals, and soaps.
- Limited value as it neither quantifies levels nor suggests a cause.

Bile salt malabsorption

SeHCAT scan

- The labelled bile acid [75]selenium homotaurocholate (SeHCAT) is administered orally. Retention is measured at 7 days by whole body counting.
- Retention >15% SeHCAT is normal (less indicates malabsorption).
- Useful second line investigation in patients with diarrhoea of unknown aetiology.

Further reading

Wildt S, Norby Rasmussen S, Lysgard Madsen J, et al. Bile acid malabsorption in patients with chronic diarrhoea: clinical value of SeHCAT test. Scand J Gastroenterol 2003; **38**: 826–30.

Tests for bacterial overgrowth

Deep duodenal/jejunal aspiration

- Samples may be collected through the biopsy channel at OGD.
- Scanty bacteria are present in normal upper small bowel.
- Numbers in excess of 10^6/mL of aspirated fluid are pathological.
- This technique may culture *Giardia* and *Strongyloides* spp.

Hydrogen breath tests

Rationale

In mammals, the only source of breath hydrogen is bacterial fermentation of carbohydrates. Hydrogen is absorbed from the intestinal lumen and expired during breathing. In bacterial overgrowth, hydrogen production can occur in the small intestine, as well as in the colon.

Method

- A mouthwash is given beforehand to reduce contamination by oral bacteria.
- Test dose of glucose (50g) and breath hydrogen measured.
- An early peak (e.g. 40 min) suggests bacterial overgrowth.

Limitations

- Sensitivity 60–90% with specificity of 80%.
- False negatives result from variations in microflora present in the small intestine or antibiotic administration within 3 weeks.
- False positives occur in patients with impaired glucose tolerance, those with rapid transit to the colon, and smokers.
- Patients should avoid eating pulses for 48 h prior to the test (normal digestion of pulses liberates excess hydrogen).

Alternative

- Lactulose 10–15g (a non-absorbable disaccharide) that ferments in the small intestine if bacterial overgrowth is present, producing hydrogen.
- Rapid transit to the colon will also produce an early peak.

^{14}C-glycocholic acid test

Rationale

- Bacteria act to deconjugate radiolabelled bile salts to produce radioactive glycine, which is metabolized in the liver to $^{14}CO_2$.
- An early peak suggests bacterial overgrowth in the small intestine or rapid transit to the colon.

Method

^{14}C-labelled bile salts given by mouth and $^{14}CO_2$ measured in expired air.

Limitations

- Difficult to distinguish between small bowel overgrowth and other causes of bile salt malabsorption, e.g. ileal dysfunction, unless faecal bile acid excretion is measured.
- Ileal dysfunction leads to a late peak in $^{14}CO_2$ and high faecal bile acids, while bacterial overgrowth results in increased and early breath excretion of $^{14}CO_2$ and low faecal bile acid excretion (<5%).

Tests of pancreatic exocrine function

Symptoms of pancreatic exocrine dysfunction include diarrhoea or steatorrhoea and weight loss. Investigations aim to determine the degree of pancreatic insufficiency; however, both biochemical and particularly radiological investigations are unreliable in mild disease. Fat malabsorption may occur in small bowel or pancreatic disease and diagnosis may prove difficult as a result (see 📖 Tests of small bowel absorption, p482). A diagnostic algorithm for investigation of diarrhoea is shown in Fig. 7.4.

Faecal testing

Elastase

Elastase is a proteinase produced by pancreatic acinar cells and remains undegraded during gut transit. Immunoassay of faeces allows measurement of elastase in a random faecal sample. Levels of >200µg/g faeces are normal, 100–200 represents mild insufficiency and <100 is diagnostic of severe disease. Specificity is 93%, while sensitivity is 63, 100, and 100% for mild, moderate, and severe disease, respectively. False positives may occur with high volume watery stools. This test is not affected by pancreatic enzyme supplements.

Chymotrypsin

This proteinase is cheaper to measure in faeces, but is less sensitive (64%) and specific (89%) than elastase, and its use is mainly in children to screen for cystic fibrosis. Result is affected by pancreatic enzyme supplements.

Direct investigations

Secretin test

Direct intubation of the duodenum allows collection of pancreatic juice following intravenous injection of a hormonal secretogogue. Secretin injection allows measurement of volume and bicarbonate content, cholecystokinin (CCK) injection allows measurement of amylase, trypsin, and lipase. This test is highly sensitive and specific, even with mild pancreatic disease, but is not widely available.

Indirect investigations

Both tests are more sensitive and specific with more advanced dysfunction.

PABA test

A synthetic peptide (N-benzoyl-L-tyrosol p-aminobenzoic acid (PABA)) is given orally. In normal patients, pancreatic chymotrypsin hydrolyses this peptide to yield free PABA, which is absorbed, metabolized, and excreted in urine. In the presence of pancreatic insufficiency, free PABA levels are reduced, and thus absorption and excretion are lower. This results in lower urinary PABA and a lower serum concentration.

Pancreolauryl test

Fluorescein dilaurate (an ester) is taken orally with a set diet. In the presence of normal pancreatic function, arylesterases release fluorescein, which is absorbed, partially conjugated in liver, and excreted in urine. A 24 h urine collection for excreted levels shows close correlation with pancreatic exocrine function.

Testing for neuroendocrine tumours

Carcinoid and carcinoid syndrome

Urinary 5-hydroxyindole acetic acid (5HIAA)

- 24 h collection of urine for 5HIAA.
- High levels imply carcinoid syndrome.
- High specificity, but false positives result from serotonin-rich bananas, tomatoes, or drugs such as phenothiazines.

Further investigations

Abdominal CT scan with biopsy of liver metastases may confirm the diagnosis. The 1° tumour is identified in only 50–70%. Radiolabelled octreotide scintigraphy establishes tumour extent in difficult cases as most carcinoid tumours express somatostatin receptors.

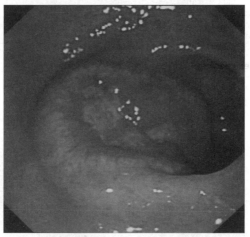

Fig. 7.6 Endoscopic image of a rectal carcinoid tumour. (☐ Colour plate 5.)

Hormone-secreting pancreatic tumours
- Pancreatic islet-cell tumours that produce vasoactive peptide hormones.
- Measured using fasting gut hormone assays: insulin (paired with a serum glucose sample), glucagon, vasoactive intestinal peptide (VIP), pancreatic polypeptide (PP), gastrin, and somatostatin.
- Single tumours often secrete more than one type of hormone.
- Up to 50% of these slow-growing tumours are thought to be non-functional.
- Several types of tumour occur as part of the multiple endocrine neoplasia syndrome type 1 (MEN-1).
- Concurrent therapy with a proton pump inhibitor will falsely raise serum gastrin levels.

Further investigations
- Abdominal CT scan.
- Endoscopic ultrasound.
- Laparoscopy.
- Radiolabelled octreotide scintigraphy.
- Rarely, selective venous sampling will confirm the diagnosis.

Further reading
Oberg K. Neuroendocrine gastrointestinal tumours—a condensed overview of diagnosis and treatment. *Ann Oncol* 1999; **10** (suppl 2), S2–8.

Gastrointestinal physiology

pH monitoring

Indications

- Assessment of gastro-oesophageal reflux disease (GORD).
- Atypical symptoms such as asthma or non-cardiac chest pain.
- Before consideration of anti-reflux surgery.
- Poorly controlled GORD to confirm diagnosis on or off treatment.

Investigation

An ambulatory 24 h test that places a pH electrode through the nose to sit 5cm above the lower oesophageal sphincter. This is connected to a portable microprocessor that records episodes where the pH dips below 4. The patient fills in a simultaneous event diary, to correlate symptoms and episodes of low pH. For most patients, H_2 receptor antagonists and proton pump inhibitors are stopped 7 days beforehand. A few patients require testing on medication to establish treatment response.

Results

Several parameters are measured:

- Frequency and duration of episodes of pH <4.
- Duration of longest episode.
- Correlation between symptoms and pH.
- Excessive oesophageal acid reflux is defined as a total duration of pH <4 of 4–6% of recording time.

Oesophageal manometry

Indications

- Diagnosis and assessment of motility disorders suggested by symptoms/ OGD/barium swallow findings.
- Defining the precise location of the lower oesophageal sphincter prior to 24 h pH monitoring.
- Before consideration of anti-reflux surgery.

Investigation

A static test using a nasogastrically-placed multiple channel, water perfused catheter, which is gradually withdrawn during a series of wet and dry swallows. Pressure is measured through the length of the oesophagus, at the upper and lower oesophageal sphincter and the duration and frequency of contractions are recorded (see Table 7.3).

Table 7.3 Results

Non-specific motility disorder	Abnormal and incomplete peristalsis with normal body contractions
Achalasia	Incomplete relaxation and high pressure of lower oesophageal sphincter with aperistalsis of the oesophageal body
Nutcracker oesophagus	High amplitude and duration of contractions, normal peristalsis
Oesophageal spasm	Disordered peristalsis with simultaneous prolonged contractions throughout

Gastric emptying

Scintigraphy using the radioactive tracer ^{99m}technetium displays gastric movements with a range of test meals (liquid to solid) to quantify gastric emptying and intestinal filling over time. This confirms dysmotility although in practice, barium and endoscopic studies provide enough information (see 📖 Gastric emptying studies, p842).

Intestinal transit studies

Intestinal transit may be established using 50 radio-opaque plastic markers inside a pH-sensitive gel capsule, which is designed to release its contents in the terminal ileum. An abdominal radiograph at 100 h should show less than 20% of markers present in the colon. A rarely used alternative is radioactive indium-labelled polystyrene pellets with gamma camera recording of the pellet's progress through the intestine. These investigations are useful to determine colonic transit in suspected slow transit constipation. Normal transit from mouth to anus is 1–3 days.

Anorectal manometry

A water-perfused catheter measures anorectal pressures to assess voluntary and involuntary sphincter squeeze pressures and reflex responses to balloon distension in the rectum. Readings allow assessment of rectal sensation, spinal reflexes, and internal and external sphincter integrity. These tests are useful for assessment of faecal soiling, incontinence and chronic constipation.

Sphincter of Oddi manometry

A water-perfused pressure catheter is used during ERCP to measure sphincter of Oddi pressures to formally diagnose SOD (a triad of abnormal liver function, biliary type abdominal pain and dilatation of the biliary tree in the absence of a physical cause such as gallstone disease). Diagnosis is confirmed by high resting pressure, retrograde peristalsis and a failure of contrast to drain from the biliary tree within 45 min. Although patients with SOD have an increased risk of pancreatitis after ERCP, biliary sphincterotomy may relieve symptoms of pain.

Non-invasive liver investigations

Basic liver function testing

These are basic serological screening tests that establish whether liver inflammation, infection, or obstruction is present.

Alanine transaminase

Alanine transaminase (ALT: cytosol enzyme specific to the liver) and aspartate transaminase (AST: mitochondrial enzyme also present in heart, muscle, kidney and brain)—both enzymes are present in hepatocytes and leak into blood with liver cell damage.

Alkaline phosphatase

Alkaline phosphatase (ALP: canalicular and sinusoidal membranes of liver but also bone, intestine, placenta)—specific isoenzymes for ALP are produced by different tissues but a simultaneously raised γ-glutamyl transpeptidase (γGT) and ALP implies a hepatic origin. Extra- and intrahepatic cholestasis may cause raised ALP, and result from benign or malignant disease with or without raised bilirubin. Highest levels result from 1° biliary cirrhosis and hepatic metastases.

γ-glutamyl transpeptidase

γGT (microsomal enzyme)—activity can be induced by drugs, such as phenytoin, rifampicin, and alcohol. Mild elevation of γGT is common with even a small alcohol intake and isolated elevation does not imply liver disease. It rises in parallel with ALP in cholestasis.

Albumin

A protein that is synthesized in the liver. Plasma concentration partially results from functional capacity within the liver. However, it has a serum half-life of 20 days and may be normal in early phases of acute liver disease. Hypoalbuminaemia may also arise from an increased volume of distribution (sepsis, overhydration, pregnancy); increased excretion or degradation (nephrotic syndrome, protein-losing enteropathy); haemorrhage; or catabolic states such as malignancy or burns.

Prothrombin time

Test of plasma clotting activity and reflects the activity of vitamin K-dependent clotting factors synthesized by the liver. Prothrombin time (PT) may be elevated in acute or chronic liver disease. In vitamin K deficiency with normal liver function, PT will return to normal within 18 h of administration of parenteral vitamin K.

Bilirubin

In liver disease, a raised bilirubin is usually associated with other liver function abnormalities. There are many causes of raised serum bilirubin. Bilirubin may be conjugated or unconjugated, although in practice, this conjugation state only differentiates congenital hyperbilirubinaemias. In Gilbert's syndrome (the most common, benign cause of an isolated raised serum bilirubin) an elevated unconjugated bilirubin, which rises during fasting and mild illness diagnoses the condition.

Immunoglobulins

- IgG ↑ in viral hepatitis, chronic autoimmune hepatitis, and cirrhosis.
- IgM ↑ in 1° biliary cirrhosis, non-biliary cirrhosis, and acute viral hepatitis.
- IgA is ↑ in alcoholic liver disease with β–γ fusion seen on electrophoresis.

Specific biochemical tests

These are summarized in Table 7.4, with serological tests, diagnosis, and definitive investigations required to confirm the diagnosis. The best investigations for an individual patient are established from history, examination, and basic biochemical parameters.

Specific virological tests

Hepatitis A

- **Acute infection**: —positive IgM antibodies to hepatitis A (HAV).
- **Chronic infection**: does not occur.
- **Markers of clearing virus**: positive IgG antibodies to HAV and anti-HAV IgM.

Hepatitis B

Acute infection with subsequent clearing of virus

- HBsAg appears in blood from 6–12 weeks after infection then disappears.
- HBeAg appears early then declines rapidly.
- Anti-HBs appears late and indicates immunity.
- Anti-HBc is the first antibody to appear and IgM anti-HBc may persist for many months as the only marker of ongoing viral replication when HBsAg has disappeared and anti-HBs is not yet detectable.
- Anti-HBe appears after anti-HBc and indicates decreased infectivity.

Acute infection leading to chronic hepatitis B

- HBsAg persists and indicates chronic carrier state.
- HBeAg persists, correlating with increased severity and infectivity.
- Anti-HBe indicates seroconversion (if this occurs) with disappearance of HBeAg and a rise in ALT.
- HBV DNA suggests continued viral replication.

Hepatitis C
- **Acute infection**: hepatitis C HCV RNA is positive 1–2 weeks after infection with HCV antibodies developing after ~12 weeks.
- **Chronic infection**: more than 50% patients with persistent HCV RNA, which can be measured as viral load.
- Hepatitis C has 6 genotypes that determine response to treatment.

Hepatitis E
- Similar to hepatitis A with no chronic or carrier state.

Investigation of liver disease
Fig. 7.7 shows an algorithm for investigation of liver disease. This differentiates obstructive from parenchymal liver disease to suggest further investigation and treatment.

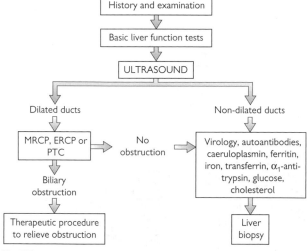

Fig. 7.7 An algorithm for investigation of liver disease.

Table 7.4 Specific biochemical tests

Test	Condition	Findings	More specific tests
Serum ferritin Serum iron Transferrin saturation	Haemochromatosis	Serum iron >30µmol/L Serum ferritin >500µg/L Transferrin sat >60%	HFE gene testing (83–90% patients have Cys 282 Tyr mutation; 25% have His 63 Asp; 187G in complete linkage disequilibrium with Cys 282 Tyr). Liver biopsy—with dry weight of iron
Urinary copper excretion Serum copper Caeruloplasmin	Wilson's disease	Serum copper and caeruloplasmin levels are usually reduced, but can be normal α_1-antitrypsin	Liver biopsy—with dry weight of copper
α_1-antitrypsin	α_1-antitrypsin def.	Levels of <10% of normal in homozygotes and 60% in heterozygotes	Liver biopsy and lung function testing for emphysema
AMA	Primary biliary cirrhosis	Antimitochondrial antibodies present in titres >1/160 specific M2 antibody (possible non-specific ↑ ANA/SMA) ↑ serum IgM and ALP	Liver biopsy
ANA/SMA	Type I autoimmune hepatitis	↑ ANA ± SMA ↑ total IgG	Liver biopsy
Anti-LKM1 or anti-liver cytosol antibodies	Type II autoimmune hepatitis	↑ Antibodies titres ↑ Total IgG	Liver biopsy
Fasting cholesterol and glucose, glycosylated haemoglobin	Non-alcoholic fatty liver disease/ non-alcoholic Steatohepatitis	Impaired glucose tolerance	Liver biopsy

Liver biopsy

- Obtains tissue for diagnosis of diffuse or localized parenchymal disease.
- Severity of histological liver dysfunction cannot be predicted from basic LFTs.
- Consent should be obtained based on risks.
- Transjugular liver biopsy overcomes many contraindications.

Indications

- Unexplained persistently abnormal LFTs.
- Staging of disease in hepatitis B or C infection, and prior to considering antiviral treatment.
- Acute hepatitis of unknown aetiology.
- Cirrhosis of unknown aetiology.
- Alcohol-related liver disease.
- 1° biliary cirrhosis/chronic active hepatitis.
- Targeted liver biopsy of lesions (not if resection/transplant is a possibility).
- Pyrexia of unknown origin.
- Haemochromatosis/Wilson's disease.
- Storage diseases.
- Post-liver transplant to rule out acute or chronic rejection.

Methods for obtaining tissue: (risks and benefits)

Percutaneous with or without ultrasound viewing (Table 7.5)

- Standard method for obtaining tissue.
- Ultrasonography of liver and biliary tree pre-procedure to identify anatomical variations increasing risk and to rule out obstruction.
- Most complications <2 h, but can occur up to 24 h.
- No evidence that direct ultrasound-guided biopsy is safer and ultrasound should be used only if a targeted biopsy is required.

Contraindications

- An uncooperative or confused patient.
- PT prolonged by >3 s, platelets <80 × 10⁹/L or bleeding diathesis.
- Ascites.
- Hydatid cysts (risks of anaphylaxis and abdominal seeding).
- Extrahepatic cholestasis.
- Higher risk of bleeding if amyloidosis present.

Minor complications

Shoulder tip pain, minor intra-abdominal bleeding, or mild abdominal pain (up to 30%)—usually settles with analgesia.

Major complications

- Perforation (0.01–0.001%: pneumothorax, gallbladder puncture, kidney, colon).
- Intra-abdominal haemorrhage; haemobilia (0.05%: a triad of biliary colic, jaundice and melaena within 3 days of liver biopsy).
- Mortality varies between 0.001–0.0001% and results from intraperitoneal haemorrhage or biliary peritonitis.
- Risk of tumour seeding if a malignant lesion is biopsied: if curative resection/transplantation is planned, needle biopsy should be avoided.

Transjugular

- Specialist technique carried out using fluoroscopic guidance.
- Catheter passes from the right internal jugular vein, through the right atrium and inferior vena cava, and into the hepatic veins.
- Patient holds his/her breath while the biopsy needle is advanced through the catheter then rapidly pushed forward by 1–2cm into the liver to obtain a small core of liver parenchyma.
- Safe technique with few complications (1.3–2% morbidity and 0.5% mortality) usually performed in higher risk patients.
- Complications range from neck haematoma, puncture of intrathoracic arteries, transient Horner's syndrome, cardiac arrhythmias, infection, and perforation of the liver capsule.
- Test of choice in patients excluded from percutaneous biopsy by coagulopathy, bleeding diathesis, ascites, portal hypertension, and amyloidosis.
- Transjugular cannulation allows measurement of portal venous pressures.

Laparoscopic

- Allows sampling of the liver when an operation is planned.
- Allows targeted biopsies, as well as parenchymal biopsies.
- Bleeding is directly controlled and perforation is avoided.
- Risks of surgery and anaesthesia should be considered.

Table 7.5 Percutaneous liver biopsy—practical procedure

Procedure	Should be carried out by an experienced doctor using aseptic precautions
Check	Clotting, FBC, and take G&S within 24 h before procedure (cancel if platelets <80 × 10^9/L or PT prolonged >3 s)
Patient	Lies flat on his/her back
Liver margins	Delineated using percussion or ultrasound
1% lidocaine	5mL injected at the point of maximal dullness down to the liver capsule through intercostal space in expiration
Menghini or Trucut needle	Used to obtain sample with patient's breath held in expiration (up to 2 passes may be used). Menghini needles use suction, have a lower rate of complications and allow more rapid biopsy, but have a lower yield for tissue than Trucut (a cutting needle)
Sample	Placed into 10% formalin (or into a dry pot to estimate dry weight of iron or copper or for culture)
Patient	Nurse in supine position or right lateral for >6 h with regular BP and pulse measurements (every 15 min for 2 h, every 30 min for the next 2 h then hourly) with urgent medical review if any sign of deterioration
If stable	At 6 h, the patient can be discharged home as long as s/he can return to hospital within 30 min and have a responsible adult with him/her overnight

Further reading

Grant A, Neuberger J, Day C, Saxseena S. Guidelines on the use of liver biopsy in clinical practice. *Br Soc Gastroenterol* 2004, 1–15. ✍ www.bsg.org.uk

Investigations of ascitic fluid

Investigation requires diagnostic aspiration

- 10mL is sent for cell count, Gram stain, Ziehl–Neelsen (ZN) stain culture (add 10mL to a pair of blood culture bottles to increase diagnostic yield).
- 10mL is sent for cytology.
- 10mL for biochemical investigation of protein, glucose, lactate dehydrogenase (LDH), triglycerides (if chylous ascites is suspected), and amylase if pancreatic ascites is suspected.

Results

Cell count

- Polymorphonuclear leucocytes (neutrophils) >250cells/mm^3 suggest underlying spontaneous bacterial peritonitis (or 2° infection).
- Total leucocytes of >500cells/mm^3 imply bacterial peritonitis (SBP) if a specific neutrophil count is not available.
- Lymphocyte count >500cells/mm^3 implies tuberculous peritonitis (with raised protein, positive ZN stain/TB culture and low glucose).

Gram stain and culture

- Gram staining for early identification of bacteria and bacterial culture allows targeting of antimicrobial therapy.

Protein

- Using ascitic fluid protein levels to aid diagnosis is best achieved using the serum ascites albumin gradient (SAAG) by subtracting ascites albumin concentration from serum albumin concentration. Levels ≥11g/L suggest cardiac failure, cirrhosis, and nephrotic syndrome, while levels <11g/L suggest malignancy, tuberculosis or pancreatitis as causes.
- Risk of spontaneous bacterial peritonitis is greatest if ascitic protein <10g/L.

Cytology

May be diagnostic in cases of peritoneal malignancy.

Amylase

↑ ascitic amylase (> 2000 IU/L) is typical of pancreatic ascites.

Triglycerides

↑ in chylous ascites.

Table 7.6 Ascitic fluid aspiration—practical procedure

Patient	Lies on his/her back tilting towards side planned for aspiration
Percussion	Used to find shifting dullness in left or right lower quadrant
Chlorhexidine	Used to clean the site
Lignocaine	2–3mL of 1% used to infiltrate a site in the left or right lower quadrant where shifting dullness is detected. It should be possible to aspirate ascitic fluid using a standard 19G needle.
50mL syringe	Sterile 19G needle placed through the same site to obtain the samples required.
Rare complications	Include bowel perforation, secondary bacterial peritonitis or haemorrhage

Respiratory medicine

Airway hyper-responsiveness test or histamine/methacholine challenge test

Clinical indications
Suspected asthma.

Patient preparation
1 Explain procedure to patient.
2 Obtain informed consent.
3 Warn that wheezing and shortness of breath may occur, and that a bronchodilator may be given.
4 Baseline FEV_1 measured.
5 Patient breathes in a nebulized aerosol of histamine (or methacholine) of increasing concentrations. This stimulates bronchoconstriction in a dose-dependent manner.
6 The FEV_1 is measured after each dose.
7 Patient must remain in department for 30 min following the procedure to observe any delayed reactions.

Possible results
The % fall in FEV_1 from baseline is plotted against the dose of inhaled histamine on a logarithmic scale. A dose–response curve is constructed and the provocation concentration (PvC) of inhaled histamine required to reduce the FEV_1 by 20% (PvC_{20}) can be derived by linear extrapolation. This figure has been arbitrarily chosen to assess degrees of bronchial reactivity for ease of comparison and safety.

Interpretation
- Asthma suggested by PvC_{20} <8mg/mL.
- A direct relationship exists between the severity of asthma and requirement for medication, and the PvC_{20} value as an index of bronchial hyper-responsiveness.
- Non-asthmatic subjects almost always have a PvC_{20} >8mg/mL.

Advantages over other tests
- Easy to do.
- Cheap.
- Non-invasive.
- Quick.
- Reproducible.
- Safe—bronchoconstriction may be reversed by inhaled β-adrenergic agonist. It is important that personnel performing the test are able to recognize severe bronchospasm and that resuscitation equipment is available.

Contraindications
- Documented cholinergic hypersensitivity, e.g. cholinergic urticaria or angio-oedema, or both.
- Allergy to histamine/methacholine (Fig. 8.1).
- Inability to perform acceptable quality spirometry.

- Unstable cardiac status, e.g. recent MI, arrhythmia, or heart failure.
- Uncontrolled hypertension (systolic BP >200 or diastolic BP >100).
- Pregnancy.
- Severe baseline obstruction with FEV_1 <80% predicted or <1.5L.

Ancillary tests
- PEFR chart: diurnal variation.
- Sputum cytology: eosinophilia.

Pitfalls
- Bronchial hyperresponsiveness in asthma is not a static phenomenon and may vary widely from day to day.
- May change quite markedly without any change in symptoms (and vice versa).
- Represents only one component contributing to the symptomatology of asthma. Others include airway oedema and mucus hypersecretion.

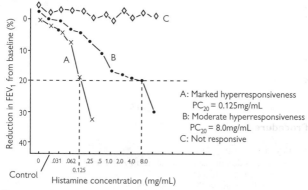

A: Marked hyperresponsiveness
PC_{20} = 0.125mg/mL
B: Moderate hyperresponsiveness
PC_{20} = 8.0mg/mL
C: Not responsive

Fig. 8.1 Differing responses to varying concentrations of histamine.

Further reading

Crapo RO, Casaburi R, Coates AL, *et al.* Guidelines for methacholine and exercise challenge testing-1999. *Am J Respir Crit Care Med* 2000; **161**: 309–29.

Joos GF, O'Connor B. Indirect airway challenges. *Eur Respir J* 2003; **21**: 1050–68.

Lotvall J, Inman M, O'Byrne P. Measurement of airway hyperresponsiveness: new considerations. *Thorax* 1998; **53**, 419–24.

Pratter MR, Irwin S. The clinical value of pharmacologic bronchoprovocation challenge. *Chest* 1984; **85**: 260–5.

Smith CM, Anderson SD. Inhalation provocation tests using nonisotonic aerosols. *J Allergy Clin Immunol* 1989; **84**: 781–90.

Arterial blood gas sampling

Clinical indications
- Breathlessness (acute or chronic).
- Cardiorespiratory failure.
- Metabolic disturbance.
- Poisoning with drugs.
- Acute asthma with O_2 saturation <92% (on air).

📖 *OHCM* 8e, p181.

Patient preparation
Informed consent (verbal usually satisfactory).

Common sites: radial/brachial/femoral arteries.

Contraindications to radial
- Absent ulnar circulation.
- Atrioventricular (AV) fistula for dialysis.
- Fractured wrist.
- Poor peripheral circulation.

Contraindications to brachial
- AV fistula.
- Fractured elbow.
- Poor peripheral circulation.

Contraindications to femoral
Presence of graft/extensive vascular disease.

Procedure
1 Identify pulse.
2 Clean skin with alcohol swab.
3 Confirm position of maximum pulsation with non-dominant hand.
4 Local anaesthetic reduces pain.
5 Insert 23G needle attached to heparinized syringe.
6 If using low-resistance syringe this will fill automatically, otherwise aspirate gently.
7 Remove needle and apply firm gentle pressure with cotton wool ball for 5 min.
8 Label hazardous specimens.
9 Expel air bubbles from sample.

Possible results
- Hypoxia with normal CO_2.
- Hypoxia with ↑ CO_2.
- Normoxia with ↓ CO_2.
- Metabolic acidosis *vs.* compensation.

📖 *OHCM* 8e, p162, p684.

Interpretation

Start by looking at pH. Next check whether CO_2 fits with pH change; if so, primary problem is respiratory. Then check for any metabolic compensation, or for combined respiratory and metabolic process. If CO_2 is not consistent with pH change, the primary disturbance is metabolic and you should check whether there is any respiratory compensation. To assess oxygenation properly, it is essential to record the patient's inspired oxygen concentration (FiO_2) at time of sampling.

Advantages over other tests

- Easy, quick, cheap.
- No real alternative for assessing CO_2 or acid–base balance.
- Greater precision in upper ranges of SaO_2 curve.

Ancillary tests

- **Pulse oximetry**: gives indication of oxygenation status, but not CO_2 levels.
- Arterialized blood sampling.

Complications

- Haematoma.
- Nerve damage.
- Inadvertent venous sampling.

Pitfalls

- If sample is to be analysed in a laboratory with >5 min transit time it should be kept on melting ice to slow the metabolic activity of the cells.
- Avoid arterial puncture if possible in patients on anticoagulant therapy, patients with bleeding disorders or who have received thrombolytics in previous 24 h.
- Failure to note FiO_2 at time of sampling will lead to difficulty in interpretation and potential therapeutic errors.

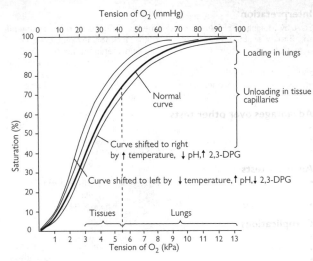

Fig. 8.2 Dissociation curve for oxyhaemoglobin.

Further reading
Carruthers DM, Harrison BD. Arterial blood gas analysis or oxygen saturation in the assessment of acute asthma? *Thorax* 1995; **50**, 186–8.

Syabbalo N. Measurement and interpretation of arterial blood gases. *Br J Clin Pract* 1977; **51**: 173–6.

Diagnostic pleural aspiration

Clinical indications
Pleural effusion detected clinically and with imaging, e.g. chest X-ray (CXR), ultrasound scan (USS), computed tomography (CT) chest.

Patient preparation
1 Informed consent (verbal usually acceptable).
2 Patient sitting with arms forward supported on table/pillows.
3 Posterior or axillary approach if effusion large (otherwise be guided by USS).
4 Clean skin with iodine solution.
5 Infiltrate area one rib space below upper level of dullness to percussion with local anaesthetic (1 or 5% lidocaine).
6 Insert 19G needle attached to 50mL syringe. **Note**: ensure needle enters immediately above rib to avoid the neurovascular bundle.
7 Aspirate fluid. If no fluid then try adjusting angle of needle.
8 Remove needle and apply plaster.
9 Post-aspiration CXR.

Possible results
- Pleural fluid is normally straw coloured.
- Pleural fluid analysed for protein, glucose, LDH, microbiology, cytology, and pH.
- If heavily bloodstained suspect malignancy, pulmonary infarction, or trauma. A traumatic tap will become progressively less bloodstained.
- If pus present: empyema.
- If creamy opalescent fluid: chylothorax (lymphoma, trauma to thoracic duct, yellow nail syndrome, lymphangioleiomyomatosis) or pseudo-chylothorax, e.g. in tuberculosis (TB) or rheumatoid arthritis (RhA).

Interpretation
See Table 8.1.

Advantages over other tests
- Quick and easy.
- Cheap.
- Relatively non-invasive.
- Provides cytological, microbiological, and biochemical data.

Ancillary tests
- Thoracoscopy (medical or surgical).
- Pleural needle biopsy.

Pitfalls
- Traumatic tap.
- Difficult to locate effusion if loculated. If in doubt or if initial tap is dry, use USS chest to guide aspiration.

Complications
- Haemorrhage.
- Pneumothorax.

Table 8.1 Interpretation

Cytology	+ve in ~60% especially carcinoma of lung/breast Increased diagnostic rate with repeated sampling
Protein	Exudate >30g/L protein Transudate <30g/L protein
pH	<7.0: empyema, oesophageal rupture >7.0 and <7.3: collagen disorders, TB, malignancy, empyema
Glucose	↓ in RhA, TB, malignancy, infection
Microbiology	Organisms, ZN stain
Eosinophilia	>10% in benign asbestos effusions, parasitic hydropneumothorax
Neutrophilia	>1.0 x 10⁹/L in acute inflammation, e.g. pneumonia, infarction
Lymphocytosis	Chronic effusions, e.g. TB, malignancy or RARhA
Amylase	↑↑↑ in pancreatitis ↑ in oesophageal rupture (salivary amylase) ↑ in malignancy
ANF	>1:160 virtually diagnostic of SLE
LDH	↑ in infection
Rheumatoid factor	+ve in RARhA
Complement	↓ in RARhA, SLE, malignancy, infection

Epworth test/Epworth sleepiness scale

Clinical indications
Screening tool for obstructive sleep apnoea. Measures general level of daytime sleepiness.

Patient preparation
1. Ask patient to fill in questionnaire.
2. Subject rates on a scale of 0–3 the chances that, as part of his usual life in recent times, he would doze in each of 8 different situations.

Use the following scale to choose the most appropriate number for each situation:
0 = Would NEVER doze
1 = SLIGHT chance of dozing
2 = MODERATE chance of dozing
3 = HIGH chance of dozing

Situation
- Sitting and reading.
- Watching TV.
- Sitting inactive in a public place (e.g. theatre or a meeting).
- As a passenger in a car for an hour without a break.
- Lying down to rest in the afternoon when circumstances permit.
- Sitting and talking to someone.
- Sitting quietly after lunch without alcohol.
- In a car, while stopped for a few minutes in the traffic.

Possible results
Epworth sleepiness scale (ESS) score is the sum of eight item scores and can range from 0 to 24.

Interpretation
Clinically normal score = 10. Each ESS item gives an estimate of sleep propensity in one of eight specific situations, whereas the total ESS score gives a measure of more general average sleep propensity. Does not measure 'subjective' sleepiness.

Advantages over other tests
- Cheap.
- Easily administered.

Ancillary tests
- Polysomnography/Visi-Lab studies.
- Stanford sleepiness scale.
- Multiple sleep latency test.
- Maintenance of wakefulness test.

Pitfalls
Limited by patient's ability to read and comprehend the questionnaire and answer questions honestly.

Exercise testing

Clinical indications

- To confirm that reduced exercise tolerance exists.
- To determine the degree of impairment and disability.
- To investigate which system appears responsible for the reduction.
- To evaluate treatment results.
- To plan rehabilitation.

Patient preparation

1 Evaluate patient's medical history for contraindications to test.
2 Warn patient of cardiovascular complications (e.g. mortality 1:10,000 tests).
3 Obtain written consent.
4 Patient to wear comfortable clothes and shoes.
5 Monitoring: ECG, O_2 saturation, BP.
6 Exercise: treadmill/bike/free run on flat surface.
7 Steady state 5–12 min walking test (usually 6 min) or stepped stress test.
8 During a maximal exercise test the patient should be able to achieve 85–90% of predicted maximum heart rate.

Contraindications to test

- Unstable myocardium (recent MI, unstable angina, arrhythmias, severe valvular heart disease, congestive heart failure).
- Acute asthma.
- Acute febrile illness.
- Uncontrolled diabetes.
- Systemic hypertension (systolic >200mmHg, diastolic >120mmHg).

Possible results

- **Cardiac response**: electrocardiogram (ECG), blood pressure (BP), cardiac output, and stroke volume response.
- **Ventilatory response**: ventilatory limitation (reduced breathing reserve), pattern of response, V_T, minute volume, respiratory rate.
- **Gas exchange**: arterial blood gases, A–a gradient, P_aCO_2.
- **Ventilatory (anaerobic) threshold**: normal or i.
- **VO_2 max (maximum oxygen uptake)**: normal or i.

Interpretation

Useful in making the distinction between exertional dyspnoea secondary to lung disease or fatigue secondary to cardiac dysfunction. In patients known to have asthma, exercise test is +ve in 75% of cases with a single treadmill run and 97% if the test is repeated in –ve responders. A fall of 10% or more from baseline in PEFR or FEV_1 suggests exercise-induced asthma.

Advantages over other tests

Best assessment of exercise capacity. Adds to diagnostic accuracy quantitatively (measurement of work capacity, maximum VO_2, and sustained work capacity) and qualitatively (identification of the cause of exercise limitation).

Ancillary tests

- Static lung function tests.
- For asthma: histamine/methacholine inhalation challenges and peak expiratory flow rate (PEFR) diary.

Pitfalls

- Dependent on patient effort and compliance.
- Not suitable for patients with severe objective measurement of respiratory impairment.

Complications

- ▶ **Bronchospasm**: usually easily reversed with an inhaled adrenergic agent.
- ▶ **Cardiac arrhythmias/arrest**: appropriate equipment and drugs should be available in the exercise testing area. Personnel should be trained in basic and advanced cardiopulmonary resuscitation.

Further reading

Hughes JMB, Pride NB (eds). *Lung Function Tests. Physiological Principles and Clinical Applications*, WB Saunders Philadelphia, 1999.

König P. Exercise challenge: indications and techniques. *Allergy Proc* 1989; **10**: 345–8.

Sue DY. Exercise testing in the evaluation of impairment and disability. *Clin Chest Med* 1994; **15**: 369–87.

Exhaled nitric oxide

Clinical indications

Asthma
- Diagnosis.
- Assessment of severity.
- Assessment of treatment response.

Patient preparation

1 Patient breathes directly into the nitric oxide (NO) analyser.
2 With this technique, gas samples from various compartments of the exhaled volume can be selectively analysed. This prevents contamination by nasal NO.
3 Perform three tests each time and record the largest value.

Possible results

Exhaled NO can be detected by chemiluminescence analysis in the range of 3–20ppb.

Interpretation

Patients with asthma have higher concentrations of NO in their expirate than do similar non-asthmatic subjects (13.9 vs. 6.2ppb in one study).

Advantages over other tests

- Simple.
- Non-invasive.
- Objective measure of response to treatment.

Ancillary tests for diagnosis of asthma

- PEFR diary.
- Histamine/methacholine inhalation challenges.
- Sputum cytology: Eosinophilia.

Pitfalls

- Exhaled NO is also elevated in bronchiectasis and upper/lower respiratory tract infections.
- Exhaled NO levels are reduced by smoking, alcohol, and caffeine.

Further reading

Kharitonov SA, Barnes PJ. Exhaled markers of pulmonary disease. *Am J Respir Crit Care Med* 2001; **163**; 1693–722.

Massaro AF, Gaston B, Kita D, Fanta C, Stamler JS, Drazen JM. Expired nitric oxide levels during treatment of acute asthma. *Am J Respir Crit Care Med* 1995; **152**: 800–3.

Fibre optic bronchoscopy & video bronchoscopy

Clinical indications

- Any patient with persistent/substantial haemoptysis.
- Suspected lung neoplasm:
  - For histology.
  - To assist with staging.
- Infection:
  - To identify organism.
  - To determine course of recurrence/persistence.
- Diffuse parenchymal lung disease (DPLD) to obtain transbronchial biopsies (useful in diagnosis of sarcoidosis, extrinsic allergic alveolitis and lymphangitis carcinomatosa).

Pre-assessment

- CXR.
- Full blood count (FBC).
- Spirometry.
- Clotting.
- Pulse oximetry.
- Arterial blood gases (ABGs) on air if hypoxia suggested by oxygen saturation.

Patient preparation

Endoscopy suite

1. Patient informed and consented.
2. Frontal approach with patient lying on couch, trunk at 45°.
3. IV access obtained.
4. Basic monitoring—pulse oximeter and cardiac monitor.
5. Supplementary O_2 via single nasal cannula.
6. IV sedation: midazolam/alfentanil.
7. Topical lidocaine spray to nose and pharynx (30–50mg of 4 or 10%).
8. Bronchoscope lubricated with 2% lidocaine gel, and passed via nostril or mouth guard.
9. Further boluses of lidocaine (4%) applied to cords and then bronchial tree (2%).

Possible results

- Direct inspection of nares, nasopharynx, and oropharynx.
- Assess movement of vocal cords (ask patient to say 'eee').
- Direct inspection of bronchial tree down to subsegmental level.
- Able to take bronchial/transbronchial biopsies and brushings. Bronchoalveolar lavage (BAL): wedge tip of bronchoscope into a subsegmental bronchus and instil 20–50mL sterile saline into the distal airway. Aspirate immediately aiming to obtain approximately 50% of instilled volume.

Interpretation (Table 8.2)

Table 8.2 Interpretation

Histology	Tumours/DPLD	Biopsy
Cytology	Tumours	Brush
Microbiology	Gram stain	Lavage
	ZN stain	
	Stain for *Pneumocystis carinii*	
	Fungi	
	Virus	

Some appearances diagnostic.

Screening: X-ray-guided biopsy of non-visible lesions.

Advantages over other tests
- Well tolerated.
- Quick, cheap.
- Provides histological and immunobiological confirmation (to back up CT/CXR diagnosis).
- Therapeutic—removal of retained secretions, mucus plugs, blood clots.

Ancillary tests
- **Endobronchial ultrasound (EBUS): allows assessment and biopsy of mediastinal lymph nodes and tumours**.
- **Rigid bronchoscopy: under GAn:**
  - Allows therapeutic interventions, e.g. laser therapy, cryotherapy, stent insertion, debulking of large tumours in the major airways, and better control of haemorrhage.
  - Preferable for removal of foreign body.

Side effects and complications
- Pneumothorax with transbronchial biopsies.
- Haemorrhage post-biopsy.
- Hypoxia.
- If performed on day case unit patient will not be able to drive home and will need a responsible adult in attendance overnight.

Pitfalls
- Only visualizes proximal airways.
- Biopsies may be inadequate or from necrotic areas.
- Not easy to biopsy submucosal tumour.
- Needs good quality cytology preparation.

Further reading
Yasufuku K, Nakajima T, Chiyo M, Sekine Y, Shibuya K, Fujisawa T. Endobronchial Ultrasonography: Current Status and Future Directions. *J Thorac Oncol* 2007; **2**: 970–9.

'Fitness to fly' assessment

Clinical indications

The following groups of patients should be referred to a chest physician for assessment before flying:
- Severe asthma or chronic obstructive pulmonary disease (COPD).
- Severe restrictive disease (including chest wall and respiratory muscle disease).
- Cystic fibrosis.
- Recent pneumothorax.
- Within 6 weeks of discharge for an acute respiratory illness.
- Pre-existing requirement for ventilator support or oxygen therapy.
- Co-morbidities with other conditions worsened by hypoxaemia (e.g. coronary artery disease).

Patient preparation

1. Take a history and examine patient with particular reference to cardi-orespiratory disease and previous symptoms during flights.
2. Perform spirometry.
3. Measure SpO_2 by pulse oximeter. ABGs should be performed if hypercapnia is suspected.
4. A hypoxic challenge test (breathing 15% FiO_2 for 20 min via a face mask followed by arterial blood gas sampling) may be necessary depending on the results of the initial assessment.

Possible results (Tables 8.3 and 8.4)

Table 8.3 Results of initial assessment

Screening result	Recommendation
Sea level SpO_2 >95%	Oxygen not required
Sea level SpO_2 92–95% and no risk factor*	Oxygen not required
Sea level SpO_2 92–95% and additional risk factor* and ABGs	Perform hypoxic challenge
Sea level SpO_2 <92%	In-flight oxygen

*Additional risk factors: hypercapnea; FEV_1 <50% predicted; lung cancer; lung fibrosis; kyphoscolosis; respiratory muscle weakness; cerebrovascular or cardiac disease; within 6 weeks of discharge for an exacerbation of chronic lung or cardiac disease.

Table 8.4 Results of hypoxic challenge test

Hypoxic challenge result	Recommendation
P_aO_2 >7.4 kPa (>55mmHg)	Oxygen not required
P_aO_2 6.6–7.4 kPa (50–55mmHg)	Borderline—seek advice
P_aO_2 <6.6 kPa (<50mmHg)	In-flight oxygen (flow rate 2L/min)

Interpretation
Identifies most patients requiring in-flight oxygen therapy.

Ancillary tests
- Exercise testing.
- In complex cases patients may require testing in a hypobaric chamber.

Pitfalls
- Infectious patients should not fly.
- Even with in-flight oxygen therapy, travel cannot be guaranteed to be safe.

Further reading
Anon. Managing passengers with respiratory disease planning air travel: British Thoracic Society recommendations. *Thorax* 2002; **57**: 289–304.
Coker RK, Shiner RJ, Partridge MR. Is air travel safe for those with lung disease? *Eur Respir J* 2007; **30**: 1057–63.

Flow volume loops/maximum expiratory flow-volume curve

Clinical indications
Patient in whom COPD/small airways disease or upper airway obstruction is suspected.

Patient preparation
- Advised to wear comfortable, loose clothing.
- Technician explains procedure to patient.
- Mouthpiece in position, patient breathes in maximally, and then out as hard and fast as possible.
- 3 acceptable manoeuvres should be performed. Patients must perform the test with maximal effort each time and the results should be similar for each of the 3 attempts.

Interpretation
Particularly useful in recognizing patients with narrowing of the central airway (larynx and trachea). Narrowing at this site has greatest effect on maximum expiratory flow and also on maximum inspiratory flow giving rise to a characteristic appearance. Also identifies patients with reduced elastic recoil (bullae, emphysema) or reduced airway lumen (asthma, chronic obstructive pulmonary disease, bronchiolitis).

Oscillation of flow gives a 'saw tooth' pattern. This usually signifies instability of the upper airway and has been observed in obstructive sleep apnoea, thermal injury to the airway, bulbar muscle weakness, extrapyramidal neuromuscular disorders, upper airway stenosis/tracheomalacia, and snoring.

Advantages over other tests
- Allows early detection of small airway disease—more sensitive than FEV_1 alone.
- Reproducible.

Ancillary tests
- Spirometry.
- Transfer factor.

Pitfalls
- Dependent on patient understanding and maximal effort.
- Infection control necessary in patients with known or suspected transmissible disease (e.g. active pulmonary tuberculosis).

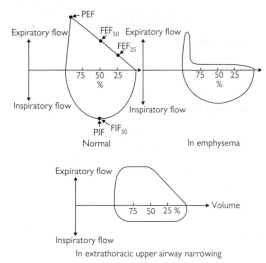

Fig. 8.3 Flow volume loops.

Nijmegen questionnaire

Clinical indications

Hyperventilation syndrome
- Diagnosis.
- Assessment of severity.
- Assessment of response to therapy.

Patient preparation

1 Ask patient to fill in questionnaire.
2 Subject rates on a scale of 0–4 the frequency of 16 different symptoms.

Use the following scale to choose the most appropriate number for each symptom:
0 = Would NEVER experience that symptom
1 = RARELY experience that symptom
2 = SOMETIMES experience that symptom
3 = OFTEN experience that symptom
4 = VERY OFTEN experience that symptom

Symptoms

- Chest pain.
- Feeling tense.
- Blurred vision.
- Dizzy spells.
- Feeling confused.
- Faster or deeper breathing.
- Short of breath.
- Tight feelings in chest.
- Bloated feeling in stomach.
- Tingling fingers.
- Unable to breathe deeply.
- Stiff fingers or arms.
- Tight feelings around mouth.
- Cold hands or feet.
- Heart racing (palpitations).
- Feelings of anxiety.

Possible results

Nijmegen score is the sum of 16 item scores and can range from 0 to 64.

Interpretation

Clinically normal score <23.

Advantages over other tests

- Cheap.
- Easily administered.

Ancillary tests
- Arterial blood gases to identify hypocapnia and respiratory alkalosis.
- Hyperventilation provocation test. (Ask the patient to over-breathe for several minutes to see if it reproduces symptoms.)

Pitfalls
Limited by patient's ability to read and comprehend the questionnaire and answer questions honestly.

Further reading
Van Dixhoorn J, Duivenvoorden HJ. (1985) Efficacy of Nijmegen Questionnaire in recognition of the hyperventilation syndrome. *J Psychosom Res* 1985; **29**: 199–206.

Peak flow charts

Clinical indications

Asthma
- Diagnosis.
- Assessment of severity.
- Assessment of treatment response to β_2 agonists.

Occupational asthma
Diagnosis.

Patient preparation
Patients need to be equipped with a peak flow meter, and peak flow and symptom diary, and have a thorough understanding of how to use them.

Guidelines to patients should include
1 Perform the test standing (if possible).
2 Hold the meter lightly and do not interfere with the movement of the marker.
3 Perform three tests each time and record the largest value.

Readings should be taken at various times throughout the day. Limiting the patient to two readings in each day may aid compliance. In occupational asthma 2-hourly peak flow readings are required during the day and evening.

Possible results
- **Diurnal variability**: as measured by the lowest PEFR value (usually on waking) and the highest PEFR value (usually in the afternoon/evening).
- Patient symptoms and PEFR can be examined together.

Interpretation
Diurnal variation is increased in patients with asthma compared with normals (amplitude >20%), i.e. peak flow falls significantly overnight and in the early morning (Figs 8.3 & 8.4).

Advantages over other tests
- Cheap.
- Saves time of respiratory physician and technician.
- Reproducible.
- Objective measure of response to treatment.

Ancillary tests for diagnosis of asthma
- Bronchoprovocation test.
- Exercise test.
- Sputum cytology: eosinophilia.
- Exhaled NO.

Peak Flow Meter Record

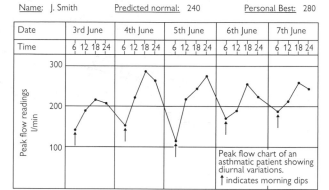

Fig. 8.4 An example of a patient's peak flow record.

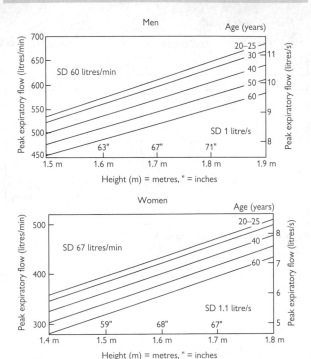

Fig. 8.5 Peak flow readings.

Pitfalls

- Not all asthma exacerbations are associated with increased diurnal variability.
- Calculating diurnal variation can be complicated and tedious.
- Time of recording or recent use of β_2 agonist drugs may result in minor changes in peak flow, but can cause large errors in diurnal variability.
- Dependent on patient understanding, cooperation and accuracy.

Further reading

Hetzel MR, Clark TJ. Comparison of normal and asthmatic circadian rhythms in peak expiratory flow rate. *Thorax* 1989; **35**: 732–8.

Reddel H, Jenkins C, Woolcock A. Diurnal variability—time to change asthma guidelines? *BMJ* 1999; **319**: 45–7.

Pleural needle biopsy

Clinical indications

Pleural effusion of unknown aetiology especially if TB or malignancy suspected. *Note*: may be combined with diagnostic and/or therapeutic pleural aspiration. In which case, obtain diagnostic fluid sample first, then do needle biopsy, then follow with therapeutic aspiration.

Patient preparation

1 Informed written consent.
2 Patient sits with arms forward supported on table/pillows.
3 Posterior or mid-axillary approach.
4 Skin cleaned with iodine solution.
5 Lignocaine (1 or 5%) infiltrated in rib interspace. Check pleural fluid aspirated.
6 Stab incision with narrow scalpel.
7 Insert closed Abrams needle (requires firm pressure to be applied until it penetrates parietal pleura: *take care not to apply too much force*).
8 Attach 50mL syringe.
9 Twist open Abrams needle.
10 Aspirate fluid to ensure needle in pleural space.
11 Withdraw needle at angle to chest wall until side hole 'snags' parietal pleura.
12 Maintain lateral pressure and rotate to close hole, thereby cutting biopsy. Remove needle and extract biopsy tissue.
13 Repeat with samples taken from 3, 6, and 9 o'clock (avoid the 12 o'clock position to avoid the neurovascular bundle).
14 May require suture to close.
15 Apply dressing.
16 Obtain CXR post-procedure.
17 Place samples in formalin for histological examination and saline for microbiological culture.

Possible results

- Slivers of white pleural tissue.
- Examine histology and culture for acid and alcohol fast bacilli (AAFB).

Interpretation

- Malignant mesothelioma may be diagnosed on histology, especially with addition of immunohistochemical methods looking at tumour cell markers.
- More sensitive than pleural fluid aspiration in diagnosing TB.
- Carcinoma cells may arise from direct spread from lung 1° or represent 2° carcinoma. In either case, management is palliative.

Advantages over other tests

- Easy, quick, cheap; more reliable than diagnostic pleural aspiration.
- Less invasive than thoracoscopy for diagnosis of TB.

Ancillary tests

- Diagnostic pleural fluid aspiration.
- Thoracoscopy.
- CT- or ultrasound-guided pleural biopsy is more sensitive than Abrams' pleural biopsy at diagnosing malignancy.

Complications

- Pneumothorax.
- Haemothorax.

Pitfalls

- Skeletal muscle biopsy—inadequate specimen.
- Damage to neurovascular bundle.
- Diagnosis of mesothelioma may remain equivocal.

Further reading

Benamore RE, Scott K, Richards CJ, Entwisle JJ. Image-guided pleural biopsy: diagnostic yield and complications. *Clin Radiol* 2006; **61**: 700–5.

Kirsh CM *et al.* (1995) A modified Abrams needle biopsy technique. *Chest* 1995; **108**: 982–6.

Kirsh CM *et al.* (1997) The optimal number of pleural biopsy specimens for a diagnosis of tuberculous pleurisy. *Chest* 1997; **112**: 702–6.

Maskell NA, Gleeson FV, Davies RJ. Standard pleural biopsy versus CT-guided cutting-needle biopsy for diagnosis of malignant disease in pleural effusions: a randomised controlled trial. *Lancet* 2003; **361**: 1326–30.

Prakash UB, Reiman HM. Comparison of needle biopsy with cytologic analysis for the evaluation of pleural effusion: analysis of 414 cases. *Mayo Clin Proc* 1985; **60**: 158–64.

Polysomnography

Clinical indications

Note: symptoms alone do not help predict which patient with sleep disturbance has obstructive sleep apnoea (OSA).

- Patients with low probability sleep disorder, e.g. snores with no other features suggestive of OSA.
- Patients with high probability sleep disorder, e.g. typical symptoms and physiognomy. Need study for diagnosis and assessment of severity.
- Known OSA—assessing treatment response.
- Assessment of nocturnal hypoventilation syndromes, e.g. scoliosis.
- Patients with unexplained sleep–wake disorders.

Patient preparation

The patient is admitted to the sleep laboratory in the early evening. Monitoring is explained and attached, using some combination shown in Table 8.5.

Table 8.5 Monitoring combinations

Sleep	Electroencephalogram	
	Electro-oculogram	
	Electromyogram	
Oxygenation	Oxygen saturation probe (ear or finger)	
Breathing pattern	Airflow by:	Thermocouples
		Thermistor
		End tidal CO_2 pressure
	Thoracoabdominal movement by	Inductance plethysmography
		Impedance
		Strain gauge
Miscellaneous	Snoring	Microphone
	Leg movement by	EMG
		Video
		Movement detector

Possible results

Original diagnosis of OSA based on polysomnography—overnight recording of sleep, breathing patterns, and oxygenation. It is relatively expensive and most centres use a combination of video to assess quality of sleep, identify transient arousals, and paroxysmal leg movement disorder (PLMD), and oximetry (to detect desaturation), plus some form of measuring the breathing pattern to detect hypopnoea.

Interpretation

OSA diagnosed in the context of multiple (typically >15/h) hypopnoeic/ apnoeic events occurring throughout the night and resulting in desaturation.

Advantages over other tests

Demonstrates number of hypopnoeic (reduction in breathing) or apnoeic (absence of breathing) events occurring per hour. May be used to monitor effectiveness of treatment.

Ancillary tests

Epworth sleepiness score.

Pitfalls

- Expensive.
- Time-consuming.
- Most sleep study systems are poorly validated; therefore, need expert interpretation of results to consider false positives and negatives.
- Patients need to sleep for >3 h/night and have rapid eye movement (REM) sleep.

Pulse oximetry

Clinical indications

- **Any acutely unwell patient**: avoids repeated blood gas measurements provided that hypercarbia is absent.
- **Monitoring of long-term oxygen therapy (LTOT)**: not suitable for initial assessment.
- **Assessment of nocturnal FiO_2 and screening for sleep apnoea syndrome**: identification of nocturnal desaturations.
- **Exercise walk test**.

Patient preparation

1 Clean probe site (ear or finger).
2 Ensure good contact of probe with warm well-perfused skin.
3 Avoid nail-varnished fingers.

Possible results

Oxygen saturations expressed as %.

Interpretation

- Respiratory failure unlikely if O_2 saturation >92% on air.
- Provides almost immediate arterial oxygen saturation data.
- Must know the FiO_2 the patient is breathing.

Advantages over other tests

- Non-invasive.
- Easy, cheap.
- Instantaneous.
- Sensitive.
- Portable.

Ancillary tests

Arterial blood gas sampling.

Pitfalls

- Does not detect carbon dioxide levels.
- If carboxyhaemoglobin or methaemoglobin are present in the blood in elevated levels, the pulse oximeter will give a falsely elevated reading for the arterial oxygen saturation.
- ↑ in jaundice.
- Erroneous information if patient poorly perfused.
- Excessive patient movement can give false readings.

Skin prick tests

Clinical indications
- To evaluate atopy in asthmatic individuals.
- To assess the possible development of allergic bronchopulmonary aspergillosis (ABPA) in patients with asthma/other long-standing lung disease.

Patient preparation
1 Explain what the test involves.
2 Use a pen to label the patient's forearm with the antigens to be tested, including positive and negative controls (alternatively, numbered adhesive tape my be used)
3 Clean the test area with an alcohol wipe.
4 Place a drop of antigen next to each corresponding label.
5 Use a lancet to puncture the skin. Repeat with other antigens using a new lancet each time.
6 Blot off excess antigen taking care not to contaminate other test sites.
7 After 10 min measure any resulting wheal reactions using a ruler. Record mean diameter in mm.

Possible results
A positive result is indicated by a wheal and flare reaction ≥3mm providing there is no reaction at the negative control site. Negative results are validated by a wheal reaction at the positive control site.

Interpretation
A positive result indicates sensitization to the allergen, but does not necessarily mean that this allergen is responsible for the patient's problems. All tests should be carefully interpreted in the light of the clinical history.

Advantages over other tests
Cheap, quick.

Ancillary tests
- Specific immunoglobulin E (IgE) to allergens (especially where the history is not supported by skin test results).
- Total IgE (affects interpretation of weak positive specific IgE results, which are less relevant if the total IgE is very high).
- Aspergillus precipitins (immunoglobulin G (IgG)).

Pitfalls
- False negative results if the patient has taken an antihistamine within 5 days of the test.
- False positive results with dermatographism or inflamed skin.

Spirometry

Clinical indications
- To evaluate symptoms, signs, or abnormal test results.
- Provide objective, quantifiable measures of lung function.
- Evaluate and monitor disease.
- Assess effects of environmental/occupational/drug exposures, both adverse (e.g. amiodarone) and beneficial (e.g. bronchodilators).
- Pre-operative assessment.
- Employment/insurance assessment.
- Early detection of bronchiolitis obliterans in lung transplant patients.

Patient preparation
1 Explain what the test involves. Most respiratory technicians demonstrate technique to ensure maximal effort and co-operation of patient.
2 Patient must inhale fully before test.
3 Exhale into breathing tube. Encourage maximal effort with no breath holding before manoeuvre.
4 No cough/glottal closure in the first second.
5 Test should last at least 6 s (may need up to 15 s with obstruction).
6 No evidence of airflow leak/obstruction of mouthpiece.

Possible results (Table 8.6)

Table 8.6 Possible results	
FEV_1	Forced expiratory volume in 1 s
	Test of mechanical function of the lungs
	Depends on size and elastic properties of the lungs, calibre of the bronchial tree and collapsibility of airway walls
FVC	Forced vital capacity

Interpretation
At least three acceptable tracings should be obtained. Examine each tracing to ensure adequate effort made by patient, that it is reproducible, and that there are no artefacts (Table 8.7).

Advantages over other tests
- Cheap, quick.
- Bedside/outpatient test.
- Reproducible.

Table 8.7 Interpretation

FEV₁/FVC ratio	Index of the presence/absence of airflow limitation Young and middle aged healthy non-smokers rate ≥75% Older normal patients ratio 70–75%
FEV/FVC ↓	Obstructive Classify severity using FEV, expressed as % of predicted value, e.g. COPD, asthma
FEV/FVC ↔ or ↑	Restrictive, but need reduced thin layer chromatography (TLC) to confirm, e.g. lung fibrosis, chest wall problems, pulmonary effusion and oedema

If used for monitoring purposes need adequate baseline study.

Ancillary tests

- **Total lung capacity**: to confirm interstitial disease with restrictive spirometry.
- **Pre- and post-bronchodilator studies**: an increase of 15% in FEV_1 and 20% in FVC suggest reversibility.

Pitfalls

- Need standardization of normal data for height, weight, age, sex, and race.
- Level at which a result may be considered abnormal is contentious, usually accepted to be outside range of 80–120% of mean predicted.
- FEV_1 may remain relatively normal in early stages of generalized lung disease.
- FEV_1/FVC ratio is good guide to presence or significant airway narrowing, but as disease progresses, both will fall and correlation with severity of disease is poor.
- Variability (noise) is greater in pulmonary function tests than in most other clinical laboratory tests because of the inconsistency of effort by patients.

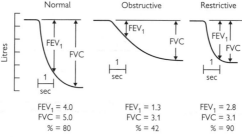

Fig. 8.6 Examples of spirograms.

See examples of spirograms 📖 *OHCM* 8e, p157.

Further reading

Crapo RO. Pulmonary-function testing. *N Engl J Med* 1994; **331**: 25–30.

Sputum microscopy & culture/ sputum cytology

Clinical indications

Microbiology
- Productive cough with sputum.
- Infective exacerbations of any chronic lung disease.
- Pneumonia.

Cytology
- Suspected lung cancer, especially in elderly/frail patients who may not be fit for invasive investigation.
- Sputum eosinophilia in asthma.

Patient preparation
- Explain need for the sputum sample.
- Provide suitable sputum pots.
- Early morning samples are best.
- Consider induced sputum—use ultrasonically nebulized hypertonic saline to facilitate sputum production in association with chest physiotherapy.

Possible results
Induced sputum results in successful sputum production in >70% of normal and asthmatic subjects who cannot produce sputum spontaneously (Table 8.8).

Table 8.8 Possible results

Gram stain	Gram +ve or –ve organisms
ZN stain	AAFB
Microscopy	Differential cell count Eosinophils in asthma
Cytology	Malignant cells Small cell, squamous cell, adenocarcinoma cells

Interpretation
- Commensal organisms common.
- *Streptococcus pneumoniae* and *Haemophilus influenzae* likely pathogens in COPD.
- *Streptococcus pneumoniae* commonest organism in community-acquired 1° pneumonia.
- *Staphylococcus aureus* and *Pseudomonas* likely in bronchiectasis.
- Nosocomial infections:
  - *Staphylococcus aureus*.
  - *Pseudomonas*.
  - *Klebsiella*.
- The sensitivity of sputum cytology varies by location of the lung cancer and is greatest in central endobronchial lesions.
- Advantages over other tests
- Cheap, easy.
- Non-invasive.

Ancillary tests
- Bronchoscopy and bronchoalveolar lavage.
- Serum serology if atypical pneumonia suspected.
- If bronchiectasis suspected consider high-resolution CT chest +/– CT sinuses and check immunoglobulins (IgG, IgA, and IgM). Other investigations depend on clinical scenario (RF, IgG subclasses, IgE, aspergillus precipitins, alpha-1-antitrypsin). Involve Respiratory team early.
- PCR for drug-resistant TB.

Pitfalls
- Sputum may be diluted by saliva.
- Diagnosis of squamous cell carcinoma is not as robust as for small cell lung cancer or adenocarcinoma. Needs careful cross-referencing to Radiology and should be confirmed if possible with biopsies.
- Negative results should not preclude further investigations if malignancy suspected.

Further reading
Rivera P, Mehta A. Initial diagnosis of lung cancer; ACCP Evidence-Based Clinical Practice Guidelines, 2nd edn. *Chest* 2007; **132**: 131S–48S.

Rosia E, Scano G. Association of sputum parameters with clinical and functional measurements in asthma. *Thorax* 2000; **55**: 235–8.

Static lung volumes/whole body plethysmography

Clinical indications
- Differentiate between obstructive and restrictive disease patterns.
- Identify and quantify trapped air (shown by ↑RV/TLC ratio).
- Assess response to therapeutic interventions (e.g. drugs, radiation, transplantation).
- Identify presence and amount of unventilated lung.
- Assess chronic lung disease (e.g. sarcoidosis, rheumatoid lung).
- Pre-operative assessment.
- Assessment of pulmonary disability.

Patient preparation
1 Ask patient to wear comfortable clothes.
2 Place mouthpiece securely in mouth with lips tight around it.
3 Breathe in a relaxed manner through spirometer system (nose clips mandatory).
4 After total of 5 tidal breaths with consistent end-expiratory levels, patient asked to maximally inspire to total lung capacity followed by exhalation with encouragement to force out the last 5–15% of air.
5 A minimum of 2 attempts should be obtained.
6 More may be needed in the young and elderly to obtain reproducible results.

Most accurate results are obtained with whole body plethysmography.

Possible results
- **Total lung capacity**: volume of air in the lungs at the end of full inspiration.
- **Residual volume**: volume of air remaining in the lungs after maximal expiration.
- **Vital capacity**: the amount of air expired (or inspired) between maximum inspiration and maximum expiration.
- **Functional residual capacity**: the amount of air in the lungs at the end-tidal position.
- **Inspiratory capacity**: the maximum amount of air that can be breathed into the lungs from the end-tidal position.
- **Tidal volume**: the volume of air inspired and expired with each breath.
- **Inspiratory reserve volume**: the volume between the peak inspiratory tidal position and maximum inspiration.

See Table 8.9.

Interpretation

- Only interpret if test is reproducible, i.e. if the 2 largest vital capacity values are within 5% or 100mL (whichever is the larger).
- VC may remain within normal range in some pulmonary disease, e.g. emphysema.
- ↓VC—restrictive pulmonary disease, neuromuscular disease, e.g. amyotrophic lateral sclerosis.
- During the testing process, the patient is enclosed in a chamber equipped to measure either pressure, flow or volume changes. Because all the gas in the thorax is accounted for, this method is particularly useful in patients with trapped gas, e.g. bullous emphysema.

Advantages over other tests

Reproducible.

Pitfalls

- Patient co-operation is essential. They must provide maximal effort and be capable of understanding instructions.
- Calibration should take place on a regular basis.
- Risk of disease transmission between patients, and between patient and technician; therefore avoid if pulmonary TB suspected.

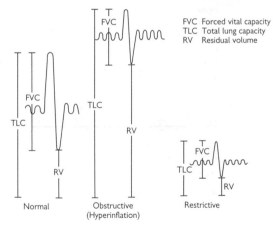

FVC Forced vital capacity
TLC Total lung capacity
RV Residual volume

Normal

Obstructive
(Hyperinflation)

Restrictive

Fig. 8.7 Lung volumes: physiological and pathological.

Table 8.9 Causes

Causes of ↑ TLC:	Generalized airway obstruction, e.g. COPD Emphysema (including bullae) Bronchiectasis Asthma Other, e.g. acromegaly
Causes of ↓ TLC:	*Intrapulmonary* pneumonectomy collapsed lung consolidation oedema fibrosis Extrapulmonary pleural disease effusion thickening pneumothorax rib cage deformity scoliosis thoracoplasty respiratory muscle weakness
Causes of ↑ RV:	Generalized airway obstruction Pulmonary vascular congestion, e.g. mitral stenosis, ASD Expiratory muscle weakness, e.g. spinal injury, myopathies
Causes of ↑ FRC:	Age, lung disease causing air trapping, e.g. asthma, emphysema, COPD
Causes of ↓ FRC:	Restrictive lung diseases, e.g. diffuse interstitial pulmonary disease of any aetiology, pneumonectomy

Sweat test

Clinical indications

Suspected cystic fibrosis (CyF) in the context of
- Bronchiectasis/recurrent chest infections.
- Pancreatic insufficiency/diabetes mellitus.
- Family history.
- Fertility problems.

Patient preparation

1 Obtain informed consent: verbal usually sufficient, but important to discuss reasons for test and possible implications. Perform two sweat tests simultaneously on each arm for greater accuracy.
2 Induce sweating by pilocarpine iontophoresis. A weak electrical current aids penetration of pilocarpine into skin, thus stimulating the sweat glands of the forearm, previously washed and dried, to secrete sweat.
3 Collect sweat on preweighed filter paper (>100mg), then measure eluted Na^+ and Cl^-.

Possible results

- 98–99% of children homozygous for CyF have sweat Cl^- and Na^+ levels well >70 and 60mmol/L, respectively.
- Sweat Na^+ concentrations tend to increase with age and show wide variability between individuals.
- Diagnostic accuracy is improved in borderline cases by a suppression test using fludrocortisone.

Interpretation

- A +ve test is virtually diagnostic of CyF. This should lead to counselling and genetic testing.
- Equivocal results are defined as Na^+ or Cl^- concentrations between 50 and 70mmol/L.
- The diagnosis should never rest on the sweat test alone, and should be considered together with the clinical findings and laboratory evidence of pancreatic insufficiency.

Advantages over other tests

- Cheaper than genetic tests.
- Assesses functional deficit, therefore capable of detecting patients who have rare variants of CyF.

Ancillary tests

- Nasal potential difference.
- Pancreatic function tests (3-day faecal collection).
- Genetic studies.

Pitfalls
- A wide discrepancy between the results from each arm suggests a problem with technique.
- Accurate interpretation of sweat tests requires knowledge of the age-related changes in sweat Na^+ and Cl^- concentrations and should be done in a specialized centre.

False negatives
- Inexperience of operator.
- Low rates of sweating.
- Poor skin preparation.
- Poor iontophoretic contact with skin.
- Faulty chemical analysis.

False positives
- Evaporation of sweat secondary to inadequate sealing during collection.
- Untreated adrenal insufficiency.
- Nephrogenic diabetes insipidus.
- Hypothyroidism.
- Glycogen storage disease.
- Nephrotic syndrome.
- Severe malnutrition.
- AIDS (some reports of abnormal sweat electrolytes).
- Faulty chemical analysis.

Further reading
Green A, Dodds P, Pennock C. A study of sweat sodium and chloride; criteria for the diagnosis of cystic fibrosis. *Ann Clin Biochem* 1985; **22**: 171–6.

Hall SK, Stableforth DE, Green A. Sweat sodium and chloride concentrations—essential criteria for the diagnosis of cystic fibrosis in adults. *Ann Clin Biochem* 1990; **27**: 318–20.

Heeley AF, Watson D. Cystic fibrosis—its biochemical detection. *Clin Chem* 1983; **29**: 2011–18.

Medical thoracoscopy

Clinical indications
- Pleural effusions when pleural fluid analysis non-diagnostic.
- Pneumothorax.
- Staging of lung cancer.
- Diagnosis of malignant mesothelioma and other pleural abnormalities, e.g. neurinomas, lipomas, plastocytomas.
- Suspected empyema.

Pre-assessment
- A recent (<1 month) CT scan of the chest is mandatory.
- FBC.
- Clotting.
- Spirometry.
- Pulse oximetry.
- ABGs on air if hypoxia suggested by oxygen saturation.

Patient preparation
Endoscopy suite
1 Patient informed and consented.
2 Intravenous access obtained.
3 Patient lying supine with affected side nearest to operator. Must be able to keep hand behind head in order to prevent arm from obscuring operating field.
4 Basic monitoring: pulse oximeter and cardiac monitor.
5 Supplementary oxygen given via face-mask or nasal cannulae.
6 Intravenous sedation—midazolam/alfentanil .
7 An absolute prerequisite for thoracoscopy is the presence of an adequate pleural space (i.e. at least 6–10cm diameter).
8 If pleural effusion: drain using 3-way tap. Replace with equal quantity atmospheric air.
9 If no effusion: create pneumothorax.
10 Insert needle connected to manometer into pleural space. Introduce 400–1000mL air.
11 Skin incision 5th intercostal space, mid-axillary line 1.5–2cm.
12 Insert 5–10mm pleural trocar and cannula.
13 Introduce thoracoscope via trocar into pleural cavity.
14 After inspection and biopsies remove trocar and insert drain.
15 CXR post-procedure.
16 Commence chest drain suction at rate of 20cmH$_2$O on ward.

Possible results
- Direct inspection of pleural surfaces.
- Biopsy of parietal pleura—histology/culture esp. AAFBs.
- Pleural fluid → microscopy, culture, & sensitivity (MC&S) → cytology.
- Therapeutic options: pleurodesis, coagulation of blebs, resection of fibrinous loculations in empyemas.
- Drainage of large pleural effusions possible without risk of re-expansion pulmonary oedema due to rapid equalization of pressures by entrance of air into pleural space.

Interpretation

Macroscopic appearance of pleura may be diagnostic, e.g. TB, RhA, scleroderma, metastatic disease.

Advantages over other tests

- Better than blind pleural biopsy.
- Able to obtain diagnosis in 70–95% of cases.
- Especially good at diagnosing TB.
- Less invasive than thoracotomy.
- Less expensive than thoracotomy. Does not require a theatre or anaesthetist.
- Done under sedation unlike video-assisted thoracic surgery (VATS), which requires a GAn and selective one-lung ventilation.

Ancillary tests

Diagnosis of mesothelioma improved with use of immunohistochemical markers.

Pitfalls

Biopsies may be inadequate or non-representative.

Contraindications

- Obliterated pleural space.
- Small pneumothorax.
- Patient short of breath at rest unless secondary to pneumothorax or pleural effusion, which can be treated during procedure.
- Disturbed haemostasis:
  - Platelets $<40 \times 10^9$/L.
  - APTT >50% normal.
- Recent MI, arrhythmias, heart failure.

Complications

- Fever 24–36 h post-procedure.
- Empyema (<1%).
- Wound infection.
- Subcutaneous emphysema.
- Air embolism.
- Bronchopleural fistula following lung biopsy.
- Seeding of metastases/mesothelioma along trocar wound. (Radiotherapy a few weeks post-thoracoscopy should be carried out to prevent this.)
- Haemorrhage.
- Arrhythmias.
- Mortality rate <0.01%.

Further reading

Blanc FX, Atassi K, Bignon J, Housset B. Diagnostic value of medical thoracoscopy in pleural disease: a 6-year retrospective study. *Chest* 2002; **5**: 1677–83.
Buchanan DR, Neville E. *Thoracoscopy for Physicians: a Practical Guide.* London: Arnold, 2004.
Colt HG. Thoracoscopy: window to the pleural space. *Chest* 1999; **116**: 1409–15.
Loddenkemper R. Thoracoscopy—state of the art. *Eur Resp J* 1998; **11**: 213–21.

Transfer factor

Clinical indications

Test for abnormalities of pulmonary gas exchange.

Patient preparation

- Avoid smoking 6 h prior and strenuous exercise 2 h prior.
- Allow 15–30 min for test.
- Usually measured by single breath inhalation technique.
- Patient breathes in air containing a known concentration of CO and holds breath for 10 s.

Possible results

- Transfer factor (TLCO).
- Transfer coefficient (KCO).
- May need to correct for anaemia:
  - Result usually standardized to Hb 14.6g/dL.
  - Effect of mild anaemia (Hb >10g/dL) slight, but becomes progressively more marked at lower values.

Interpretation

↓ *in DLCO*

- Obstructive lung disease, e.g. COPD, emphysema.
- Diffuse interstitial lung disease, e.g. CFA, amiodarone lung.
- Pulmonary involvement in systemic disease, e.g. systemic lupus erythematosus (SLE), RhA, Wegener's.
- Cardiovascular disease, e.g. pulmonary oedema, mitral stenosis, pulmonary embolism (PE).
- Others: anaemia, cigarette smoking.
- ↑ in DLCO
- Diseases associated with polycythaemia.
- Pulmonary haemorrhage.
- Diseases associated with increased pulmonary blood, such as from left to right intracardiac shunts.
- Exercise.
- Asthmatics (reasons not clear).

Advantages over other tests

- Quick.
- Relatively easy to perform.
- Reproducible.

Pitfalls

- Breath holding time may be difficult for some patients to achieve.
- Calculation of TLCO is based on assumption that ventilation and diffusion are homogeneous in the entire lung. With unequal distribution of ventilation and diffusion, the TLCO will be underestimated on the alveolar level.
- With extrapulmonary lung restriction and consequent inability to achieve full inspiration, KCO tends to be higher than normal.

Neurology

Lumbar puncture

Indications

- Meningitis.
- Encephalitis.
- Polyradiculitis, polyneuritis.
- Multiple sclerosis.
- Myelitis.
- Vasculitis.
- Suspected subarachnoid haemorrhage (SAH).
  - Note: In general, a −ve computed tomography (CT) does not exclude a SAH.
- Suspected malignancy with meningeal involvement.
- Assessment of cerebrospinal fluid (CSF) pressure:
  - High (e.g. idiopathic or 'benign' intracranial hypertension, IIH).
  - Low (e.g. 'low pressure' headache).
- Therapeutic trials, e.g.
  - IIH.
  - Normal pressure hydrocephalus, NPH (not particularly helpful).
- To seek specific antibodies/markers in CSF, e.g.
  - Human immunodeficiency virus (HIV).
  - Lyme (*Borrelia*).
  - Syphilis.
  - Angiotensin converting enzyme (ACE; for neurosarcoid).
  - Tumour markers.
  - Lactate in mitochondrial cytopathies.

Preparation

- Decide exactly what investigations you want. If necessary, alert the appropriate laboratories and organize transport of samples. In particular, samples for xanthochromia and cytology should be rapidly taken to the laboratory to be spun down.
- If the patient is also due to have a neuroradiological investigation with contrast and lumbar puncture (LP) is not urgent, delay LP until after scan as there may be diffuse meningeal enhancement after the LP.
- If the patient is extremely anxious, s/he may benefit from 5–10mg of oral diazepam prior to the LP.

Procedure

1. Explain to the patient what you are about to do.
2. Arrange all your equipment on a sterile tray, including assembled CSF manometer.
3. Position patient on his side, with back perpendicular to bed, at the edge of a firm bed. Place head on one pillow. Draw knees up and place one pillow between them.
4. Adjust height of bed so that you are comfortable.

5 Identify the bony landmarks. L3/L4 space is in line with the iliac crests, and is most commonly used. L2/L3 to L5/S1 are also used. If you like, mark the target space with the imprint of your thumb nail. Take time over these first four stages.

6 The insertion of the needle should be a sterile procedure. Clean the skin over the lower back. Don sterile gloves and mask.

7 Insert a little (0.25–0.5mL) local anaesthetic—too much can obscure the bony landmarks.

8 Pass LP needle horizontally into the space, with tip angled at about 10–15° (toward the umbilicus), in the midline horizontal plane. At all times, stylet should be fully inserted and bevel of needle facing up.

9 Slight resistance should be felt as needle passes through ligamentum flavum and the dura, and then a 'give' as it enters the subarachnoid space.

10 Slowly withdraw the stylet. CSF drops should appear.

11 If CSF does not appear, reinsert the style and slightly rotate the needle—this sometimes frees it of obstructing nerve roots. A gentle cough from the patient can also help.

12 If the needle encounters bone, or the patient complains of pains shooting down the leg, check the position of the needle (is it in the midline? Is it angled correctly?) and then withdraw it entirely.

13 Insert a fresh needle, correcting for any error noted above.

14 If this second pass is unsuccessful, withdraw needle and inform patient. If he is happy for you to proceed, then attempt LP in another space, repeating all steps from 4 down. Use a fresh needle.

15 If you fail again, explain to patient and seek a more experienced operator to perform the LP. Multiple failed attempts are painful and discouraging (to both you and your patient).

16 If a more experienced operator fails, ask your friendly radiologist to do it under X-ray guidance, but give him the help he requests and precise instructions about the samples required.

17 When CSF collection is complete, gently pull out the needle and place a sterile dressing over the insertion site.

18 Allow the patient to mobilize shortly after the LP.

Measuring the cerebrospinal fluid pressure

As soon as the CSF starts to flow, attach the pre-assembled manometer. Wait until the CSF stops rising. If the patient is very anxious, or uncomfortable, a falsely raised opening pressure may be recorded. Sometimes having the patient slightly relax his legs will help. Using the 3-way tap, let the CSF run into your first pre-labelled tube (do not waste the CSF!). Having collected all the CSF you require, if the opening pressure was elevated, note the closing pressure. If the opening pressure is expected to be very raised, e.g. in suspected or confirmed idiopathic (benign) intracranial hypertension, then two or more manometers should be pre-assembled, as the pressure may exceed 40mm CSF.

Collecting samples

- As always, tailor your investigations to the clinical picture. If you are just checking the CSF pressure, then no samples need necessarily be collected. If you suspect a subarachnoid haemorrhage, collect three samples in sequentially labelled bottles and promptly hand carry to the laboratory for quantitative estimation of xanthochromia and haemoglobin breakdown products. If you are looking for evidence of malignant cells, then at least one sample should be sent to the laboratory promptly for cytology.
- To avoid contamination, allow the Microbiology laboratory to split samples, rather than attempting this yourself.
- Collect at least 10 drops in each bottle. The microbiology and cytology laboratories in particular will thank you for greater volumes.
- As soon as the CSF is collected, a blood sample should be obtained (if necessary) for glucose and oligoclonal band detection.

Alternative positioning of patient

Sometimes there is a dry tap if the CSF pressure is too low to distend the lumbar cistern. This can sometimes be overcome by performing the LP with the patient sitting on a firm reversed chair, leaning forward to bend over its back. This manoeuvre maximizes the separation of the vertebrae. Again, the needle should be angled slightly (10°) upward relative to the spine at that point. This position does not allow precise measurement of CSF pressure.

Which needle to use?

22G usually appropriate. Needles with larger bores tend to cause a greater CSF leak (and thus more headache). Some advocate even finer needles, but these make the collection of CSF take too long. 'Blunt' anaesthetists' needles probably also reduce the risk of post-LP headache.

Clinical record keeping

Record what you did in the notes after the procedure (e.g. if more than one pass was required; which space you used), the opening and closing CSF pressure, and what investigations you have requested. Note the appearance of the CSF (if normal, it will be clear and colourless). If the CSF appears bloody, record this and whether the final bottle collected is clearer than the first.

When *NOT* to attempt a lumbar puncture

- Risk of herniation:
  - Space-occupying lesions.
  - Non-communicating hydrocephalus.
  - Cerebral oedema (if in doubt, cranial imaging should be performed first).
- Uncorrected bleeding diathesis/anticoagulant use.
- *Caution* if previous lumbar spine surgery or known anatomical abnormalities.
- Local skin sepsis.

- **Note**: it is usually safe and *appropriate* to perform an LP in suspected meningitis, *unless* there are specific clinical features to suggest raised intracranial pressure, in which case cranial imaging should be performed first.

Complications and what to do about them

Headache

- Usually starts within 24h of LP.
- May last from a few hours to 2 weeks, but typically several days.
- Probably related to persistent CSF leak via the dural tear; therefore, tends to have 'low pressure' characteristics (frontal, worse on sitting up, better on lying down). There may be mild meningism and nausea.

Treatment has traditionally involved bed rest, analgesia, and the encouragement of plenty of fluids.

- If nausea is a major problem, the patient may require IV fluids.
- Rarely, if the headache is severe and persistent, then an anaesthetist may place an autologous blood patch to 'plug' the dural tear. Surgical intervention is very rarely required.

Low backache

A variety of causes of post-LP backache exist; these may usually be treated conservatively.

Infection

Very rare if sterile technique is used. Occasionally may occur if the needle passes through a region of infection. Meningitis typically develops within 12 h. Very rarely there may be an epidural abscesses or vertebral osteomyelitis. Treat with appropriate antibiotics and if necessary surgery.

Herniation

- Uncal or cerebellar herniation may occur, particularly in the presence of a posterior fossa mass. ▶▶ **An LP should not be performed if there is suspicion of raised intracranial pressure without first obtaining cranial CT or magnetic resonance (MR) imaging**.
- Should the CSF pressure be found to be very high (300mm of CSF), even after relaxing patient, and in the absence of idiopathic (benign) intracranial hypertension, manage as follows:
  - Nurse patient prone with no pillow.
  - Raise foot of bed.
  - Start infusion of 20% mannitol at 1g/kg over 20min.
  - Start neurological observation chart.
  - Arrange urgent CT of brain and notify neurosurgeons.

▶▶ **Do not instil saline into the subarachnoid space**.

Haemorrhage

A 'traumatic' tap may cause a little local bleeding that is rarely of clinical significance. Patients with impaired clotting (remember warfarin) or platelet function are at risk of more extensive bleeding, and LP should not be attempted unless the coagulopathy is corrected. An arachnoiditis, or spinal subdural, or epidural haemorrhage may develop. A spinal subdural haematoma (SDH) is otherwise rare, and an intracranial SDH very rare.

Cerebrospinal fluid constituents: normal values
- **White cells**: 0–4/mm^3.
- **Red blood cells**: ideally none!
- **Protein**: 0.15–0.45g/L.
- **Glucose**: ~1/2 to 2/3 of simultaneous blood glucose.
- **Opening pressure**: 10–25cm CSF.

Note: If there is a traumatic 'bloody' tap, there may be hundreds or thousands of red blood cells/mm^3. If so, then white cells should be expected in the CSF, but in similar proportions to the peripheral blood.

Rules of thumb
1 Pressure:
- ↑ by space-occupying lesions within the cranial vault, such as oedema, masses, chronic inflammation.
- ↑ by increased central venous pressure, e.g. in the anxious patient with tensed abdominal muscles.
- ↓ if the spinal subarachnoid space is obstructed, thus impeding CSF flow.

2 Cells:
- **Polymorphs (neutrophils)**: suggest acute bacterial infection.
- **Lymphocytes & monocytes**: viral and chronic infections or tumours.
- **Eosinophils**: tumours, parasites, foreign body reactions.

3 Glucose— ↓ by non-viral processes causing meningeal inflammation.
4 Total protein— ↑ by breakdown of the blood–brain barrier.
5 Immunoglobulins (Igs) specific to the CSF, i.e. without matching Igs in a simultaneous blood sample: inflammation within the theca, e.g. multiple sclerosis (MS), infection, tissue damage.

Common patterns
These are shown in Table 9.1.

📖 *OHCM* 8e, p782.

Table 9.1 Common patterns

Condition	Glucose	Protein	Cells	Comments
Acute bacterial meningitis	↓	↑	Often >300/mm^3	Polymorphs; lactate ↑*
Acute viral meningitis	N	N or ↑	<300 mononuclear	Culture, antigen detection may be possible
Fungal meningitis	↓	↑	<300 mononuclear	Culture and antigen detection
Tuberculous meningitis	↓	↑	Mixed pleocytosis <300	ZN stain organisms, culture PCR
Herpes simplex encephalitis	N	Mildly ↑	5–500 lympho	PCR
Guillain–Barré syndrome	N	↑	Normal	
Subarachnoid haemorrhage[†]	N	May be ↑	Erythrocytes	Look for bilirubin pigments on spectrophotometry; xanthochromia unreliable.
Malignant meningitis	↓	↑	Mononuclear	Rapid cytospin and look for malignant cells
HIV	N	N or ↑	Mononuclear pleocytosis	Culture, antigen detection, antiviral antibodies
Neurosyphilis	N or ↓	↑	<300 lymphocytes	VDRL
Neurosyphilis –early	↑		Treponema pallidum	
Neurosyphilis –late			Immobilization tests	

[†]LP should be done >12 h after onset of headache; the CSF should be spun down within 45 min; decreasing numbers of red blood cells (RBCs) in successive bottles are compatible with SAH.

*Taken from Kleine et al. (2003).[1]

Further reading

Hasbun R, et al. Computed tomography of the head before lumber puncture in adults with suspected meningitis. New Engl J Med 2001; **345**: 1227–33.

Thomas SR, et al. Randomised controlled trial of atraumatic versus standard needles for diagnostic lumbar puncture. BMJ 2000; **321**: 986–90.

Whiteley W, et al. CSF opening pressure: reference interval and the effect of body mass index. Neurology 2006; **67**: 1690–1.

1 Kleine TO, et al. New and old diagnostic markers of meningitis in cerebrospinal fluid (CSF). Brain Res Bull 2003; **61**: 287–97.

Skull radiograph

Indications
Usually more modern imaging techniques are much more informative, but there are occasions when these may not be speedily available. However, the plain SXR has quite low specificity and sensitivity for detecting many abnormalities of neurological importance.

Used in (suspected) cases of
- Skull fracture.
- Pituitary fossa abnormalities.
- Tumours involving bone.
- Bone changes related to meningiomata.

Procedure
Lateral view in the first instance.

Consider
- Occipitofrontal.
- Towne's (half axial).
- Basal (submentovertical).
- Specific views (e.g. orbits).

What to look for (what you see will depend on the pathology)
See 📖 Radiology, Chapter 13.
- Shape and symmetry of vault.
- Pituitary fossa.
- Position of calcified pineal (midline shift?).
- Bone density changes (e.g. tumour, meningioma, Paget's).
- Fractures.
- Evidence of neurosurgical procedures.
- Intracranial air.
- Post-nasal space.
- Craniocervical junction.

Indications for SXR after head injury (but see section on cranial CT below; in general, CT is the preferred imaging modality)
In an orientated adult patient
- Loss of consciousness or amnesia.
- Fall >60cm.
- Full thickness scalp laceration.
- Scalp haematoma.

If a skull fracture is detected, proceed to CT.

Ultrasound

Ultrasound may be used in a variety of modes.

Mostly commonly used in neuroradiology

- **B mode**: gives 2-dimensional images.
- **Doppler** effect is used to assess alterations in the pattern (especially velocity) of flow in vessels.
- **Duplex** scanning combines B mode and Doppler.

Extracranial vessels

B mode

- Can image from clavicle (common carotid bifurcation), and internal and external carotids to angle of jaw.
- Can image proximal and distal subclavian, and vertebral arteries.
- Supraorbital artery (anterior circulation).
- Fibrofatty plaques and thrombus on plaques not very echogenic therefore missable.
- Fibrous plaques more echogenic.
- Calcification in plaque is highly echogenic.
- Can sometimes detect intraplaque haemorrhage or ulceration.

Note: requires patient co-operation and considerable operator skill. High grade stenosis can appear as total occlusion.

Doppler mode

Stenosis alters the normal pattern of velocities recorded.

Duplex

Combination of anatomic and flow imaging more sensitive and specific for clinically significant stenoses.

Comment

Use of carotid ultrasound: most commonly in the assessment of patients with carotid territory ischaemic strokes or TIAs, who might be candidates for carotid endarterectomy. Such surgery should be performed as soon as possible, so carotid Doppler studies should be arranged promptly after the first event. If a patient has neurological signs or symptoms suggestive of posterior circulation events, there is little point in organizing carotid (that is, anterior circulation) studies. Both the degree of stenosis and the morphology of the plaque (irregular plaques are more pathogenic) are important.

Intracranial vessels

Transcranial Doppler

- 2mHz to penetrate thinner bone.
- Flow velocity in anterior, middle, and post cerebral, ophthalmic and basilar arteries; carotid siphon.

What it shows
- Intracranial haemodynamics.
- Vasospasm in SAH.
- Monitoring of microemboli.
- This is an area of active research with new clinical indications being described frequently.

Further reading
Rothwell PM, *et al*. Analysis of pooled data from the randomised controlled trials of endarterectomy for symptomatic carotid stenosis. *Lancet* 2003; **361**: 107–16.
Tegeler CH. Ultrasound in cerebrovascular disease. In: Greenberg JO (ed.) *Neuroimaging*. New York: McGraw-Hill, 1995; 577–95.

Angiography

Indications
- Strongly suspected or confirmed SAH.
- Suspected cerebral vasculitis.
- Delineation of other vascular abnormalities (e.g. arteriovenous malformations, AVM).
- Delineation of tumour blood supply (occasionally).

Procedure
1 Catheter passed via femoral artery to carotid or vertebral artery under image intensification.
2 Contrast is given.
3 In digital subtraction angiography (DSA), subtraction of pre- from post-contrast images (pixel by pixel) is used to help remove signals from bone density.

Arch angiography (aortography)
- Visualizes aorta, major neck vessels, and sometimes circle of Willis.
- No venous imaging.

Selective intra-arterial angiography
Later images show venous system.

Carotid artery
Antero-posterior (AP), lateral, and oblique views—anterior and middle cerebral, and internal carotid arteries.

Vertebral artery
Towne's (half axial) and lateral views—vertebral, basilar, posterior cerebral arteries.

What can be demonstrated?
- Occlusion, stenosis, plaques.
- Aneurysms.
- Arteriovenous and other blood vessel abnormalities.
- Abnormal tumour circulation.[1]

- Displacement or compression of vessels.[1]
- Experimental role in acute stroke analysis.

Complications

- Sensitivity to the contrast medium.
- Cerebral ischaemia, e.g. secondary to dislodgement of embolic fragments by catheter tip or thrombus in the catheter lumen.
- The rate of transient or permanent neurological defect following angiography depends on the operator.

Further reading

Larsen DW, Teitelbaum GP. Radiological angiography. In: Bradley WG, et al. (eds) *Neurology in Clinical Practice*, 3rd edn. Boston: Butterworth-Heinemann, 2000; 617–43.

Osborne AG. *Diagnostic Cerebral Angiography*, 2nd edition, New York: Lippincott, Williams & Wilkins, 1999.

---

1 Although CT and MRI give finer spatial details, angiography is still useful, e.g. delineating blood supply of a tumour.

Myelography

Indications
- Largely superseded by CT and especially MRI.
- Still used in subjects in whom MRI is contraindicated (e.g. cardiac pacemaker, metallic implants, claustrophobia).
- Can screen whole spinal cord and cauda equina for compressive or expanding lesions.
- Can visualize roots.
- Spinal vasculature abnormalities.

Procedure
5–25mL of (usually water-soluble) radio-opaque contrast medium is injected via an LP needle in the usual location (occasionally cisternal puncture is used). By tipping the patient on a tilt table, the whole spinal subarachnoid space may be visualized.

Complications
- Those of LP.
- Spinal arachnoiditis (after months or years), now rare with water-soluble contrast.
- Acute deterioration if there is cord/root compression.
- Direct neurotoxicity (3 in 10,000):
  - Seizures, encephalopathy.
  - Usually resolves in 48 h.
- Allergic reaction to contrast. Give dexamethasone 4mg 12 and 2 h prior to investigation if known allergy.

Note: Send CSF for usual investigations (📖 Lumbar puncture, p546).

Radionuclide scans

Positron emission tomography (PET)

Unstable positron-emitting isotopes (produced locally by a cyclotron or linear accelerator) are incorporated into biologically active compounds. The distribution of isotope shortly after IV administration is plotted. A range of compounds may be labelled, such as ligands for specific neurotransmitter receptors, or 18F fluorodeoxyglucose (FDG). Commonly, PET is used to determine regional cerebral blood flow.

Single photon emission computed tomography (SPECT)

- Stable radioactive isotopes are incorporated into biologically active compounds.
- Their distribution after IV administration is plotted.
- These images often lack fine spatial detail.

Although the range of ligands available is limited, SPECT has certain advantages over PET:
- Isotopes are stable and therefore a cyclotron or linear accelerator need not be on site.
- A labelled ligand can be given after a clinically important event, e.g. can give agent and scan within 20 min of the occurrence of a seizure.

Uses of PET and SPECT

PET is not widely available as a clinical tool. With the advent of functional MRI (FMRI), the uses of PET in both clinical practice and in neuroscience research may well become more restricted. SPECT is more widely available in clinical centres.

Clinical/research applications of PET and SPECT have included

- Determination of regional cerebral blood flow, glucose metabolism, and oxygen utilization
- Hypometabolism may be seen following a stroke. The affected area may exceed that with a demonstrable lesion on conventional CT or MR imaging.
- The epileptogenic focus may show interictal hypometabolism (ictal hypermetabolism may be demonstrated with SPECT).
- Regional hypometabolism may be seen in Alzheimer's, Parkinson's, and related degenerative conditions.
- 'Pseudodementia' secondary to psychiatric disease such as depression (with normal SPECT scans) may sometimes be differentiated from dementia due to 'organic' neurological disease (with regional hypoperfusion), although psychiatric diseases may themselves be associated with regional hypoperfusion.
- Whole body FDG-PET may be useful in demonstrating occult malignancy in paraneoplastic syndromes.
- Assessment of Parkinsonism.

The functional integrity of the nigrostriatal system can be assessed, e.g. by the use of SPECT ligands for the dopamine transporter (e.g. FP-CIT). Such direct antibody test (DAT) scans can be used to differentiate true Parkinsonism from other causes of movement disorders.

• *In vivo* pharmacology (e.g. distribution of neurotransmitter receptors).

📖 Nuclear medicine, Positron Emission tomography, p819.

Further reading

Marshall V, Grosset D. Role of dopamine transporter imaging in routine clinical practice. *Mov Disord* 2003; **18**: 1415–23.

Younes-Mhenni S, *et al.* FDG-PET improves tumour detection in patients with paraneoplastic neurological syndromes. *Brain* 2004; **127**: 2331–8.

Computed tomography

Cranial computed tomography

Now widely available; it should be considered a basic neurological tool.

Look for

- Disturbances in the normal anatomy of the ventricular system.
- Skull base and vault.
- Width of cortical fissures/sulci.
- Midline shift.
- Areas of abnormal tissue density.
- Opacity or lucency of sinuses.
- Normal flow voids.

High density ('white') signal

- Fresh blood.
- Calcification:
  - Slow growing tumour.
  - AVM/aneurysm.
  - Hamartoma.
  - In pineal/choroid plexus/basal ganglia, may be normal.

Low density ('black') signal

- Infarction.
- Tumour.
- Abscess.
- Oedema.
- Encephalitis.
- Resolving haematoma.

Mixed density

- Tumour.
- Abscess.
- AVM.
- Contusion.
- Haemorrhagic infarct.

After administration of IV contrast medium, areas with a breakdown in the blood–brain barrier may 'enhance' (appear 'white'). This may reveal previously 'invisible' lesions (isodense with the surrounding tissue). Especially useful for tumour and infection.

Common patterns of enhancement include

- Ring enhancement of tumours and abscesses.
- Solid enhancement of meningiomas.
- Meningeal enhancement with meningeal disease involvement.

Indications for head CT after head injury

CT imaging of the head in adults
Request CT brain scan immediately for adult patients with any of the following risk factors:
- Glasgow coma score <13 on initial assessment in the Emergency department
- Glasgow coma score <15 2 h after the injury on assessment in the Emergency department
- Suspected open or depressed skull fracture
- Any sign of basal skull fracture
- Post-traumatic seizure
- Focal neurological deficit
- One or more episodes of vomiting
- Amnesia for events more than 30 min before impact.

CT imaging of the head in children
Request computed tomography of the brain immediately for children with any one of the following risk factors:
- **Age over 1 year**: Glasgow coma score (GCS) <14 on assessment in the Emergency department
- **Age under 1 year**: GCS paediatric <15 on assessment in the Emergency department
- Age under 1 year and presence of bruise, swelling, or laceration (>5 cm) on the head
- Dangerous mechanism of injury
- Clinical suspicion of non-accidental injury
- Loss of consciousness lasting more than five min (witnessed)
- Post-traumatic seizure but no history of epilepsy
- Abnormal drowsiness
- Suspected open or depressed skull injury, or tense fontanelle
- Any sign of basal skull fracture
- Focal neurological deficit
- Three or more discrete episodes of vomiting
- Amnesia (antegrade or retrograde) lasting more than 5 min.[1,2]

CT angiography
CT, especially rapid image acquisition with helical CT, can allow imaging of the intracranial vasculature. This technique is particularly used in the detection of aneurysms, and is increasingly widely available.[3]

1 🖰 www.nice.org.uk/CG056 (2007)

2 Yates D, et al. Assessment, investigation, and early management of head injury: summary of NICE guidance. BMJ 2007; **335**: 719–20

3 Karamessini MT, et al. CT angiography with three-dimensional techniques for the early diagnosis of intracranial aneurysms. Comparison with intra-arterial DSA and the surgical findings. Eur J Radiol 2004; **49**: 212–23.

CT of spine

MRI is usually preferable, but plain CT can give information about the discs and bony architecture. After myelography compressive lesions can be demonstrated.

Indications for cervical spine imaging after trauma

Plain radiograph is the initial investigation, but CT preferred when:

- **Age >9 years**:
  - GCS <13 on initial assessment.
  - Inbubated patient.
  - Technically inadequate plain radiographs.
  - Clinical suspicion of injury despite normal radiograph.
  - Patient being scanned for multi region trauma.
- **Age <10 years**:
  - GCS <9.
  - Strong clinical suspicion of injury despite normal radiograph.
  - Technically inadequate plain radiographs.[1,2]

📖 *OHCM* 8e, p405.

1 🖱 www.nice.org.uk/CG056 (2007).
2 Yates D et al. (2007) Assessment, investigation, and early management of head injury: summary of NICE guidance. BMJ 335:719-20

Magnetic resonance imaging or nuclear magnetic resonance imaging

For most applications, MRI is superior to CT, but has more restricted availability.

Note: MRI is not safe in the presence of ferromagnetic materials (e.g. certain prostheses, metal filings in the eye).

Most common sequences are T1 and T2, but increasingly other sequences are being used clinically, such as FLAIR, proton density, diffusion-weighted imaging (Table 9.2).

In general
- T1 CSF is hypo-intense ('black'); fat and mature blood clot white.
- T2 CSF is hyperintense ('white').

Magnetic resonance imaging with enhancement
Intravenously administered gadolinium leaks through areas of damaged blood–brain barrier to give a marked enhancement.
- Ischaemia.
- Infection.
- Tumour (may help differentiate from surrounding oedema).
- Active demyelination.

Magnetic resonance venography and angiography
MR may be used to obtain non-invasive images of blood vessels by using special MRI sequences and image reconstruction. While standard angiography remains a 'gold standard' for many purposes, MR angiography has the advantage of being non-invasive and, therefore, 'safe'. MRA images flow, rather than structure and therefore may fail to 'pick up' low flow abnormalities, such as cavernous angiomas. ▶ **Caution**: congenital abnormalities in the venous sinuses may be misinterpreted as thrombosis on MRV.

Uses
- Assessment of patency of major arterial and venous vessels.
- Visualization of large (~3mm diameter) aneurysms.

Functional magnetic resonance imaging (FMRI)
A recent development allows certain (indirect) indices of neural activity (most commonly changes reflecting regional perfusion) to be imaged with sufficient temporal resolution to be useful for both research and clinical applications (although FMRI has been largely a research tool to date). As a conventional MRI machine, albeit with special software, is required, it is likely that FMRI will become a widely used clinical tool.

Clinical and research applications have included

- Demonstration of the language areas prior to epilepsy surgery.
- Demonstration of the functional anatomy of cognitive, sensory, and motor processes.

Table 9.2 Comparison of T1 and T2 MRI

T1	T2	Tissue or lesion
Good anatomical detail	Reveals most pathology better than T1	
Hypo-intense	Hyperintense	CSF
Hyperintense	Iso-intense	Fat, e.g. dermoid, lipoma, some metastases (melanoma), atheroma
Very hypo-intense	Very hyperintense	Cyst, hygroma
Hypo-intense	Hyperintense	Ischaemia, oedema, demyelination, many malignant tumours
Hyperintense	Moderately hyperintense	Subacute or chronic haemorrhage
Iso	Hypo-intense	Acute haemorrhage
Iso	Iso	Meningioma

Further reading

Powell HW, *et al*. The application of functional MRI of memory in temporal lobe epilepsy: a clinical review. *Epilepsia* 2004; **45**: 855–63.

White PM, *et al*. Intracranial aneurysm: CT angiography and MR angiography for detection prospective blinded comparison in a large patient cohort. *Radiology* 2001; **219**: 739–49.

Nerve conduction studies

Please give your neurophysiologists as much information as possible about your case and, if necessary, discuss it with them. They will then be in the position to organize the most appropriate neurophysiological investigations. In certain circumstances, you may need to specifically ask for unusual investigations, such as repetitive stimulation in suspected Lambert–Eaton myasthenic syndrome (LEMS, 📖 Nerve conduction studies, Repetitive stimulation, In Lambert–Eaton myasthenic syndrome, p568).

Sensory nerve action potential and sensory conduction velocity

Procedure
Orthodromic conduction velocity: electrically stimulates distal sensory branches (e.g. index finger) and records the evoked sensory nerve action potential (SNAP) proximally (e.g. over median nerve at wrist). The distance between the two sites (D) and the latency (L) of the onset of the SNAP determine the sensory conduction velocity (D/L). The SNAP amplitude is also useful.

Antidromic conduction velocity: supramaximal electrical stimulation proximally; records distally (e.g. by a ring electrode on little finger). By varying the position of the stimulating electrode, the conduction velocity in various portions of the nerve may be ascertained.

What does it mean?
- ↓ SNAP amplitude or SNAP absence altogether imply a lesion distal to the dorsal root ganglion.
- ↓ Velocity/↑ latency (Table 9.3). Motor velocities are more commonly measured.

Table 9.3 Typical values

	Latency	Amplitude
Median nerve (index finger to wrist)	2–3 ms	9–40mV
Ulnar nerve (little finger to wrist)	2–2.6 ms	6–30mV
Sural nerve (midcalf to below med. mall.)	2–4 ms	5–40mV

med. mall. = medial malleolus.

Motor conduction velocity

Procedure
Supramaximally stimulate a peripheral nerve trunk at a proximal (p) and a more distal (d) site. Record the time to the onset of the evoked muscle response (compound motor action potential (CMAP)) from each (Tp and Td), and the distance between them (D). The motor conduction velocity between p and d is therefore $D/(Tp–Td)$.

Typical values
- Median nerve in forearm (to abductor pollicis brevis) >48m/s.
- Ulnar nerve in forearm (to abductor digiti minimi) >48m/s.
- Common peroneal nerve (to extensor digitorum brevis) >40m/s.

What does it mean?
See Table 9.4.

Table 9.4 Typical patterns

	Conduction velocity	AP amplitude	AP dispersion
Axonal neuropathy	Late stage: ↓ distally > proximally (loss of fastest conducting axons)	Late stage: ↓	Not seen
Demyelinating neuropathy	Marked slowing		Greater dispersion, perhaps especially in acquired not inherited demyelination
Ganglionopathies	Slowing proportional to loss of large fibres; often not marked	↓ Proportional to loss of large fibres; often not marked	not seen

Note: Limbs should be warm; look for asymmetries. What are your laboratory's current values?

Distal motor latency
Latency from stimulation of most distal site on nerve to CMAP.

Typical values
- Median nerve (wrist to abductor pollicis brevis) <4.1m/s.
- Ulnar nerve (wrist to abductor digiti minimi) <3.8m/s.
- Radial nerve (spiral groove to brachioradialis) <5m/s.

Note: These latencies include time taken for impulses to pass along the most distal (unmyelinated) portion of the nerve and for transmission at the neuromuscular junction (therefore they may not be used to calculate nerve conduction velocities). Compare with velocities elsewhere in the nerve being studied.

What does it mean?

↑ *DML seen in*
- Conditions in which the very distal segment of a nerve is compromised (most commonly carpal tunnel syndrome).
- Early demyelinating neuropathy (e.g. Guillain–Barré syndrome).
- Chronic demyelinating neuropathy.

Compound motor action potential

The waveform, amplitude and area-under-the-curve of the CMAP reflect the number of depolarized muscle fibres (e.g. reduced in axonal neuropathy and denervated muscle) and the temporal dispersion of conduction velocities in the motor neurones to them (e.g. increased in demyelinating neuropathy).

Late responses

F wave

If a motor nerve is stimulated, there are orthodromically directed action potentials that may cause a response in the muscle (CMAP). However, antidromically directed action potentials will also pass proximally towards the cell body. If these result in sufficient depolarization of the axon hillock, then a second orthodromic volley will pass down the nerve. This may cause a second motor action potential (the F wave). Therefore, the F wave (i) does not involve synapses (other than the neuromuscular junction of course) and (ii) depends on the integrity of the whole axon.

It may be difficult to elicit.

Delay or absence of the F wave may reflect a lesion proximal to the site of stimulation, in parts of the nerve that may be inaccessible to electrodes, e.g. brachial plexopathy or thoracic outlet syndrome. May also be an early feature in GBS.

H wave

- This is 'an electrical ankle jerk': submaximal stimulation of posterior tibial nerve in the popliteal fossa causes trans-synaptic activation of soleus, recorded as a CMAP.
- Amplitude may be ↓ by afferent or efferent problems, e.g. neuropathy or radiculopathy.

Repetitive stimulation

- Procedure: stimulate a motor nerve with 3–5 supramaximal stimuli at 2–4Hz while recording evoked CMAPs.
- **Normal response**: no change in CMAP amplitude.
- **In myasthenia gravis**: >10% decrement in CMAP amplitude after 2 stimuli.
- **In Lambert Eaton myasthenic syndrome (LEMS)**:
  - After voluntary contraction, or after rapid stimulation (20–50Hz) for 2–10 s, the CMAP amplitude, often initially small, increases by 25% (suggestive) or 100% (diagnostic).
  - At a slow (3Hz) rate of stimulation, there is a response decrement.

Electromyogram (EMG)

Procedure
- A concentric needle electrode is usually used.
- It is inserted into the muscle to be studied.
- The difference in potential between the inner part of the electrode and the outer core is amplified and displayed on an oscilloscope or computer screen.
- It is also 'displayed' as an auditory signal, and experienced electromyographers as much listen to as watch the pattern of electrical activity.

Normal muscle is 'silent' (electrically inactive) at rest (there is no 'spontaneous activity'), although there will be a brief burst of activity when the electrode is first inserted (the 'insertional activity').

The electrode can pick up electrical activity from muscle fibres within about 0.5mm of its tip; therefore, muscle fibres from several motor units (each innervated by a different motor neurone) in this volume can contribute to the signal. However, with care, potentials from a single motor unit may be recorded when a co-operative subject tries to exert the muscle a little (the 'motor unit potential'). With increasing muscular effort, more muscle fibres are recruited, giving rise to the 'interference pattern'.

Various nerve and muscle problems cause characteristic alterations to these four patterns of activity
1 Insertional.
2 Spontaneous.
3 Motor unit potential.
4 Recruitment.
5 In addition, certain other patterns may be observed in certain diseases (in particular, myotonia).

1. Insertional activity
- Usually there is a brief burst of potentials which lasts <1 s.
- Insertional activity is normal in upper motor neurone (UMN) lesions and most non-inflammatory myopathies.
- It may be longer lasting in lower motor neurone (LMN) lesions, inflammatory myopathies and acid maltase deficiency.
- In myotonia, myotonic discharges occur, see ▢ Electromyogram p571).

2. Spontaneous activity
- Normal muscles at rest are silent.
- This is also the case in UMN lesions, non-inflammatory myopathies (unless 2° denervation has set in) and myotonia.
- Fibrillation potentials and +ve sharp waves are seen in LMN lesions and inflammatory myopathies. They occur in regular bursts of constant amplitude (unlike activity related to voluntary contraction).
- Fibrillation potentials are spontaneous APs in irritable, acutely denervated, muscle fibres. They are low amplitude brief −ve potentials.
- Positive sharp waves are brief +ive potentials, followed by a −ve wave. Typically, they can be seen for 2–3 weeks after denervation, but may persist.

3. Motor unit potentials (MUPs)

- If the electrode is positioned quite close to the fibres of a motor unit which is active during slight voluntary contraction, then a motor unit potential may be recorded. In normal muscle (and in UMN lesions), this waveform is triphasic, 5–10 ms and has an amplitude of 0.5–1mV (larger muscles have larger motor units).
- In myopathies and muscular dystrophies, the motor units are smaller and polyphasic. They tend to be briefer, but in some cases last longer than usual.
- In denervated and then reinnervated muscles (typically LMN lesions), the size of individual motor units increases (as the surviving motor neurones 'take over' the muscle fibres previously innervated by now absent other motor neurones). MUPs therefore are of greater amplitude and duration, and are polyphasic.
- In myotonia, myotonic discharges are seen.

Note: Up to 15–20% of MUPs in 'normal' muscle may be polyphasic.

4. Recruitment

- Normally, as the strength of voluntary contraction increases, increasing numbers of motor units are recruited, and these units tend to be larger (Heinneman's size principle). The potentials due to these active units overlap, and become difficult and finally impossible to tell apart—a full 'interference pattern', usually well below maximum voluntary contraction.
- In muscle diseases, a full interference pattern may be produced, but it is of low amplitude. In weak muscles, there may be 'early recruitment' (i.e. recruitment of many motor units at low levels of voluntary contraction).
- In denervated muscles, a full interference pattern may not be achieved, because of the decreased number of motor units.
- In UNM lesions, there is a lower frequency of 'normal' MUPs.

5. Myotonia

High frequency repetitive discharges occurring after voluntary movement or provoked by moving the electrode. The amplitude and the frequency wax and wane, giving the auditory signature likened to the sound of a Second World War dive bomber (or a motor cycle).

Note: Following the onset of a neuropathy, it may take at least 10–14 days for evidence of denervation to appear in the EMG. Therefore, a repeat study after this time is often useful.

Single fibre EMG

A recording electrode with a smaller recording surface than usually used samples a few muscle fibres from a single motor unit (supplied by a single motor neurone). The variability ('jitter') in the timing of action potentials from different muscles should be less than 20–25 ms. Conduction block during voluntary contraction may also be shown. These techniques are used to investigate neuromuscular disorders and reinnervation in neuropathies.

Electroencephalogram (EEG)

The standard electroencephalogram (EEG) is non-invasive. Electrodes are attached to the scalp with collodion adhesive. Stable recordings may be made for days. Usually they are arranged according to the international 10–20 system. This is a method for positioning electrodes over the scalp in an orderly and reproducible fashion. Additional electrodes can be applied to the scalp, depending on the region of interest.

Standard recording conditions

- Rest.
- Hyperventilation for 3–5 min can activate generalized epileptiform changes (and precipitate absence seizures):
  - Can ↑ frequency of focal discharge.
  - Can ↑ slow wave abnormalities.
- Photic stimulation (a strobe light at 30cm with a frequency of 1–50Hz); this can produce several patterns of activity:
  - *Photoparoxysmal response*—bilateral spike or spike and wave discharges not time-locked to the visual stimulus, which may outlast the visual stimulus by hundreds of milliseconds. Generalized, but may have frontal or occipital predominance.
  - Commonly seen in idiopathic generalized epilepsies.
  - High voltage occipital spikes, time-locked to the stimulus.
  - Weakly associated with epilepsy.
  - *Photomyogenic (photomyoclonic) responses*—non-specific mostly frontal spikes due to muscle activity.
  - Associated with alcohol and some other drug-withdrawal states.
- Sleep studies:
  - Subject either stays awake the night before the recording or is given a small dose of choral prior to the recording (sometimes both).
  - Subjects tend to show the earlier stages of non-rapid eye movement (REM) sleep.
  - These studies increase the yield of EEG abnormalities, including epileptiform ones.
  - By capture of 'natural sleep': certain seizure types are more common in sleep (e.g. juvenile myoclonic epilepsy).
  - Sleep deprivation itself increases the number of seizures and epileptiform changes.

📖 Polysomnography, p579.

Table 9.5 EEG rhythms

Activity	Frequency (Hz)	Amplitude (mV)	Scalp location	Behavioural state
Alpha	8–12	20–60	Usually occipital	Maximum relaxed, awake, eyes close
Beta	>13	10–20	Frontocentral	Wakeful, drowsy; REM and slow wave sleep 1 and 2
Theta	4–8	Variable diffuse	Frontocentral, temporal	Minimally awake, drowsy, SWS (slow wave sleep)
Delta	<4	Variable	Diffuse	Awake; drowsy
Mu	8–10	20–60	Central	Awake, suppressed in voluntary movements

The terms alpha, beta, theta and delta are often used to describe the background activity but are also used to describe the frequency of EEG activity.

Sharp activity may be a normal phenomenon.

Electroencephalogram: abnormalities

The normal electroencephalogram

There is a wide range of normal EEG phenomena. Some of the common patterns in the awake adult are listed in Table 9.5.

EEG abnormalities (not peri-ictal or ictal)

- A variety of EEG abnormalities may be seen outside the peri- or per-seizure period.
- Abnormalities in the EEG are not restricted to the appearance of abnormal waveforms.
- The loss, or redistribution in the scalp location, of normal background activities is abnormal.

The classification of EEG abnormalities is complex. Below is a highly simplified guide

1 General excess of slow waves: commonly seen in:
- Metabolic encephalopathy.
- Encephalitis.
- Post-ictal states.

2 Focal slow waves: commonly seen in:
- Large cerebral lesions (e.g. tumour, haematoma).
- Post-ictal states.
- Migraines.

3 Localized intermittent rhythmic slow waves: may be seen in Idiopathic generalized and localization related epilepsies.

4 Epileptiform abnormalities:
- Spikes (if last <80ms) or sharp waves (80–200ms) may be associated with slow waves.
- Consistently focal spikes suggest epilepsy with a focal seizure onset.

Note: 2–4% of non-epileptics have occasional spikes or sharps.

5 Repetitive stereotyped 'periodic' complexes.

EEG patterns may show periodicity. These patterns may be epileptiform or not, and may be focal or generalized. They are an abnormal EEG feature, the interpretation of which depends on the clinical context.

Examples include

- **Burst suppression**: bursts of generalized high voltage mixed waveforms, alternating with generalized voltage suppression:
  - Coma.
  - Late stage status epilepticus (both convulsive and non-convulsive).
- **Triphasic waves over one or both temporal lobes**: common in herpes simplex encephalitis.
- Periodic lateralized epileptiform discharges (PLEDs) are localized sharp or slow wave complexes 0.2–1 s long, every 1–5 s:
  - Non-specific but suggest localized cerebral insult (stroke, haematoma, tumour).
  - Occasionally seen in migraine and focal epilepsies.
- **BIPLEDs are bihemispheric PLEDs**: suggest more widespread insults, e.g. anoxia, encephalitis. to use the EEG.

- **Bilateral or generalized high voltage complexes for 0.5–2 s every 4–15 s**: characteristic of subacute sclerosing panencephalitis.
- **Triangular waves**:
  - Characteristic of Creutzfeldt–Jakob disease (CJD).
  - Not seen in vCJD; may see a 'disorganized' EEG without repetitive complexes).
- **Runs of broad triphasic waves (1.5–3Hz)**: severe metabolic encephalopathy (e.g. renal or hepatic failure).
- **Periodic spikes or sharp waves**: bi- or multiphasic morphology (0.5–2Hz); usually generalized—suggest severe encephalopathy, e.g.
  - Herpes encephalitis.
  - CJD (in setting of rapid dementia and myoclonus).
  - Lithium intoxication.
  - Post-anoxic brain injury.
  - Tricyclic antidepressant overdose.

Electroencephalogram: in epilepsy

Idiopathic (primary) generalized epilepsy (IGE)
- Generalized, bilaterally synchronous epileptiform discharges with virtually normal background.
- Absence epilepsy: 3Hz spike and wave.
- Juvenile myoclonic epilepsy (JME): 6Hz multiple spike and wave.

Symptomatic (secondary) generalized epilepsy
- More variable.
- **Inter-ictal background activity**: excess slow.
- **Inter-ictal epileptiform activity**: irregular spikes or sharp and slow waves 1.5–4Hz. Usually generalized, but may show asymmetry or (multi) focal features.

Localization-related partial epilepsy
- Inter-ictal EEG is often normal, particularly if the focus is located deeply (especially common with frontal foci).
- There may be lateralized or localized spikes or sharp waves.

Electroencephalogram: how to use

In suspected epilepsy

- Routine EEG with photic stimulation and hyperventilation gives about up to a 50% detection rate for interictal epileptiform abnormalities in a subject with epilepsy (higher 'yield' in 1° generalized epilepsies than in localization-related epilepsies).
- Sleep-deprived or choral-induced sleep recording may increase the yield of EEG abnormalities to up to 60–70%.
- Consider 24 h or longer ambulatory EEG, ideally with audio/video monitoring. Most useful in helping to determine the nature of the seizure in a subject with frequent (e.g. daily) attacks.

In general, avoid reduction in anti-epileptic drugs or drugs such as pentylenetetrazole to induce seizures, except in exceptional circumstances, e.g. videotelemetry as part of work-up for epilepsy surgery.

Note:

- No interictal spikes does not imply no epilepsy.
- Similarly, interictal spikes do not always imply epilepsy.
- A –ve ictal EEG does not necessarily imply a non-epileptic ('pseudo') seizure, especially in simple partial and some brief complex partial seizures. Scalp electrodes may fail to record deep, esp. frontal, activity.
- However, a tonic-clonic seizure with loss of consciousness should be associated with an epileptiform EEG during the ictus. This EEG activity may be obscured by muscle artefact, but post-ictal slowing may be seen.
- The EEG may be slow after a tonic-clonic seizure for many tens of minutes.

Note: The diagnosis of epilepsy is mainly clinical! Remember that most episodes of altered consciousness are not epileptic in origin. In many cases, cardiological investigations are appropriate. Have a low threshold for ordering a 12-lead ECG. Ambulatory ECG monitoring, particularly with cardiac memo devices, can be very useful.

In established epilepsy

- Classification (e.g. complex partial seizure (CPS) *vs.* absence).
- Assessment of frequency of seizures (e.g. ambulatory EEG to assess frequency of absence seizures).
- Reduction in inter-ictal discharges in some syndromes (e.g. absence, photosensitive epilepsy) correlates with AED efficacy.

In focal cerebral dysfunction

Often not particularly helpful. Modern imaging studies usually provide more information.

- Small, deep, or slow growing lesions often cause no effects.
- Asymmetric voltage attenuation may be caused by a subdural haematoma (or other fluid collection) overlying the cortex.
- Direct grey matter involvement may cause alteration/loss of normal EEG, or cause epileptiform discharges.
- Subcortical white matter changes can cause localized polymorphic slow waves.
- Deeper subcortical lesions tend to produce more widespread slow wave disturbances.

In CNS infections

- CJD and subacute sclerosing panencephalilits (SSPE) have relatively characteristic EEG associations.
- Meningitis and encephalitis cases may show diffuse background disturbances and polymorphic or bilateral intermittent slow wave abnormalities.
- Encephalitis usually causes more changes than meningitis.
- Focal changes may be seen over abscesses and in cases of herpes simplex encephalitis.

In dementia

- To exclude some conditions such as toxic encephalopathy, non-convulsive status epilepticus (NCSE).
- A few dementing conditions have characteristic EEGs (CJD, SSPE).
- Slowing of background frequency occurs in Alzheimer's disease, but values may overlap with those of the normal aged; therefore, not very helpful clinically.

In confusional states

- Helpful in diagnosing NCSE (absence and complex partial status).
- To exclude cerebral dysfunction.
- Not very useful in psychiatric diagnosis *per se*, but an abnormal EEG in a confusional state may help exclude psychogenic causes for an apparent reduction in level of consciousness.

In toxic-metabolic encephalopathies

- EEG always abnormal.
- Diffuse slowing in mild cases.
- Other abnormalities may develop in later stages.
- Specific patterns may be seen in certain aetiologies.
- **Excess fast activity**: barbiturate and benzodiazepine toxicity.
- **Triphasic waves**: hepatic and renal failure, anoxia, hypoglycaemia, hyperosmolality, lithium toxicity.
- **Periodic spikes or sharp waves**: anoxia, renal failure, lithium and tricyclic antidepressant toxicity.

In coma

- EEG, especially serial EEGs, provides an indication of degree of cerebral dysfunction.
- In general, any 'normal'-looking EEG, spontaneous variability, sleep–wake changes, and reaction to external stimuli are relatively good prognostic signs.
- An invariant, unreactive EEG is a poor prognostic sign; the pattern, however, is not uniform, it may include periodic spikes of sharp waves, episodic voltage attenuation, alpha coma, burst suppression.
- May give some diagnostic clues, e.g. localized abnormality—supratentorial mass lesion; persistent epileptiform discharges—status epilepticus.
- 'Alpha coma': monotonous unresponsive alpha with anterior distribution seen after cardio/respiratory arrest is a poor prognostic feature.
- Monotonous but partially reactive alpha may follow brainstem infarcts.

Electroencephalogram: invasive techniques

These are generally restricted to specialist centres, most commonly used in the pre-surgical workup of patients.

Foramen ovale electrodes, corticography (usually done by laying strips of electrodes on the surface of the brain) and depth EEG (electrodes implanted into the parenchyma of the brain) may be used, depending on the region of interest. Sphenoidal electrodes are rarely used today, but can give useful EEG information about the medial temporal structures.

Polysomnography

- This is the multimodal recording used in the analysis of sleep-related disorders.
- There is concurrent recording of electromyogram (EMG), EEG, and electro-oculography (EOG—eye movements), often with audiovisual channels. Other physiological parameters may also be recorded, e.g. nasal air flow, chest expansion.

Sleep is classically divided into 4 stages (1–4), of progressively 'deeper' slow wave sleep (SWS), and a fifth stage of REM sleep (Table 9.6), characterized physiologically by bursts of rapid eye movements (saccades).

Table 9.6 Sleep stages

Stage	Behaviour	Main EEG pattern	Comments
1	Drowsy	Diffuse alpha → theta	Flat to medium
2	Light sleep	High theta	K complexes
3	Medium sleep	Delta	Broad K complexes delta activation
4	Deep sleep	Continuous delta	None

REM: rapid eye movements.

There is progression through stages 1 to 4, and several episodes of REM during a typical night's sleep. Polysomnography can be important in understanding the pathophysiology of the insomnias, parasomnias and other sleep patterns.

Multiple sleep latency test

This is a diagnostic test for narcolepsy. Following a good night's sleep, normal subjects typically enter REM sleep with a latency of >>10 min (usually ~90 min). In narcolepsy the latency is <10 min.

Sodium amytal (Wada) test

Sodium amytal is injected into the R or L internal carotid artery. It is a short-acting barbiturate and temporarily causes hemispheric dysfunction on the injected side. If injected into the left in most right-handers, the ability to speak and continue to hold up the R arm is temporally impaired. If speech is preserved following R-sided injection, it suggests normal left-lateralization for language function. More complex testing may also be undertaken during the period of hemispheric dysfunction, but it is usually used to determine language dominance prior to certain neurosurgical procedures.

Sensory evoked potentials or responses

While many techniques and protocols have been developed in research laboratories, there are only a few techniques in widespread clinical use. A stimulus is delivered to the periphery, thus activating a sensory system and evoking an electrical response over a more central, often cortical, area. Multiple surface electrode recordings time-locked to the peripheral stimulus are recorded and averaged, to help eliminate ongoing random background 'noise' from the sensory stimulus-evoked 'signal'. Deviations of this evoked potential or response (EP or ER) from the norm (especially in latency and waveform) suggest pathology in the sensory pathway tested.

Visual evoked potentials

Pattern-evoked visual evoked potentials

An alternating chequerboard pattern (temporal frequency 1–2Hz) is presented to each eye individually (Fig. 9.1). The EP is recorded over the occipital (1° visual) cortex. Most commonly the first large +ve wave, called P1 or P100 (as it typically occurs at about 100ms), is studied.

A delayed, smaller or dispersed visual evoked potentials (VEP) indicates disease in the retino-geniculo-striate pathway (if severe refractive errors or cataracts have been excluded), but most commonly affecting the optic nerve (a uni-ocular deficit implies a lesion anterior to the optic chiasm) or at the chiasm.

Flash-evoked VEP

In subjects with very poor vision or fixation, and in the very young, a bright flash may be used as the stimulus. This gives less reproducible results, particularly in the P100 latency.

Common uses

The VEP is used in general to document intrinsic, inflammatory, or compressive lesions of the optic nerve (or chiasm).

1 Suspected optic or retrobulbar neuritis.
2 In a patient with suspected MS, evidence of a VEP abnormality in an asymptomatic eye would suggest a previous episode of an optic neuritis.
3 Evaluation of hysterical blindness (may need to use a strobe light stimulus if patient non-cooperative).
4 Evaluation of optic nerve function in compressive lesions, such as dysthyroid eye disease, optic nerve glioma.
5 Follow-up after surgery to decompress the optic nerve or chiasm.
6 Assessment of poor visual acuity in patients unable to co-operate with usual testing. Vary the size of the chequerboard squares; subjects with poor acuity will only have a VEP to the coarser patterns.

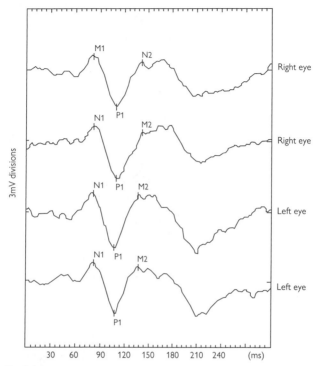

Fig. 9.1 Visual evoked potential (to chequerboard stimulus).

Somatosensory EPs

- Stimulation site over a peripheral nerve, e.g. ulnar or median at wrist, common peroneal at knee, posterior tibial at ankle (Fig. 9.2).
- Record over Erb's point (above the medial end of the clavicle), C7 or C2 vertebra, parietal cortex for arm stimulation; L1, C7, C2, or vertex for leg stimulation.
- Calculate absolute and interpeak latencies.
- Need to show with nerve conduction studies (NCS) that distal parts of the somatosensory pathways are conducting normally.
- Assesses dorsal column not anterolateral (spinothalamic) tract pathways:
  - E.g. stimulate median nerve at wrist, prolonged latency to Erb's point; suggests brachial plexus (or more distal) lesion.
  - Prolonged Erb's point to C2 latency suggests spinal cord lesion.

Uses
- Diagnosis of plexopathies.
- Evaluation of subclinical myelopathy in possible MS.
- Evaluation of hysterical sensory loss.
- Per-operative monitoring (e.g. during scoliosis surgery).

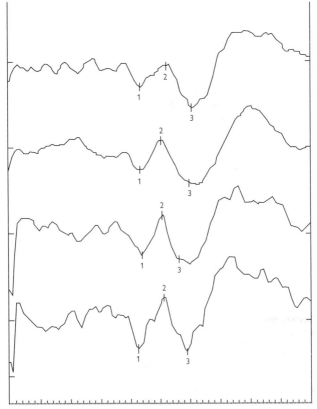

Fig. 9.2 Leg somatosensory potentials.

Brainstem auditory evoked potentials (BAEPs, BAERs, BSAEPs, Fig. 9.3)

- Stimulus: rarefaction clicks of 50 or 100 ms duration, presented mono-aurally at 10Hz at 60–70DB above threshold (masking noise to other ear).
- Record over mastoid and vertex of skull.
- Classic waveform has seven peaks, said to be generated by sequential auditory nuclei:
    - **I** VIIIth nerve (must be present to interpret subsequent waves).
    - **II** Cochlear nucleus (may be absent in normals).
    - **III** Superior olive.
    - **IV** Lateral lemniscus (may be absent in normals).
    - **V** Interior colliculus (should be 50% or more of wave I's amplitude).
    - **VI** Medial geniculate (too variable for regular clinical use).
    - **VII** Auditory thalamocortical radiation (too variable for regular clinical use).

Latency I–V (central conduction time) should be no more than 4.75 ms. The difference between left and right central conduction times should be <0.4 ms.

Uses

- Hearing assessment, especially in children.
- Evaluation in suspected MS and other myelinopathies (e.g. adreno-leukodystrophy; MRI more important now).
- Evaluation and detection of posterior fossa lesions (e.g. acoustic neuromas; MRI more important now).
- Evaluation of brainstem function (e.g. tumour, cerebrovascular accident (CVAs)).
- Evaluation of brainstem function in coma and brain death.
- Per-operative, e.g. acoustic neuroma excision.

The use of EPs in the diagnosis of MS

Traditionally, trimodal EPs (VEPs, SSEPs and BAEPs) have been requested to look for evidence of a disturbed conduction in multiple sensory systems. Modern practice however is to request only VEPs, if any at all. MRI is much more useful in demonstrated dissemination of central nervous system lesions.[1]

1 Polman CH, et al. (2005) Diagnostic criteria for multiple sclerosis: revisions to the 'McDonald criteria'. Ann Neurol **58**: 840–6.

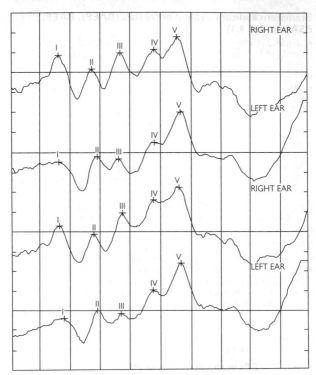

Fig. 9.3 Brainstem auditory evoked potentials.

Transcranial magnetic stimulation

- Brief, high-current pulse produced in a circular or figure-of-eight-shaped coil held over the scalp.
- This induces a magnetic field with flux perpendicular to the coil.
- This in turn produces an electric field perpendicular to the magnetic field.

The result is excitation or inhibition of the subjacent cortex (depending on stimulus parameters).

- TMS has been used for diagnostic purposes in a number of ways, although as yet it is not in widespread clinical use.

Measurement of central motor conduction time

- TMS over the motor cortex indirectly (presumably via synaptic activation of corticospinal neurones) causes a volley of activity in the corticospinal tracts. The latency of the EMG in, say, the abductor digiti minimi may be measured.
- May be used in cervical myelopathy and MS to show increased latency of EMG in hand muscles evoked by transcranial magnetic stimulation (TMS) over the motor cortex. If the EMG latency to more distal stimulation (e.g. at C7 over the spinal cord and in the ulnar nerve) is normal, then an increased central motor conduction time may be inferred.
- Latency may also be increased in other neurogenerative conditions.

Motor evoked potentials

Abnormalities in the amplitude of the motor evoked potentials (MEP) may reflect abnormalities anywhere in the pathway form the motor cortex to the muscles.

Silent period

- If a subject maintains muscle contraction and a single suprathreshold TMS pulse is applied to the contralateral motor cortex, ongoing EMG activity ceases for a few hundred milliseconds after the MEP (the 'silent period').
- Silent period may be long in, e.g., stroke, MS, spinal cord injury.
- Silent period may be short in, e.g., motor neuron disease (MND), Parkinson's disease (PD).

Interhemispheric conduction

- Interhemispheric inhibition may be decreased in MS or MND.
- It may be absent following lesions to the corpus callosum.

Motor cortex excitability

- High thresholds may be seen in stroke or MS.
- Low thresholds and increased intracortical inhibition may be seen in MND.
- Decreased intracortical inhibition may be seen in PD.

Psychogenic limb weakness

Some authorities have used TMS to evoke muscle activity in 'paralysed' limbs in patients with psychogenic paralysis. This needs to be done in the context of an 'holistic' approach to the patient, aimed at dealing with any psychological pathology.

Potential clinical applications

There have been many TMS studies; some that may prove useful as clinical tests, e.g.

- Determination of lateralization of language function by repetitive TMS (rTMS) prior to surgery for epilepsy.
- Assessment of cortical excitability in certain epilepsy syndromes.
- Assessment of decreased intracortical inhibition in dystonia.
- Assessment of recovery from stroke.[1]

Further reading

Curra A, et al. Transcranial magnetic stimulation techniques in clinical investigation. *Neurology* 2002; **59**: 1851–9.

Kobayashi M, Pascuel-Leone A Transcranial magnetic stimulation in neurology. *Lancet Neurol* 2003; **2**: 145–56.

1 Devlin JT, Watkins KE (2007) Stimulating language: insights from TMS. Brain 130: 610-622

Neurological investigation of sphincter disturbance

Electromyogram

- Of pelvic floor muscles may be helpful in faecal incontinence, stress urinary incontinence, and cauda equina syndrome.
- Pelvic floor and sphincter muscle EMGs may reflect pudendal nerve damage.
- Anal sphincter EMG abnormalities may reflect damage to Onuf's nucleus, e.g. in multi-system atrophy. It is characteristically unaffected in MND.

Magnetic resonance imaging

In suspected sacral spinal cord, conus medullaris, and equina equina lesions.

Urodynamics

Flowmetry

- Measurement of rate and amount of urine flow over time.
- Allows calculation of parameters, such as time to maximal flow, maximum and mean flow rate, volume voided.
- Post-micturition ultrasound can determine residual volume.

Cystometry (needs urinary catheterization)

- Measurement of intravesicular pressure during filling (usually at 50mL/min) or emptying. Typically, bladder filling sensation starts at about 100mL and the bladder is full at 400–600mL (with no more than a 15cm of water rise in pressure). Detrusor instability may cause sharp rises in the pressure during filling.
- During voiding, flow rate should be >15mL/min (♂) or >20mL/min (♀) with pressures of <50cmH$_2$O (♂) or 30 cmH$_2$O (♀).

Further reading

Fowler CJ. Investigational techniques. *Eur Urol* 1998; **34**(suppl): 10–12.

Edrophonium (Tensilon®) test

Procedure

- Explain the test to patient.
- Select weak and/or fatiguable muscles to be assessed.
- Attach ECG monitor.
- Draw up 0.6mg atropine (for use if extreme bradycardia develops), 10mg of edrophonium in 5mL normal saline (A), 5mL normal saline (B), and saline flush.
- Administer 1mL of test solution (A or B, ideally patient and administrating physician should be blinded to the nature of the solution).
- If no adverse reaction, administer remaining 4mL.
- Repeat with other solution (B or A).

Note: if the diagnosis of MG is clinically obvious, and the patient has responded to pyridostigmine given empirically, there is little point in stopping this and performing an edrophonium test.

Interpretation

- In myasthenia gravis, there should be a response within 30–60 s, which should wear off in 2–4 min.
- There may be a response in Lambert Eaton myasthenic syndrome, polymyositis, and motor neurone disease (MND).

Biopsies

- Always liaise with those taking the biopsy and those processing it!
- A biopsy should be undertaken to answer specific questions, in the light of a differential diagnosis formulated following history, examination, and other investigations.

Skeletal muscle

Indications

- Primary muscle disease, e.g. metabolic myopathy, polymyositis, muscular dystrophy.
- Neurogenic atrophy.
- Mitochondrial cytopathies (even in the absence of clinical muscle involvement).
- Multi-organ disease, e.g. vasculitides.

Which muscle to biopsy?

- An involved, but not end stage muscle.
- One that has not been used for EMG recording or had an injection for >1 month.
- Quadriceps and deltoid often used.

Open or needle biopsy?

Open biopsy
- Larger specimen.
- Can fix specimen at *in situ* length.
- Especially for inflammatory myopathy and in vasculitis.

Needle biopsy
- Smaller scar.
- Multiple biopsies possible.
- However:
  - Smaller biopsies.
  - Difficulties in orientating the sample.

What may be done to the tissue?

- Routine histology.
- Examination of small blood vessels.
- Histochemistry.
- Electron microscopy.
- Tests of muscle metabolism.
- Mitochondrial DNA studies.

Nerve

Indications
- Distinction between segmental demyelination and axonal degeneration (if not already determined).
- Certain neuropathies with characteristic histological features, e.g. due to amyloid deposition, sarcoid, vasculitis, neoplastic involvement.
- Certain myelinopathies (e.g. leukodystrophies) with peripheral nervous system (PNS) and central nervous system (CNS) involvement.

Which nerve to biopsy?
- The cutaneous branch of the sural nerve at the ankle (usually).
- Superficial peroneal (sometimes).
- Superficial radial (occasionally).
- Occasionally, small motor nerve twigs are obtained in muscle biopsy.
- Overlying skin may be co-biopsied.

What is done?
2–3cm of full-thickness nerve or fascicle.

What may be done to the tissue?
- Routine light microscopy (morphometry, structural survey; amyloidosis).
- Frozen section light microscopy (immunochemistry).
- Electron microscopy (ultrastructure).
- Teased out single fibres (to examine sequential myelin internodes).

Brain/meningeal biopsy

Indications
- Diagnosis and management of suspected 1° and some metastatic brain tumours.
- Differential diagnosis of other mass lesions (inflammatory and infective).
- Differentiation of radiation necrosis and tumour regrowth.
- Differentiation of neoplastic and non-neoplastic cysts (and their drainage).
- Diagnostic biopsy of a suspected infectious lesion that has not responded to a trial of therapy.
- Diagnosis of cerebral vasculitis or vasculopathy.

What is done?
- High quality cranial CT/MRI, possibly with contrast, to delineate lesion.
- If no discrete lesion, generally an area of non-dominant, non-eloquent cerebrum is taken.
- Stereotactic needle biopsy with image guidance:
  - Deep, small, lesions in 'eloquent' areas.
  - Multiple biopsies along needle track (useful in heterogeneous lesions such as some gliomas).
- And/or open biopsy:
  - Accessible lesions.
  - When resection considered during procedure.

- Intra-operative evaluation of frozen samples:
  - E.g. can a biopsy be made?
  - E.g. is the sample adequate?

Note: Caution in suspected CJD!!

Skin

- Some storage diseases:
  - Lafora body.
  - Batten's disease.
- Mitochondrial cytopathies.

Bone marrow

- Niemann–Pick type C.
- Haematological and other malignancies.

Rectal and appendicectomy

- Most neuronal storage diseases affect the autonomic nervous system, so evidence can be sought in neurones of the gut's intrinsic plexi.
- Amyloid in rectal biopsy.

Tonsillar biopsy

Research tool in vCJD.

Oligoclonal bands

- Electrophoresis of serum and CSF separates protein components by size and charge.
- OCBs may be present in serum and CSF. Bands in the CSF not seen in the serum suggest intrathecal-specific synthesis of immunoglobulins.
- This pattern is seen in most (95%) cases of established MS, but may also occur in other conditions, such as chronic meningitis, neurosyphilis, SSPE, and neurosarcoid (although uncommonly).

Further reading

Thompson EJ. Cerebrospinal fluid. In: Hughes RAC (ed.) *Neurological Investigations*, London: BMJ Publications, 1997. 443–66.

Diagnostic & prognostic antibodies, and other markers in blood & urine

Multi-system disorders

PNS and CNS are affected in many multi-system disorders; markers in blood, and other fluids and tissues for these are therefore commonly requested in neurology patients.

Vasculitides, e.g.
- Extractable nuclear antigens in SLE.
- ANCA in Wegener's.
- Rheumatoid factor in rheumatoid arthritis (RhA).

Enteropathies, e.g.
Gliadin and endomysial antibodies in coeliac disease (an area of controversy).

Systemic infections, e.g.
- Serology for many diseases, e.g. *Borrelia* in Lyme disease, HIV.
- Polymerase chain reaction (PCR) for tuberculosis (TB).

Disorders of coagulation: thrombophilia screen currently commonly includes
- Protein S and C levels.
- Antithrombin III levels.
- Screening for the Leiden mutation in factor V.
- Lupus anticoagulant.
- Tumour markers, e.g.
  - CEA for gut neoplasia.
  - Serum and urinary paraproteins in haematological disorders like myeloma.

Sarcoid
ACE and ACE genotype.

Endocrinopathies, e.g.
TSH, FT4, and FT3, thyroid autoantibodies in thyroid dysfunction.

Other metabolic disorders, e.g.
- **Wilson's disease**: blood copper and caeruloplasmin; some authorities also request 24 h urinary copper excretion. **Note**: Slit lamp examination performed by an experienced ophthalmologist reveals Kayser–Fleischer rings in most cases of Wilson's disease with neurological involvement.
- **Phaeochromocytoma**: catecholamine metabolites in three 24 h urine collections.

Disease-specific markers
Myasthenia gravis: anti-acetylcholine receptor and muscle specific kinase (MuSK antibodies).

Paraneoplastic antibodies

Certain neurological syndromes are 'paraneoplastic', i.e. due to remote, but non-metastatic effects of non-nervous system cancers. These paraneoplastic syndromes are rare, but important to recognize. In perhaps 50% of cases, the neurological symptoms may predate those of the cancer. This is an area of intensive research. Antibody tests that are well-described include those in Table 9.7.

Table 9.7 Paraneoplastic antibodies

Antibody	Paraneoplastic syndrome	Associated tumour
Anti Hu (ANNA1)	Encephalomyelitis Sensory neuronopathy Cerebellar degeneration Chronic GI pseudo-obstruction Limbic encephalitis	Small cell lung cancer (SCLC)
Anti Yo (PCA1)	Cerebellar degeneration	Breast, ovary
Anti Ri (ANNA2)	Brainstem encephalitis	Breast, SCLC
CV2 (CRMP5)	Encephalomyelitis Chorea Sensory neuronopathy Sensorimotor neuropathy Cerebellar degeneration Limbic encephalitis Chronic GI pseudo-obstruction	Thymoma, SCLC
Anti Ma2 (Ta)	Limbic/diencephalic encephalitis Cerebellar degeneration Brainstem encephalitis	Testis, lung
Anti-amphiphysin	Stiff person syndrome Other syndromes	Breast, SCLC
CAR	Retinopathy	Breast, SCLC
Tr	Cerebellar ataxia	Hodgkin's

Further reading

Graus F, et al. Recommended diagnostic criteria for paraneoplastic neurological syndromes. J Neurol Neurosurg Psychiat 2004; **75**: 1135–40.
Honnorat J, Antoine, J-C Paraneoplastic neurological syndromes. Orpahanet J Rare Dis 2007; **2**: 22.

Biochemical markers

Many 'inborn errors of metabolism' cause neurological disease. A variety of investigations, including tests on blood, urine and CSF, biopsies and genetic analyses, is used in their diagnosis (see 📖 Diagnostic & prognostic antibodies, and other markers in blood & urine, p592; 📖 Genetic tests, p595; for an accessible review see Gray et al).

Biochemical tests

Some basic principles

Many autosomal recessive and X-linked metabolic diseases are caused by reduced or absent activity of a specific enzyme, in turn due to a single gene defect.

In some there is a tissue-specific deficit:
e.g. McArdle's (glycogen storage disease V): demonstrates absence of phosphorylase activity in muscle biopsy (as only the myophosphorylase isozyme is affected).

In other conditions, notably the lipidoses, the enzyme is deficient in many tissues:
e.g. in Niemann–Pick diseases A and B, sphingomyelinase is deficient in brain and spinal cord, but also in the gastrointestinal tract, liver, spleen, and bone marrow. Abnormal lipid metabolism can, therefore, be demonstrated in relatively easily accessible tissue such as fibroblasts.

Not only may the absence or lower activity of an enzyme reduce the amount of the product of the reaction it catalyses, it may lead to the accumulation of precursors in the metabolic pathway:

$$A \text{---}(1) \to B \text{---}(2) \to C \text{---}(3) \to D$$

If enzyme (3) is reduced, A, B, and C may accumulate, with lower levels of D than usual being produced

- e.g. in acute intermittent porphyria, there is increased urinary excretion of δ haeminolevulinic acid and porphobilinogen (intermediates in the haem- synthetic pathway) during an acute attack.
- Decreased levels of porphobilinogen deaminase may be demonstrated in erythrocytes, leucocytes, and cultured fibroblasts.

Ischaemic forearm exercise test (ischaemic lactate test)

Procedure

1. Rest patient supine for 30 min.
2. Draw a baseline lactate sample from a catheter in an antecubital vein.
3. Inflate sphygmomanometer cuff on that arm to above arterial pressure.
4. Subject squeezes a rubber ball in that hand until exhaustion.
5. Rapidly deflate cuff.
6. Take further venous samples at 30, 60, and 240 s.

Results

Normally the venous lactate will rise by 2-, 3-, or even 4-fold; if it fails to rise by 1.5-fold, then there is likely to be a glycogenolysis or glycolysis defect (or the patient has not exercised sufficiently!).[1]

---

1 Gray RG et al. Inborn errors of metabolism as a cause of neurological disease in adults: an approach to investigation. *J Neurol Neurosurg Psychiat* 2000; **69**: 5–12.

Genetic tests

The list of diseases for which we have specific genetic tests grows each month. Rather than give a necessarily incomplete compendium, we discuss some general principles.

Several important neurological conditions may today be diagnosed by (relatively) simple genetic tests, whereas in the past biopsy was necessary. For example, Duchenne, Becker, and oculopharyngeal muscular dystrophies are associated with well defined genetic abnormalities. Similarly, several mitochondrial cytopathies (such as myoclonic epilepsy and ragged red fibres—MERRF, and mitochondrial myopathy, lactic acidosis and stroke-like episodes—MELAS) may now often be diagnosed by finding common mutations or deletions in mitochondrial DNA.

When might a neurologist refer to a clinical geneticist?
- Genetic counselling of an index patient and his family.
- Cytogenetic or molecular diagnosis.
- Long-term follow up of family:
  - Notification of advances.
  - Counselling family members as they become adult.
  - Co-ordinating care with paediatric and adult neurologists.

Cytogenetics: when to do it
- Female with an X-linked disorder.
- Unexplained developmental delay.
- Unexplained major CNS malformation.
- The coexistence of two genetic diseases in a patient.

What is done?
- Conventional karyotype.
- Fluorescent *in situ* hybridization (FISH) for suspected submicroscopic chromosomal aberrations: e.g. a p13.3 deletion may cause lissencephaly.

Molecular genetics: when to do it
- Confirming a clinical diagnosis.
- Identify carriers in the family.

What is done?
An ever-increasing range of diseases may be tested for. Some of these tests may be routinely available at your local clinical Genetics laboratory; others at regional, national, or even supranational centres. Other tests may be available on a 'research' basis. It is clear, however, that tests for genetic 'lesions' or risk factors will become increasingly available. Rather than give an, at best, partial list of readily available tests, we give a few examples below of the kinds of tests that are available. The astute reader will spot that different mutations within a given gene can give rise to different clinical phenotypes. Indeed, recent work has shown that the same mutation in some genes can give rise to more than one phenotype: we clearly have a great deal yet to learn about the genetics of neurological diseases!

Detection of deletions
- e.g. in mitochondrial (mt)DNA in MELAS and MERRF.
- e.g. of dystrophin gene in Duchenne and Becker muscular dystrophies.

Detection of DNA rearrangement
e.g. PMP22 gene duplication in some cases of Charcot–Marie–Tooth disease type 1 (or hereditary motor-sensory neuropathy type 1, (HMSN1); deletions within this gene cause hereditary neuropathy with liability to pressure palsies (HNPP).

Detection of trinucleotide repeats
- Found in >10 neurological diseases (see Table 9.8).
- So far, there in no overlap in the number of repeats in controls and affected patients (except rarely in Huntington's, in the region of 33 to 36 repeats).
- Anticipation (more severe phenotype and earlier onset) often reflects in increased number of repeats in the most recent generations (especially myotonic dystrophy).

Table 9.8 Trinucleotide repeat diseases

Disease	Gene	Triplet repeats	Transmission
Fragile X	FMR1	CGG	X-linked
Myotonic dystrophy	DM	CTG	AD
Friedreich's ataxia	FRDA	GAA	AR
Spinobulbar muscular atrophy	Androgen receptor	CAG	X-linked
Huntington's disease	IT15	CAG	AD
Spinocerebellar atrophy			
• SCA 1	SCA 1	CAG	AD
• SCA 2	SCA 2	CAG	AD
• SCA 3	SCA 3	CAG	AD
• SCA 6	SCA 6	CAG	AD
• SCA 7	SCA 7	CAG	AD
Dentorubropallidoluysian atrophy	DRPLA	CAG	AD

Note: SCA 6 is a CAG triplet expansion in the CACNL1A4 calcium channel gene. Other (non-triplet repeat) mutations in the gene cause other conditions: episodic ataxia type 2 and familial hemiplegic migraine.

Detection of single base mutations

This involves fragmenting the DNA of the gene into manageable pieces, then amplifying these so that there are multiple copies. Subsequently, various methods may be used to detect fragments with abnormal sequences, even if only differing at a single base from 'wild type'. There are several such techniques, constantly being refined, and many are restricted to research laboratories.

- However, molecular genetics is proceeding at a tremendous pace, both in terms of the number of conditions with identified genetic lesions and the laboratory techniques for analysis.
- High speed DNA sequencing will facilitate sequencing large pieces of DNA.
- e.g. point mutations in the MPZ gene, which encodes for P0, a component of the myelin sheath, have been found in some families with Charcot–Marie–Tooth disease type 1B.

Genetic risk factors

Another area of clinical genetics which is likely to become more important is the detection of genetic 'risk factors' for diseases. Certain allelic variants, whilst not 'causing' a disease in the traditional sense, may predispose an individual to exhibiting a certain clinical phenotype, or alter the age at which it might become apparent.

e.g. there are three allelic variants in the apolipoprotein E (APOE4) gene, e2, e3, e4. Homozygosity for e4 is likely to be a risk factor for developing Alzheimer's disease, and for developing it at an earlier age. However, the majority of e4 homozygotes do not develop the condition (therefore it is not 'causative').

Detection of the presence of abnormal protein or altered levels of normal protein

Immunocytochemistry and immunoblotting (Western blots) on tissue samples from the patient allow direct visualization of the presence of abnormal protein, or absence or reduced levels of normal protein, in a variety of conditions. (These techniques are not genetic in the strictest sense, but are often useful in 'genetic' conditions.)

e.g. Duchenne and Becker muscular dystrophies have absent or reduced levels of dystrophin in muscle biopsy samples.

Useful website

Online Mendelian Inheritance in Man (OMIM) is a continually updated catalogue of 'genetic' diseases in man, giving data about the genotype, mode of inheritance and the clinical phenotype of thousands of disorders (not just neurological).

Further reading

Young AB. Huntington's disease and other trinucleotide repeat disorders. In: Martin JB (ed.) *Scientific American Molecular Neurology*. New York: Scientific American, 1998; 35–54.
⅏ http://www.ncbi.nim.nih.gov/Omim/

Neuro-otology

Pure tone audiometry

Measure threshold for air and bone conduction at frequencies from 250 to 8000Hz.

Typical patterns

- Conduction deafness BC > AC at all frequencies.
- Sensorineural deafness AC = BC at all frequencies, but increasing deafness as frequency rises.

AC = air conduction; BC = bone conduction

More specialized tests

- Tone decay.
- Loudness discomfort.
- Speech audiometry.
- Acoustic impedance.

Caloric testing

Procedure

1 Inspect eardrum; if intact, proceed.
2 Place patient supine with neck flexed 30° (on pillow).
3 Irrigate external auditory meatus with 30°C water (ice water if testing for brain death).
4 Observe for (or record[1]) nystagmus.
5 Repeat after 5 min with 44°C water.

What should happen

1 Cold water induces convection of fluid in ipsilateral lateral semicircular canal (LSCC).
2 There is less output from ipsilateral LSCC.
3 Imbalance of signals from the two LSCCs results in eye drift towards the irrigated ear.
4 Fast phase contraversive movements correct for eye drift (hence, nystamus with fast phase away from irrigated ear).
5 This nystagmus starts in about 20 s and persists for 1 min.
6 Warm water reverses the nystagmus.

---

1 There are various techniques for recording eye movements. Although quite crude, electronystography has the advantage that it requires no instrumentation of the eyeball directly, allows recordings in the dark or with closed eyes (thus abolishing visual fixation and other responses that can interfere with the vestibulo-ocular reflex) and is relatively cheap.

Common pathological responses

Canal paresis

1 Reduced duration of nystagmus following irrigation on one side (with cold or warm water).
2 Suggests ipsilateral peripheral or central lesion.

Directional preponderance

1 Prolonged nystagmus in one direction.
2 Suggests central lesion on side of preponderance or contralateral peripheral lesion.

Combination of clinical examination, audiometry and caloric testing of the vestibulo-ocular reflex will help localize a lesion (peripheral *vs.* central; L *vs.* R).

Brainstem auditory evoked responses

📖 Sensory evoked potentials or responses, Brainstem auditory evoked responses, p580.

Further reading

Troost BT, Arguello LC. Neuro-otology. In: Bradley WG *et al.* (eds) *Neurology in Clinical Practice*, 3rd edn. Boston: Butterworth-Heinemann, 2000.

Renal medicine

Estimation of kidney function

Estimates based on serum creatinine

Measurement of serum creatinine concentration is the most commonly used way of assessing the excretory function of the kidneys, which is mostly dependent on glomerular filtration rate (GFR). Creatinine is the non-enzymatic breakdown product of creatine and phosphocreatine (almost exclusively found in skeletal muscle). Its production rate is proportional to muscle mass—the average individual produces around 10mmol/day. Endogenous production of creatinine is usually constant, but ingestion of cooked meat and severe exercise cause a rapid, temporary rise in production of creatinine, and thus in creatinine concentration. It is excreted mainly by glomerular filtration, but tubular secretion of creatinine also occurs, and contributes a significant proportion of overall excretion when GFR falls, resulting in overestimation of GFR at low GFR. Drugs, e.g. cimetidine, trimethoprim, can block the secretory component and elevate serum creatinine without any change in true GFR.

Because of the reciprocal relationship between clearance and serum creatinine, serum creatinine does not rise outside the normal range until there has been a substantial fall in GFR, particularly in patients with low muscle mass (Fig. 10.1). However, in an individual patient, a progressive increase in serum creatinine over time, even within the normal range, indicates declining GFR. Wide variation between individuals based on muscle mass, sex, and age makes serum creatinine an imperfect screening test for renal failure. Estimation of 24 h urine creatinine excretion allows measurement of creatinine clearance, but is beset with difficulties largely related to the timing and completeness of urine collections. For these reasons, use of creatinine clearance in clinical practice has been superseded by the use of prediction formulae.

The 4-variable Modification of Diet in Renal Disease formula

GFR may be estimated by the 4-variable Modification of Diet in Renal Disease (MDRD) formula. This is the simplest of several formulae derived from the MDRD dataset and gives an estimate of GFR normalized to a body surface area of 1.73 m²:

GFR (mL/min/1.73m²)
$= 175 \times \{[\text{serum creatinine (mmol/L)}/88.4]^{-1.154}\} \times \text{age (years)}^{-0.203}$
$\times$ 0.742 if ♀ and
$\times$ 1.21 if Afro-Caribbean

This formula does not give an accurate estimate of GFR at extremes of muscle mass, including amputees, and is not validated in the paediatric population. Most laboratories in the UK now measure creatinine with an assay calibrated to an isotope dilution mass spectrometry (IDMS) standard, and are able to report an estimated GFR alongside creatinine results using this formula.

▶Where the laboratory report a value for estimated GFR, this should be used, rather than any value subsequently derived.

The formula previously used a constant of 186, rather than 175, as it was developed using a creatinine assay that gave higher values than the standard; it remains important to check which assay is being used before using this or any other formula to estimate GFR.

The Cockroft and Gault formula and other estimates of eGFR

The Cockroft and Gault formula gives an estimate of creatinine clearance, using age, weight and serum creatinine as input variables. For simplicity of reporting, because weight is not required, and because the MDRD formula gives an estimate of GFR, which is normalized to body surface area (and thus gives an estimate of how well kidney function is matched to body size) the MDRD formula is now preferred.

Creatinine clearance

$= ((\{[140 - \text{age (years)}] \times \text{weight (kg)}\}/\text{serum creatinine (mmol/L)}))$

$\times$ 1.23 if ♂ or

$\times$ 1.04 if ♀

See ♖ http://www.kidney.org/professionals/kdoqi/guidelines_ckd/p5_lab_g4.htm for a discussion of these and other formulae, including those that can be used to estimate GFR in children. Note that there is also a 6-variable MDRD equation in use that also requires urea and albumin values: because of interlaboratory differences in albumin estimations, *this equation is not recommended*.

Where estimation of GFR is made the formula used should be stated. There are important differences between the two estimates, particularly as GFR declines at extremes of body size, but either formula is a major advance on the use of serum creatinine alone.

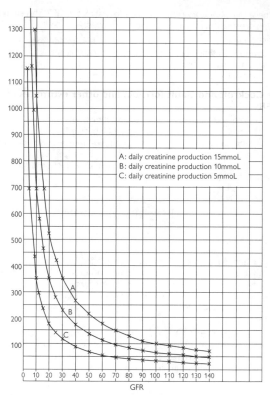

Fig. 10.1 Creatinine production is dependent on muscle mass, which varies widely. Graph illustrates the theoretical relationship between GFR and plasma creatinine, ignoring effects of tubular secretion of creatinine, which results in over-estimation of GFR from plasma creatinine or measurement of creatinine clearance. Note that in a patient with low muscle mass, creatinine does not rise outside the normal range until the GFR has fallen <30mL/min, whereas a patient with higher muscle mass will reach the same level of creatinine at a GFR of 90mL/min.

Classification of kidney disease

The following classification of chronic kidney disease (CKD) is now commonly used in the UK and elsewhere. It is based on the classification proposed by the National Kidney Foundation Kidney Disease Outcomes Quality Initiative (K-DOQI).[1]

- **CKD 1**: normal GFR; GFR >90mL/min/1.73m^2 with other evidence of chronic kidney damage.[2]
- **CKD 2**: mild decrease in GFR; GFR 60–89mL/min/1.73m^2 with other evidence of chronic kidney damage.[2]
- **CKD 3a**: moderate decrease in GFR 45–59mL/min/1.73m^2.
- **CKD 3b**: moderate decrease in GFR 30–44mL/min/1.73m^2.
- **CKD 4**: severe decrease in GFR 15–29mL/min/1.73m^2.
- **CKD 5**: established renal failure (ERF) GFR <15mL/min/1.73m^2 or on dialysis.

The suffix (p) can be used to indicate the presence of proteinuria (albumin:creatinine ratio (ACR) >30mg/mmol or protein:creatinine ratio (PCrR) >50mg/mmol). For more information see the section on proteinuria. Classification of CKD in this way allows identification of those with severe disease in need of specialist assessment, and can be used to guide blood pressure targets and frequency of monitoring in those with less severe disease.[3]

Serum urea

Urea is the product of protein catabolism in the liver. Production is increased by high protein intake, catabolic states, breakdown of blood in the gut lumen in gastrointestinal (GI) bleeding and tetracycline treatment, and may decreased in liver disease. Urea is freely filtered at the glomerulus with variable reabsorption, which is influenced by extracellular volume status. Intravascular volume depletion, diuretics, congestive cardiac failure (CCF), GI bleeding, tetracyclines, and renal failure cause elevated levels. Disproportionate rise in serum urea compared to creatinine occurs in hypovolaemia and GI bleeding. Reduced levels are seen in chronic liver disease and alcohol abuse. By itself, serum urea is a very poor marker of excretory kidney function.

---

1 ℘ http://www.kidney.org/professionals/kdoqi/guidelines_ckd/p4_class_g1.htm

2 Other evidence of chronic kidney disease may include persistent microalbuminuria, proteinuria, or glomerular haematuria, structural abnormalities, including renal scarring and polycystic disease, and biopsy proven chronic glomerulonephritis. An estimated GFR of >60 in the absence of other evidence of kidney damage should be considered normal.

3 See ℘ http://www.nice.org.uk/Guidance/CG73 for the latest NICE guidance

Cystatin C

Cystatin C, a 13kDa protein of the cystatin superfamily of cysteine protease inhibitors, is produced by all nucleated cells at a relatively constant rate and excreted nearly exclusively by glomerular filtration. It can be assayed using efficient, enzyme-linked immunoassays. Preliminary studies suggest serum cystatin C may be a more sensitive and specific marker than creatinine for assessing impaired excretory renal function. Minor reductions in GFR cause cystatin C concentrations to rise above normal when serum creatinine is still within normal range.

Measurement of glomerular filtration rate

Occasionally, it is necessary to measure renal excretory function accurately, e.g. in clinical research:

- When using drugs with a narrow therapeutic index and which are excreted by the kidney.
- When accurate measurement of kidney function is required in patients with abnormal muscle mass, e.g. paraplegics with bilateral lower limb muscle wasting.

The 'gold standard' for measurement of GFR is measurement of inulin clearance: inulin is freely filtered, not protein bound, and not reabsorbed or secreted. However, measurement of inulin is difficult.

Radionuclide studies

Radionuclide studies are contraindicated during pregnancy and women of child-bearing age need to have a negative pregnancy test before proceeding with the test.

A variety of radioisotope markers are available for estimating GFR. An ideal marker should be safe, not extensively protein-bound, be freely filtered, but not secreted or reabsorbed by the tubule, and should be excreted only by the kidney.

- The commonly used markers are ^{51}Cr EDTA, ^{99m}Tc DTPA, and ^{125}I iothalamate. Iothalamate is also available without radiolabelling and can be measured by fluorimetry.
- These substances are injected intravenously (SC in ^{125}I iothalamate) and after allowing for equilibration, plasma levels are measured at predetermined intervals. Plasma clearance and, hence, renal elimination is calculated from the rate of fall of the substance from circulation.
- ^{51}Cr ethylenediamine tetra-acetic acid (EDTA) has been the most extensively studied marker and is extensively used in Europe as a single injection technique followed by plasma sampling at 0, 90, 120, 150, and 240 min. ^{51}Cr EDTA is reliable even at low levels of renal function. Studies in humans suggest renal clearance estimated by this method is ~10% lower than that of inulin.
- ^{125}I iothalamate is only slightly protein-bound and studies suggest clearance values similar to that of inulin. Unlike other markers it can also be administered SC, and this allows for slow equilibration with stable plasma concentrations. It is considered safe, but potential problems of thyroid uptake necessitate pre-treatment with oral iodine.
- ^{99m}Tc DTPA is used in renal isotope scanning, which allows anatomical correlation to renal function, such as information on relative contribution from each kidney, can be obtained. ^{99m}Tc has a very short half-life, and radiation exposure is minimized. Protein binding can result in diminished renal clearance.

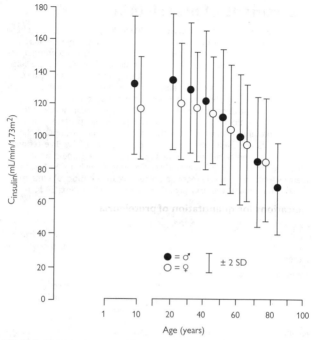

Fig. 10.2 Glomerular filtration rate, measured by insulin clearance ($C_{insulin}$), in apparently healthy individuals according to age.

Assessment of proteinuria

Proteinuria may result from increased glomerular permeability or tubular disease, causing decreased reabsorption of filtered protein or increased excretion of tubular enzymes. Glomerular proteinuria is commoner and more likely to signal potentially progressive kidney damage. Disease states influence the absolute amount of protein excreted, so protein excretion should be assessed either by measurement of excretion over 24 h (the 'gold standard', but highly inconvenient), or after correction for the degree of urine concentration. Because total daily urine creatinine excretion is constant, the ratio of albumin: creatinine (ACR) or protein: creatinine (PCrR)in the urine can allow correction for urine concentration. Although dipstick tests are useful, they can be misleading, with false +ve (concentrated urine) and false –ve (dilute urine) results. Assuming an average creatinine production of 10mmol/day (ignoring inter-individual variation due to variation in muscle mass), a protein:creatinine ratio of Nmg/mmol allows estimation of the daily protein excretion as $10 \times$ Nmg/24 h.

Indications for quantitation of proteinuria

Diagnosis of nephrotic syndrome

Nephrotic syndrome is defined as triad of *oedema*, *hypoalbuminaemia* and *proteinuria* >3g/24 h. Hyperlipidaemia and lipuria are also commonly present.

Prognosis of progressive renal disease

Proteinuria is one of the most potent risk markers for progressive loss of renal function in renal disease, e.g. diabetic nephropathy, chronic glomerulonephritis, and reflux nephropathy. In addition, treatments that reduce proteinuria (e.g. antihypertensive drugs, particularly angiotensin converting enzyme (ACE) inhibitors) decrease rate of progression. Presence of significant proteinuria should result in adoption of lower blood pressure targets and preferential use of ACE inhibitors or ARB drugs. Because reduction of proteinuria is an important therapeutic aim, regular assessment of the severity of proteinuria is also important in monitoring the effects of treatment. Annual measurement of albumin:creatinine ratio is now recommended in the UK for all patients with stage 3–5 chronic kidney disease.

Diagnosis of early diabetic nephropathy

Diabetic nephropathy is most treatable in its early stages—characterized by an *increase* in GFR, increased albumin excretion, and then by hypertension. 'Microalbuminuria' is the term for pathologically increased albumin excretion below the limit of detection of standard dipstick tests for proteinuria. Microalbuminuria without diabetic retinopathy should raise suspicion of non-diabetic kidney disease.

Quantitation of proteinuria

Urine protein and creatinine concentrations should be measured in an early morning urine sample (because protein excretion increases with activity).

Detection of proteinuria in glomerular disease should be by ACR. This allows for detection of proteinuria and thus CKD at lower levels of protein excretion than either reagent strips or PCrR. Microalbuminuria is present if urine ACR is ≥2.5mg/mmol (in ♂) or >3.5mg/mmol (in ♀) in repeated samples. Reagent strip testing for albuminuria is not recommended although strips that detect and even quantify microalbuminuria are now available.[1]

Measurement of total protein in urine is cheap, but does not differentiate between the various proteins present in urine. Proteinuria >30mg/mmol creatinine is usually defined as pathological, but patients with early diabetic nephropathy have total protein excretions below this limit, hence the preferred use of ACR in the identification of early renal disease. Although less sensitive than ACR at detection of low levels of proteinuria and less precise at all degrees of proteinuria, PCrR can still be used for quantification and monitoring of established proteinuric renal disease if ACR cannot be used for reasons of cost.

Diagnosis of postural proteinuria

Protein excretion increases with activity and upright posture. In some individuals this increase is exaggerated, resulting in +ve dipstick tests for proteinuria and even increased 24 h urine protein excretion. This 'postural proteinuria' has a nearly completely benign prognosis. In patients with proteinuria who have no other evidence of renal disease, it is worth quantifying proteinuria separately in urine collected while the patient has been recumbent overnight and in a daytime specimen. This can be done by measuring ACR on both early morning urine and a sample taken after a period of activity. Normal protein excretion during the night with increased protein excretion during the day indicates postural proteinuria.

Assessment of tubular proteinuria

This is occasionally of value to detect the relatively low grade proteinuria that results from tubular disease, e.g. Dent's disease (a rare genetic disorder caused by mutation in a tubular chloride channel), which causes calcium stone formation and tubular proteinuria. Other examples include screening for generalized tubular dysfunction and for drug toxicity, e.g. during treatment with platinum derivatives. Tubular proteinuria is best diagnosed by measurement of specific proteins whose presence in the urine result from tubular disease, e.g. retinol binding protein (RBP), N-acetyl-D-glucosaminidase (NAG) or β2-microglobulin, either in 24 h urine specimens or as ratios between the protein concentration and creatinine concentration.

1 ⅋ http://www.nice.org.uk/Guidance/CG73

Assessment of selectivity of proteinuria

The more severe the damage to glomerular permeability, the larger the protein molecules that pass through the glomerulus in glomerular disease. Measurement of the ratio of clearance of transferrin or albumin (a small molecule) to immunoglobulin G (a large molecule) can therefore be used as a measure of selectivity, and is calculated as follows:

Albumin/IgG clearance = {(urine [IgG] × serum [albumin])/ (serum IgG × urine [albumin])} × 100%

Transferrin/IgG clearance is calculated similarly.

A ratio of <0.16 indicates highly selective proteinuria.

In children, minimal change nephropathy causes selective proteinuria, whereas non-selective proteinuria raises the possibility of an alternative type of renal disease and might lead to a recommendation of renal biopsy to avoid steroid treatment when this would be unlikely to be of benefit. Measurement of selectivity in adults rarely influences clinical decision making.

Detection and quantitation of urinary light chains (Bence–Jones protein)

Measurement of urinary light chains requires specific immunoassays for light chains and is performed on 24 h urine samples as part of the regular assessment of disease activity in multiple myeloma. These tests are probably a less reliable marker of disease activity in the presence of severe renal impairment. Plasma free light chain assays are increasingly available; these have improved disease detection rates in comparison with urinary light chain quantification and may obviate the need for such tests in the future.

Assessment of renal tubular function

There are two main types of renal tubular diseases: those due to a single defect, usually genetic, in solute secretion or reabsorption, and those due to generalized tubular damage.

Screening tests for generalized tubular dysfunction: test for

- **Renal glycosuria**: dipstick or laboratory test for glucose in urine plus normal plasma glucose.
- **Hypophosphataemia**: can be followed by estimation of phosphate reabsorption, (🕮 Assessment of phosphate reabsorption, p614).
- **Low molecular weight proteinuria**: due to failure of tubular reabsorption plus increased release of proteins derived from tubular cells.
- **Normal anion gap metabolic acidosis**: serum bicarbonate, plus sodium potassium and chloride to permit calculation of the anion gap (followed by tests to confirm renal tubular acidosis, 🕮 Assessment of urinary acidification, p620).
- **Aminoaciduria**: detected by amino acid electrophoresis on a random urine sample.
- **Hypouricaemia**: plasma urate may be low due to decreased tubular reabsorption. (This can be followed by measurement of fractional urate excretion; see 🕮 Assessment of renal urate handling, p615).

Assessment of phosphate reabsorption

This is occasionally useful in the differential diagnosis of hypophosphataemia, e.g. in confirming the diagnosis of X-linked hypophosphataemic rickets.

Procedure
- The patient is asked to fast overnight.
- The overnight urine is discarded.
- The next urine sample is obtained, together with a blood sample.
- Both are analysed for phosphate and creatinine.

Fractional phosphate excretion is calculated as:

$FE_{PO_4} = C_P/C_{Cr}$ = [serum creatinine × urine phosphate]/[urine creatinine × serum phosphate]

This is the fraction of filtered phosphate, which appears in the urine

Fractional tubular reabsorption of phosphate (TRP) is calculated as

$1 - FE_{PO_4}$

TmP/GFR, the tubular maximum for phosphate reabsorption can be read off a nomogram[1], or can be calculated as follows:

If TRP <0.86,

TmP/GFR = TRP × plasma phosphate

If TRP >0.86,

TmP = {0.3 × TRP/[1 − (0.8 × TRP)]} × plasma phosphate

Interpretation

The adult reference range for TmP/GFR is 0.80–1.35mmol/L. Higher values of normal are seen in infancy and childhood[2]. Low values are seen in X-linked hypophosphataemic rickets and in osteogenic osteomalacia, both of which are thought to be due to overproduction or failure of inactivation of phosphatonins (a group of phosphaturic hormones including FGF-23 and FRP4). TmP/GFR is raised in hypoparathyroidism and reduced in hyperparathyroidism and by PTH-related peptide secretion.

Reduced phosphate reabsorption may also be seen in hypercalciuric stone formers, but it remains difficult to be certain whether this is the 1° disorder, causing increased production of 1, 25-$(OH)_2$ vitamin D, or 2° to tubular damage as a result of renal stones.

Reduced phosphate reabsorption is also seen in a number of 1° and 2° disorders of renal tubular function.

Assessment of tubular urate handling

The relative contributions of production rate, glomerular filtration, pre-secretory reabsorption, secretion and post-secretory reabsorption to control plasma urate concentration cannot be dissected out without complex tests involving selective pharmacological blockade of some of these processes. However, it is possible to determine whether an abnormal plasma urate concentration is due to abnormal production or abnormal renal handling.

24 h urinary urate excretion is increased in over-production, but normal in patients whose hyperuricaemia is due to decreased excretion. In the latter case urate excretion is normal, not decreased, because in under excretion the steady state is maintained at the expense of a raised plasma level. If 24 h urinary urate is raised, the collection should be repeated on a low purine diet.

Fractional excretion of urate is calculated as:

{(urinary [urate] × plasma [creatinine])/

(plasma [urate] × urinary [creatinine])} × 100%

Normal values are dependent on age and sex, but in adults are of the order of 10%. High fractional excretion is a cause of hypo-uricaemia in syndrome of inappropriate antidiuretic hormone (SIADH) and several other conditions; low fractional excretion occurs in 1° gout, but also in a familial syndrome of hypo-uricaemia with early-onset gout and progressive renal failure.

1 Walton RJ, Bijvoet OLM. Nomogram for derivation of renal threshold phosphate concentration *Lancet* 1975; **ii**: 309–10.
2 Payne RB. Renal tubular reabsorption of phosphate (TmP/GFR): indications and interpretation *Ann Clin Biochem* 1998; **35**: 201–6.

Assessment of acid–base balance

Plasma HCO_3^- and Cl^- are the two major anions in extracellular fluid. The major reason for measuring them is to assess acid–base status. Changes in serum $[HCO_3^-]$ concentration reflect changes in acid–base balance, with a decrease in $[HCO_3^-]$ reflecting metabolic acidosis and an increase reflecting alkalosis. Plasma Cl^- is helpful in assessing the cause of acidosis or alkalosis.

There is no justification at all for performing an arterial puncture to measure arterial pH as part of the assessment of metabolic acidosis or alkalosis—it can be adequately assessed from serum $[HCO_3^-]$. Arterial samples are needed when it is unclear whether the acid–base disturbance is respiratory or metabolic in origin or in mixed disturbances.

Plasma bicarbonate

The most reliable way to interpret plasma HCO_3^- is to use the acid–base diagram (Fig. 10.3), which allows assessment of how much the change in $[HCO_3^-]$ concentration is due to changes in CO_2 excretion via the lungs and how much to changes in $[H^+]$ or HCO_3^- wasting. In the absence of significant respiratory disease it can often safely be assumed that any change is due to metabolic causes, in which case low plasma HCO_3^- indicates increased H^+ production (or, occasionally, increased HCO_3^- loss) and vice versa. If arterial blood gases are obtained, the 'standard bicarbonate' is a calculated value which indicates what the plasma HCO_3^- would be if CO_2 excretion were normal, and is thus a way of allowing assessment of whether there is a metabolic component to an abnormal HCO_3^- concentration or whether it is solely due to the respiratory disturbance.

Remember that the kidneys compensate for respiratory disease and the lungs for metabolic disease: for instance, metabolic acidosis causes hyperventilation, resulting in lower PCO_2 and lessening the acidosis seen. However, overcompensation does not occur.

Plasma chloride

Many laboratories omit plasma Cl^- assays from 'routine' serum chemistry measurements, but this measurement is helpful if a systemic acid–base disturbance is suspected. As a useful over-simplification, low bicarbonate with high chloride can be seen as accumulation of hydrochloric acid, which can only result from altered renal handling of acid, as in renal tubular acidosis. If HCO_3^- is low with a normal or low Cl^-, some other acid must be accumulating. More precision in deciding the cause of metabolic acidosis can be obtained by calculating the anion gap.

The anion gap

The anion gap is the difference between the sum of the concentrations of the positively charged ions routinely measured in plasma and the negatively charged ions:

$$\text{Anion gap} = ([Na^+] + [K^+]) - ([Cl^-] + [HCO_3^-])$$

Obviously, the total positive charges in plasma must be balanced by the same number of negative charges. The normal anion gap is caused by the fact that there are more unmeasured anions in plasma (mostly albumin, but including lactate, sulphate, and others) than cations (including calcium and magnesium). The concentrations of all of these unmeasured ions can vary, so the normal range for the anion gap is wide, e.g. hypoalbuminaemia reduces the anion gap by 2.5mEq per 1g/dL fall in serum albumin.

The main use of calculation of the anion gap is in the differential diagnosis of metabolic acidosis.

A high anion gap acidosis is caused by an abnormally high concentration of an unmeasured anion, such as
- L-lactate (reflecting anaerobic metabolism or hepatic dysfunction).
- Salicylate (in aspirin poisoning).
- β-hydroxybutyrate (in diabetic ketoacidosis).
- Glycolate and oxalate (in methanol poisoning).
- Hippurate (in toluene poisoning, e.g. glue-sniffing).
- D-lactate (from gut bacterial fermentation in blind-loop syndrome).

A normal anion gap acidosis may be caused by loss of bicarbonate or failure of renal H^+ excretion, for instance
- Renal tubular acidosis.
- High ileostomy losses (bicarbonate wasting).
- Carbonic anhydrase inhibitors.
- Urinary diversions, e.g. ureterosigmoidostomy (Cl^-/ HCO_3^-) exchange and NH^+_4 reabsorption in the colonic segment).

▶*Beware*: in North America the anion gap is usually calculated as $[Na^+] - \{[Cl^-] + [HCO_3^-]\}$, not including $[K^+]$ in the measured cations. This results in a lower reference range for the anion gap. In addition, different laboratories use different assays for chloride. For these reasons, the local laboratory reference range for anion gap should be used.

In general, the anion gap is only useful when very high, confirming high concentrations of an unmeasured anion. If the diagnosis is not already obvious, this then justifies further investigation, including assay of plasma lactate concentration.

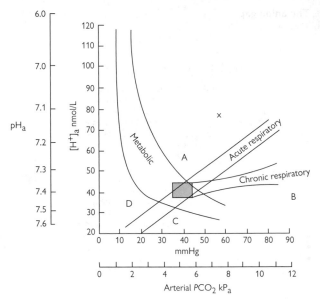

Fig. 10.3 Acid base diagram.

Assessment of urinary acidification

Indications
Unexplained hyperchloraemic metabolic acidosis.

Defects in the kidneys' ability to excrete acid in the urine may lead to permanent systemic acidosis, or to systemic acidosis at times of increased acid generation, depending on the severity of the defect. Acidification defects may occur as part of generalized tubular disease or as isolated, often genetically determined, alterations in function, most commonly of cell surface ion pumps.

Ammonium chloride loading test
This test is regarded as the 'gold standard' for the diagnosis of distal ('type 1') renal tubular acidosis, where there is impaired excretion of 'fixed acid' into the distal tubule.

Procedure
- The patient attends after an overnight fast, but is allowed to drink water.
- At the start of the test, a urine sample is sent to the laboratory for measurement of pH, and a plasma or serum sample is sent for measurement of bicarbonate. Because pH changes rapidly in urine exposed to the air, the urine container should be filled to the top or the urine sent in a stoppered syringe, and sent to the laboratory without any delay.
- If the urine pH is <5.4, this indicates normal acidifying ability, and there is no need to continue with the test.
- If the venous blood bicarbonate is low, with a urine pH >5.4, the diagnosis of renal tubular acidosis is confirmed.
- If neither of these conditions is met, then proceed to give the patient ammonium chloride, 0.1g/kg body weight. Ammonium chloride is given as capsules, is unpalatable, and frequently causes nausea and vomiting, but this can be reduced if the capsules are taken slowly, or with bread and honey. Even if the patient vomits, it is worth proceeding with the test as acidosis is often achieved; no more ammonium chloride should be given.
- Urine samples are then collected hourly for the next 6–8 h and sent, protected from the air (as above), for pH analysis in the laboratory. If any sample has a pH of ≤5.4 the test can be stopped, as this indicates normal acidifying ability of the distal tubule.
- At 3 h after ingestion of ammonium chloride, a venous sample should be sent for plasma bicarbonate measurement to ensure that acidaemia has occurred.

Alternative tests of distal acidification

Rationale

The distal tubule reabsorbs sodium ions in exchange for hydrogen ions. Furosemide, by increasing delivery of sodium to the distal tubule, therefore causes a fall in urine pH, particularly in 'salt-avid' states produced by sodium restriction or fludrocortisone.[1]

Procedure

- No need to fast or fluid restrict.
- Collect a baseline urine sample for pH.
- Administer furosemide 40mg and fludrocortisone 1mg orally.
- Collect urine for pH measurement hourly for 4 h or until urine pH<5.3.
- Urine pH persistently >5.3 at 4 h implies distal renal tubular acidosis (RTA).

Bicarbonate infusion test

This is the 'gold standard' for the diagnosis of proximal ('type 2') renal tubular acidosis, which is characterized by impaired bicarbonate reabsorption. In this condition, urine pH may be <5.5 in untreated patients, because at steady state serum bicarbonate levels fall to the point at which filtered bicarbonate is reabsorbed and distal acidification mechanisms are intact.

Procedure

- Sodium bicarbonate is infused IV at 0.5–1.0mmol/kg/h. After 60 min plasma bicarbonate is measured to confirm that this has risen to >20mmol/L. Urine pH is measured hourly and urine bicarbonate measured, to allow calculation of the fractional excretion of bicarbonate:

$$FE_{HCO_3} = \{(\text{urine } [HCO_3^-]) \times \text{plasma } [\text{creatinine}]\}/(\text{plasma } [HCO_3^-] \times \text{urine } [\text{creatinine}]) \times 100\%$$

- Fractional excretion of bicarbonate is normally <15%.
- A level of >20% confirms type 2 renal tubular acidosis.

1 Walsh SB, *et al.* Urinary acidification assessed by simultaneous furosemide and fludrocortisone treatment: an alternative to ammonium chloride. *Kidney International* 2007; **71**: 1310–16

Plasma potassium

Although most of the body's potassium is intracellular, small changes in extracellular potassium concentration can cause major changes in membrane excitability. Hypokalaemia causes increased excitability, causing atrial and ventricular cardiac arrhythmias; hyperkalaemia decreases excitability, causing a characteristic pattern of ECG changes and eventually causing asystole. Both hypokalaemia and hyperkalaemia may be associated with skeletal muscle paralysis.

Plasma K^+ concentration is influenced both by distribution across cell membranes, and the balance between intake and excretion. Renal excretion is dependent on renal function, urine flow rate, and aldosterone.

Pseudohyperkalaemia

Caused by excessive release of K^+ from cells after venepuncture and should be considered when hyperkalaemia 'doesn't fit' with the clinical picture. The laboratory should report the presence of visible haemolysis (usually due to RBC trauma during difficult venepuncture), but pseudohyperkalaemia can also occur in the absence of visible haemolysis, e.g.:

- Haematological malignancies causing a high white cell or platelet count.
- Other causes of leucocytosis and thrombocytosis, e.g. leukaemoid reactions, rheumatoid arthritis.
- Familial pseudohyperkalaemia: rare disorder of RBC cation transport leading to an increased rate of release of K^+ from red cells at low temperatures.

Diagnosis can be confirmed by showing that plasma $[K^+]$ is normal in a heparinized sample analysed immediately and then by demonstrating that delayed separation results in higher values being obtained. Pseudohyperkalaemia with a normal WBC and platelet count can be further investigated by measuring the rate of rise of plasma $[K^+]$ in samples incubated at 37°C and at 22°C, and studying the effects of drugs that affect cation exchange, e.g. thiazide diuretics and quinine. Artefactual hyperkalaemia can be caused by fist clenching plus a venous tourniquet during phlebotomy: plasma K^+ can rise by as much as 2mmol/L.

Hyperkalaemia due to redistribution across cell membranes

Hyperkalaemic periodic paralysis is an autosomal dominant genetic muscle disorder caused by mutations in the voltage-gated sodium channel SCN4A. It presents in early infancy with attacks of paralysis associated with hyperkalaemia.

Other causes of release of potassium from tissues
(including muscle) include

- Exercise.
- Acidosis (particularly inorganic acidosis).
- Muscle damage (rhabdomyolysis), e.g. crush injury, revascularization of ischaemic limb, prolonged unconsciousness following drug intoxication.
- Burns.
- Tumour lysis, e.g. after initiation of chemotherapy for haematological malignancy.

- Drugs, e.g. digoxin, depolarizing muscle relaxants, β-blockers.
- Malignant hyperthermia.

Hyperkalaemia due to altered external balance

- Increased ingestion is seldom able to cause hyperkalaemia on its own, but can contribute to hyperkalaemia when combined with impaired excretion of a potassium load.
- Decreased excretion may be due to decreased glomerular filtration rate, decreased urine flow rate, decreased aldosterone production, drugs which inhibit renal tubular K^+ excretion, or genetic defects in renal potassium excretion (pseudohypoaldosteronism, Liddle's syndrome).
- In most cases the cause is obvious.

Investigation of unexplained hyperkalaemia

- Serum creatinine, creatine kinase, bicarbonate.
- Urine K^+, creatinine, osmolality, allowing calculation of transtubular K^+ gradient (see 📖 p624). Occasionally useful, for instance in confirming trimethoprim-induced inhibition of K^+ secretion.
- Tests for type IV renal tubular acidosis:
  - Normal synacthen test (to exclude Addison's disease).
  - 24 h urinary aldosterone (low in type IV RTA).
  - Plasma renin and aldosterone response to upright posture and 40mg furosemide (subnormal levels of both suggest hyporeninaemic hypoaldosteronism).
  - Correction of hyperkalaemia with oral fludrocortisone 0.1mg/day.

Pseudohypokalaemia

Can be caused by delayed separation of samples kept at warm ambient temperatures and is caused by continued uptake of K^+ into cells. This occurs more in heparinized samples than in those allowed to clot.

Hypokalaemia due to redistribution across cell membranes

- Alkalosis.
- Insulin treatment.
- β_2-adrenergic stimulation (e.g. high dose nebulizers).
- B_{12} therapy of pernicious anaemia.
- Rapid cell division, e.g. acute leukaemia.
- Hypokalaemic periodic paralysis. Mutations in the CANCL1A3 and SCN4A voltage gated ion channels can lead to this rare condition. Carbohydrate intake or rest after exercise typically precipitates hypokalaemia.
  - Confirm diagnosis (under strict supervision) by infusing 2g/kg glucose and 0.1u/kg insulin; consider referral for mutation analysis of relevant ion channels.
  - Consider thyrotoxic hypokalaemic periodic paralysis in non-familial patients, particularly of oriental background: check thyroid function tests.

Hypokalaemia due to increased renal loss

📖 Chapter 2.

Urine potassium, chloride, & magnesium measurements

Measurement of urine potassium concentration is occasionally useful in the differential diagnosis of hyperkalaemia. The proportion of potassium filtered at the glomerulus which is excreted in the urine is extremely variable, and is modulated by the distal tubule in response to aldosterone, plasma potassium concentration, acid–base balance, urine flow rate, sodium status, and other factors. The final concentration of potassium in the urine also depends on urine dilution, controlled independently by factors (e.g. antidiuretic hormone (ADH)) controlling water excretion.

Low urinary K^+ (<20mmol/L) with hypokalaemia is seen in
- Gastrointestinal potassium loss, e.g. diarrhoea, laxative abuse, villous adenoma, high ileostomy output, enterocutaneous fistula, ureterosigmoidostomy.
- Dietary deficiency
- Skin losses, e.g. burns, severe eczema.

High urinary K^+ (>20mmol/L) with hypokalaemia and normal blood pressure is seen in
- Vomiting (K^+ is exchanged for hydrogen ions: acid–base preservation takes precedence)—**Note**: urinary chloride will be low.
- Diuretic use, abuse, and conditions, which mimic diuretic use, e.g. Bartter's syndrome, Gitelman's syndrome.
- Tubular damage causing potassium wasting, e.g. renal tubular acidosis types 1 and 2.
- Diabetic ketoacidosis.

High urinary K^+ (>20mmol/L) with hypokalaemia and high blood pressure is seen in
- **Hyperaldosteronism**: adrenal adenomas, bilateral adrenal hyperplasia.
- Apparent mineralocorticoid excess.
- Liddle's syndrome.

Transtubular potassium gradient

This is a calculation that is promoted in the USA, but not widely used in the UK or Europe. The main purpose is to distinguish hyperkalaemia caused by decreased aldosterone action from hyperkalaemia due to effective volume depletion. The principle is that correcting for urine dilution, by using the ratio of plasma and urine osmolality, allows estimation of the urine potassium gradient in the cortical collecting duct, after the main site of potassium secretion (which is influenced by aldosterone), but before the main site of urine dilution or concentration (which is influenced by ADH). The index is only valid when the urine is concentrated, i.e. the urine osmolality exceeds the plasma osmolality, and when urine sodium concentration is >25mmol/L. It is calculated as follows:

$$TTKG = \{urine\ [K^+]/plasma\ osmolality)/(urine\ osmolality \times plasma\ [K^+])$$

TTKG can vary widely in healthy subjects, but is commonly around 7–9

- Values <7 in a patient with hyperkalaemia suggest hypoaldosteronism.
- Values >7 in a hyperkalaemic patient suggest that aldosterone is acting normally, and that hyperkalaemia is due to low urine flow, limiting the rate at which potassium can be excreted.
- Values <7 in hypokalaemic patients suggest extrarenal potassium loss.
- Values >9 in hypokalaemic patients suggest renal potassium loss.

Urine chloride

This measurement is helpful in the differential diagnosis of otherwise unexplained normotensive hypokalaemia. Urine chloride is low if hypokalaemia is being caused by extrarenal sodium chloride or hydrogen chloride losses, as seen in diarrhoea or vomiting, respectively. In these conditions potassium is exchanged in the distal tubule for sodium or hydrogen, respectively, but chloride is conserved. Urine chloride is high when the cause of hypokalaemia is inappropriate loss of potassium chloride, as in diuretic use and in Bartter's syndrome (the genetic equivalent of being on permanent high dose loop diuretics) and Gitelman's syndrome (the genetic equivalent of being on permanent high dose thiazide diuretics).

The distinction between the drug-induced and genetic causes can be very difficult to make, but temporary withdrawal from diuretics causes intense chloride retention and a very low urinary chloride concentration, which is never seen in Bartter's or Gitelman's syndromes. Repeated measurements of urine chloride are, therefore, helpful in this situation, together with screens for the presence of diuretics in the urine when urine chloride is high.

Urine magnesium

This measurement can be helpful in identifying the cause of hypomagenesaemia by distinguishing inappropriate tubular magnesium loss (e.g. from diuretics, aminoglycosides, Gitelman's syndrome) from GI magnesium loss.

$$FE_{Mg} = \{(\text{urine } [Mg^{2+}] \times \text{plasma } [\text{creatinine}])/((0.7 \times (\text{plasma } [Mg^{2+}]) \times \text{urine } [\text{creatinine}])\} \times 100\%$$

The plasma magnesium is multiplied by 0.7 as only 70% of magnesium is non-albumin bound and thus freely filtered.

Fractional magnesium excretion >2% in a subject with normal renal function indicates renal magnesium loss.

Urine sodium concentration

In health, serum electrolyte concentrations are kept constant because intake of electrolytes is balanced by excretion in the faeces and urine. Renal excretion is tightly regulated to achieve this balance. These basic principles imply that the urinary excretion of, for instance, sodium, is nearly totally dependent on dietary intake of sodium. Because this is very variable, there is no 'normal range' of urinary sodium, or any other urinary electrolyte. Measurements of urinary electrolytes therefore have to be interpreted with great caution.

24 h urine sodium excretion is a good marker, at steady state, for dietary intake, and has been used in epidemiological studies of the relationship of salt intake to blood pressure. Dietary sodium intake varies from as little as 10mmol/day in the Amazon rainforest to >400mmol/day in Westerners living on processed foods. Current UK advice is to restrict sodium intake to around 100mmol/day.

In clinical practice there are several reasons for measuring sodium output, including

- **Calcium stone formers**: sodium and calcium excretion are linked, and reduction of excessive salt intake results in a reduction in calcium excretion.
- **Cystine stone formers**: similarly, cystine excretion is reduced by reduction of dietary salt intake.
- **During antihypertensive and antiproteinuric treatment**: salt restriction amplifies the effects of ACE inhibitors in reducing not only systemic blood pressure but also protein excretion in renal disease, and may be more tolerable than diuretic treatment.

24 h urine sodium is usually measured on a sample collected in a plain container. However, it can also be measured, by flame photometry, in a sample collected into an acid container, and this is useful if calcium and oxalate excretion are also being measured, for instance in stone formers.

Spot urine sodium concentration is of very limited value, because sodium excretion varies considerably through the day and because it is normally influenced by urine dilution and, hence, by recent water intake. However, there are two situations in which it may be of value:

Acute kidney injury

The normal response of the kidneys to under-perfusion from hypovolaemia or hypotension is to retain salt avidly, urine sodium concentration dropping to <10mmol/L. If urinary sodium concentration is this low in acute renal failure, this indicates normal ability of the renal tubules to retain salt. Low urine sodium concentration is seen in 'pre-renal' renal failure; acute tubular necrosis results in loss of tubular salt reabsorption and a higher urine sodium concentration. The problem is that conditions other than under perfusion cause low urine sodium (e.g. contrast nephropathy, rhabdomyolysis). High urine sodium does not necessarily indicate acute tubular necrosis; indeed, it is seen in normal people. In any case, the measurement seldom has a useful impact on management, which both in pre-renal failure and in acute tubular necrosis is to restore renal perfusion by correcting hypovolaemia, hypotension, and sepsis as quickly as possible.

Syndrome of inappropriate ADH

This diagnosis cannot be made in a hypovolaemic patient, because hypovolaemia is a physiological stimulus to ADH secretion. For this reason, the diagnosis cannot be made if the urine sodium concentration is low (📕 Hyponatraemia (including syndrome of inappropriate anti-diuretic hormone), p132).

Fractional excretion of sodium is calculated as

{(urine [sodium] × plasma [creatinine])/(plasma [sodium] × urine [creatinine])} × 100%

This gives an index of avidity of sodium reabsorption independent of changes in overall renal function. An FE_{Na} of <1% is seen in pre-renal failure and >1% in acute tubular necrosis. However, this measurement is prone to some of the same criticisms as that of urine sodium excretion.

Sodium wasting and sodium retaining states

Sodium wasting is caused by diuretics, Bartter's syndrome, Gitelman's syndrome, and occasionally by renal tubular disease. It cannot be diagnosed by measurement of urine sodium excretion alone, as at steady state this equals sodium intake, but is diagnosed by finding clinical evidence of hypovolaemia without avid renal sodium retention.

Sodium retention is caused by diseases causing effective hypovolaemia (e.g. congestive cardiac failure), in which case the diagnosis is suggested by oedema and the clinical signs of the underlying disease. However, sodium retention can also cause hypertension without oedema, as in hyperaldosteronism, pseudohyperaldosteronism, chronic renal failure, and inherited disorders of renal tubular sodium excretion (e.g. Liddle's syndrome). Again, measurement of sodium excretion alone is not helpful in the diagnosis of these conditions.

Urine dipstick testing

Urine analysis has been used for many years for screening patients with potential renal disease and for serial assessment of patients with known renal pathology. However, the results of dipstick testing are dependent on urine dilution and, for this reason, laboratory measurement of albumin:creatinine ratio is the preferred screening test for proteinuria. Reagent strips should only be used for the detection of microalbuminuria if they are specifically capable of detecting low concentrations of albumin and expressing the result as an ACR.

Many commercially available dipsticks rapidly test the urine for multiple chemical contents. The sticks use reagent strips, which change colour following a chemical reaction with an active constituent depending on the presence (or absence) of a particular component.

Depending on the type of dipstick used, urine can be tested for

- pH.
- Protein.
- Haemoglobin.
- Glucose.
- Leucocyte esterases and nitrites.
- Specific gravity.
- Ketones.
- Urobilinogen.

The reagent strip is fully immersed in urine obtained by voiding or, if a 1% risk of iatrogenic urine infection is warranted, by urethral catheterization, and the excess shaken off. The change in colour, if any, is read after the time specified by the manufacturer—usually 30 s.

pH

Dipstick testing only gives a rough estimate of pH, because of the effects of storage and reaction on exposure to atmospheric air on urine pH *in vitro*. The dipstick contains a polyionic polymer bound with H^+, which is released on reaction with the cations in urine. Release of H^+ causes change in colour of a pH-sensitive dye. Normal pH varies between 4.5 and 8.0, depending on diet: vegetarians, in whom fixed acid ingestion is low, commonly have alkaline urine. Urine infection with urease-producing organisms also causes alkaline urine.

Urine pH >5.5 in spite of metabolic acidosis is seen in renal tubular acidosis. Urine pH is important in some recurrent stone formers. For instance, uric acid solubility in urine is critically dependent on urine pH, and many uric acid stone formers are found to have normal 24 h urinary urate, but highly acidic and concentrated urine (e.g. as a result of high losses from an ileostomy). In patients with triple phosphate stones, alkaline urine is commonly seen due to infection with urea splitting organisms.

Protein

Binding of proteins to the dye indicators is highly pH dependent and the indicators undergo a sequential colour change based on the concentration of protein in the sample. Albumin binds at a pH of 5–8 and has the highest affinity, so most commercially available dipsticks almost exclusively detect only albumin. Dipsticks are thus cheap, reliable, and give rapid semiquantitative assessment of proteinuric renal disease. However, these tests measure concentration of protein, rather than absolute excretion; false negative tests are therefore possible in dilute urine caused by a high fluid intake, and false positive tests may be obtained in highly concentrated urine. At pH <5 or >8 results obtained by dipsticks are not accurate. Immunoglobulin light chains (Bence Jones proteins) do not result in positive dipstick tests for proteinuria even when present in high concentrations. Sticks able to detect low concentrations of albumin and give a 'near patient' quantification of ACR are available, but not in universal use

Haemoglobin

Reagent strips use peroxidase-like activity of haemoglobin to induce a colour change in a dye linked to organic peroxide. This reaction does not distinguish haemoglobinuria from erythrocyturia or from myoglobinuria. False +ve results are obtained with myoglobin, contamination with menstrual blood and iodine. Positive dipsticks for blood with absence of RBC on microscopy suggest lysis of RBCs due to prolonged storage, myoglobinuria or haemoglobinuria. False –ve results are seen with high dose vitamin C and rifampicin.

Glucose

Most strips use the glucose oxidase/peroxidase method and can estimate levels as low as 50mg/dL. Ketones, salicylate, and ascorbic acid can interfere with results. These strips estimate all reducing sugars, including fructose and lactose. In the absence of concomitant hyperglycaemia, glycosuria is suggestive of proximal tubular disorders or, rarely, reduced renal threshold for glucose. When associated with glomerular disease, glycosuria with a normal serum glucose may be a marker of worse prognosis.

Leucocyte esterases and nitrites

The esterase method relies on esterases released from lysed WBC. Esterases release pyrroles, which react with a diazonium salt on the dipstick resulting in a colour change. False +ve results seen in vaginal contamination. Presence of glucose, albumin, ketones, tetracyclines, and cephalosporins in the urine can give false –ve results.

Most, but not all, uropathogenic bacteria convert nitrates to nitrites, which react with a diazonium compound resulting in a colour change. False –ve results are due to frequent bladder emptying, prolonged external storage and ascorbic acid. Some bacteria including *N. gonorrhoea* and *Mycobacterium tuberculosis* do not convert nitrates.

Sensitivity and specificity of the above tests vary, and are not useful for screening low-risk populations. However a –ve test is useful in excluding UTI in a patient with a high pre-test probability of infection. Further guidance on diagnosis of urinary tract infections is available at: ॐ http://cks.library.nhs.uk/clinical_topics/by_clinical_specialty/urology

Specific gravity

Dipstick testing for specific gravity is not accurate; non-ionic constituents including albumin, glucose, and urea are also estimated. Normal values are between 1003 and 1030, but vary with the patient's hydration status and, hence, urinary concentration. Specific gravity (SG) decreases with age as the kidney loses its concentrating ability. Fixed SG of 1010 is seen in chronic renal failure.

Ketones

Acetoacetic acid is detected by the nitroprusside test. Ascorbic acid results in false +ve result. Dipsticks do not detect β-hydroxybutyrate, which comprises the largest ketone fraction in blood.

Urine culture

There are numerous situations in which accurate diagnosis of UTI is important. 'Sending an MSU' is not, however, quite as simple as it sounds and is not always the most appropriate test.

Obtaining a mid-stream urine sample

The aim is to obtain a sample of bladder urine, avoiding contamination by cells or organisms on perineal skin. Men should retract the foreskin prior to micturition; women should hold the labia well apart with the parted fingers of one hand to allow the urine to exit directly from the urethral meatus. The patient should be asked to begin to pass urine, and then, without stopping passing urine, pass a sterile container into the path of the urinary stream and collect a sample, before finishing passing urine normally. If a sterile foil container has been used to catch the specimen, the specimen is then transferred into a specimen container and sent to the laboratory.

Suprapubic aspiration of urine

In patients suspected of having bladder infection, but in whom the results of culture of mid-stream urines are equivocal, it may be necessary to proceed to suprapubic aspiration (widely performed in paediatrics, but not in adults). After skin preparation a fine needle (e.g. a lumbar puncture needle) is introduced into the bladder by direct puncture just above the symphysis pubis and urine aspirated. Ultrasound can be used to confirm that the bladder is full prior to the procedure.

'In–out' catheter urine specimens

Although bladder catheterization carries a small (1–2%) risk of introducing new infection into the bladder, this risk is sometimes justified by the importance of obtaining urine direct from the bladder. A urethral catheter is passed into the bladder, the first few millilitres discarded, and sample collected.

Obtaining urine specimens from ileal conduits

Urine in ileal conduit bags is always contaminated by skin organisms and the culture of 'bag urine' is not a useful way of diagnosing upper urinary tract infection in patients with conduits. In patients suspected of having ascending infection, a urine specimen should be obtained by passing a catheter as far into the conduit as it will go.

'Two glass test'

This is a test for urethritis, and is performed when a patient presents with dysuria or urethral discharge, and a sexual history suggesting possible recent infection. Culture of a urethral swab or of the urethral discharge should also be obtained and sent for gonorrhoea testing (requires attendance at a sexual health clinic). Two urine samples are collected—the first 10mL passed and a mid-stream sample. Each is sent for culture; urethritis is diagnosed when the bacterial count is highest in the first sample. The first sample should also be sent for *Chlamydia* testing.

'Stamey–Mears test'

This test is performed for the diagnosis of prostatitis. A mid-stream urine (MSU) sample is obtained, and then the patient is asked to stop passing urine. The pro-state gland is massaged per rectum and 'expressed prostatic secretions' collected, followed by a final urine sample. In prostatitis, bacterial counts are higher in the expressed prostatic secretions or the post-massage urine sample than in the mid-stream sample.

In-dwelling catheter urine specimens

Colonization of the bladder is nearly inevitable within a fortnight of insertion of an in-dwelling urethral or suprapubic catheter. Unnecessary antibiotic treatment increases the selective pressure for the emergence of antibiotic-resistant organisms, and increases the risk of antibiotic associated diarrhoea and hospital acquired infection. Antibiotic therapy must therefore be reserved for symptomatic infection. There is no point in sending catheter specimens unless there is a suspicion of symptomatic infection at the time. 'Surveillance' samples sent to predict which antibiotics should be used if the patient becomes symptomatic at a later time are unjustified, because the colonizing organisms may change over time. A fresh specimen of urine is obtained from the collection port into the collection pot. Samples should NOT be collected from the reservoir into which the catheter drains.

Localization tests

- On rare occasions it is justified to attempt to localize the site of infection to the bladder or to one or other kidney.
- The 'gold standard' is to obtain samples from each ureter and from the bladder during rigid cystoscopy under general anaesthesia.
- The 'Fairley test' requires passage of a urethral catheter followed by a bladder washout with a wide spectrum antibacterial and a fibrinolytic enzyme. Sequential samples of urine are then obtained. If infection is present in the upper tracts, this will not have been affected by the bladder washout, and organisms will be detected in the first specimen obtained after washout, whereas if infection was confined to the bladder, subsequent samples will be sterile.
- Infection may be confined to one or other kidney as a result of ureteric obstruction or may be present within a renal cyst. In these situations, direct aspiration of urine under ultrasound control in the radiology department is necessary.

Microscopy and culture of urine

Once a sample has been obtained it is sent to a Microbiology laboratory for microscopy and culture.

Microscopy is required to assess pyuria (white blood cells (WBCs) in the urine) and contamination.

- Significant pyuria indicates inflammation within the urinary tract; if this persists, despite negative urine cultures the patient has 'sterile pyuria', for which there are a number of causes, including infection with an organism which does not grow on conventional culture media, e.g. *Chlamydia*.
- Pyuria plus a positive culture confirm the diagnosis of urinary tract infection.
- The absence of pyuria makes a urinary tract infection less likely, but can occur in the early stages of infection or in the presence of a very high fluid intake.
- Contamination (in the female) is indicated by the presence of large numbers of squamous cells, which usually come from the vaginal wall; however, squamous cells can occasionally come from the bladder.

Culture and sensitivity are necessary to decide what treatment is necessary and to differentiate contamination of the urine sample by organisms outside the bladder from true infection.

- A 'pure growth' of a single organism to $>10^5$ colony-forming units (cfu)/mL is the conventional criterion for urinary tract infection. However:
- Low counts of 10^2–10^4 cfu/mL can be associated with early infection, and should be taken seriously in the presence of suggestive symptoms in women.
- Low counts in men are likely to represent true infection, because contamination is uncommon.
- Genuine mixed growth may occur, in the presence of impaired urinary drainage or a foreign body within the urinary tract.

Urine microscopy

Urine microscopy is a useful, quick, reliable, cheap, and under-used investigation—the 'liquid renal biopsy'! Far more information can be obtained by careful microscopy than is usually obtained in the Microbiology laboratory, where the priority is detection of significant urine infection.

Indications

- Suspected urinary tract infection.
- Suspected acute glomerulonephritis.
- Suspected acute interstitial nephritis (requires staining for eosinophils).
- Unexplained acute or chronic renal failure.
- Haematuria (with or without proteinuria) on urine dipstick test.
- Suspected urinary tract malignancy.

Procedure

A freshly voided, clean catch, mid-stream, early morning specimen is ideal. The sample should be centrifuged and re-suspended in a small volume. Although bright field microscopy will allow identification of most formed elements in the urine sediment, phase contrast microscopy is useful for detection of red cell ghosts, 'glomerular' red cells, and some other constituents. Staining of the urine sediment is not necessary for most purposes, but is useful for identification of eosinophils and malignant cells—this is usually performed in the cytology laboratory.

Haematuria

RBCs appear as non-nucleated biconcave discs. Even when urine is red in colour or dipsticks positive for blood it should be examined for the presence of red cells. The differential diagnosis of haematuria is broad, but it is broadly classified into glomerular (renal) and infrarenal causes. Transit of red cells through the renal tubules causes osmotic changes in their shape and size; 'dysmorphic' or 'crenated' red cells are best seen using phase contrast microscopy, and may be missed altogether if bright field microscopy is used. In experienced hands, detection of these glomerular red cells strongly suggests a glomerular origin for haematuria, although failure to detect these changes does not reliably indicate a lower urinary tract cause of bleeding—heavy haematuria in IgA nephropathy, for instance, can result in large numbers of normal red cells in the urine. Urine pH, concentration, and storage can affect red cell morphology.

Leucocyturia

The presence of significant numbers of polymorphs (pyuria) in urine is highly suggestive of urinary tract infection, but can also occur in glomerulonephritis, interstitial nephritis, and peri-ureteric inflammation, for instance in acute appendicitis. The presence of leucocyte casts is diagnostic of renal parenchymal infection ('acute pyelonephritis'). Eosinophiluria is associated with acute allergic interstitial nephritis and athero-embolic renal disease.

Other cells

Squamous epithelial cells are usually taken as indicative of vaginal contamination, but may also derive from the bladder and urethra. Occasionally malignant cells arising from the lower urinary tract are picked up on routine microscopy. Spermatozoa are also rarely seen.

Micro-organisms

Identification of bacteriuria, in association with leucocyturia is very suggestive of infection. Organisms may be in chains or clusters, and some are motile. Fungi including yeast and protozoans, including *Trichomonas* can also be readily identified.

Casts

Casts are cylindrical bodies, which usually form in the distal tubule and collecting duct. They consist of cells or cell debris held together by Tamm–Horsfall protein. Staining and phase contrast microscopy improves identification and characterization of casts, but results are operator dependent. Extreme shaking or agitation can disintegrate casts.

- **Hyaline casts** appear translucent and homogeneous and are present in normal urine. Number may be increased in dehydration and proteinuria.
- **Cellular casts** especially red cell casts, always indicate significant parenchymal renal disease. Red cell casts are strongly suggestive of acute glomerulonephritis, but may occur in interstitial nephritis and acute tubular necrosis as well.
- **White cell casts** are seen in acute pyelonephritis and acute interstitial nephritis.
- **Granular casts** are formed from cell debris and are seen in a wide variety of renal diseases.
- **Waxy broad casts** form in atrophic renal tubules and are seen in chronic renal failure.

Crystals

A variety of crystals can be visualized and are of importance in stone formers. A freshly voided sample should be examined as storage and temperature changes can affect type and number of crystals found. A large number of calcium oxalate crystals are seen in hypercalciuria, hyperoxaluria, and ethylene glycol poisoning. Presence of a single crystal of cystine is diagnostic of cystinuria as cystine is not a constituent of normal urine. Phosphate crystals can form in normal urine as it cools and are of no pathological significance.

Investigations in patients with renal or bladder stones

Not all renal tract stones are formed because of abnormal urine chemistry. They may also be formed because of stasis, e.g. in calyceal or bladder diverticula. Infection ('struvite') stones are the result of chronic infection in the urinary tract with urease-producing organisms, which metabolize urea to form an alkaline urine in which struvite readily precipitates.

Indications

Although up to 75% of patients who present with renal stones eventually form a second stone, this may not be for 20 yrs. Most urologists therefore only refer patients for metabolic evaluation if there is a heightened suspicion of an underlying metabolic cause.

Situations in which evaluation is definitely indicated include
- Formation of stones in childhood or adolescence.
- Recurrent stone formation.
- Nephrocalcinosis (calcification in the renal parenchyma) as well as stone formation in the collecting systems.

Radiology

Intravenous urography or unenhanced helical CT will usually have been performed during the patient's presentation with stone disease, but the films should be reviewed to look for evidence of any cause of stasis within the collecting systems, and in particular for medullary sponge kidney. Radiolucent stones can be detected using ultra-sound, intravenous urography or CT scanning, and can be made of cystine, uric acid or xanthine. 'Staghorn' calculi filling the collecting systems are most often struvite (infection) stones, but not always—calcium oxalate stones can grow to similar size and shape, particularly in hyperoxaluria.

Stone analysis

Depending on the facilities in the laboratory, this may be qualitative or semiquantitative. The purpose of analysis is to distinguish calcium stones from cystine, urate, and struvite stones, to pick up the rare types of stone, and in addition to distinguish calcium oxalate from calcium phosphate stones. The result of stone analysis should be used to guide further investigation. Stones can be obtained for analysis either at surgery, including percutaneous nephrolithotomy, or by asking a patient to pass urine through a fine sieve.

'Spot' urine tests

Amino acid analysis on a random sample of urine shows increased excretion of cystine, ornithine, lysine, and arginine in cystinuria, and this finding is sufficient to confirm a suspected diagnosis. However, measurement of 24 h urinary cystine excretion is necessary for optimal management of this condition.

Random urine calcium:creatinine and oxalate:creatinine ratios are used in children to diagnose hypercalciuria and hyperoxaluria, but are not as reliable as 24 h urine collections, which are preferred in adults.

24 h urine collections

Collections must be made into an acidified container for measurement of calcium and oxalate, and into a plain container for measurement of urate (because acidification is necessary to prevent calcium binding to the plastic surface of the urine container and to prevent *in vitro* generation of oxalate, and because acidification precipitates uric acid crystals). Measurement of sodium and citrate excretion can be made on either type of collection.

- **Calcium excretion** is not a good predictor of stone formation (calcium activity is less than concentration due to the presence in urine of anions that form soluble complexes with calcium). However, marked increase of urinary calcium is a risk factor for stone formation.
- **Oxalate excretion** correlates well with the risk of recurrent calcium oxalate stone formation, even within the normal range. Marked hyperoxaluria may result from enteric hyperoxaluria (increased colonic oxalate absorption resulting from small bowel resection, jejunoileal bypass or malabsorption), acute ethylene glycol poisoning, excess dietary oxalate, or as a result of 1° hyperoxaluria (one of several metabolic defects causing increased endogenous oxalate production).
- **Glycolate and L-glycerate** should be measured in patients suspected of having 1° hyperoxaluria to allow differentiation between type 1 and type 2 hyperoxaluria. This investigation is only available in a few laboratories; raised urine glycolate suggests type 1 disease and raised L-glycerate suggest type 2 disease, but neither test is 100% sensitive or specific. Liver biopsy or genetic testing may be necessary to confirm the diagnosis.
- **Citrate excretion** should be measured because citrate is a potent inhibitor of calcium stone formation; correction of hypocitraturia with, for instance, oral potassium citrate, reduces stone recurrence rate.
- **Sodium excretion** (a good marker for dietary sodium intake) should be measured in calcium stone formers and in patients with cystinuria, because reduction of dietary sodium intake results in decreased excretion of calcium and cystine, respectively.
- **Cystine excretion** should be measured in cystine stone formers. The aim of treatment is to maintain the cystine concentration well below the solubility limit for cystine (~1mmol/L at urine pH of 7). Rather than a single 24 h collection, it is worth asking the patient to split the urine collection into daytime and night-time aliquots to ensure that this target is met at night, when urine tends to become more concentrated, as well as during the day.
- **Urinary phosphate** measurement is of no proven value in the management even of calcium phosphate stone formers.

Tests of urinary calcium excretion

Tests performed after calcium restriction and following a high calcium test meal have been used widely in the USA to differentiate 'absorptive' from 'renal' hypercalciuria. These tests are necessary to define different phenotypes associated with hypercalciuria for research studies, but there is no evidence that management strategies based on them have any advantage over those based on simpler tests of urine chemistry.

Renal biopsy

Percutaneous renal biopsy is a valuable tool to establish diagnosis, suggest prognosis and guide therapy in renal diseases. It also has a major role in the management of a renal transplant recipient.

Definite indications (result likely to change management)

- Nephrotic syndrome (in adults).
- Steroid-unresponsive nephrotic syndrome in children.
- Acute nephritic syndrome.
- Rapidly progressive glomerulonephritis.
- Unexplained renal failure with normal-sized kidneys relative to body size and age.
- Renal involvement in multi-system disorders.
- Diagnosis of renal transplant dysfunction.

Relative indications (result may change management or help to define prognosis)

- Non-nephrotic range proteinuria with or without haematuria.
- Isolated haematuria (only rarely does biopsy change management: sometimes justified for potential live kidney donors, or for employment or insurance purposes).
- Unexplained chronic kidney disease.
- Diabetic patient with renal dysfunction, particularly with features not typical of diabetic nephropathy.

Absolute contraindications

- Uncontrolled severe hypertension.
- Bleeding diathesis including platelets $<50 \times 10^9$/L, uncorrected familial bleeding/clotting disorders and patient on anticoagulation with prolonged clotting times.

Relative contraindications

- Single kidney.
- Kidney size small compared to patient's body size and age.
- Renal tumour/mass—risk of abdominal seeding.
- Unco-operative patient (can be done under sedation or under general anaesthetic (GA)).
- Multiple renal cysts.

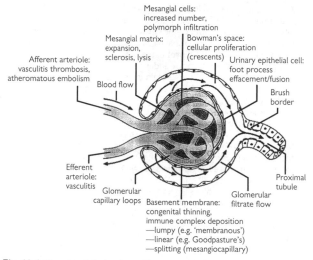

Fig. 10.4 The normal glomerulus and its repertoire of response to injury. Reprinted from Tomson (1998).[1]

For an excellent patient information sheet on renal biopsy see ℜ http:// renux.dmed.ed.ac.uk/EdREN/EdRenINFObits/RenalBiopsyShort.html

Procedure

1 Recent imaging of kidneys to document size and rule out obstruction is mandatory. A recent normal platelet count, clotting profile, and informed consent is necessary.
2 The procedure is performed where proper ultrasound facilities are available and usually done under local anaesthesia. Sedation can be given to an unco-operative or tense patient.
3 An attending pathologist or technician at the time of sampling to comment on adequacy of tissue is very useful.
4 Biopsy can be performed with either a spring-loaded disposable device or biopsy gun, depending on local practice
5 The patient lies prone and the kidney is identified with ultrasound.
6 The skin over the target area is prepared and anaesthetized with lidocaine.

1 Tomson CRV. Essential Medicine, 2nd edn. London: Churchill Livingstone, 1998.

7 A small cut in the skin is made using a scalpel. The kidney is localized with a fine bore 21G lumbar puncture needle and local anaesthetic infiltrated up to the level of the renal capsule. Either kidney can be biopsied: all parenchymal renal diseases are bilateral. After suitably protecting the ultrasound probe, the biopsy needle/gun is inserted along the anaesthetized track under real-time ultrasound guidance to the level of the renal capsule, aiming to obtain a sample from the cortex of the lower pole. The patient is asked to hold their breath while the biopsy is taken.

8 The needle/gun is fired and subsequently withdrawn. The patient is then allowed to breathe normally.

9 Two cores of tissue are usually taken; this may require three or four 'passes' with the biopsy needle. If an attending pathologist or technician is present, they can comment on the adequacy of tissue by examining the core for glomeruli using a hand held magnifying glass or a simple microscope. If immunofluorescence is to be performed, part of one core is placed in saline; the remainder is placed in formalin.

10 Following the biopsy the patient is turned supine and strict bed rest enforced for a minimum of 6 h. Vital signs are monitored every 15 min for 2 h, every 30 min for 2 h and hourly thereafter. If no complications are encountered at 6 h the patient is allowed to mobilize. Most bleeding complications occur within the first 8h, but bleeding can start up to 72 h after the biopsy. If macroscopic haematuria is present and does not resolve within the observation period, discharge should be delayed.

Renal imaging

Contrast nephropathy

Renal toxicity due to radiocontrast agents may cause or exacerbate renal impairment. Nephrotoxicity is due to a combination of local vasoconstriction and direct tubular injury. There is an increased risk in patients with pre-existing renal impairment, diabetes, myeloma, hypovolaemia, or effective hypovolaemia (e.g. congestive cardiac failure), and concurrent administration of nephrotoxic medication including non-steroidal anti-inflammatory drugs and angiotensin converting enzyme inhibitors. The Royal College of Radiologists recommends discussion with the referring clinician before contrast is given to any patient taking metformin, given the theoretical risk of precipitating lactic acidosis, but it is no longer recommended that metformin is routinely discontinued in this setting.[1]

Although usually reversible, contrast nephropathy can precipitate the need for dialysis in patients whose renal function is already seriously impaired. Non-ionic media, adequate hydration and acetylcysteine (given by mouth) administered prior to the examination might reduce the risk in high-risk patients.

Details of the radiological investigation of the urinary tract appear on 📖 Renal imaging, p644. 📖 Radiology of the urinary tract, p744. 📖 Static cortical renography: DMSA imaging, p836. 📖 Dynamic renography, p838. 📖 Captopril renography, p839.

Gadolinium-based contrast media

An association between exposure to gadolinium-based contrast media and nephrogenic systemic fibrosis (NSF) was established in 2006. NSF manifests as fibrosis of the skin and connective tissue, causing contractures and joint immobility, and can cause visceral fibrosis, in some cases leading to a fatal outcome. With relatively few cases reported so far the risks are hard to quantify, but patients with CKD 4–5 can be considered high risk and CKD 3 low risk. No cases have been reported with eGFR>60ml/min/1.73m^2. Post-exposure dialysis is recommended for patients already established on renal replacement therapy, but dialysis is not recommended for those not established on renal replacement; the risks of temporary vascular access and dialysis initiation outweigh the benefits of gadolinium removal. The risk of developing NSF seems to relate to the extent to which the contrast medium releases free Gd^{3+} ions, with cyclic agents less likely to release Gd^{3+}.[2]

1 ℘ http://www.rcr.ac.uk/docs/radiology/pdf/bfcr(09)7_metformin.pdf
2 ℘ http://www.mhra.gov.uk/Safetyinformation/Safetywarningsalertsandrecalls/
Safetywarningsandmessagesformedicines/CON2031543

Choice of investigation

Unexplained renal impairment

When a patient first presents with renal impairment it is important to decide whether this is acute—and therefore potentially reversible—or chronic. Although the history, examination, and blood tests may give some clues, considerable doubt may remain.

All patients presenting with renal impairment should therefore undergo

• **Ultrasound**:
   • Hydronephrosis suggests obstructive nephropathy.
   • Small, smooth, kidneys with increased echogenicity and decreased corticomedullary differentiation suggests chronic parenchymal renal disease, e.g. chronic glomerulonephritis.
   • Irregular cortical scarring can be caused by reflux nephropathy, previous obstructive nephropathy (e.g. complicating renal stones) and renal infarction from vascular disease or embolism.
   • Renal asymmetry, particularly in a patient with known atherosclerosis elsewhere, suggests renal artery stenosis, although this can just as commonly be bilateral.
   • Renal enlargement can occur in acute tubular necrosis, renal vein thrombosis and renal infiltration, e.g. in haematological malignancy.
• Plain abdominal film (kidneys, ureters, bladder—KUB) if renal stones or nephrocalcinosis suspected: nephrocalcinosis and urinary tract stones, particularly if outside the renal pelvis can be missed on ultrasound.

Further radiological investigations, including renal angiography and isotope scanning, are sometimes helpful.

Suspected nephrolithiasis

Unenhanced helical CT is increasingly the investigation of first choice, and is more useful than IVU particularly if the GFR is reduced or radiolucent stones present. IVU remains readily available, and may be the preferred investigation in some centres.

Investigation of haematuria

In patients over 40 and possibly in some younger patients, it is important to exclude urinary tract malignancy. Ultrasound is the investigation of choice for the detection of renal cell carcinoma, but will miss some transitional cell carcinomas of the renal pelvis, which are best detected using CT or IVU.

Investigation of suspected renal artery stenosis

In younger patients in whom fibromuscular dysplasia is suspected, conventional angiography should be performed. Atherosclerotic renal artery stenosis can be reasonably assessed by contrast CT angiography or by gadolinium-enhanced MR angiography, with direct angiography reserved for interventional procedures.

Reflux nephropathy

Confirming this diagnosis can be important in counselling patients, as reflux nephropathy is often inherited as an autosomal dominant trait. Cortical scarring is best detected using a static DMSA renal scan. However, there are other causes of cortical scarring. The diagnosis is best confirmed by showing the combination of cortical scarring with underlying calyceal deformity on IVU. Demonstration of vesicoureteric reflux on direct or indirect micturating cystourethrography is useful in infants and small children, but reflux commonly resolves with growth, so these tests are seldom used in adults.

Obstructive uropathy

Although hydronephrosis demonstrated on IVU or ultrasound is usually sufficient to confirm obstruction, it is possible to have obstruction without much dilatation (e.g. complicating encasement by tumour). More commonly, there is uncertainty over whether dilatation of the collecting system and pelvis is due to previous obstruction, now resolved, or continuing obstruction. Diuretic MAG3 renography may be useful, but gives less reliable results as GFR falls. Insertion of nephrostomy, or retrograde insertion of ureteric stents may be useful for both diagnosis and treatment of obstruction. If doubt persists, a Whitaker test may be performed: this involves infusion of saline at a constant rate through a nephrostomy tube, and measuring the relationship between pressure and flow down the ureter.

Renal transplant dysfunction

The differential diagnosis usually lies between obstruction, ureteric leak, rejection, acute tubular necrosis, nephrotoxicity, and renal vein thrombosis. Depending on the centre, ultrasound with Doppler assessment of renal blood flow (giving resistance index) or isotope renography may be the investigation of first choice.

Renal bone disease

Parathyroid hormone

Indications

Diagnosis of 1° hyperparathyroidism in patients with hypercalcaemia. Diagnosis of 2° or 3° hyperparathyroidism in patients with stage 4 or 5 chronic kidney disease.

Procedure

A serum sample is sent and separated within 4h of venepuncture. Alternatively, parathyroid hormone (PTH) remains stable for 24 h if the sample is taken into EDTA, allowing samples to be sent from primary care. Check with local laboratory.

Other markers of bone biochemistry

Serum calcium is often normal even in patients with significant renal disease, because a fall in serum calcium caused by reduced $1,25-(OH)_2$ vitamin D production results in an increase in parathyroid hormone secretion, returning serum calcium towards normal. Hypocalcaemia occurs after parathyroidectomy or after treatment with bisphosphonates. Hypercalcaemia occurs when the parathyroid hormone release loses sensitivity to serum calcium in 3° hyperparathyroidism.

If PTH is raised in the presence of CKD 3, check 25–(OH) vitamin D; vitamin D deficiency should be corrected before treatment of hyperparathyroidism.
- **Serum phosphate** is often increased in patients with renal impairment due to impaired renal excretion of phosphate.
- **Serum total alkaline phosphatase** rises in severe hyperparathyroidism and in osteomalacia.
- **Serum bone alkaline phosphatase** is a more sensitive marker of bone turnover, but quantitative measurement is not widely available. If total alkaline phosphatase is raised, alkaline phosphatase isoenzymes can be measured as an indicator of whether the increase is of bone origin.

Serum aluminium and the desferrioxamine test

Patients with renal disease may be exposed to aluminium from contaminated water used for preparation of dialysate or by ingesting aluminium hydroxide as an antacid or, rarely nowadays, as a phosphate binder taken with meals. Because of the effects of aluminium on the brain, bone marrow, and bones it is important to monitor patients at risk for evidence of aluminium accumulation.

Serum aluminium has to be taken into an aluminium-free glass tube. Serum aluminium levels reflect current exposure and do not give any information about cumulative exposure. Serum aluminium levels may be increased by iron deficiency. Levels above 60µg/L (2.2µmol/L) are considered indicative of a dangerous level of exposure and should lead to a review of treatment.

The increment in serum aluminium 24 or 48 h after IV desferrioxamine is a marker of aluminium 'load'. The original protocol requires the use of 40mg/kg desferrioxamine; a rise in serum aluminium of >200μg/L correlates well with the presence of aluminium-related bone disease on bone biopsy. Low dose protocols have also been described and validated.

Skeletal survey

Severe hyperparathyroidism causes erosion of the terminal phalanges, sub-periosteal erosions and, in rare cases, brown tumours and pathological fractures. Severe osteomalacia causes loss of bone density and Looser zones (pseudo-fractures). These radiological signs are not commonly seen in modern renal patients because biochemical monitoring allows earlier detection of bone disease.

Transiliac bone biopsy

This is the 'gold standard' for the diagnosis of renal bone disease, but is not commonly used in clinical (as opposed to research) settings. However, it can be useful particularly for the confirmation of aluminium-related bone disease. For the maximum information to be gained from this invasive test, double tetracycline labelling should be performed.

Procedure

14 and 13 days before the procedure the patient takes a tetracycline antibiotic, e.g. oxytetracycline 250mg qds, and 4 and 3 days before the procedure a different tetracycline, e.g. demeclocycline 300mg bd. Under general anaesthetic a transiliac core of bone, including both cortical surfaces, is taken and placed in absolute alcohol. The sample should be sent to a laboratory specializing in the interpretation of bone biopsies in patients with metabolic bone disease.

Immunological tests in renal medicine

Immune-mediated diseases can affect the kidney in isolation or as part of a systemic disorder. Immunological tests commonly used to diagnose or monitor progress of renal disease are discussed here.

Complement

Indications

Acute nephritic syndrome, renal failure with skin ± neurological involvement and suspected SLE, endocarditis or cryoglobulinaemia. The normal complement system, its activation pathways and assay methods are discussed elsewhere (📖 p322). In relation to renal disease, hypocomplementaemia is important and relative deficiencies of various components can point to certain disorders.

Table 10.1 Complement levels in selected diseases

	C3	C4
Post-streptococcal GN	Low	Normal
SLE	Low	Low
Cryoglobulinaemia	Low/normal	Very low
Membranoproliferative GN	Low	Low/normal
Subacute endocarditis	Normal/low	Low

GN, glomerulonephritis

Successful treatment normalizes complement levels in endocarditis, and in SLE except when SLE results from congenital complement deficiency.

C3 nephritic factor (C3Nef) is an IgG autoantibody that binds to and stabilizes alternative pathway C3 convertase—C3bBb. This results in continuous activation of the alternative pathway with C3 depletion. It is detected by ELISA. C3Nef is classically associated with type 2 membranoproliferative glomerulonephritis.

Immunoglobulins and serum electrophoresis for paraproteins

Indications

- Suspected myeloma or other clonal B cell disorders.
- Unexplained renal failure, with or without proteinuria, particularly in patients >50 years.
- Renal failure in association with hypercalcaemia.

Serum electrophoresis to identify a monoclonal immunoglobulin band may be useful, but should always be combined with tests for urinary light chains (Bence–Jones protein), as some types of myeloma cause light chain proteinuria without a monoclonal band in the serum. Serum free light chain assays are also now available and should be used to monitor myeloma in patients with kidney disease. Routine measurement of serum and urine electrophoresis in the absence of clinical features to suggest a B cell disorder will identify many patients with MGUS incidental to their renal disease and seldom identifies treatable disease.

Measurement of serum immunoglobulin concentrations is of value in patients with known myeloma, but is otherwise not useful in the assessment of patients with renal disease. Polyclonal hypergammaglobulinaemia is seen in chronic infections, connective tissue disorders (e.g. rheumatoid arthritis, Sjögren's syndrome), neoplasms, and chronic liver disease. Measurement of serum IgA concentration is of no value in the diagnosis of IgA nephropathy.

Paraproteins are products of abnormal B cell clones and can be detected in serum as monoclonal bands on immunoglobulin electrophoresis or in urine as Bence–Jones proteins. Paraproteins may be whole immunoglobulins or heavy or light chains in isolation. Light chains are sufficiently small to be filtered at the glomerulus, are not reabsorbed and are not picked up on routine dipsticks. Bence–Jones proteins are light chains excreted in the urine. Bence–Jones proteins precipitate on heating to 45°C and redissolve on boiling, but are now detected by electrophoretic techniques.

Paraproteins can cause a number of different renal lesions, including

- Myeloma cast nephropathy.
- Light chain nephropathy.
- AL amyloidosis.
- Fibrillary/immunotactoid glomerulopathy (although this appearance is more frequently not associated with a plasma cell dyscrasia).

Cryoglobulins

Cryoglobulins are immunoglobulins, which precipitate on cooling and redissolve on warming.

Cryoglobulinaemia should be suspected in

- Renal failure with otherwise unexplained hypocomplementaemia or positive rheumatoid factor.
- Renal failure in association with skin and neurological involvement.
- Unexplained proteinuria/renal failure in patients with clonal B cell disorders.

Meticulous attention to collection, transportation, and assessment of the sample is required: a serum sample must be kept at 37°C and sent to the laboratory for analysis immediately, having warned the laboratory that the sample is on the way. False negative results are common due to improper handling of the specimen.

Once a cryoglobulin has been found, further electrophoresis and immunofixation allows identification of three distinct types:

- Type 1 has a single monoclonal immunoglobulin (IgG, IgA, or IgM) and is associated with monoclonal B cell disorders.
- Type 2 has a monoclonal IgM directed against the Fc portion of IgG, and the cryoprotein therefore consists of monoclonal IgM with polyclonal IgG. Tests for rheumatoid factor (i.e. anti-IgG antibodies) are positive. This may be associated with haematological malignancy, chronic hepatitis C infection or may be unexplained ('essential').
- Type 3 has polyclonal IgG and polyclonal IgM and occurs in chronic infections (e.g. bacterial endocarditis, viral hepatitis), autoimmune disorders (e.g. rheumatoid arthritis, SLE) or may be unexplained ('essential').

Hypocomplementaemia, especially very low C4 levels due to classical complement pathway activation, is characteristic and helpful in diagnosing active cryoglobulinaemic disorder. Renal disease can present as an acute nephritic disorder or as nephrotic syndrome, and is usually seen in association with skin and systemic involvement.

Antineutrophil cytoplasmic antibody (ANCA)

These are autoantibodies directed against enzymes present in the cytoplasm of human neutrophils. They are present in nearly all patients with small vessel vasculitis (including Wegener's granulomatosis, microscopic polyangitis, renal limited crescentic GN and Churg–Strauss syndrome). ANCA and its pattern of distribution is conventionally detected by indirect immunofluorescence, with pANCA having a characteristic perinuclear staining pattern, and cANCA a cytoplasmic staining pattern. Changing titres can reflect changing disease activity. ELISA is now readily available for the two most common ANCA protein targets; proteinase 3 (PR3) which is the most common target of cANCA, and myeloperoxidase (MPO), the most common target of pANCA. Low-titre positive ANCA is unlikely to reflect underlying disease if the ELISA is negative. However, a negative ANCA does not rule out vasculitis, and false positive tests occur, so the test is not a substitute for renal biopsy.

Anti-glomerular basement membrane antibody

Circulating anti-GBM antibodies are present in Goodpasture's Disease and may also be positive in ANCA-positive vasculitis, where 'double positivity' confers a worse prognosis than ANCA positivity alone. ELISA and radio-immunoassays are available. Confirmatory renal biopsy in Goodpasture's Disease shows linear deposition of anti-GBM IgG along the glomerular basement membrane, detectable by immunofluorescence or immunoperoxidase staining.

Poisoning & overdose

General principles

Many poisoned patients recover without specific management other than supportive care. A minority have life-threatening toxicity. In assessing the poisoned patient it is important to ensure adequate airway, breathing and circulation, take a thorough history, and undertake a full clinical examination. Tablets, bottles, syringes, aerosol containers, and other items found with or near the patient should be retained, although it is usually best to analyse biological specimens (usually blood and/or urine) if analytical confirmation of toxin exposures is required.

The role of blood and urine tests in toxicology

Close collaboration between analytical staff and clinicians is required if anything other than the simplest toxicological analysis is to be useful.

Toxicological analysis using blood or urine is used to confirm:
- The diagnosis of poisoning when this is in doubt or for medicolegal purposes.
- To help in the management, or in the diagnosis of brain death.
- To work out the time to restart chronic drug therapy.

Few centres have full analytical toxicology services and a 'toxicology screen' rarely influences acute in-patient management, with the exception of paracetamol, salicylate, lithium, digoxin, and iron poisoning, and on occasions a drugs of abuse screen. Toxicological analysis of blood plasma or serum is also of value if an extracorporeal method of elimination such as haemodialysis or MARS® (Molecular Absorbance Recirculating Systems)[1] is being contemplated. Any toxicology analysis should be tailored to that patient's circumstances and the poisons commonly encountered in that country. In Western Europe and North America, most patients will have taken drugs, but pesticide poisoning, for example, is common in less well developed countries.

Plasma paracetamol, salicylate, lithium, digoxin, and iron measurements in blood are usually available on an urgent basis. For other patients, particularly those who present a complex clinical picture or who are unconscious, a 50mL sample of urine and a 10mL sample of heparinized blood should be collected on admission and stored at 4°C (refrigerated). This can be analysed later if it is felt the result will influence your management, or is needed for medicolegal purposes (🕮 Samples of medicolegal importance, p656). Urine is useful for screening, especially for drugs of abuse, as it is often available in large volumes, and often contains higher concentrations of poisons and their metabolites than blood. The samples should be obtained as soon as possible after admission, ideally before any therapeutic drugs are administered. Urine samples usually provide qualitative results, e.g. detect the presence of amphetamines or benzodiazepines. Quantitative measurements in urine are of little use because some compounds, such as benzodiazepines, are extensively metabolized prior to excretion in urine.

Sample requirements

Plasma or serum is normally used for quantitative assays for drugs and drug metabolites, and in general there are no marked significant differences in concentration between these fluids. Evacuated blood tubes and containers containing gel separators or soft rubber stoppers are not recommended if a toxicological analysis is to be performed, as the plasticizers (phosphates and phthalates) used in many such tubes may interfere with chromatographic methods, and volatile compounds such as carbon monoxide or ethanol may be lost.

EDTA tubes are preferred for carboxyhaemoglobin assays and for measurement of lead, and some other metals as these are concentrated in red blood cells. A fluoride/oxalate tube should be used if ethanol, cocaine or benzodiazepines are being assayed, although special tubes containing 1% (w/v) fluoride are needed if enzymic hydrolysis of these and other compounds is to be completely prevented.

The use of disinfectant swabs containing alcohols should be avoided, as should heparin, which contains phenolic preservatives (chlorbutol, cresol) and preservatives containing mercury salts (see Table 11.1).

Table 11.1 Sample requirements for metals/trace elements analysis

Metal	Sample needed
Aluminium	10mL whole blood in plastic (not glass) tube—no anticoagulant/beads*
Antimony	5mL heparinized whole blood; 20mL urine
Arsenic	5mL heparinized whole blood; 20mL urine
Bismuth	5mL heparinized whole blood
Cadmium	2mL EDTA whole blood*; 10mL urine*
Chromium	2mL heparinized whole blood*; 20mL urine*
Copper	2mL heparinized or clotted whole blood, or 1mL plasma; 10mL urine
Iron	5mL clotted blood or 2mL serum (avoid haemolysis)
Lead	2mL EDTA whole blood
Lithium	5mL clotted blood or 2mL serum (NOT lithium heparin tube!)
Manganese	1mL heparinized whole blood or 0.5mL plasma*
Mercury	5mL heparinized whole blood; 20mL urine
Selenium	2mL heparinized whole blood or 1mL plasma/serum
Thallium	5mL heparinized whole blood; 20mL urine
Zinc	2mL whole blood (not EDTA) or 1mL plasma/serum

*Send unused container from the same batch to check for possible contamination.

1 ✆ http://www.teraklin.com/eng/mars.html

Samples of medicolegal importance

A toxicology screen is helpful if murder, assault, or child abuse is suspected. Samples collected in such cases are often so important that they should be kept securely at −20°C or below, until investigation of the incident is concluded. Legal requirements mean that all specimens should be clearly labelled with the patient's family or last name, and any forenames, the date and time of collection, and the nature of the specimen, if this is not obvious. Strict chain of custody procedures should be implemented, and the doctor or nurse taking the sample should seal the bag with a tamper-proof device, and sign and date the seal. A chain of custody form must accompany the sample, and should be signed and dated by every person taking possession of the sample. The sample should be secured in a locked container or refrigerator if left unattended before arrival at the laboratory.

Methods used in analytical toxicology

A range of chromatographic and other methods, such as radioligand immunoassays, are available for toxicological analyses. Plasma concentrations associated with serious toxicity range from mcg/L ($\equiv$ μg/L) in the case of drugs such as digoxin to g/L in the case of ethanol. Specialized laboratories use a combination of solvent extraction and thin layer chromatography (TLC) together with gas–liquid chromatography (GLC) using either flame-ionization or selective detectors such as nitrogen/phosphorus detectors or mass spectroscopy (MSp) as the basis for a poison screen. It is unwise to use TLC without corroboration of results by another method, e.g. GLC, because the resolution power of TLC is limited and interpretation of chromatograms is subjective. A commercial kit for TLC (Toxi-lab, Marion Laboratories) is supplied with a compendium of colour plates, but even so problems can arise in differentiation of compounds with similar mobility and colour reactions. The kit is aimed at the US market and some common UK drugs are not included.

Spectrophotometry is commonly used to measure salicylates, iron, and carboxyhaemoglobin. However, UV spectrophotometry and spectrophotofluorimetry are often used as detectors for high-performance liquid chromatography (HPLC) and in immunoassays. Spectrophotometric methods and immunoassays often suffer from interference from metabolites or other drugs. Immunoassays have the advantage of long shelf life and simplicity, but all require confirmation with a chromatographic method if the results are to stand scrutiny. This is because immunoassays for small molecules are often not specific, e.g. some urine amphetamine immunoassays give positive results with proguanil, isoxsuprine, labetalol, tranylcypromine, and phenylethylamine. The Syva Emit antidepressant assay cross-reacts with phenothiazines after overdose. Chromatographic methods have the advantage of selectivity and sensitivity and ability to perform quantitative measurements, but are expensive. Generally, GLC is still used to measure basic drugs although modern high pressure HPLC, such as UPLC, or even better alternative if coupled with a tandem MSp (i.e. LCMS-MSp). Acidic or neutral moieties can also be analysed by LCMS/MSp. For screening very large numbers of compounds simultaneously or sequentially, then the Applied Biosystems Q-Trap technology is one of the most versatile—this is a LCMS/MSp where one of the quadruples of the triple quadrupole is use as an ion trap. Most laboratories that aim to be as versatile as possible have a fast GLC in addition to the LC-MSp/MSp.

Modern methods of assay for heavy metals vary enormously. Inductively coupled plasma mass spectroscopy (ICPMS) is the most modern method used. Here, ICPMS is used instead of the flame or electrothermal furnace for atomization of the elements and mass is the detector. Atomic absorption spectrophotometry, with either flame or electrothermal atomization is the older method. In the case of iron, reliable kits based on the formation of a coloured complex are available.

There is wide variation in the units that various laboratories use to report results. This has caused confusion and errors in treatment and great care is needed to ensure that clinical interpretation is undertaken in full knowledge of the units used. Particular care is also required in interpretation and application of analytical techniques in post-mortem toxicology.

Further reading

Baselt RC, Cravey RH. *Disposition of Toxic Drugs and Chemicals in Man*, 7th edn. Chemical Toxicology Institute, San Francisco, California, 2004.

Drummer OH. Requirements for bioanalytical procedures in post-mortem toxicology. *Anal Bioanal Chem* 2007; **23**: Epub ahead of print.

Flanagan RJ. The poisoned patient; the role of the laboratory. *Br J Biomed Sci* 1995; **52**: 202–13.

Brainstem death testing & organ donation

Brain death cannot be diagnosed in the presence of drugs that mask central nervous system (CNS) activity. There is a rule of thumb, based on the pharmacological principle that most drugs need five half-lives to be effectively eliminated from the circulation, to allow four half-lives of any drug to elapse before declaring death, or to allow at least 2–3 days for drug effects to wear off. Whether this is satisfactory for patients with organ failure and, hence, impaired drug elimination is unclear and often in such patients measurement of plasma concentrations of residual drugs is required to determine whether brainstem death tests are valid or whether a drug could be interfering with the results.

Selected donor organs from those who have died from poisoning by tricyclic antidepressants, benzodiazepines, barbiturates, insulin, carbon monoxide, cocaine, methanol, and paracetamol have been used in transplantation. It is important to identify which organs act as reservoirs for drugs and either not consider such organs, e.g. a liver from a paracetamol-poisoned patient, or take prophylactic precautions like N-acetylcysteine administration in the case of donation of a heart from a paracetamol-poisoned patient.

Further reading

Baselt RC, Cravey RH. *Disposition of Toxic Drugs and Chemicals in Man*, 7th edn, Chemical Toxicology Institute, California, 2004.

Jones AL, Simpson KJ. Drug abusers and poisoned patients: a potential source of organs for transplantation? *Q J Med* 1998; **91**: 589–92.

Interpretation of arterial blood gases in poisoned patients

Interpretation of blood gas values may be found in 📖 *OHCM* 8e, p156, p684. Essentially four patterns emerge, which may be mixed together.

Respiratory acidosis

Hypoventilation results in retention of carbon dioxide. This can occur after an overdose with any drugs that depress the CNS, e.g. tricyclic antidepressants, opioids, and barbiturates.

Respiratory alkalosis

Hyperventilation with respiratory alkalosis is classically caused by aspirin (commonly measured as salicylate). It can also occur in response to hypoxia, drugs, and CNS injury.

Metabolic alkalosis

Metabolic alkalosis is very uncommon in poisoning. Rarely, it may result from excess administration of alkali, e.g. deliberate alkali ingestion.

Metabolic acidosis

This is the most common metabolic abnormality in poisoning. If acidosis is particularly severe (e.g. pH <7.2), this should raise the question of poisoning by ethanol, methanol, or ethylene glycol. Measuring the anion gap and osmolal gaps are helpful in further differentiation (📖 Ethylene glycol, ethanol & methanol poisoning, p668).

Amphetamines & derivatives

E.g. MDMA (ecstasy), MDEA, MDA (adam)

The following investigations should be considered in patients presenting to hospital with acute amphetamine(s) intoxication.

Plasma urea and electrolytes and glucose

It is critical that at least one set of U&E are checked in every patient. Most are profoundly dehydrated and require vigorous rehydration. Some patients develop hyponatraemia, often after drinking excess water and antidiuretic hormone secretion may be responsible for this (📖 OHCM 8e, p688). Hypoglycaemia may occur.

Dipstick test of urine for myoglobin and subsequent serum creatine kinase

A hyperthermic (serotonin-toxicity) syndrome with autonomic instability and rigidity, can develop leading to rhabdomyolysis. Dipstick testing of urine is positive for blood as myoglobin is detected by the haemoglobin assay. This is an indication that serum CK should be then be measured. If found to be elevated, adequate rehydration is needed to avoid deposition in renal tubules and incipient renal failure.

Full blood count

Rarely, aplastic anaemia (📖 OHCM 8e, p358) has been reported after ecstasy (MDMA) ingestion.

Clotting studies

Disseminated intravascular coagulation (📖 OHCM 8e, p346) can occur, often in the context of hyperthermia. Once liver damage ensues the international normalized ratio/prothrombin time (INR/PT; 📖 OHCM 8e, p340) will rise.

Temperature

Hyperpyrexia can lead to rhabdomyolysis, disseminated intravascular coagulation and hepatocellular necrosis. Risks relate to the time in hours spent above 39°C. A rectal thermometer is the most accurate measure of temperature.

Liver function tests

Acute liver injury can occur with a rise in aspartate aminotransferase (AST) or alanine aminotransferase (ALT), often of several thousands.

▶▶ **Note**: Don't miss a hidden paracetamol overdose—check paracetamol levels in blood, from the earliest sample you have on that patient!

ECG

Cardiac arrhythmias are common and deaths, which occur soon after ingestion, may be due to these. Arrhythmias are often supraventricular, though ventricular arrhythmias also occur.

Urine tests

Urine tests, e.g. EMIT dipstick system or by immunoassay in the laboratory, are sensitive and group-specific for amphetamines and can confirm an amphetamine has been ingested if that is in doubt, e.g. agitated patient in A&E. *Note*: amphetamine, MDMA, MDEA and MDA concentrations in blood are of no value in determining management.

Further reading

Greene SL, Dargan PI, O'Connor N, Jones AL, Kerins M. Multiple toxicity from 3,4-methylenedi-oxymethamphetamine ("ecstasy"). *Am J Emerg Med* 2003; **21**(2): 121–4.

Benzylpiperazine

Clinical features

This original anti-helminthic agent has recently been reported as a drug of abuse, and is sold as ecstasy or amphetamines. Patients have presented with recurrent seizures, collapse, and cardiovascular features,

Serum tests

GCMS is used to analyse serum. Previous case report of toxicity at 2.5 mg/L.

Further reading

Wood DM, Dargan PI, Button J, Holt DW, Ovaska H, Ramsay J, Jones AL. Collapse, reported seizure—and an unexpected pill. *Lancet* 2007; **369**: 1490.

Anticonvulsants

For most anticonvulsants LCMS/MSp will be the analytical method of choice. Some like valproic acid are difficult to assay by LCMS/MSp and GC may be more appropriate.

Carbamazepine toxicity

Plasma concentrations of carbamazepine and its active metabolite 10, 11-epoxide can be measured by HPLC, but do not correlate well with the degree of toxicity. They are seldom performed unless the diagnosis is in doubt or there is concern about a therapeutic excess. The therapeutic range is between 8 and 12mg/L. Toxicity has been seen with carbamazepine concentrations above 20mg/L (85mmol/L). Coma, fits, respiratory failure, and conduction abnormalities have been seen with concentrations in excess of 40mg/L (170mmol/L).

An ECG should be performed in all but the most trivial carbamazepine over dosage

The urea & electrolytes (U&E) should be checked as hyponatraemia and syndrome of inappropriate antidiuretic hormone (SIADH; 📖 *OHCM* 8e, p687) have been reported. Hypoglycaemia has also been reported.

Lamotrigine toxicity

Plasma concentrations of lamotrigine can be measured for compliance purposes (therapeutic range 1–4mg/L; upper limit may be as high as 10mg/L), but are not of value in the overdose situation.

An ECG should be performed in all but the most trivial lamotrigine over dosage.

Valproate toxicity

Plasma concentrations of sodium valproate can be measured by HPLC, but do not correlate well with either with depth of coma or risk of seizures after overdose. The therapeutic range is 40–100mg/L. U&E and glucose should be measured as hypernatraemia, hypoglycaemia, and hypocalcaemia have been reported after over dosage.

Phenytoin toxicity

Most patients with acute phenytoin poisoning do not require measurement of the plasma phenytoin concentration. An urgent phenytoin measurement may help in severe phenytoin poisoning where charcoal haemoperfusion is contemplated if the plasma phenytoin concentration is rapidly rising towards or exceeds 100mg/L.

Patients with suspected chronic phenytoin toxicity as a result of therapeutic dosing should have their plasma phenytoin concentration measured. The 'therapeutic range' is 10–20mg/L. Routine measurements may be useful to monitor anticonvulsant therapy or to time re-institution of chronic therapy after overdose.

Benzodiazepines

Most patients who have taken an overdose with benzodiazepines just sleep off the drug without sequelae within 24 h. However, more severe effects can occur when benzodiazepines are mixed with other drugs, especially in patients with pre-existing cardiovascular or respiratory disease. Pulse oximetry is useful for monitoring the adequacy of ventilation if significant CNS depression is present.

Generally, measuring benzodiazepine concentrations in blood or urine is not of value in the management of benzodiazepine overdose patients. Rarely a urine screen by EMIT (immunoassay) is undertaken to confirm ingestion. LCMS/MSp is the method of choice for analysis of diazepam and its metabolites. Liquid chromatography simultaneously assays diazepam and its polar metabolites, and post-mortem blood concentrations of 5 and 19mg/L have been found in fatalities.

Carbon monoxide

Carbon monoxide (CO) is the most common cause of death by poisoning in the UK. Those particularly at risk include patients with pre-existing cardiac or respiratory disease.

Carboxyhaemoglobin

A carboxyhaemoglobin (COHb) concentration in blood confirms recent exposure and should be measured urgently in all patients with suspected carbon monoxide poisoning, including those with smoke inhalation. The space above the blood in the sample tube (headspace) should be minimized. Normally expected values for COHb are up to 5% in non-smokers and up to 10% in smokers. However, after acute exposure ceases the blood COHb concentration does not indicate the severity of poisoning because COHb begins to dissociate from the moment of removal from the source of CO, and the rate of dissociation is also dependent on factors such as oxygen administration in the ambulance. Thus the use of nomograms to 'back-extrapolate' to find the initial highest COHb is meaningless. Management of the patient is determined by the clinical condition and also on circumstantial evidence such as the intensity and duration of exposure, rather than a COHb concentration *per se*, although a level of >40% has been used as one criterion to guide the use of hyperbaric oxygen. A patient should be administered high flow oxygen (e.g. 12L/min through a tight-fitting, e.g. CPAP, mask) until the COHb is <5% and clinical signs of carbon monoxide poisoning such as impaired heel–toe walking and finger–nose inco-ordination have resolved.

Arterial blood gases

Any patient with suspected poisoning by carbon monoxide requires arterial blood gas analysis. Oxygen saturation monitors are misleading as they read carboxyhaemoglobin as oxyhaemoglobin (HbO) and the true oxygen saturation of the patient can only be determined by arterial blood gas analysis.

Electrocardiogram

An electrocardiogram (ECG) should be performed in anyone severely poisoned (e.g. drowsiness or any neurological abnormality, chest pain or breathlessness) or with pre-existing heart disease. ECG changes such as ST segment depression, T-wave abnormalities, ventricular tachycardia or fibrillation, and arrest can occur. If ischaemia/infarction is seen on the ECG or suspected clinically, the patient should also have cardiac enzymes sent.

Further reading

Greene SL, Dargan PI, Jones AL. Acute poisoning: understanding 90% of cases in a nutshell. *Postgrad Med J* 2005; **81**: 204–16.

Cocaine

Cocaine is snorted into the nose or injected intravenously.

Blood pressure monitoring

Patients with cocaine intoxication should have frequent measurements of their blood pressure, as hypertension is a significant risk, and strokes and chest pain have been widely reported. A Dynamap or equivalent advice for repeated measurements is suitable.

ECG and cardiac enzymes

Cocaine-induced angina and myocardial infarction are common. ECG monitoring is advised for all but the most trivial exposure to cocaine. Appropriate cardiac enzyme activity, i.e. creatine kinase (CK), AST, lactate dehydrogenase (LDH), and troponin T should also be performed in any patient with chest pain or ECG abnormalities.

Diagnosis of cocaine related myocardial infarction is difficult as 84% of patients with cocaine related chest pain have abnormal ECG's even in the absence of myocardial infarction (MI). Half of all cocaine users have elevated creatinine kinase concentrations in the absence of myocardial infarction. Troponin T is the most sensitive indicator of myocardial damage due to cocaine.

Urine or blood testing

Cocaine can be detected in urine by simple 'drugs of abuse' screening tests, e.g. EMIT testing. This may help identify if a body-packer (who has swallowed packets containing cocaine) is either a pre-existing cocaine user or is leaking cocaine from the packets. Gas chromatography (GC)–MSp is more specific and can be carried out on blood or urine. Metabolites of cocaine (benzoylecgonine) can be detected in urine 2–3 days after exposure. Cocaine is unstable in blood and samples are best taken into 1% w/v fluoride oxalate tubes if medicolegal sequelae are a possibility. Nasal insufflation of 106mg of the drug to six volunteers produced mean peak plasma concentrations of 0.22mg/L at 0.5 h and 0.61mg/L for the metabolite benzoylecgonine at 3 h. Smoking 50mg in six volunteers produced mean peak plasma concentrations of 0.2mg/L at 0.08 h and 0.15mg/L for benzoylecgonine at 1.5 h. Patients have survived plasma concentrations of 5.2mg/L, but usually fatalities are associated with cocaine/benzoylecgonine concentrations in excess of 5mg/L, depending on the route of use. The IV route is the most dangerous.

Further reading

Hollander JE, et al. Acad Emerg Med 1994; **1**: 330–59.
Gitter MJ et al. Ann Intern Med 1990; **115**: 277–82.

Cyanide

Cyanide poisoning can occur by deliberate inhalation of gas, ingestion of salts, or by exposure in industrial fires.

Arterial blood gas estimation

Such measurements are essential to determine the oxygen saturation and acid–base status of the patient.

Serum lactate

This is helpful in confirming suspected toxicity and can be used clinically as a surrogate for the cyanide assay. It is likely to exceed 7mmol/L in cases of significant exposure.

Electrocardiogram

All patients should have an ECG. It should be examined for evidence of ischaemic damage, e.g. ST depression, ST elevation, T-wave inversion.

Cyanide assay

Blood cyanide concentrations are rarely of use in emergency management because they cannot be measured quickly enough. However, a sample should be taken before antidote administration for assay at a later stage. Cyanide concentrations of <0.2mg/L are 'normal'; 1.0–2.5mg/L causes obtundation and coma; and more than 2.5mg/L is potentially fatal.

▶▶ **Note**: The antidote of choice for cyanide poisoning is hydroxocobalamin together with oxygen; these are antidotes that can safely be given without certainty of cyanide ingestion. An alternative is to give sodium thiosulphate and sodium nitrite, and dicobalt edetate. However, note that dicobalt edetate should only be given if cyanide poisoning is certain, i.e. a proper history is available; otherwise you may kill your patient with cardiotoxicity of the antidote. Excessive administration of sodium nitrite, can cause significant methaemoglobinaemia.

Further reading

Borron SW, Baud FJ, Megarbane B, Bismuth C. Hydroxocobalamin for severe acute cyanide poisoning by ingestion or inhalation. *Am J Emerg Med* 2007; **25**(5): 551–8.

Borron SW, Baud FJ, Barriot P, Imbert M, Bismuth C. Prospective study of hydroxocobalamin for acute cyanide poisoning in smoke inhalation. *Ann Emerg Med* 2007; **49**: 794–801.

Jones AL, Dargan PI. *Churchill's Pocketbook of Toxicology*, Edinburgh: Churchill-Livingstone, 2001.

Digoxin

Patients who are already taking digoxin and those with pre-existing cardiovascular disease are more susceptible to digoxin toxicity after over dosage. Digoxin toxicity can also result from progressive renal impairment or due to interactions with other drugs, as well as overdoses.

Electrocardiogram

All patients with suspected digoxin poisoning should have a 12-lead ECG and all symptomatic patients should be attached to a cardiac monitor. Digoxin poisoning can cause virtually any type of cardiac arrhythmia. The combination of heart block with tachyarrhythmia is very common.

Plasma digoxin concentration

Absorption of digoxin often peaks at 4–6 h after ingestion. Its half-life is in excess of 30 h. Digitoxin is a structurally-related drug that has an even longer plasma half-life (6 days). A digoxin measurement is a useful, but not absolute, guide to toxicity as plasma digoxin concentrations correlate poorly with the severity of poisoning, particularly early in the course of acute poisoning. However it is desirable (although not essential) if anti-digoxin Fab antibody fragments are to be used, as it is useful in calculating the dose of fragments (☐ Digoxin, Indications for Fab fragments and doses of Fab fragments, p666), as well as confirming exposure. Plasma digoxin concentrations cannot be interpreted after administration of digoxin antibody fragments using normal assay procedures. Samples taken to investigate probable chronic digoxin intoxication should be taken at least 6h after dosing. They are not normally analysed urgently unless life-threatening features of toxicity are present and use of antibody fragments (Fab) is being considered. The therapeutic range for digoxin is 0.8–2.0 mcg/L.

Urea and electrolytes

It is important to ascertain if the patient has any renal impairment and plasma creatinine and urea are helpful, although of course do not exclude renal impairment completely. Hyperkalaemia is common in acute digoxin overdose and may be severe, e.g. >7mmol/L. If possible a magnesium level is helpful to exclude hypomagnesaemia, which contributes to risk of cardiotoxicity and is easily corrected.

Indications for Fab fragments and doses of Fab fragments

- Severe hyperkalaemia (>6.0mmol/L) resistant to treatment with insulin/ dextrose infusion.
- Bradycardia or heart block associated with hypotension.
- Tachyarrhythmias associated with hypotension, especially ventricular arrhythmias.

Fab antibody fragment administration should be considered in less severe stages of poisoning in older patients and those with pre-existing cardiovascular disease.

The dose of Fab fragments to give can be calculated from either the dose of digoxin ingested or the plasma digoxin concentrations. If in doubt 10 ampoules of Digibind® can be given.

> Number of 40mg vials of Fab =
>
> plasma digoxin concentration (ng/mL) × body weight × 0.0084
>
> *or*
>
> ingested dose (mg) × 1.2
>
> *or*
>
> best guess of 10–20 vials

📖 *OHCM* 8e, p854.

Further reading

Dasgupta A. Therapeutic drug monitoring of digoxin: impact of endogenous and exogenous digoxin-like immunoreactive substances. *Toxicol Rev* 2006; **25**: 273–81.

Flanagan RJ, Jones AL. Fab antibody fragments: some applications in clinical toxicology. *Drug Safety* 2004; **27**: 1115–33.

Ethylene glycol, ethanol, & methanol poisoning

A history of ingestion or the presence of a metabolic acidosis raises suspicion of poisoning with these substances. Calculation of the anion gap and osmolal gaps is helpful in the assessment of such patients.

Anion gap

Calculating the anion gap = $([Na^+] + [K^+]) - ([Cl^-] + [HCO^-_3])$

The normal anion gap is 12 ± 2

Many toxins cause a high anion gap acidosis and these include

- Ethanol.
- Methanol (*Note*: The high anion gap is due to metabolites and may take several hours to develop).
- Ethylene glycol (*Note*: The high anion gap is due to the metabolites and may take 6–24 h to develop).
- Metformin.
- Cyanide.
- Isoniazid.
- Salicylates (aspirin).

This list can be further reduced by measuring the osmolal gap.

Osmolal gap

This is the difference between the laboratory estimation of osmolality (Om) and calculated osmolality (Oc).

Calculating the osmolal gap

The osmolal gap is measured osmolality (Om) minus calculated osmolality (Oc)

$Oc = 2([Na+] + [K+]) + [urea] + [glucose]$

The osmolal gap is normally <10

Toxic causes of a raised osmolal gap include

- Methanol.
- Ethylene glycol.
- Diethylene glycol.
- Isopropanol.
- Ethanol.

The acronym 'MEDIE' can be a helpful mnemonic.

Ethylene glycol and methanol plasma concentrations

Often the diagnosis of ethylene glycol or methanol poisoning can be difficult because assays for these substances are not widely available. If possible, their measurement can help manage severe intoxication. Other parameters may have to be used, i.e. anion gap, osmolal gap, and arterial blood gas analysis. A normal osmolal gap does not exclude poisoning with ethylene glycol or methanol, but if the osmolal gaps and anion gaps are both normal, and the patient is not symptomatic, then significant ingestion is unlikely to have occurred. In general, ethylene glycol or methanol measurements should not be carried out unless metabolic acidosis is present and there is an anion gap.

Ethylene glycol and methanol concentrations in blood are useful to confirm ingestion, and indicate when to stop antidotal treatment (with ethanol or 4-methylpyrazole) and/or when haemodialysis is needed (>500mg/L, 📖 'Indications for haemodialysis in methanol or ethylene glycol poisoning are', p670). However, a low concentration may just mean that most of the parent compound has been metabolized. Formate (i.e. the methanol metabolite) levels can also be checked in patients who may have taken methanol.

Microscopy of urine for oxalate crystals

In suspected ethylene glycol poisoning, microscopy should be performed to look for oxalate crystals. However, they are only present in 50% of cases and often only many hours after ingestion. Treatment of a patient should not be delayed or dependent upon looking for crystals.

Plasma ethanol concentrations

Plasma ethanol concentrations are usually not needed in patients who are drunk unless there is doubt about the diagnosis, e.g. patients with a widening osmolar gap or the patient is so severely poisoned that haemodialysis is being considered for the ethanol poisoning. They are, however, essential to guide appropriate use of ethanol as an antidote in ethylene glycol or methanol poisoning (📖 Ethylene glycol, ethanol, & methanol poisoning, Indications for haemodialysis in methanol or ethylene glycol poisoning p670). Rarely, a plasma ethanol measurement will be needed in child protection cases and such sampling will need chain of custody and a specific (GLC) method by a specialist laboratory. The need for frequent monitoring of ethanol concentrations is avoided by use of the alternative antidote 4-methylpyrazole (a competitive alcohol dehydrogenase antagonist).

Antidotal therapy with ethanol

The dose of ethanol for treatment of ethylene glycol and methanol poisoning can be very difficult to predict because ethanol metabolism is variable and unpredictable. It is therefore important to frequently recheck the blood ethanol concentrations on patients receiving an ethanol infusion. The dose should be adjusted to achieve a blood ethanol concentration of 1–1.5g/L to achieve competitive inhibition of alcohol dehydrogenase.

Indications for continued ethanol therapy are
- Methanol or ethylene glycol poisoning with blood concentrations >200mg/L.
- Metabolic acidosis with pH <7.3.
- Osmolal gap >10mOsmol/kg water.
- Formate concentration >10mg/L.
- Urinary oxalate crystals.
- Severe symptoms.

Indications for haemodialysis in methanol or ethylene glycol poisoning are
- Methanol or ethylene glycol concentration >500mg/L.
- Severe metabolic acidosis (pH <7.3) unresponsive to therapy, i.e. arterial blood gases are needed in all cases of high anion gap poisoning.
- Renal failure—hence, it is essential to check plasma urea and electrolytes in all patients.
- Presence of visual problems in methanol poisoning.
- Formate concentration >500mg/L in methanol poisoning.

▶ Haemodialysis should be continued until the methanol/ethylene glycol concentration is well below 200mg/L.

Further reading
Megarbane B, Borron SW, Baud FJ. Current recommendations for treatment of severe toxic alcohol poisonings. *Intens Care Med* 2005; **31**: 189–95.

Iron

Serum iron concentrations
Serum iron concentrations should be measured urgently in all patients who may have ingested more than 30mg/kg of elemental iron. One 200mg tablet of ferrous sulphate contains 65mg elemental iron. If a sustained-release preparation of iron has been taken, a later serum iron concentration should be taken. A blood sample taken late after ingestion may underestimate the iron as it may have already started distributing to tissues, i.e. in a late presenting patient a low concentration cannot be interpreted, but a high one indicates toxicity. If the antidote desferrioxamine is given before 4 h have elapsed, it interferes with the colorimetric assay for iron and so a serum sample for iron should be taken off before it is given. If atomic absorption spectrophotometry is available for measurement of serum iron, there is no interference from desferrioxamine.

It is essential to interpret the serum iron concentration result in the context of the clinical state of the patient. If <55µmol/L (<300mg/dL), mild toxicity is expected. If above 90µmol/L (500mg/dL), severe toxicity is expected and treatment with desferrioxamine is necessary. Antidotal treatment is also indicated for patients with iron concentrations >55µmol/L if there is additional clinical evidence of toxicity, e.g. gastrointestinal symptoms, leucocytosis, or hyperglycaemia. Antidotal therapy with desferrioxamine is indicated without waiting for the serum iron concentration in patients with severe features (e.g. fitting, unconscious, or hypotensive). Desferrioxamine is usually continued until the urine has returned to a normal colour, symptoms have abated and all radio-opacities of iron tablets on abdominal X-ray have disappeared. Urine free iron estimation is the best test of when to stop chelation therapy with desferrioxamine, but is not widely available.

Working out if the patient needs a serum iron level checked

If a patient has ingested <30mg/kg body weight of elemental iron (a 200mg ferrous sulphate tablet ≡ 65mg elemental iron), then no serum iron level is required. If in doubt a plain abdominal X-ray will usually indicate if lots of tablets are present. A serum concentration of <55μmol/L (<300mg/dL) also indicates low risk (📖 Iron, Serum iron concentrations, p670).

Abdominal X-ray

This is required in patients who have ingested in excess of 30mg elemental iron/kg body weight. The AXR determines the need for gut decontamination either by gastric lavage or whole bowel irrigation with polyethylene glycol. Undissolved tablets appear radio-opaque, but they disappear once dissolved, so the absence of radio-opacities does not exclude the possibility of toxicity.

Full blood count

This is needed in all cases of iron poisoning. A leucocytosis (>15 × 10^9/L) is common with significant toxicity.

Blood glucose

Hyperglycaemia is common in serious poisoning.

Arterial blood gases

These should be checked in symptomatic or severely poisoned patients. Metabolic acidosis is common.

Total iron binding capacity

This has no role in the assessment of acute iron poisoning.

What to do if estimation of serum iron concentration is unavailable

If serum iron assay is not available, the presence of nausea, vomiting, leucocytosis (>15 × 10^9/L) and hyperglycaemia (>8.3mmol/L) suggests significant ingestion and the need for treatment with desferrioxamine.

📖 *OHCM* 8e, p854.

Lead poisoning

Blood lead concentrations

Blood lead concentrations are used to confirm the diagnosis and decide on whether chelation therapy is required. Samples are not 'urgent' (except in the case of suspected acute lead encephalopathy) and must be taken into an ethylenediamine tetra-acetic acid (EDTA) tube. 'Normal' concentrations are <100mcg/L. Lead causes changes in red cell and urinary porphyrins, but these are not measured routinely. A plain AXR should be performed in all children, particularly if there is a history of pica, to exclude ingested paint or lead foreign bodies, such as curtain pulls. Long bone X-rays in children may show lead lines.

Zinc protoporphyrin (ZPP) estimations can be helpful in individuals with moderate (>200 µg/L)–high (>400 µg/L blood lead concentrations in whom one is trying to determine the chronicity of exposure. There is a poor correlation between ZPP and blood lead at lower blood lead concentrations. There are other conditions (e.g. iron deficiency) that can increase ZPP and there is significant inter-individual variation. It has been proposed as a surrogate marker for blood lead but blood lead is the best marker and should not be replaced by ZPP.

There are two agents used for chelation therapy in lead poisoning—intravenous EDTA (disodium calcium edetate) and oral DMSA (2,3-dimercaptosuccinic acid). Before use, chelation therapy should be discussed with a poisons centre. In general patients with a blood lead concentration >450µmg/L should be treated with chelation therapy and removal from further exposure. Children with encephalopathy or a blood lead concentration of >750mcg/L require admission to hospital for urgent chelation therapy.

Other essential investigations

Patients should also have a full blood count and blood film (for basophilic stippling), urea and electrolytes, liver function tests, and serum calcium measured. Patients who are pale should have their serum iron measured as iron deficiency is an important diagnosis. When corrected, it reduces the amount of iron absorbed by the gut.

Lithium

Blood lithium concentration

Lithium is available as sustained-release, non-sustained-release tablets and liquid. After ingestion of liquid preparations, plasma lithium concentrations peak at 30 min. With sustained-release preparations peak concentrations occur at 4–5 h. The plasma half-life is often in excess of 24 h. Interpretation of plasma lithium concentrations depends on the clinical circumstances of exposure (see Acute overdose in lithium naive patient, Chronic excess of lithium, Acute on chronic lithium poisoning). Do not take blood for lithium levels into a lithium heparin tube!

Acute overdose in lithium naive patient

A single overdose in a lithium naive patient is of low risk. However, onset of toxicity may be delayed for as much as 24 h. Samples for lithium assay should be taken at 6 h post-ingestion and measured urgently. Consider haemodialysis if plasma lithium concentration is >7.5mmol/L.

Chronic excess of lithium

Lithium toxicity can occur if the patient has been taking too high a dose, is dehydrated, or if an interaction with thiazide diuretics, non-steroidal anti-inflammatory drugs (NSAIDs), angiotensin converting enzyme (ACE) inhibitors, or tetracycline has occurred. Risk of toxicity is further enhanced by the presence of hypertension, diabetes, cardiac failure, renal failure or schizophrenia. Blood for plasma lithium assay should be taken at presentation. Often good IV hydration suffices to clear the lithium; rarely haemodialysis is needed. Consider haemodialysis if the plasma lithium exceeds 2.5mmol/L.

Acute on chronic lithium poisoning

A patient taking lithium chronically who takes an acute overdose is at risk of serious toxicity, because tissue binding of lithium is already high. The plasma lithium levels should be measured urgently at 6h post-ingestion. Lithium measurements should be repeated 6–12-hourly in symptomatic patients until clinical improvement occurs. Consider haemodialysis if plasma concentrations exceed 4mmol/L.

Indications for haemodialysis

Lithium is effectively removed by haemodialysis. It is indicated in all patients with severe lithium poisoning, i.e. coma, convulsions, respiratory failure or acute renal failure. Plasma lithium concentrations can also guide the need for haemodialysis. Each hour of dialysis will reduce the plasma lithium by 1mmol/L, but plasma lithium often rebounds after haemodialysis so the assay should be repeated at the end of dialysis and again 6–12 h later.

Urea and electrolytes

Hyponatraemia is common in lithium toxicity. It is also important to check the serum potassium concentration and urea, as lithium is renally excreted and renal failure delays its elimination.

Methaemoglobinaemia

Oxidizing agents convert haemoglobin to methaemoglobin (MetHb) and this renders it incapable of carrying oxygen. Common agents causing methaemoglobinaemia include: dapsone, sulphonamides, chlorates, nitrites, nitrates, and local anaesthetic including lidocaine. The onset and duration of symptoms will depend on the agent. Nitrites cause breathlessness and flushing within minutes of exposure, but dapsone may cause a methaemoglobinaemia several hours after ingestion and the methaemo-globinaemia may then persist for days.

Essential investigations

Patients with suspected methaemoglobinaemia should have the following

- Arterial blood gases.
- BC (especially if dapsone has been taken → haemolytic anaemia).
- Blood methaemoglobin concentration.

Methaemoglobin can produce a normal PO_2 in the presence of reduced oxygen saturation. Pulse oximetry measures both methaemoglobin and oxygenated haemoglobin, so can give false results.

Methaemoglobin estimation in blood

Measurement of blood methaemoglobin is required to confirm the diagnosis and assess the severity of poisoning. The measurement must be done urgently when administration of the antidote (methylene blue) is contemplated. Samples for methaemoglobin estimation need to be analysed as soon as possible after collection, as if left to stand around the methaemoglobin will be falsely low owing to a reduction by endogenous methaemoglobin reductase. The severity of symptoms correlates roughly with the measured methaemoglobin concentrations. Anaemia, cardiac or pulmonary disease will lead to more severe symptoms at a lower methaemoglobin level (Table 11.2).

Table 11.2 Clinical effects

MetHb conc. (%)	Clinical effects
0–15	None
15–30	Mild: cyanosis, tiredness, headache, nausea
30–50	Moderate: marked cyanosis, tachycardia, dyspnoea
50–70	Severe: coma, fits, respiratory depression, metabolic acidosis, arrhythmias
>70%	Potentially fatal

If the patient has severe clinical features of toxicity or if the blood methaemoglobin concentration is >30% the patient should be given methylene blue. Methylene blue can be given at lower blood methaemoglobin concentrations in those who are symptomatic.

Opioids

Classic features of opioid poisoning
- Depressed respiration.
- Pin-point pupils.
- Coma.
- Signs of parenteral drug use, e.g. needle marks.

Toxicity can be prolonged for 24–48 h, particularly after ingestion of methadone, which has a long half-life. The life-saving measure is prompt administration of adequate doses of naloxone, before waiting for results of any investigations.

Adequacy of ventilation
Oxygen saturation monitoring and/or arterial blood gas analysis demonstrates the adequacy of ventilation in those whose respiration is depressed, together with the respiratory rate.

Drug screening
Qualitative screening of the urine (group-specific immunoassay) confirms recent use. This may not detect fentanyl derivatives, tramadol, and other synthetic opioids.

Measuring opioids in blood with gas chromatography-mass spectroscopy
This is sometimes required for medicolegal purposes, particularly where a fatality or a child-care issue is involved. Plasma morphine levels as high as 0.3mg/L were observed in addicts taking IV doses of heroin (diamorphine) of 150–200mg. Post-mortem morphine levels in heroin overdose deaths vary depending on prior narcotic history, but in general exceed 0.3mg/L. Following a single oral dose of 15mg of methadone, plasma concentrations peaked at 4 h at 0.075mg/L and declined slowly ($t\frac{1}{2}$ = 15 h) until 24 h when the concentration was still 0.03mg/L. Plasma methadone concentrations in maintenance patients increase by approximately 0.26mg/L for every 1mg/kg increase in oral dose. Deaths are due largely to reduced tolerance and blood concentrations of 0.4–1.8mg/L have been found post-mortem, although live patients with tolerance exceed these values. 8.75mg/70kg IV morphine given to adults produces mean serum concentrations of 0.44mg/L at 0.5 min, with rapid decline to 0.02mg/L by 2 h. Average morphine concentrations in fatalities range from 0.2 to 2.3mg/L, depending on tolerance.

Paracetamol screening
Opioid tablets are frequently combined with paracetamol. All unconscious patients should, therefore, have a plasma paracetamol measured.

Organophosphorus insecticides

Measurement and interpretation of AChE

Measurement of red cell cholinesterase (AChE) is useful in confirmation of exposure to organophosphorus compounds, such as insecticides or nerve warfare agents, where this is suspected, e.g. restlessness, tiredness, headache, nausea, vomiting, diarrhoea, sweating, hypersalivation, chest tightness, miosis, muscle weakness, and fasciculation. In general, clinical features are more helpful than red cell cholinesterase measurements in determining the severity of intoxication and, hence, the prognosis. There is a wide degree of intersubject variation in cholinesterase activity and clinical effects (see Table 11.3).

Table 11.3 Clinical effects

Cholinesterase activity	Clinical effects
Approx. 50% of normal	Subclinical poisoning
20–50% of normal	Mild poisoning
<10% of normal	Severe poisoning

The need for treatment with cholinesterase reactivators, such as pralidoxime is largely judged by the occurrence of convulsions, fasciculation, flaccid paralysis and coma. Such features rapidly reverse within 20–30 min of pralidoxime administration, together with atropine. The need for further therapy is guided by clinical improvement, together with monitoring of cholinesterase activity. It may take 90–120 days for red blood cell cholinesterase to recover to normal values.

Other vital investigations

An ECG should be carried out in all organophosphorus poisoned patients, and urea and electrolytes, and glucose should also be monitored. In those with respiratory embarrassment or muscular paralysis, frequent assessment of tidal volume/peak flow rates and oxygen saturations is essential in anticipating the need for intubation.

📖 OHCM 8e, p855.

Paracetamol (acetaminophen) poisoning

Overview

▶▶ Paracetamol is the most common drug taken in overdose in the UK. Measurement of a plasma paracetamol concentration is essential for assessing the need for antidotal treatment within 16 h of a paracetamol overdose and should be performed urgently in all patients with known or suspected paracetamol overdose. It can be measured by a variety of assay methods, but HPLC is less susceptible to interference than some enzyme-based assays. It should also be done urgently in patients with undiagnosed coma, or where a history is unreliable. Routine measurement of para-cetamol concentrations in awake patients who deny taking paracetamol is unnecessary. For most patients, only a single measurement of paracetamol concentration is indicated. It is important to err on the side of caution and to give the antidote N-acetylcysteine if the blood paracetamol concentra-tion lies near or just below the treatment line (Fig. 11.1) as stated timing of the overdose may be inaccurate and other agents such as opioids may slow gastric emptying.

If N-acetylcysteine is given within 12 h of the overdose, it provides complete protection against liver injury and renal failure. Beyond 12 h after ingestion the protection is less complete and assessment of liver damage is required. Paracetamol poisoning can be deceptive, as there is a latent phase of many hours, where the patient remains well before liver damage develops.

INR/PT

The most sensitive marker of prognosis in paracetamol poisoning is the prothrombin time (PT) or INR. This often starts to increase within 24–36 h of the overdose and peaks at 48–72 h. Once the INR/PT starts to improve, this is a sign that hepatotoxicity is starting to improve and the patient will not go on to develop acute liver failure. Approximately half of patients with a PT of 36 s at 36 h post-ingestion will develop acute liver failure.

Plasma alanine and aspartate aminotransferases (ALT and AST)

These may begin to rise as early as 12 h post-ingestion but usually peak at 72–96 h. AST or ALT values in excess of 10,000IU/L are not unusual and a plasma ALT>5000IU/L is very suggestive of paracetamol poisoning (Fig. 11.2). Serum bilirubin may peak after the aminotransferase and this should not lead to concern for patients in whom the INR or PT have begun to fall.

▶▶ Do not correct abnormalities in PT or INR with FFP, or cryopre-cipitate unless life-threatening bleeding is taking place; otherwise the most sensitive marker of how the patient is progressing will be lost.

Other blood test abnormalities in paracetamol poisoning

Hypoglycaemia and metabolic acidosis are common. Early metabolic acidosis is often associated with very high plasma paracetamol concentrations, e.g. >400mg/L. Later, development of acidosis indicates incipient acute liver failure and the need to urgently check ABGs, liver function tests and INR/PT.

Pancreatitis with ↑ serum amylase has been reported. Five cases of thrombocytopenia have been reported.

Renal failure can occur in the context of hepatic failure, but also in its absence (in 1 in 100 patients). It is treated with N-acetylcysteine and supportive measures, e.g. haemodialysis, if needed. Full recovery with supportive care is common.

Investigating the patient who has taken a paracetamol overdose <4 h ago

Ingestion of >150mg/kg paracetamol or a paracetamol-containing product should be recognized as a hepatotoxic dose for most people. If ingestion of this amount or more has occurred within the last 1 h, activated charcoal should be given orally (50g for an adult). Chronic alcohol ingestion (>14 units per week for ♀, >21 units per week for ♂), regular use of enzyme-inducing drugs (e.g. anticonvulsants) or the presence of eating disorders have been reported to reduce the ceiling of toxicity of paracetamol to 75mg/kg.

A plasma paracetamol should then be checked at 4h from the time of ingestion, to determine the need for N-acetylcysteine treatment from the treatment curve (Fig. 11.1). Very rarely, e.g. after ingestion of 4 × 500mg tablets by an adult, a confirmatory plasma paracetamol level is not needed, but in general it is cheap (approx £1) and safer to be certain by checking a blood concentration.

Investigating the patient who has taken a paracetamol overdose between 4 and 8 h ago

A plasma paracetamol level should be checked as soon as possible to determine the need for N-acetylcysteine antidote treatment from the treatment curve (Fig. 11.1). ▶▶ Use high-risk treatment line for patient with induced enzymes (e.g. anticonvulsants) or glutathione depletion (e.g. eating disorders).

Investigating the patient who has taken a paracetamol overdose between 8 and 24 h ago

Start treatment with N-acetylcysteine straight away. Take blood for a paracetamol level, INR/PT, creatinine, and plasma venous bicarbonate (if plasma venous bicarbonate is abnormal, check arterial blood gases). Check results and refer to graph to determine whether treatment with N-acetylcysteine needs to be continued (i.e. is the plasma level above the treatment line?) or can be stopped (below the line). ▶▶ Beyond 16 h after ingestion the sensitivity of the assay for paracetamol may be too low to detect a treatable level—check and, if in doubt, treat the patient with N-acetylcysteine! On completion of N-acetylcysteine, check blood INR/PT, creatinine, and plasma venous bicarbonate (if abnormal check ABGs). If the patient is asymptomatic and the INR or creatinine is normal or falling discontinue the N-acetylcysteine. If the patient has symptoms (abdominal pain or vomiting) or the INR or creatinine is rising, continue maintenance N-acetylcysteine (50mg/kg in 500mL dextrose every 4h) until the INR improves. ▶▶ Contact a poisons centre/liver unit.

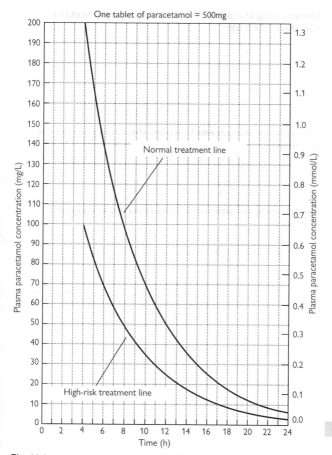

Fig. 11.1 *N*-acetylcysteine treatment graph. Patients whose plasma paracetamol concentrations are above the **normal treatment line** should be treated with acetylcysteine by IVI (or, provided the overdose has been taken **within 10–12 h**, with methionine by mouth). Patients on enzyme-inducing drugs (e.g. carbamazepine, phenobarbitone, phenytoin, rifampicin and alcohol) or who are malnourished (e.g. in anorexia, in alcoholism, or those who are HIV-positive) should be treated if their plasma paracetamol concentrations are above the **high-risk treatment line**. *Note:* if paracetamol ingestion has been staggered (over some hours) serum levels may mislead: treat regardless, if significant amounts have been taken. Reproduced with permission from Dr Alun Hutchings and the *Oxford Handbook of Clinical Medicine*, 5th edition, Oxford University Press.

Investigating the patient who has taken a paracetamol overdose >24 h ago

It is too late for plasma paracetamol level estimation to be of any value. Start treatment with the antidote *N*-acetylcysteine straight away, unless a trivial amount has been taken. Take blood for baseline INR/PT, creatinine and venous bicarbonate (if abnormal check ABGs).

If the patient is asymptomatic and the lab tests normal, discharge the patient and advise to return if vomiting/abdominal pain develops. If the blood results are abnormal, phone a liver unit/poisons centre for advice.

Investigating the patient in whom the timing of overdose is unknown

Err on the side of treating the patient with the antidote *N*-acetylcysteine, checking an INR/PT, creatinine, plasma venous bicarbonate (ABGs if abnormal) at baseline and at the end of the first full course of treatment. If abnormal contact liver unit/poisons centre for further advice.

Investigating the patient who has taken a staggered overdose

Determine if the patient is in an at-risk group (i.e. enzyme induction or glutathione depletion) as discussed above. If the patient is not in an at-risk group but has ingested >150mg/kg body weight over 24 h they should receive a full course of IV *N*-acetylcysteine. If they are in an 'at-risk' group and have ingested more than 75mg/kg body weight of paracetamol over 24 h, they should receive a full course of *N*-acetylcysteine. There is no point measuring a plasma paracetamol level in this group of patients, unless the substance ingested is in doubt and a 'not detected' result may be falsely reassuring. At admission and at the end of the course of *N*-acetylcystine a blood INR/PT, creatinine, and venous bicarbonate should be checked. If abnormal at any stage, consult the poisons centre/liver unit.

📖 *OHCM* 8e, pp854–5.

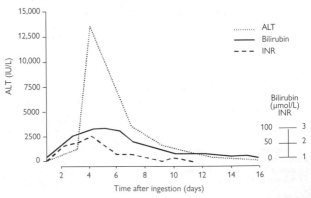

Fig. 11.2 Time course of liver function tests in paracetamol poisoning.

Salicylate[*] poisoning

Features of severe poisoning

Ingestion of >150, 250, and 500mg/kg body weight of aspirin, respectively, produces mild, moderate, and severe poisoning, respectively. Signs of serious salicylate poisoning include metabolic acidosis, renal failure and CNS effects such as agitation, confusion, coma, and convulsions. Death may occur as a result of CNS depression and cardiovascular collapse.

▶▶ The development of metabolic acidosis is a bad prognostic sign as it also indicates increased CSF transfer of salicylate.

Plasma salicylate concentration

Plasma salicylate should be measured urgently in all, but the most trivial overdose, i.e. all those thought to have ingested >150mg/kg of aspirin or any amount of oil of wintergreen. It should be performed at 4 h post-ingestion, because delayed absorption of the drug renders such levels uninterpretable before this time. As salicylates may form concretions in the stomach, which delay absorption, it is recommended that a salicylate level is rechecked 3–4 h after the first sample, to catch the peak salicylate concentration. There is no evidence for indiscriminate requesting of salicylate concentrations in every unconscious patient (unlike paracetamol), or in conscious patients who deny taking aspirin and who have no features suggesting salicylate toxicity. The plasma salicylate concentration is not an absolute guide to toxicity, as paracetamol levels are in paracetamol poisoning, but should be interpreted together with clinical features and acid–base status of the patient.

Urinary alkalinization (📖 OHCM 8e, p856) is indicated for patients with salicylate concentrations of 600–800mg/L in adults and 450–700mg/L in children and the elderly. Metabolic alkalosis is not a contraindication to bicarbonate therapy as patients may have high base deficit in spite of an elevated serum pH.

Haemodialysis is very effective at salicylate removal, and correction of acid–base and electrolyte abnormalities. It should be considered if the plasma salicylate levels are >700mg/L in children and >800mg/L in adults. Other indications for haemodialysis include resistant metabolic acidosis, severe CNS effects, such as coma, convulsions, pulmonary oedema, and acute renal failure.

Arterial blood gases

Acid–base problems are common in salicylate poisoning. Respiratory centre stimulation causes respiratory alkalosis. Uncoupled oxidative phosphorylation and interruption of glucose and fatty acid metabolism by salicylates often causes a concurrent metabolic acidosis. Serial ABGs are needed in severe salicylate poisoning.

[*]Aspirin, oil of Wintergreen.

Theophylline

Acute theophylline poisoning can carry a high mortality and its management is best guided by the Shannon severity grading scheme,[1] bearing in mind that delayed effects tend to occur after sustained-release formulations have been ingested. The adult therapeutic range is 10–20mg/L. Serious toxicity occurs at >100mg/L (770mmol/L).

Urea and electrolytes

It is vital to check the plasma K^+ concentration frequently, as hypokalaemia is a life-threatening complication and the serum K^+ concentration is a useful guide to severity. If >2.5mmol/L the patient is less severely poisoned (grade 1) than if it falls <2.5mmol/L (grade 2). Check blood glucose since hyperglycaemia is a common complication.

Arterial blood gases

In potentially serious poisoning (e.g. ingestion of >20mg/kg body weight) ABG analysis is helpful in optimizing the acid–base status of the patient. An initial phase of hyperventilation with respiratory alkalosis can be followed by a further stage of metabolic acidosis.

Plasma theophylline concentrations

Measuring plasma theophylline concentrations confirms theophylline ingestion where this is in doubt and is usually undertaken by HPLC. It is also helpful in deciding when to employ charcoal haemoperfusion in seriously poisoned patients, particularly if plasma concentrations are >100mg/L (770mmol/L). Charcoal haemoperfusion can be considered at lower concentration, e.g. 80mg/L, in the elderly or those with pre-existing ischaemic heart disease. Charcoal haemoperfusion can also be decided on the basis of grade 3 or 4 severity grading alone, especially if administration of multiple doses of activated charcoal is not possible. However, for the vast majority of poisoned patients, obtaining a plasma theophylline concentration does not guide their management.

Therapeutic levels rarely exceed 20mg/L (155mmol/L). Theophylline peak concentration in plasma may occur at 1–3 h after ingestion of a standard-release formulation. However, overdose is often with sustained-release products and delayed absorption can result in delayed peak plasma concentration and toxicity, often 12–24 h later.

Urine testing for myoglobinuria & measuring serum creatine kinase

Theophylline poisoning can be accompanied by rhabdomyolysis. Hence, the urine should be dip-sticked and if found positive for blood a serum CK should be obtained. This will then indicate that renal function should be closely monitored and the urine should undergo alkalinization.

1 Shannon M. Predictors of major toxicity after theophylline overdose. *Ann Intern Med* 1993; **119**, 1161–7.

Tricyclic antidepressants

The main risks of overdose with these drugs are cardiovascular system (CVS) and CNS toxicity.

Electrocardiogram

An ECG should be performed in all but the most trivial cases of overdose.

ECG abnormalities are common in moderate–severe poisoning and include

- **QRS prolongation**: >110 ms in adults predicts the risk of ventricular cardiac arrhythmias (and the need for IV sodium bicarbonate) and QRS >160 ms predicts the risk of fits. In children a QRS >110 ms is predictive of the risk of arrhythmias, but not fits.
- *Note*: ECG criteria are not the only factors assessing risk of arrhythmias, fits, and acidosis—electrolyte disturbances contribute. Supraventricular and potentially fatal ventricular arrhythmias can occur.

Cardiac monitoring

This is essential if ingestion of >10mg/kg body weight has taken place. It is seldom necessary beyond 24 h after ingestion.

Arterial blood gas analyses

These should be done on all patients with marked symptoms and signs, particularly those with a reduced Glasgow Coma Score. It should also be performed on those with widened QRS or seizures, not least because such patients are receiving intravenous sodium bicarbonate therapy and a pH of 7.5 should not be exceeded.

Plasma concentrations

This is of no value as plasma concentrations of tricyclic antidepressants correlate poorly with clinical features of toxicity.

Table of conversion factors between mass & molar units

See Table 11.4.

Table 11.4 Conversion factors between mass and molecular units

Drug	Mass units	Molar (SI) units	Conversion factor
Carbamazepine	mg/L	µmol/L	4.23
Digoxin	mg/L or ng/mL	nmol/L	1.28
Ethanol	g/L	mmol/L	1.28
Iron	mg/L	mmol/L	0.179
Lead	mg/L	mmol/L	0.0048
Paracetamol	mg/L	mmol/L	0.0066
Phenytoin	mg/L	mmol/L	3.96
Salicylate (aspirin)	mg/L	mmol/L	0.0072
Theophylline	mg/L	mmol/L	7.7

Rheumatology

Rheumatological investigations

Investigations in rheumatology are important not only in diagnosis, but also in assessing disease activity and monitoring treatment. They are complementary to a careful history and physical examination, and should only be requested in the correct clinical context where results are likely to affect management. In isolation, 'abnormal' results can lead to unwarranted anxiety, investigations and treatment.

Inflammatory markers

Inflammatory rheumatic disease is usually associated with an acute phase response. This is reflected in blood tests by raised markers of inflammation. The most commonly used are erythrocyte sedimentation rate (ESR), which is a good screening test for the presence of an acute phase response and C-reactive protein (CRP), a common reactant. They are entirely non-specific and alternative causes for their elevation, e.g. infection, should always be considered. Conversely, a normal ESR or CRP does not exclude rheumatic disease, e.g. psoriatic arthritis.

Erythrocyte sedimentation rate

ESR is measured by observing how fast red blood cells fall through a column of blood in 1 h. It is dependent upon many variables including serum immunoglobulins, fibrinogen, and haematocrit. Therefore, raised ESR may not reflect inflammation, but other factors, e.g. hypergammaglobulinaemia. Normal ESR levels also increase with age. In some centres plasma viscosity is preferred as a screening for acute phase response rather than ESR as it is independent of age, sex and Hb (📖 Erythrocyte sedimentation rate, p233).

C-reactive protein

CRP production is driven by interleukin-1 (IL-1) and IL-6 on hepatocytes. It generally provides a more accurate reflection of inflammatory or infective processes than ESR as it changes more rapidly and is independent of the variables that complicate ESR interpretation.

ESR and CRP in diagnosis and monitoring

Although ESR or CRP are not specific, the degree of elevation and relationship of ESR to CRP may suggest a diagnosis. For example CRP and ESR may be very high in infection and gout but are usually only moderately raised in rheumatoid arthritis (RhA; Table 12.1). Isolated elevation of CRP may also reflect systemic amyloidosis where there has been longstanding inflammation or infection.

In cases where ESR/CRP are increased in active disease, they are extremely useful in monitoring disease activity and response to treatment.

Other acute phase markers

In general, it is not helpful to measure other acute phase reactants, e.g. caeruloplasmin, α-1-antitrypsin, fibrinogen, and haptoglobin. Two exceptions are serum ferritin and complement, which can be useful in diagnosis. Other common biochemical and haematological tests discussed below also reflect levels of inflammation e.g. albumin and Hb fall whilst alkaline phosphatase (ALP) and gamma glutamyl transferase (GGT) rise.

Serum ferritin

Although primarily used as a surrogate marker to assess body iron stores ferritin is also an acute phase reactant. In the presence of active inflammation or infection a normal or high serum ferritin may be found even if the patient has true iron deficiency (Assessment of iron status, p226). Serum ferritin may be particularly helpful in the diagnosis of adult Still's disease, where levels can be very high. Elevated ferritin is also seen in haemachromatosis arthropathy.

Complement

Complement components C3 and C4 usually rise in the presence of active inflammation or infection. However in systemic lupus erythematosis (SLE) they are commonly low. In some, but not all, SLE patients they are abnormal when disease is active and normalize on treatment, making them useful in monitoring disease activity, especially lupus nephritis. Low levels of C1 can be associated with development of SLE.

Table 12.1 ESR and CRP in diagnosis

Diagnosis	ESR	CRP
Infection	++ or +++	++ or +++
Malignancy	Normal to ++	Normal to +
Rheumatoid arthritis	++	++
SLE*	+	Normal to +
SLE with serositis	+	Normal to ++
Gout/CPPD**	++ or +++	++ or +++
Sjogrens Syndrome	+ or ++	+
Vasculitis	++ or +++	++ or +++
Osteoarthritis	Normal	Normal
Psoriatic arthritis/spondyloarthropathy	Normal to ++	Normal to ++

*Systemic Lupus Erythematosus ** Calcium Pyrophosphate Disease

Haematology

Haemoglobin

There are three common scenarios for anaemia ($\downarrow$ Hb) in patients with rheumatic symptoms.

- Often it is 'anaemia of chronic disease'.
- It may be a manifestation of an underlying systemic disorder that presents with arthralgia (e.g. coeliac disease/leukaemia).
- It may be a result of drug side-effects e.g. gastrointestinal (GI) bleeding due to non-steroidal anti-inflammatory drugs or pancytopenia caused by immunosuppressive agents (e.g. methotrexate).

The degree and type of anaemia, as well as changes in level should therefore be assessed, taking into account the global clinical picture. Trends in haemoglobin (Hb) are useful in monitoring disease activity and treatment.

Microcytic hypochromic anaemia

The major differential diagnoses are:

- Chronic iron deficiency anaemia.
- Thalassaemia trait.
- Anaemia of chronic disease (typically associated with normal mean cell volume (MCV), but if *chronic* the MCV may reduce).

Iron deficiency related to acute or chronic blood loss (e.g. due to non-steroidal anti-inflammatory drugs (NSAID) ingestion), nutritional or 1° bowel disease, such as Crohn's disease or coeliac-related arthritis, should be considered.

Macrocytic anaemia

Vitamin B_{12} or folate deficiency related to nutritional deficiency, e.g. scleroderma causing jejunal diverticulosis, Whipple's disease causing malabsorption, or due to drug therapy, such as methotrexate, sulphasalazine, and azathioprine. Excessive alcohol consumption may also cause macrocytosis without significant anaemia.

Normocytic normochromic anaemia

Usually reflects chronic disease and the degree of anaemia may vary with the severity of the disease, e.g. RhA, crystal arthritis, vasculitis.

Dimorphic anaemia (large and small red cells)

This picture is seen in mixed deficiency, e.g. iron deficiency + vitamin B_{12} or folate deficiency, post-transfusion, or during iron replacement therapy in a patient with iron deficiency. A feature of malabsorption associated with coeliac related arthritis, scleroderma of the gut, and jejunal bypass arthritis.

White cell count

White cell count may be helpful in diagnosis and monitoring disease activity in certain circumstances, and is essential for monitoring immunosuppressive therapies. Diagnoses to consider where levels are elevated/decreased levels are listed.

Increased
- **Neutrophilia**: septic arthritis, crystal arthropathy (gout and pseudogout), and systemic corticosteroid administration.
- **Lymphocytosis**: consider lymphocytic leukaemia with joint symptoms and viral infection.
- **Eosinophilia**: Churg–Strauss syndrome and other 1° vasculitides, hypereosinophilic syndromes, eosinophilic fasciitis, and also Addison's disease (can complicate rheumatological diseases). Newly raised eosinophils should heighten awareness of potential adverse reactions to disease modifying drugs.

Reduced
- **Neutropenia**: consider autoimmune neutropenia, e.g. associated with SLE and Felty's syndrome in RhA. May be drug-induced (especially sulfasalazine, methotrexate, azathioprine, cyclophosphamide, ciclosporin, mycophenolate, leflunomide, and other cytotoxics).
- **Lymphopenia**: is common in SLE.

Platelet count
- *Thrombocytosis*: Reflects active inflammation e.g. RhA, or can be due to underlying polycythaemia rubra vera (associated with gout).
- *Thrombocytopenia*: Autoimmune thrombocytopenia, may also be related to connective tissue disease including SLE, RhA (Felty's Syndrome) and 1° antiphospholipid syndrome (APS).
- Can also reflect drug toxicity including those listed under neutropenia.

Biochemistry tests

Although biochemical tests do play a role in the diagnosis of rheumatic disease in some cases (e.g. metabolic bone disease) their major use is in the assessment of systemic involvement of disease, e.g. renal or hepatic. In addition they are essential for monitoring treatment.

Renal function

Renal function is measured in the diagnosis and monitoring of systemic disease. A wide range of diseases may involve the kidney including vasculitis, SLE, Sjogren's syndrome, and gout.

Dose of immunosuppressive treatments should be adjusted according to renal function e.g. cyclophosphamide, ciclosporin, methotrexate. Drug treatment should also be considered as a reversible cause for decline in renal function in rheumatology patients, e.g. NSAIDs, sulphasalazine.

Uric acid

90% cases of gout will have a raised serum urate. However it may also be elevated in normal health and be increased by diuretic treatment. Definitive diagnosis can only be made by identification of urate crystals by polarizing light microscopy of joint fluid or in biopsy.

γ-globulins

γ-globulins are often elevated in active inflammatory disease. They are usually globally increased in Sjögren's syndrome, but may also be raised in RhA, sarcoidosis, SLE, and other connective disease.

Liver function tests

These are measured in the monitoring of many disease modifying agents, e.g. methotrexate and sulphasalazine. Elevated GGT and ALP can reflect also reflect active inflammation. They may be relevant in considering underlying diagnoses of arthralgia, e.g. haemachromatosis.

Bone function

Serum calcium

Hypercalcaemia should raise suspicion of malignancy, metabolic bone disease, and sarcoidosis. In metabolic bone disease/hyperparathyroidism calcium is not always elevated and a 'high normal' result may be significant in the correct clinical context. Hypocalcaemia may indicate hypoparathyroidism (Ⅲ Hypercalcaemia, p176; Ⅲ Hypercalcaemia/osteomalacia, p178).

Alkaline phosphatase

ALP may be elevated due to bone, liver, or GI disease. If GGT is concomitantly raised one would suspect it originates from the liver. In isolation it is more likely to be related to bone and further investigation, e.g. parathyroid hormone (PTH), vitamin D, urinary calcium should be considered. ALP is high in Paget's disease, hyperparathyroidism, fractures, and bony mets. Low ALP may be the only biochemical clue to hypophosphatasia.

Phosphate

Hypophosphataemia occurs in hyperparathyroidism, hereditary, and acquired hypophosphatasia.

Serum parathyroid

Where bone biochemistry is abnormal, PTH should be measured. It is elevated in hyperparathyroidism and vitamin D deficiency. In cases of hypocalcaemia, low PTH suggests 1° parathyroid disease whereas normal or raised PTH suggests PTH resistance (Ⅲ Hypercalcaemia, p176; Ⅲ Hypercalcaemia/osteomalacia, p178).

Urine calcium

Urinary calcium is useful in the investigation of hypercalcaemia and elevated PTH. In hyperparathyroidism urinary excretion is increased. If it is low, familial hypocalciuric hypercalcaemia should be considered. Hypercalciuria may also be associated with renal calculi.

Autoantibodies

Autoantibody tests are an integral part of rheumatological investigation. Detection of antibodies against specific antigens is useful for both diagnostic and prognostic purposes and occasional monitoring disease activity. However, these tests have their limitations. Most autoantibodies are not specifically associated with a single diagnosis, but can occur in a range of diseases and in healthy individuals.

Rheumatoid factor

Rheumatoid factor (RF) is an antibody to Fc portion of IgG immunoglobulins, forming immune complexes, first described in the 1940s. Although included in the American College of Rheumatology criteria for rheumatology RF it is not specific to RhA. It can be found in 4–16% healthy individuals (prevalence increases with age). It may also be positive in other autoimmune diseases, malignancy and chronic infection. However the rheumatoid arthritis particle agglutination test (RAPA) remains useful in confirming a diagnosis of rheumatoid disease in the presence of an appropriate clinical picture of symmetrical inflammatory polyarthritis. A high titre, e.g. 1:320 is of more relevance than a borderline result, e.g. 1:20. It is less helpful in early diagnosis compared to established disease with RF being positive in around one-third of rheumatoid patients at three months post diagnosis and two thirds at 6 months.

Anti-cyclic citrullinated peptide antibodies

The importance of anti- cyclic citrullinated peptide (CCP) antibodies in the diagnosis of RhA is being increasingly recognized. First described in 1998, they are high affinity IgG class antibodies that react with the amino-acid citrulline and measured by enzyme-linked immunosorbant assay (ELISA). They are found in sera of about 75% rheumatoid patients and are about 96% specific for RhA. They appear earlier than RF, are unaffected by treatment and predict the development of erosions.

Anti-nuclear factor

Antinuclear antibodies (ANA), commonly detected by ELISA, is often thought of as a screening test for SLE or other connective tissue disease. Although ANA is positive in 99% case of lupus it is not specific and can be positive in numerous situations including healthy individuals, hepatic disease, e.g. 1° biliary cirrhosis, pulmonary disease, e.g. 1° pulmonary hypertension, chronic infections, malignancy, or may be drug-induced. It should, therefore, be interpreted only in the context of clinical symptoms.

The fluorescent ANA test is another method of detecting ANA and results may be present as patterns of fluorescence, e.g. homogenous, speckled, nucleolar. Although not specific some clinicians may use these in determining relevance of the test, e.g a strong positive homogenous ANA is more likely to be associated with SLE than a weak speckled pattern.

Anti-DNA antibody (dsDNA)

In contrast to ANA antibodies, double-stranded DNA (dsDNA) is less sensitive (50–80% cases), but highly specific for SLE. They are seen only exceptionally rarely in healthy individuals and rarely in disorders, such as chronic active hepatitis and Sjögren's syndrome. Therefore, they are thought to be virtually diagnostic for lupus erythematosus. They are also useful in monitoring disease activity in some, but not all individuals with SLE.

Extractable nuclear antigen antibodies (ENA)

Where ANA is positive ENA antibodies should be measured as there presence can indicate certain clinical scenario.

- **Anti-Ro and anti-La (SSB)**: occur in Sjogren's syndrome and SLE, but also other autoimmune diseases. They have been associated with fetal heart-block when they are present in the mother.
- **Anti-Scl-70 and anti-centromere antibodies**: these antibodies are associated with scleroderma. Anticentromere is particularly associated with limited cutaneous scleroderma and anti-Scl-70 with diffuse systemic sclerosis. They may be a marker of pulmonary hypertension.
- **Anti-Jo-1 antibodies**: a marker of polymyositis.
- **Anti-RNP antibodies**: have been associated with 'mixed connective tissue disease' where features of several clinical syndromes can occur in combination.
- **Anti-histone antibodies**: have been associated with drug-induced lupus.

Antiphospholipid antibodies

Primary antiphospholipid syndrome (thrombosis, thrombocytopenia, and fetal loss) and other connective tissue diseases are associated with APL antibodies. They should only be requested in the correct clinical context as they can also be detected in normal health. IgG and IgM anti-cardinolipin antibodies (ACL) are most commonly measured, via ELISA. A single positive result should be interpreted with caution and the test should be repeated after 6 weeks to determine relevance. A high titre ACL antibody and IgG ACL may be of greater clinical relevance.

VDRL tests and lupus anticoagulant are also available although less specific for APS.

Anti-β2-glycoprotein is not commonly available, but has been investigated in specialist centres in an attempt to improve disease characterization.

Anti-neutrophil cytoplasmic antibody (ANCA)

First described in 1982 classical ANCA (cANCA) gives a characteristic bright central granular cytoplasmic staining of ethanol-fixed human neutrophils by immunofluorescence (IIF). pANCA was later described to give a perinuclear IIF pattern. ELISA is used to identify antigen-specific ANCA and proteinase 3 (PR3) and myeloperoxidase (MPO) are now usually tested routinely.

ANCA is often thought to be a screening test for vasculitis. Indeed the presence of c ANCA and PR3 in combination has been reported to be 99% specific (and ~55% sensitive) for Wegener's Granulomatosis. Similarly

(~ 90% specific) the presence of p ANCA and MPO together is associated with microscopic polyangiitis. However like other autoantibodies ANCA (especially p ANCA) may be positive in many other situations including infection, malignancy and inflammatory bowel disease. Therefore the full clinical picture must be used in making treatment decisions and reliance should not be put on ANCA alone.

HLA B27

HLA B27 has been strongly associated with ankylosing spondylitis (present in 90% patients) and is also linked to other diseases, including reactive arthritis, inflammatory bowel disease, and uveitis. However, as it occurs in about 8% of the population it is not helpful as a screening test in such a common symptom as back pain (approximately two-thirds of HLA B27 positive individuals with back pain would not have ankylosing spondylitis).

Reactive and infection related arthritis

Where reactive arthritis is suspected appropriate serology and swabs should be sent. These may include anti streptolysin O titre and anti-DNAse for streptococcus, serology for *Campylobacter*, *Salmonella*, *Yersinia*, and Epstein–Barr virus (EBV), stool samples for culture and urethral swab for *Chlamydia*. Investigations chosen and results depend upon clinical presentation. Where an infection related arthritis is suspected specific investigations should be requested, e.g. Borrelia for lyme disease, leptospirosis for Weils disease, etc.

Urinalysis

Where systemic disease is a possibility, e.g. vasculitis and SLE urinalysis should be tested both in diagnosis and routine monitoring of disease. The presence of red blood cells and casts are early indicators of renal disease. Proteinuria in long-standing inflammatory disease should raise the suspicion of amyloidosis.

Urinalysis is also used in monitoring of drugs including gold, ciclosporin, and penicillamine.

Arthrocentesis

This refers to the aspiration of fluid from a joint. Examination of the fluid can be helpful in diagnosis and is essential in septic arthritis, crystal arthropathy, and haemarthrosis. Where infection is excluded, the joint may be therapeutically injected with steroid (e.g. Depo-Medrone® or trimancinolone).

Synovial fluid examination

Physical characteristics

Observation of the colour and consistency of synovial fluid is helpful in diagnosis. In general inflammatory arthritis, e.g. sepsis/RhA/gout, is associated with turbid fluid with low viscosity whilst osteoarthritis or normal joint fluid is clear with higher viscosity. Crystal arthropathies are often associated with blood stained fluid.

Microscopy

White cell count and % polymorphonuclear cells should be measured in synovial fluid. They are higher in inflammatory arthritis e.g. RhA (5000–75,000/mm^3, >50%) and septic arthritis (>50,000/mm^3, >75%) than normal (<200/mm^3, <25%) or osteoarthritis (200–10,000/mm^3, <50%). A Gram stain and culture should be performed to detect organisms in suspected septic arthritis. Culture for less common organisms such as tuberculosis may also need to be considered.

Polarized light microscopy should be used to detect the presence of crystals. Urate is associated with characterisitic negatively birefringent crystals whilst calcium pyrophosphate crystals are positively birefringent. Other crystals may also be observed, e.g. hydroxyapatite in Milwaukee shoulder.

Arthroscopy

Arthroscopy and synovial biopsy may occasionally be required for the diagnosis of chronic indolent infections, such as tuberculosis, or unusual slow growing organisms, such as *Coxiella* (fever polyarthritis). Arthroscopy is essentially a diagnostic procedure used by orthopaedic surgeons where direct visualization of the affected joint is required.[1]

---

1 ℰ www.orthoinfo.aaos.org/

Neurophysiology

These are dynamic electrical nerve and muscle tests that are performed in the context of appropriate clinical history and examination. They may be considered in rheumatology include:

- Assessment of muscle disorders, e.g. to distinguish inflammatory muscle disease (polymyositis/dermatomyositis) and other 1° muscle disease, e.g. muscular dystrophy.
- Where mononeuritis multiplex/peripheral neuropathy is suspected as part of a rheumatological diagnosis, e.g. vasculitis, RhA, amyloidosis.
- Nerve entrapment syndromes, e.g. carpal tunnel syndrome, tarsal tunnel, or ulnar nerve compression where clinical diagnosis is uncertain.
- Spinal cord/nerve root compression.

Diagnostic imaging

Imaging techniques are essential tools in the management of rheumatological conditions and are useful if performed under appropriate indications. It is not a substitute for clinical examination and findings should be interpreted in the context of clinical abnormalities. It is important to follow the guidelines for radiological investigations published by the Royal College of Radiologists.

Inflammatory arthritis

It is important to diagnose inflammatory arthritis as early as possible as timely treatment with disease modifying anti-rheumatic drugs improves outcomes in terms of function, joint damage, quality of life, and costs to health service usage. Although conventional X-rays can be useful in diagnosis, this is generally only when disease is established and structural damage to the joints has already occurred. The challenge to identify early arthritis has led to wider spread use of alternative imaging techniques including musuloskeletal ultrasound and magnetic resonance imaging (MRI).

Plain radiography

Arthropathy

Hand and feet radiographs are useful in diagnosis. Soft tissue changes can show swelling, effusions, and specific abnormalities, such as calcification, which can be helpful even in early disease. Bony changes occur in more established arthritis. The pattern and type of radiological damage can suggest diagnosis. (Table 12.2) and serial films can be used to assess disease progression. Other findings may suggest specific diseases, e.g. calcinosis in limited cutaneous scleroderma and chondrocalcinosis in calcium pyrophosphate disease.

Radiographs of the lumbar spine and sacroiliac joints may be utilized in distinguishing mechanical and inflammatory (e.g. ankylosing spondylitis/ psoriatic arthritis) back pain. Changes seen in inflammatory back disease include sacroiliitis (sclerosis and joint space loss), squaring of the vertebrae, bony proliferation along vertebrae (syndesmophytes), and spondylodiscitis. However, changes do not occur early in disease and it can be difficult to distinguish changes from degenerative disease (osteophytes, loss of disc height). Evidence of bony change elsewhere, e.g. enthesitis is helpful in diagnosis. Isotope bone scan or MRI may be appropriate further investigations.

Other joints should be imaged according to an individual's clinical needs. For example, a knee or hip would be required if joint replacement surgery may be appropriate, a shoulder if calcific tendinitis is considered. Plain radiography is also useful in assessing complications of rheumatic disease, e.g. rheumatoid lung disease. Limitations of plain films are that only limited information is provided about soft tissues and bone texture and early joint damage is missed.

Bone lesions

Osteopenia should be further investigated with dual-energy X-ray absorptiometry (DXA) scanning (below) and appropriate blood tests e.g. PTH, immunoglobulins and vitamin D. Underlying diagnosis can be suggested by typical bony appearances e.g. Looser's zones are lucent lines visualized at

90° to the bony cortex in osteomalacia (vitamin D deficiency). Periosteal reactions and, in more advanced disease, bone resorption, can be seen in hyperparathyroidism and renal osteodystrophy. Hypertrophic osteoarthropathy is another cause of periostitis, which can signify underlying disease e.g bronchial carcinoma.

Sclerotic bone lesions (increased bone density) can also be seen in renal osteodystrophy.

Paget's disease is characterized by focal excessive bone resorption (osteolytic phase) followed by excessive bone formation (osteoblastic phase). Radiological features are of radiolucent areas associated with bone widening, then subsequent coarsening of trabeculae and areas of increased radiodensity/sclerosis. In advanced disease there may be bowing of the bone, pathological fracture and increased risk of osteosarcoma.

Other causes of sclerotic bone lesions include neoplasms (1° and metastases), osteomyelitis, fluoride toxicity, and haemangiomas. Myeloma and other neoplasms should be considered in osteolytic lesions.

Figs 12.1–12.4 show the use of plain radiology in a variety of rheumatological disorders.

Table 12.2 X-ray appearance in arthritis of the hands.

Diagnosis	Pattern	Joints involved	Radiographic features
Osteoarthritis	Asymmetrical	DIPs, PIPs	Joint space loss Peri-articular sclerosis Bone cysts Osteophytes
Rheumatoid arthritis	Symmetrical	MCPs, PIPs	Joint space loss Peri-articular osteopenia Erosions Psoriatic
Psoriatic arthritis	Asymmetrical/ Symmetrical	DIP, PIPS (MCPs)	Periostitis Resorption terminal phalanx Bony proliferation Ivory digit Peripheral erosions Pencil in cup deformity Soft tissue dactylitis
Gout	Asymmetrical	DIPs, PIPs (MCPs)	Juxta-articular erosions – can be 'punched out' Soft tissue tophi
Calcium pyrophosphate disease	Asymmetrical	DIPs, PIPs, MCPs	Erosions Chondrocalcinosis

Fig. 12.1 Hands in rheumatoid disease.

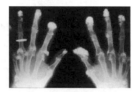

Fig. 12.2 Hands showing calcinosis, especially prominent distally.

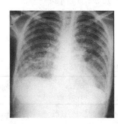

Fig.12.3 Plain CXR showing pulmonary fibrosis in rheumatoid disease.

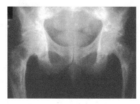

Fig.12.4 X-ray of pelvis showing avascular necrosis of the femoral heads.

Ultrasound

Ultrasound scanning is ideally suited to rheumatology. It is a non-invasive, 'X-ray free' technique that can be used dynamically in a clinic setting as an extension to clinical examination. Grey scale ultrasound can be used in inflammatory arthritis to detect synovial thickening, joint effusions and bony erosion in RhA, entheseal changes in spondyloarthropathy, and crystal deposition in calcium pyrophosphate.

Ultrasonography

Ultrasound may have an important role in the diagnosis of early arthritis because erosions can be identified before they are visible on radiograph and subclinical synovitis can be detected. It can also be helpful in monitoring disease progression/treatment response. Power Doppler can be used to assess joint activity in addition to joint damage.

Ultrasound is also ideal for imaging tendon pathology, including tendinitis, tenosynovitis, calcific tendinitis, and tears. It has been reported to be highly sensitive and specific for rotator cuff tears, and the dynamic nature of examination means that a tendon/joint can be examined, whilst in motion. Bursae, fluid filled cysts, and ganglia are also readily identified.

More advanced ultrasound assessments include soft tissue and muscle disorders, assessment of masses, and nerve entrapment. Imaging of temporal arteries in giant cell arteritis is also reported to show diagnostic changes in experienced hands with a hypoechoic halo being demonstrated due to artery oedema and stenosis. This may potentially be used to guide biopsy. Ultrasound has also been used to assess blood flow in vasculitis e.g. brachial and axillary arteries.

Limitations of ultrasound include difficulty in imaging less accessible areas, e.g. carpal bones and no information beyond the bony cortex.

Figs 12.5–12.8 show the use of ultrasound in a variety of rheumatological disorders.

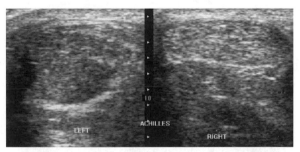

Fig. 12.5 Achilles tendinosis.

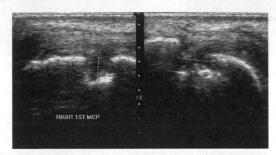

Fig. 12.6 Erosion of MCP joint.

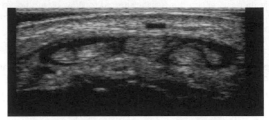

Fig. 12.7 Extensor tenosynovitis of wrist.

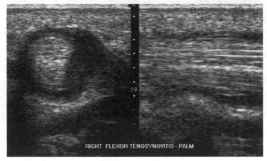

Fig. 12.8 Flexor tenosynovitis of middle finger.

Magnetic resonance imaging
In contrast to plain films and ultrasound, MRI imaging has the strength that all components of a joint can be visualized at once. Not only can the bony cortex be appreciated, but also the composition of the bone. Use of MRI is limited by accessibility and presence of metal implants e.g. pacemakers preclude its use.

Inflammatory arthritis
Not only can MRI detect erosions earlier than X-ray, it is also able to identify 'pre-erosion'—areas of bony oedema, which proceed to erosions in time. This suggests that patients with erosive arthritis could be identified prior to any damage and potentially early treatment could prevent structural damage. Similarly areas of bony inflammation can be seen at points of enthesitis in spondyloarthropathy and lesions have been described to resolve on treatment. Unfortunately, MRI appearances are not entirely specific to inflammatory arthritis with similar self-resolving appearances being seen in some healthy joints, bone cysts, and ganglia. Further study is therefore required into clinical utility of MRI findings, but as evidence mounts it is likely that MRI will have an expending role in rheumatology.

Muscle disease
MRI is useful in identifying abnormal areas of muscle. In the context of myositis an MRI scan can be used to guide a muscle biopsy to ensure sampling of abnormal tissue.

Soft tissue and back disorders
MRI is able to visualize tendon and cartilage lesions, and bone tumours. It is of particular clinical use in the assessment of orthopaedic 'soft-tissue' lesions, such as mensical tears in the knee, especially prior to surgery. MRI is particularly useful in assessment of the back, identifying inflammatory lesions, sacroilitis, spinal stenosis, myelopathy, discitis, disc prolapse disease, and nerve compression.

Bone lesions
Other bony disorders, such as avascular necrosis and transient osteoporosis of the hip may also be identified. Bone change can also be seen in regional chronic pain syndrome ('reflex sympathetic dystrophy')

Vasculitis
MR angiography is used in the investigation of vasculitis including large vessel vasculitides, e.g. giant cell arteritis and Takayasu's arteritis, and smaller vessel disease, e.g. Buerger's Disease.

Computed tomography scans

CT scans are rarely used in imaging of the musculoskeletal system, especially as associated radiation dose is high. CT/high resolution computed tomography (HRCT) does, however, have a role in the confirmation of diagnosis in bony lesions, e.g. infiltrative lesions, haemangiomas, lipomas, osteoid osteomas, and other bone lesions. Sacro-iliac inflammation, erosions, and calcification are also well visualized. HRCT has been used in the assessment of osteoporosis, but is largely superseded by DXA scanning (below).

The major role for CT is in identifying complications of rheumatic disease, e.g. pulmonary fibrosis associated with RhA.

Nuclear medicine imaging

Bone scan

Radionuclide imaging with ^{99m}technetium or ^{67}gallium is relatively easy to perform, and gives information about the whole body. In rheumatology it is used to assess the pattern of joint involvement in arthritis and to detect other causes of bony pain including Paget's disease, metastases, stress fractures, and other specific diagnoses, e.g. chronic regional pain syndrome. Although bone scans are sensitive to abnormalities, they have poor specificity so should be used in clinical context and may be a guide to further additional investigation e.g. MRI

Positron emission tomography (Fig. 12.9)

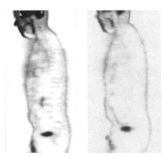

Fig. 12.9 PET scanning in aortitis pre- (L) and post- (R) treatment.

Newer techniques including single photon emission computed tomography (SPECT) and positron emission tomography (PET) are becoming more widely used in the assessment of inflammatory disorders and early pathology. Fluoro-18-decarboxyglucose PET has been shown to be useful in the assessment of activity in blood vessels in vasculitic disorders, e.g. Aortitis, Takayasu's arteritis, and giant cell arteritis. They are also used in the detection of neoplastic lesions.

Dual-energy X-ray absorptiometry scan

Osteoporosis is usually not recognized clinically unless a fracture occurs. DXA is a non-invasive assessment of bone density for patients at risk of developing osteoporosis. Potential fracture sites (lumber spine, hip, neck of femur, and wrist) are imaged and the result is compared with that expected in a normal population. For every standard deviation below the mean of the normal population the fracture risk is increased by two to three times. DXA is offered to patients at risk of developing osteoporosis (Table 12.3).

Table 12.3 Risk factors in osteoporosis

Osteoporosis	Diseases associated with osteoporosis/bone fragility
Primary	
Menopause <45(+<5 yr HRT)	Rheumatoid arthritis
Secondary amenorrhoea	Ankylosing spondylitis
Radiological osteopenia	Lupus
History of maternal hip fracture	Hyperparathyroidism
Previous fragility fracture*	Hyperthyroidism
Heavy long-term smoking	Male hypogonadism
Low BMI (kg/m^2) < 19	Chronic liver disease
Prolonged immobilization, e.g MS	Chronic inflammatory bowel disease
Excessive alcohol consumption	Malabsorption
	Chronic renal failure
Secondary	Hypopituitarism
Oral steroids	Haemachromatosis
Aromatase Inhibitors	Organ transplant patients
Androgen deprivation treatment for prostate cancer	Anorexia/Bulimia
Excessive thyroxine/anticonvulsants	

*Fracture sustained with no trauma or fall from standing height.

Radiology

Radiology & the role of imaging

The effective use of the Radiology department relies on good communication between radiologists and their clinical colleagues. The overall aim must be to target investigations efficiently in order to provide answers to clinical dilemmas at minimal cost and radiation dose (Table 13.1). The investigation of neurological problems has been transformed by the advent of CT and MRI. Local availability varies and CT in particular can add considerably to the radiation burden. Conversely, if a CT is likely to provide the best answer and minimize overall costs by resulting in an early discharge then it should be the investigation of choice. It is helpful to consider plain films, contrast studies, ultrasound and then CT/MRI as a hierarchy where plain films are requested as an initial investigation. This hierarchy may be circumvented if a more expensive investigation is likely to produce the definitive result.

The following are important points to consider:
1 **Will the investigation alter patient management?** i.e. is the expected outcome clinically relevant? *Do you need it?*
2 **Investigating too often or repeating investigations before there has been an adequate lapse of time to allow resolution or to allow treatment to take effect**. *Do I need it now?* Especially relevant when investigations may have been performed elsewhere. Make every effort possible to obtain prior studies. Transfer of digital data through electronic links will assist in this process. *Has it been done already?*
3 **Would an investigation that does not use ionizing radiation be more appropriate**, e.g. ultrasound scan (USS)/magnetic resonance imaging (MRI)?
4 **Failure to provide accurate clinical information and questions that you are hoping will be answered by the investigation may result in an unsatisfactory outcome**. *Have I explained the problem?*
5 **Would another technique be more appropriate?** The advances in radiology mean that discussion with a radiologist may be helpful in determining the best possible test. *Is this the best investigation?*
6 **Over investigating**: are you taking comfort in too many tests or providing reassurance to the patient in this way?

Table 13.1 Typical effective doses from diagnostic medical exposures

Procedure	Typical effective dose (mSv)	Equivalent number CXRs	Equivalent period background radiation
Chest (P-A)	0.02	1	3 days
Lumbar spine	1.0	50	5 months
Abdomen	0.7	35	4 months
IVU	2.4	120	14 months
Barium enema	7.2	360	3.2 yrs
CT head	2.0	100	10 months
CT abdomen	10.0	500	4.5 yrs
Bone scan (Tc-99m)	4.0	200	1.8 yrs
PET head (F-18 FDG)	5.0	250	2.3 yrs

UK average background radiation = 2.2mSv/yr.[1]

Table adapted from Royal College of Radiologists (2007) Guidelines for Doctors. Making the best use of clinical radiology services. Doses for conventional X-ray examinations are based on data compiled by the National Radiological Protection Board (NRPB) between 1990 and 2000. The doses for CT examinations and radionuclide studies are compiled from surveys conducted by the NRPB and the British Nuclear Medicine Society.

1 Royal College of Radiologists (2007) *Guidelines for Doctors. Making the Best Use of Clinical Radiology services*, 6th edn. London: RCR.

Plain X-rays

Wilhelm Roentgen discovered X-rays in 1895. X-rays form part of the electromagnetic spectrum with microwaves and radio waves lying at the low energy end, visible light in the middle, and X-rays at the high-energy end. They are energetic enough to ionize atoms and break molecular bonds as they penetrate tissues, and are therefore called ionizing radiation. Diagnostic X-rays are produced when high-energy electrons strike a high atomic number material. This interaction is produced within an X-ray tube. A high voltage is passed across two tungsten terminals. One terminal (cathode) is heated until it liberates free electrons. When a high voltage is applied across the terminals the electrons accelerate towards the anode at high speed. On hitting the anode target X-rays are produced.

The X-ray picture is a result of the interaction of the ionizing radiation with tissues as it passes through the body. Tissues of different densities are displayed as distinct areas depending on the amount of radiation absorbed. There are 4 basic densities in conventional radiography: gas (air), fat, soft tissue, and fluid, and calcified structures. Air absorbs the least amount of X-rays and, therefore, appears black on the radiograph, whereas calcified structures and bone absorb the most, resulting in a white density. Soft tissues and fluid have a similar absorptive capacity, and therefore appear grey on a radiograph.

Digital radiology

X-ray film is exposed by light photons emitted by intensifying screens sensitive to radiation transmitted through the patient. Storage phosphor technology uses photostimulatable phosphor screens to convert X-ray energy directly into digital signals. The increased dynamic range and image contrast of digital radiography compared with conventional film screen combinations and the facility to manipulate signal intensity after image capture reduce the number of repeat exposures. This increases efficiency and minimizes patient radiation dose. Digital images can be made available on a local network for reporting by a radiologist or for review on a ward-based computer. Picture archiving and communication systems (PACS) are efficient at image production and manipulation and in the storage, retrieval, and transmission of data. PACS facilitates remote radiology reporting and alleviates workflow pressures. Currently, all acute hospitals have PACS installations since December 2007 and current focus is on image sharing between locations.

Chest X-ray: useful landmarks

In order to interpret a plain posteroanterior (P-A) or lateral CXR some knowledge of chest anatomy and the major landmarks on the film is required. We have highlighted the major bony and soft tissue structures visible on the plain film in order to make it easier to spot abnormalities. Patient positioning for a postero-anterior CXR (Fig. 13.1) and lateral CXR (Fig. 13.2) is illustrated below.

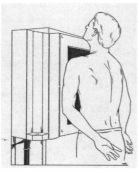

Fig. 13.1 Patient position for P-A CXR.

Fig. 13.2 P-A CXR.

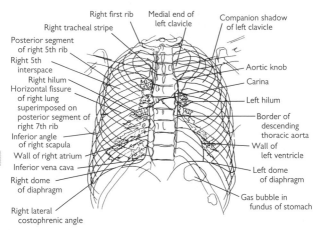

Fig. 13.3 P-A CXR landmarks.

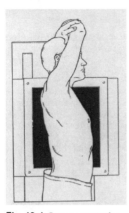

Fig. 13.4 Patient position for lateral CXR.

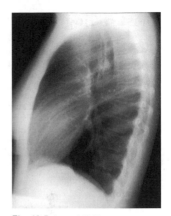

Fig. 13.5 Lateral CXR.

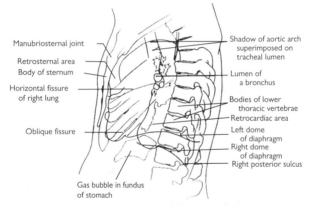

Fig. 13.6 Lateral CXR landmarks.

Chest radiograph

The chest film is the most widely requested, yet most easy to misinterpret, investigation. Using a logical approach will avoid most pitfalls. This should be the initial imaging modality in all patients with suspected thoracic pathology.

Points to consider

- Always obtain prior imaging if available; temporal changes assist greatly in image interpretation and differential diagnosis.
- Standard projections of the chest are PA (postero-anterior) *vs.* AP (antero-posterior). See section Projection below.
- Additional views to aid problem solving include lordotic, oblique, and decubitus projections.
- Initially assess technical quality.

Projection

P-A *vs.* AP will determine whether assessment of cardiac size is reliable.

Posture

Erect films enable a more accurate assessment of the mediastinum, since the lungs are more expanded, and allow detection of air–fluid levels, pleural thickening, and comment on the size of pulmonary vasculature.

Rotation

Look for the relationship of the medial ends of the clavicles to spinous process at the same level; a common cause of unilateral transradiancy is rotation.

Degree of inspiration

Ideally, 6 ribs should be seen anteriorly and 10 ribs posteriorly. If more, this suggests hyperinflation (does the patient have asthma or chronic obstructive pulmonary disease (COPD)?). If less (e.g. poor inspiratory effort, obesity, or restrictive chest disorders) there will be apparent cardiomegaly, increased basal shadowing, and less commonly tracheal deviation.

Quality of image can be assessed by degree of penetration. The thoracic disc spaces should be just visible through the heart. Absence of respiratory or motion artefact.

The heart and mediastinum

Sequentially consider the heart, mediastinum, lungs, diaphragms, soft tissues (breast shadows), and bones. Remember to assess your review areas—the lung apices, behind the heart, under the diaphragm, and the costophrenic angles.

Diaphragm

This should lie between the 5th and 7th ribs. If flattened, consider hyperinflation. In 90% of cases the right is higher than the left by 3–4cm. Effacement of the interface between lung and diaphragm suggests pleural or pulmonary pathology. Loss of smooth contour suggests localized herniation (eventration). Peaks laterally may be due to subpulmonary effusion.

Root of neck and trachea

The upper trachea is central with slight displacement to the right inferiorly due to the oesophagus. Thickening of the paratracheal line (>5mm) may imply nodal enlargement.

Mediastinum

The mediastinum should be central. The heart is normally <50% of thoracic width. Mediastinal enlargement or widening is a non-specific finding. The silhouette sign may help, but a lateral film is helpful for localization. Table 13.2 gives a list of distinguishing features that enable distinction of mediastinal masses from intra-pulmonary masses.

Normal variants mimicking a wide mediastinum are:
- AP projection (not P-A)
- Mediastinal fat (steroids, obesity)
- Vascular tortuosity

Table 13.2 Differentiating mediastinal from pulmonary masses

Mediastinal mass	Pulmonary mass
Epicentre lies in mediastinum	Epicentre in lung
Obtuse angles with lung	Acute angles
No air bronchograms	Air bronchograms possible
Smooth and sharp margins	Irregular margins
Moves on swallowing	Moves with respiration
Bilateral	Unilateral

Based on location of mediastinal abnormality, possible pathologies include:
- **Superior mediastinum**: thymoma, retrosternal thyroid, and lymphoma.
- **Anterior mediastinum** (anterior line formed by anterior trachea and posterior border of heart and great vessels): lymphoma (Hodgkin's disease (HD) & non-Hodgkin's lymphoma (NHL)), germ cell tumours, thymoma, retrosternal goitres, and Morgagni hernias (low).
- **Middle mediastinum** (extends behind anterior mediastinum to a line 1cm posterior to the anterior border of the thoracic vertebral bodies): aortic aneurysm, bronchial carcinoma, foregut duplication cysts (including bronchogenic/oesophageal) and hiatus hernia.

Posterior mediastinum (posterior to line described above)

Neurogenic tumours, Bochdalek hernia, dilated oesophagus, or aorta.

Enlarged lymph nodes

May be seen in any compartment.

Pleural disease

- Pleural and extra-pleural masses generally form obtuse angles with adjacent pleura.
- Pulmonary or intra-parenchymal masses form acute angles with the pleura.

Common pleural abnormalities

Effusion

- The lateral view is more sensitive as accumulation of fluid occurs first in the posterior recess.
- May cause mediastinal/tracheal shift to the contralateral side or adjacent atelectasis.
- Ultrasound invaluable (and better than plain film) in evaluation of small effusions and guiding thoracocentesis.
- If blunting of the costophrenic angles is present it indicates the presence of fluid of at least 200mL (P-A) or 75mL (lateral view) or may be secondary to thickening of pleura.
- Pleural thickening most commonly a sequela of inflammatory change.
- Asbestos exposure results in a spectrum of pleural abnormality ranging from benign plaques to fibrosis, and malignant mesothelioma (obtain occupational history).

Pneumothorax

- On an erect film the partially collapsed lung is delineated from pleural air as a curvilinear line (visceral pleura) paralleling the chest wall.
- On a supine film the changes are more subtle; look for the deep (costophrenic) sulcus sign, double diaphragm sign (dome and anterior portions of diaphragm outlined by lung and pleural air respectively, hyperlucent thorax and sharpening of mediastinal structures
- Subtle pneumothorax will be more readily apparent on an expiratory film or lateral decubitus film (accumulation of air superiorly).
- If the air is under tension there may be mediastinal shift (tension pneumothorax). This can result in vascular compromise. On imaging
  - The lung appears over expanded.
  - Depression of the diaphragm.
  - Mediastinal shift and of heart to contralateral side.

Thoracic intervention

Diagnostic thoracocentesis

- **Indication**: exclude malignancy, obtain sample for culture.
- **USS used to determine skin entry site**: 18–22G needle advanced into pleural fluid. Angle over superior border of rib to avoid inadvertent neurovascular injury.
- **Complications**: pneumothorax (when blind 1–3%).

Therapeutic thoracocentesis

Usually if respiratory compromise from large effusion. Similar technique as above, but place 8–12Fr catheter. Potential risk of expansion pulmonary oedema if evacuate in excess of 2–3L or aspirate both lungs in one sitting. Also potential for pneumothorax—always obtain post-aspiration chest X-ray (CXR).

Percutaneous lung biopsy

True positive rate of 90–95%. False positive results usually related to mal-placement of biopsy needle, necrotic tumour. Contraindications (relative) include severe coad, pulmonary hypertension, coagulopathy, and contral-ateral pneumonectomy. Tumour seeding is extremely rare (1:20,000).

Complications include pneumothorax and haempotysis.

Hila

Density should be equal, left is higher than the right by 5–15mm. If more disparity consider elevation due to fibrosis (e.g. tuberculosis (TB), radiotherapy) or depression by lobar or segmental collapse. Hilar enlargement may be vascular (e.g. pulmonary arterial or venous hypertension) or due to lymphadenopathy (e.g. sarcoidosis, lymphoma or TB). Hilar calcification is seen in silicosis, sarcoidosis and treated lymphoma.

Lung disease

Lung opacities may be subdivided into several basic patterns.

Alveolar

Air space shadowing: ill defined, non-segmental and with air bronchograms. No associated volume loss Large variety of causes:
- Fluid → pulmonary oedema (cardiogenic and non-cardiogenic).
- Fat → fat embolism.
- Haemorrhage → trauma, coagulopathies, pulmonary haemosiderosis.
- Cells → pulmonary alveolar proteinosis, sarcoidosis, alveolar cell carcinoma and infection (bacterial, fungal and viral).

Reticular

Linear opacities: associated obscuration of vessels and late appearance of CXR signs:
- Collagen disorders.
- Extrinsic allergic alveolitis.
- Sarcoidosis, pneumoconiosis.
- Cryptogenic fibrosing alveolitis.
- Early left ventricular failure (LVF).
- Malignancy (lymphangitis carcinomatosis).

Nodular shadows

Characterize according to their size and distribution:
- If solitary exclude tumour.
- Multiple:
  - Granulomas (TB, histoplasmosis, hydatid).
  - Immunological (Wegener's, rheumatoid arthritis).
  - Vascular (arteriovenous malformations).
  - Inhalational (PMF, Caplan's syndrome).

Primary signs of a malignancy
- Mass or nodule with speculated or irregular borders.
- Unilateral hilar enlargement or mediastinal widening.
- Cavitating nodule with thick rind of soft tissue.
- Cavitation most common in SCC.
- Malignancy can simulate air space disease (e.g. bronchoalveolar carcinoma, lymphoma).

Secondary signs of malignancy
- Atelectasis.
- Obstructive pneumonia.
- Pleural effusion.

- Interstitial patterns(lymphangitic spread of disease).
- Hilar and mediastinal adenopathy.
- Metastatic disease(including to ipsilateral or contralateral lung parenchyma).

Further reading

Corne J, Carroll M, Delaney D. *Chest X-ray Made Easy*, 2nd edn. Edinburgh: Churchill Livingstone, 2002.

Hansell DM, Armstrong P, Lynch DA, McAdams P. Imaging of Diseases *of the Chest*, 4th edn. London: Mosby, 2005.

Patterns of lobar collapse

Lobar collapse may be complete or incomplete. The commonest cause is obstruction of a central bronchus. The primary signs are opacification due to lack of aeration and displacement of the interlobar fissures. Typical patterns of lobar collapse are illustrated in Fig. 13.7.

Secondary signs include

- Elevation of the hemi-diaphragm (more prominent in lower lobe atelectasis than upper).
- Mediastinal displacement (tracheal displacement with upper lobe and cardiac displacement with lower lobe atelectasis).
- Hilar displacement more prominent with upper lobe atelectasis than lower.
- Crowded vessels in the affected lobe.
- Compensatory hyperinflation of remaining lung.

Silhouette sign

- In a normal CXR the interface between the diaphragm and the mediastinum are visible due to a difference in density between the lung and these structures.
- The silhouette sign refers to loss of normal interfaces implying there is opacification due to consolidation (the most common cause), atelectasis or a mass in the adjacent lung.
- Silhouetting helps to localize the site of the pathology and both pleural and mediastinal disease produce the silhouette sign (Table 13.3).

Table 13.3 Localization using the silhouette sign

Interface lost	Location of lung pathology
Superior vena cava	Right upper lobe
Right heart border	Right middle lobe
Right hemi-diaphragm	Right lower lobe
Aortic knob/left superior mediastinum	Left upper lobe
Left heart border	Lingula
Left hemi-diaphragm	Left lower lobe

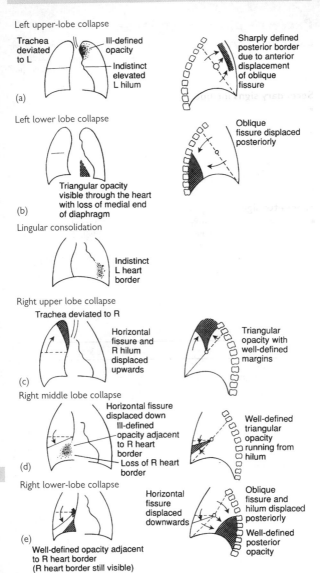

Fig. 13.7 (a) Left upper lobe collapse. (b) Left lower lobe collapse. (c) Right upper lobe collapse. (d) Right middle lobe collapse. (e) Right lower lobe collapse.

Cardiac enlargement

Increase of cardiothoracic ratio beyond 50% is considered abnormal if the P-A film is of good quality.

Aetiologies to consider
- Cardiomegaly (hypertrophy or dilatation of cardiac chambers).
- Pericardial effusion (globular heart).
- Poor inspiratory effort/decreased lung volumes.
- Pectus excavatum.

Location of cardiac valves may be relevant when determining the location of calcification. On a lateral projection draw a line from the xiphisternum to the carina and divide the heart into thirds. The location of the cardiac valves will be as demonstrated in Fig. 13.8.

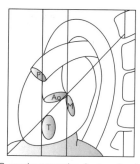

P = pulmonary valve   Ao = aortic valve
M = mitral valve   T = tricuspid valve

Fig. 13.8 Schematic diagram showing the relations of the cardiac valves on a lateral film of the chest.

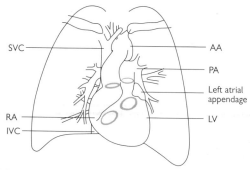

Fig. 13.9 Schematic diagram depicting a normal cardiac silhouette as seen on a plain CXR.

Normal plain film anatomy

Fig. 13.9 shows a P-A view. The right cardiac margin comprises three segments:

- Superior vena cava (SVC).
- Right atrium (RAt).
- Inferior vena cava (IVC).

The left cardiac margin comprises four segments:

- Aortic arch (AA) becomes more prominent with age).
- Main pulmonary artery (PmA) at level of left main stem bronchus.
- Left atrial appendage (may not be visible in normal hearts).
- Left ventricle (LV).
- RV is not usually seen in frontal projection.

Line positions

Endotracheal tube

- Tip of endotracheal tube (ETT) should be above carina and below thoracic inlet.
- The inflated cuff should not bulge the tracheal wall.
- Neck position can change impact location of tip
- **In neutral**: tip should be 4–6cm above carina.
- **Flexed**: moves tip inferiorly by 2 cm.
- **Extended**: moves tip superiorly by 2 cm.
- **Complications**: malpositioned results in atelectasis or collapse due to bronchial obstruction. Tracheomalacia if over-inflated cuff, tracheal rupture may result in pneumothorax.

Nasogastric tube

- Tip should be in stomach.
- Potential complications include placement in airway or gastric/duodenal erosion.

Swan Ganz catheter

Tip should be located in left or right PA within 1 cm from hilum. Loops in RA or RV may cause arrythmias. There are 2 types of Swan Ganz catheters

1 Used to measure wedge pressure.
2 With integrated pacemaker.

Complications include pulmonary infarct, haemorrhage, PmA pseudoaneurysm, and infection.

Intra-aortic balloon pump

Tip should be located just distal to the origin of the left subclavian artery and be 2–4cm below aortic knuckle.

Complications include aortic dissection, low position associated with mesenteric or renal ischaemia, high position with cerebrovascular accident (CVA).

Central venous line

Tip should end in the SVC below the anterior first rib.

Pacemaker

Typical position should be in apex of RV. Can be located in atrial appendage for atrial pacing and in coronary sinus for atrial left ventricular pacing

Complications include electrode displacement, perforation, infection, or venous thrombosis.

Chest tube
- Side port should lie within thoracic cavity.
- Tip of tube should not abut the mediastinum.

CT angiography of the coronary vessels

CT is very sensitive at:
- Detecting and quantitating calcification in coronary arteries.
- Non-invasively depicting the entire coronary tree.
- Determining luminal diameter.

For calcium scoring the examination is performed without intravenous contrast and there are various algorithms available that provide a measure of total coronary plaque burden.

Magnetic resonance coronary angiography

Also has potential for non-invasive diagnosis of coronary artery disease. The in-plane image resolution for current magnetic resonance (MR) techniques is about 1mm, sufficient for assessment of large coronary vessels, but inadequate for detecting disease in smaller side branches.

Computed tomography of the thorax

Indications include

- Evaluation of an abnormal finding on plain film.
- Staging of 1° or metastatic malignancies.
- Evaluation of suspected mediastinal or hilar mass.
- Detection of thromboembolic disease by computed tomography pulmonary angiography (CTPA). See Fig. 13.10 and 13.11.
- Detection and assessment of aortic dissection.
- Distinguishing empyema from lung abscess.
- Computed tomography (CT) guided percutaneous needle biopsy of focal lung lesion or mediastinal abnormality.
- CT guided pleural biopsy.

High resolution computed tomography (HRCT) comprises thin section images that are reconstructed using a special algorithm.

Indications include

- Evaluation of a diffuse lung disease. (Fig. 13.12).
- Characterization of a solitary pulmonary nodule.
- Haemoptysis.
- Lung disease in a patient with abnormal pulmonary function tests but apparently normal CXR (Table 13.4).
- Assessment of emphysema.

Table 13.4 HRCT patterns of interstitial lung disease

Pattern	Description	Causes
Ground glass opacity	Increased haze	Hypersensitivity Acute interstitial disease(active idiopathic fibrosis), viral PCP, pulmonary oedema, eosinophilic pneumonia
Reticulonodular	Peri-bronchovascular thickening(equivalent of cuffing on CXR) Thickened interlobular septa(Kerley lines)	Pulmonary oedema, viral, mycoplasma pneumonia, PCP Lymphangitic spread of tumours, fibrosis due to drugs, radiation, asbestos
Nodular opacities	1–2 mm interstitial nodules	Haematogenous infection, metastases, sarcoid, pneumoconiosis, histiocytosis
Cystic spaces	May or may not have walls	Lymphangioleiomyomatosis Histicytosis, honeycombing End stage interstitial disease

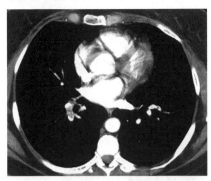

Fig. 13.10 Single slice from CT pulmonary angiogram showing the presence of thrombus within the lower lobe PmA.

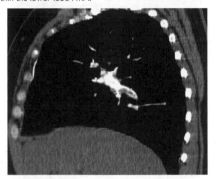

Fig. 13.11 Sagittal reformatted image confirms the extent of the thrombus and its relationship to the lumen.

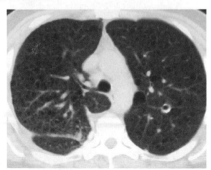

Fig. 13.12 HRCT image of the chest in a patient with cystic lung disease due to tuberose sclerosis.

Abdominal X-ray: useful landmarks

Interpretation of the abdominal X-ray (AXR), like the CXR, requires experience. In order to make things slightly easier we have provided a rough guide to the various bony, soft tissue and gas shadows seen on a 'typical' AXR (Fig. 13.13). Fig. 13.14 provides a normal abdominal XR for correlation with the diagram.

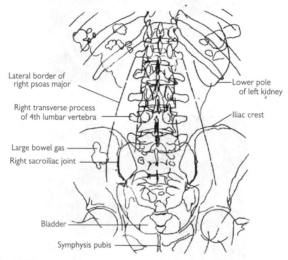

Lateral border of right psoas major

Right transverse process of 4th lumbar vertebra

Large bowel gas

Right sacroiliac joint

Lower pole of left kidney

Iliac crest

Bladder

Symphysis pubis

Fig. 13.13 P-A AXR landmarks.

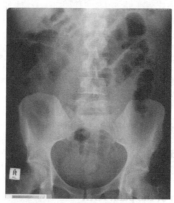

Fig. 13.14 P-A AXR.

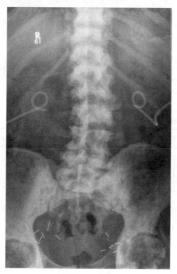

Fig. 13.15 Diffuse sclerotic metastases in a patient with a prostatic carcinoma. Note the presence of bilateral ureteric stents.

Plain abdominal X-ray

The standard plain film is a supine AXR. Erect views have largely been superseded and in the acute setting have been replaced by the erect chest to show free subphrenic air. Furthermore, chest diseases, such as myocardial infarction or pneumonia may simulate an acute abdomen. If there is doubt regarding the presence of a pneumoperitoneum, consider a lateral decubitus film (displays as little as 1mL of air).

Indications

Suspected obstruction, perforation, renal colic and toxic megacolon, and bowel ischaemia.

Contraindications

None, but where abdominal pain is non-specific and not attributable to the conditions listed above, an AXR is unlikely to be helpful.

Interpretation of the plain AXR

A normal patient will have variable amounts of gas in the stomach, small bowel, and colon. You can identify the stomach as it lies above the transverse colon, has an air/fluid level in the erect view and has rugae in its lumen. Large bowel calibre is variable; 5.5cm is considered the upper limit for the transverse colon in toxic megacolon and 9cm for the caecum in obstruction. Short fluid levels are normal. Fluid levels are abnormal when seen in dilated bowel or if numerous. If the bowel is dilated distinguish between small and large bowel by the features listed below (Table 13.5). Thickening of the bowel wall may be seen in a variety of aetiologies most notably ischaemia, but also in inflammatory bowel disease.

Table 13.5 Distinguishing features between small and large bowel

	Small bowel	Large bowel
Haustrae	Absent	Present
Valvulae conniventes	Present in jejunum	Absent
Number of loops	Many	Few
Distribution of loops	Central	Peripheral
Diameter of loops	30–50mm	>50mm
Solid faeces	Absent	May be present
Maximum diameter	3cm	65.5cm (9cm in caecum)
Maximum fold thickness	3mm	5mm

Causes of bowel dilatation include mechanical obstruction, paralytic ileus or a localized peritonitis (meteorism), e.g. adjacent to pancreatitis or appendicitis (Table 13.6).

Table 13.6 Distinguishing mechanical obstruction from a paralytic ileus

Feature	Ileus	Obstruction
Bowel calibre	Normal or dilated	Dilated
Air fluid levels	Same level in a single loop	Differential levels (stepladder)
Other distinguishing features	Air seen throughout the GI tract (diffuse ileus) or in localized ileus may be confined to a short segment	Distension seen to level of transition. Beyond this level no air in bowel

Look for extraluminal gas

- **Gas in the peritoneal cavity**: look for air under the hemidiaphragm, outlining the falciform ligament or both sides of the bowel wall (Rigler's sign). If there is any doubt consider a lateral decubitus film. Causes include perforation (ulcer, neoplasm), post-operative, following peritoneal dialysis or tracking down from the mediastinum.
- **Air in the biliary tree**: following sphincterotomy, gallstone ileus, or following anastomosis of common bile duct (CBD) to bowel. This has a linear morphology and is seen centrally within the liver
- **Portal vein gas**: pre-morbid sign in the context of bowel infarction, but less sinister in neonates with necrotizing enterocolitis (NEC) or following umbilical catheterization. In contrast to air in the bile ducts, its location is peripheral
- **Intramural gas**: linear streaks of air in the bowel wall again usually a sinister finding implying ischaemia, but may be seen due to benign causes, such as in patients with chronic obstructive pulmonary disease (COPD), where its configuration is more rounded and cystic.
- **Air in the retroperitoneum**: delineates the renal shadows and the psoas muscle; common causes are trauma, iatrogenic (e.g. after colonoscopic perforation) and after perforation of a duodenal ulcer.
- **Gas in an abscess**: look for displacement of adjacent bowel and an air/fluid level. Other causes include air in the urinary tract, and within necrotic tumours. In this scenario the gas is mottled and does not display features consistent with bowel
- **Look for any soft tissue masses or ascites**: the latter is detectable on plain films if gross. There will be displacement of the ascending and descending colon from the side walls with loops of small bowel seen centrally.

- **Look for abdominal or pelvic calcification**: first localize the site. This may require another view. The vast majority are clinically insignificant, i.e. vascular calcification, pelvic phleboliths and calcified mesenteric nodes. In the abdomen there may be pancreatic calcification (chronic pancreatitis) or hepatic calcification (old granulomas, abscesses or less commonly hepatomas and metastases from mucinous primaries). Gallstones are less commonly calcified and may contain central lucency (e.g. Mercedes Benz sign), while renal and ureteric calculi commonly calcify. Renal tumours and cysts rarely calcify and more widespread renal calcifications may be seen in nephrocalcinosis due to a wide variety of causes. In the pelvis, ovarian calcification (less common with malignant masses and seen more often in association with benign pathologies such as dermoids) is uncommon whilst uterine calcifications due to fibroids commonly occur. Bladder wall calcifications may be seen with bladder tumours, TB, and schistosomiasis. Prostatic calculi and calcifications are common and of no significance. Vas deferens calcifications are seen in patients with diabetes.
- **Soft tissues**: look at renal outlines (normally smooth and parallel to psoas, should be between 2–3 vertebral bodies). Absence of psoas margins may indicate retroperitoneal disease and haemorrhage.
- **Bones of the pelvis and lumbar spine**: look for osteoarthritis, metabolic bone disease (hyperparathyroidism, sickle cell anaemia), the rugger jersey spine of osteomalacia and Paget's disease (📖 Spinal imaging, p768. 📖 Pelvis, p770). Bony metastases may be lytic or sclerotic.

Barium studies

Barium suspension is made up of small particles of barium sulphate in a solution. Due to its high atomic number it is highly visible on X-rays. The constituents of individual suspensions vary depending on the part of the gastrointestinal (GI) tract being examined. The particles are coated to improve flow and aid mucosal adhesion. When made up it comprises a chalky (sometimes unpalatable!) suspension. Advantages include low cost, easy availability, and good assessment of mucosal surface.

Risks are more common in the context of

- **Perforation**: if leakage occurs into the peritoneal cavity it can produce pain and hypovolaemic shock (50% mortality). Long-term sequelae include peritoneal adhesions.
- **Aspiration**: in small amounts unlikely to have any clinical significance, but if pre-existing respiratory impairment or aspiration of larger amounts (i.e. more than a few mouthfuls) the patient will need physiotherapy.
- **Obscuration**: CT examination in the presence of a recent barium examination will result in a poorly diagnostic study as high-density barium results in streak artefacts.
- **Barium impaction**: rarely may exacerbate obstruction if barium collects and is concentrated above a point of obstruction.

Water-soluble contrast media

These are more expensive, and provide inferior coating and contrast. They include iodinated agents gastromiro and gastrograffin.

Indications for their use include

- Suspected perforation especially into the peritoneal cavity.
- Meconium ileus.
- To opacify bowel during CT examinations.

Risks include pulmonary oedema if aspirated and hypovolaemia, especially in children. Both are a result of hyperosmolar effects. If aspiration is likely use water-soluble non-ionic contrast, which causes less shift of body fluid compartments. Non-ionic contrast should be used in all infants (especially neonates) and pre-operative patients requiring water-soluble contrast.

Contrast agents

For studies other than when barium is being utilized the contrast media are non-ionic iodinated agents that are given orally, endoluminally or intravenously. Non-ionic contrast agents are higher in cost than their ionic counterparts (rarely used currently), but have a lower incidence of adverse reactions (by a factor of 9 for severe reactions). They are typically excreted by glomerular filtration. Half-life is dependent on the dose given, distribution, and renal function. Contrast reactions can be idiosyncratic or anaphylactoid or non-idiosyncratic.

High-risk patients are those with prior contrast reactions, a history of allergy or atopy, sickle cell disease, phaeochromocytoma, and multiple myeloma (to name a few). Contrast-induced nephropathy is more common if creatinine is elevated at time of administration or if the patient has a pre-existing renal impairment, e.g. diabetes mellitus.

Pre-medication can be administered to patients with prior contrast reactions. Protocols vary, but typically include a corticosteroid and anti-histamine. Consider the use of alternate modalities if risk is high, e.g. USS or MRI instead of CT with contrast.

Extravasation of contrast typically treated symptomatically with ice pack and elevation. Plastic surgery consult should be obtained if concern regarding compartment syndrome in patients who have in excess of 100 mL in extremity or severe pain/discolouration or altered perfusion.

Gadolinium is a MR-based contrast agent that is paramagnetic. It is also excreted by glomerular filtration.

Its safety profile is favourable in that it does not have any of the nephrotoxicity associated with the iodinated contrast media and is more commonly associated with minor reactions, such as headaches. Since 2006 there is an established association between the use of gadolinium containing contrast agents and nephrogenic systemic fibrosis (NSF). NSF involves fibrosis of skin, joints, eyes and other viscera. Subsequent to this finding the use of gadolinium is contraindicated in patients with an estimated glomerular filtration rate (GFR) under 60 and particularly if below 30.

Table 13.7 Pharmacological agents used in barium studies

Agent	Dose	Advantages	Disadvantages
Buscopan®	20mg IV	Reduced bowel peristalsis due to smooth muscle relaxant action Immediate onset Short duration of action (15 min)	Anticholinergicside-effects Contraindicated with cardiovascular disease and glaucoma
Glucagon	0.3mg IV for barium meal. 1.0mg IV for barium enema	More potent smooth muscle relaxant than buscopan. Short duration of action, no interference with small bowel transit	Contraindicated with insulinomas or phaeochromocytomas Relatively expensive
Metoclopramide	20mg po or IV	Gastric peristalsis enhances barium transit during a follow-through study	Possible extrapyramidal side-effects

Barium swallow

Plain films do not usually demonstrate the oesophagus unless it is very distended, e.g. achalasia. They may be useful in identifying an opaque foreign body within the lumen. The barium swallow is the usual contrast examination to visualize the oesophagus (Fig. 13.18). Rapid sequence films are taken with a fluoroscopy unit while the patient swallows barium (usually in the erect position). Films are taken in an anteroposterior (AP) and oblique projection (to throw the oesophagus clear of the spine) with the oesophagus distended with barium (to demonstrate its outline) and empty to show the mucosal folds.

Normal anatomy

The oesophagus commences at C5/6. There are normal indentations on its outline by the cricoid cartilage, the aortic arch, left main bronchus, and left heart.

Indications

These include the assessment of dysphagia, pain, reflux disease, tracheo-oesophageal fistulae (in children), and post-operative assessment, where there has been gastric or oesophageal surgery.

Contraindications

No absolute contraindications exist, but in all barium studies the quality of the study relies heavily on patient co-operation and, therefore, immobile patients who are unable to weight bear may only be suitable for limited studies. The post-operative oesophagus is usually assessed with gastromiro or a non-ionic contrast.

Common disorders and patterns

- **Diverticulae**: these include pharyngeal pouches (a midline diverticulum), traction diverticulae (due to adhesions), or pseudodiverticulae; dilated mucous glands seen in reflux or infective oesophagitis.
- **Luminal narrowing**: strictures may be benign (e.g. oesophagitis, shown in Fig. 13.16, scleroderma, pemphigus, corrosives or infection), or malignant.
- **Webs**: mucosal structures, which may be seen, anywhere in the oesophagus: seen with skin lesions, e.g. epidermolysis or pemphigus, graft-versus-host disease, and the Plummer Vinson syndrome.
- **Mega-oesophagus**: can be with associated obstruction as in malignant strictures or without as in achalasia, diabetic neuropathy, or Chagas' disease (Fig. 13.17a–c).
- **Ulceration/oesophagitis**: may be due to gastro-oesophageal reflux disease, infection, corrosives, or iatrogenic. Findings include lack of distensibility, fold thickening, and mucosal irregularity.
- **Oesophageal tears**: spontaneous, neoplastic, post-traumatic, iatrogenic and following prolonged emesis. Look for pneumomediastinum, left pleural effusion and features of mediastinitis.
- **Filling defects**: foreign bodies, varices (proximal due to SVC obstruction), distal (in association with portal hypertension), neoplasms

that may be benign as in leiomyoma or malignant. Most commonly squamous cell carcinoma (95%).

- **Fold thickening**: may be due to oesophagitis, varices or infiltration by lymphoma.
- **Air/fluid level**: commonest in hiatal hernias, but also seen with a pharyngeal pouch.

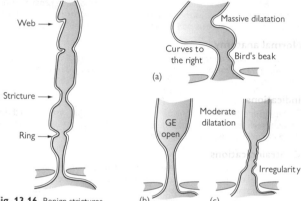

Fig. 13.16 Benign strictures.

Fig. 13.17 Obstruction in: (a) achalasia, (b) scleroderma, and (c) cancer.

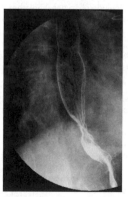

Fig. 13.18 Lateral oblique projection during a barium swallow series shows a feline oesophagus. This can be a normal variant, but is often associated with gastro-oesophageal reflux disease (GORD).

Barium meal

About 200mL of a high density (85% weight/volume barium sulphate), low viscosity barium is used for a double contrast study, which gives good coating without obscuration of mucosal detail. An effervescent agent is given to provide adequate luminal distension. The gastric mucosa is characterized by rugae (parallel to the long axis, 3–5mm thick) and area gastricae (nodular elevations 2–3mm wide). The patient is fasted for about 6 h to avoid food residue, which may cause diagnostic uncertainty. The techniques for coating the stomach and projections are variable. A smooth muscle relaxant may be given as part of the routine, particularly to assess the pylorus and duodenum.

Indications

Dyspepsia, weight loss, abdominal masses, iron deficiency anaemia of uncertain cause, partial outlet obstruction, and previous GI haemorrhage.

Contraindications

Complete large bowel obstruction.

Abnormal findings

- **Filling defects**: these may be intrinsic or extrinsic. Carcinoma remains the commonest cause of a filling defect in an adult (irregular, shouldered with overhanging edges). If there is antral involvement there may be associated outlet obstruction. Diffuse mucosal thickening and failure to distend is seen with linitis plastica. Other causes include gastric lymphoma, polyps (histology difficult to predict) and bezoars. Smooth filling defects are seen in conjunction with leiomyomas, lipomas and metastases. Extrinsic indentation by pancreatic tumours or an enlarged spleen may cause an apparent filling defect.
- **Fold thickening** (>5mm): seen in association with hypersecretion states, such as Zollinger–Ellison syndrome, gastritis, and Crohn's disease. It may also be secondary to infiltration by carcinomas, lymphomas or eosinophilia.
- **Outlet obstruction**: may be diagnosed by failure of the stomach to empty <50% of the barium ingested at 4 h. This may be seen in carcinomas, but also in scarring caused by chronic duodenal ulceration.
- **Hiatal hernia**: herniation of the stomach into the chest occurs via the oesophageal hiatus in the diaphragm. There are two types—in a sliding hernia (more common) there is incompetence of the sphincter at the cardia, often associated with reflux. Other sequelae include oesophagitis, ulceration or stricture. In a rolling hernia the fundus herniates through the diaphragm but the gastro-oesophageal junction remains competent and lies below the diaphragm.

- **Gastritis and ulceration**: gastritis is characterized by small shallow barium pools with surrounding lucent rings due to oedema. There are features that may be used to distinguish benign from malignant ulcers on barium studies. Ulcers are seen either as a crater or as a projection from the luminal surface (Fig. 13.19). Benign ulcers are commonly seen on the lesser curve with smooth radiating folds, which reach the edge of the ulcer crater. Malignant lesions may have an associated mass, have a shallow crater and an irregular contour. With the ease of availability of endoscopy, the use of barium meals in diagnosing ulceration has declined. Endoscopy has the advantage of being able to diagnose gastritis more accurately, assess ulcer healing, make a histological diagnosis and more accurately assess the post-operative stomach. However, early assessment of the post-operative stomach is radiologically performed to exclude complications such as anastomotic leaks. A water-soluble contrast agent is preferred in the early post-operative phase.

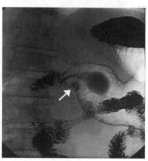

Fig. 13.19 Double contrast barium meal shows an ulcer crater.

Small intestine

Small bowel studies are performed for indications such as occult bleeding, recurrent obstructive symptoms, malabsorption and to confirm and define the extent of small bowel disease in Crohn's.

Small bowel follow-through: The patient drinks 200–300mL of barium (with metoclopramide to speed transit time). The single contrast column is followed by films at regular intervals until the barium reaches the colon. Transit time is variable, but the entire process may take 1–6 h depending on adequacy of bowel preparation. Films are taken at intervals of approximately 20 min initially, in the prone position, which aids separation of the loops. When the barium reaches the caecum spot views of the terminal ileum are taken.

Small bowel enema (enteroclysis): This technique provides better demonstration and mucosal detail, as there is rapid infusion of a continuous column of barium directly into the jejunum. Methylcellulose is administered following the barium to provide double contrast. This is achieved via a weighted nasogastric tube which is positioned at, or distal to, the duodendojejunal (DJ) flexure. Disadvantages include poor patient tolerance (related to intubation) and a relatively high screening dose.

Both techniques require the patient to be on a low residue diet beforehand.

Indications

The indications are the same for both techniques and include pain, diarrhoea, bleeding, partial obstruction, malabsorption, over-growth syndromes, assessment of Crohn's disease activity and extent, and suspected masses. The small bowel enema may be preferred for assessment of recurrent Crohn's disease or complex post-operative problems, but the small bowel follow-through is otherwise routinely used.

Contraindications

Complete obstruction and suspected perforation.

Normal findings

The small intestine measures ~5m and extends from the DJ flexure to the ileocaecal valve. The proximal two-fifths is the jejunum; the distal three-fifths is the ileum. Normal calibre is 3.5cm for the jejunum and 2.5cm for the ileum (up to 1cm more on enteroclysis). The valvulae conniventes are circular in configuration and ~2mm thick in the jejunum and 1mm thick in the ileum (Fig. 13.20).

Abnormal findings

- **Dilatation** is indicative of malabsorption, small bowel obstruction (SBO), or paralytic ileus. There may be accompanying effacement of the mucosal pattern. When seen with fold thickening it may be due to Crohn's, ischaemia or radiotherapy. Mucosal thickening may be due to infiltration by lymphoma or eosinophilia, adhesions, ischaemia, or radiotherapy.

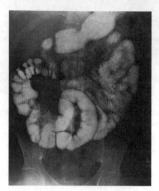

Fig. 13.20 30-min film in a small bowel follow-through series shows a normal mucosal fold pattern.

- **Strictures** are seen in Crohn's disease and in lymphoma. There is usually dilatation of the bowel proximally. Crohn's disease causes skip lesions, ulceration, strictures of variable length and a high incidence of terminal ileal involvement. There may be associated ulceration, fold thickening, and fistulation (Fig. 13.21).
- **Malabsorption**: radiological investigation may reveal an underlying structural abnormality. The findings in malabsorption include dilatation, fold thickening, and flocculation of barium.

CT enteroclysis

This is a hybrid technique that combines fluoroscopic intubation and small bowel infusion with an abdominal CT. This can be performed with positive enteral contrast or neutral enteral contrast.

The advantage of this technique is that both intra- and extra-luminal/extra enteric information is obtained rendering it superior to many of the per-oral small bowel studies. Disadvantages include the minimally invasive nature and the radiation associated with a CT examination. CT enteroclysis is complementary to capsule endoscopy in the elective investigation of small bowel disease and should be particularly considered in Crohns' disease, small bowel obstruction, and unexplained GI bleeding.

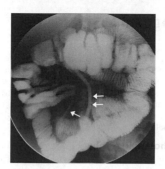

Fig. 13.21 Small bowel enema shows at least 2 strictures (arrows) in this patient with Crohn's disease. Compare the mucosal detail with the SBFT.

Cholangiography

Ultrasound

This is the 1° modality for assessment of the biliary tree and for exclusion of pancreatic pathology. With current scanner resolution the sensitivity for stone disease is in the range of >95% for stones exceeding 2mm in diameter. For choledocholithiasis(stones in the common duct) the sensitivity falls to around 50%, and magnetic resonance cholangiopancreatography (MRCP) or endoscopic retrograde cholangiopancreatography (ERCP) is more helpful.

Intravenous cholangiography

This is rarely performed, but may be useful in patients with biliary symptoms post-cholecystectomy or with a non-functional gallbladder. It is contraindicated in the presence of severe hepatorenal disease, as the side effects related to the contrast media are considerable. CT cholangiography uses a similar contrast agent, but offers the advantage of cross-sectional assessment of the bile ducts. It is often used when MRCP has not helped delineate anatomy in donors prior to liver transplantation or when MR is contraindicated or simply not available.

Endoscopic retrograde cholangiopancreatography

The biliary and pancreatic ducts are directly filled with contrast following endoscopic cannulation and during X-ray screening. This has both a diagnostic and therapeutic role. It is particularly of value in the demonstration of ampullary lesions and to delineate the level of biliary tree obstruction in patients with obstructive jaundice. It allows sphincterotomy to be performed to facilitate the passage of stones lodged in the common bile duct.

Percutaneous transhepatic cholangiography

The biliary tree is directly injected with contrast following percutaneous puncture of the liver. This is both diagnostic in defining a level of obstruction and therapeutic in biliary duct obstruction, as it may be used as a precursor to a biliary drainage procedure or prior to insertion of a stent. Contraindications include bleeding diatheses and ascites.

Other cholangiographic techniques

- **Per-operative cholangiogram** in which the CBD is filled with contrast during cholecystectomy to exclude the presence of CBD stones.
- **T-tube cholangiogram**: after operative exploration a T-tube is left in the CBD for a post-operative contrast study to exclude the presence of retained stones.

- **Magnetic resonance cholangiopancreatography (MRCP)**: this is a non-invasive, technique where heavily T2-weighted (T2W) images are obtained without contrast administration. The bile acts as an intrinsic contrast agent and stones are visualized as filling defects. The entire biliary and pancreatic ductal system can be visualized (Fig. 13.22). Common indications for this technique include unsuccessful ERCP, a contraindication to ERCP, as well as evaluation of the post-surgical biliary tree.

MRCP
- Non-invasive.
- Cheaper.
- Uses no radiation.
- Requires no anaesthesia.
- Less operator-dependent.
- Allows better visualization of the ducts proximal to the level of obstruction.
- When combined with conventional sequences allows detection of extra ductal disease.

Disadvantages
Decreased spatial resolution for peripheral intra-hepatic ducts and for pancreatic ductal side branches (e.g. as in pancreatitis).

Subtle ductal lesions may be difficult to appreciate as ducts are imaged in the non-distended physiological state.
- Inability to perform therapeutic endoscopic or percutaneous intervention of obstructing bile duct lesions.
- MRCP is comparable with ERCP in detection of obstruction with a sensitivity and specificity of 91 and 100%, respectively.
- Causes of filling defects are usually stones, air, tumours, blood, or sludge.

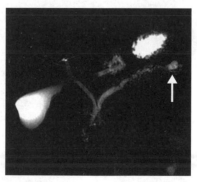

Fig. 13.22 Heavily T2W slab image shows an irregular beaded pancreatic duct in this patient with chronic pancreatitis. There is a small pseudocyst in the tail (arrowhead).

Liver disease

Ultrasound is the modality of choice for initial screening whether assessing the parenchyma for diffuse disease or trying to evaluate and/or characterize focal liver lesions. Although ultrasound is sensitive in depicting focal lesions it is not specific and there can be overlap in the imaging characteristics of benign and malignant lesions. CT and particularly MRI are more tissue specific in characterizing liver lesions. The liver is supplied predominantly by the portal venous system (80%). On CT we utilize the differing phases of enhancement to assess a lesion.

Arterial phase images (20–30s after injection) increase conspicuity of lesions that are hypervascular such as hepatocellular carcinoma or focal nodular hyperplasia. Portal venous phase images are acquired at 50–70 s and provide maximum enhancement of background hepatic parenchyma. Lesions that are relatively hypovascular on this phase stand out such as metastases.

Delayed imaging (equilibrium phase) minutes after contrast administration allows lesions that demonstrate relative washout of contrast (i.e. appear hypo-attenuating) relative to background liver, such as hepatocellular carcinomas to stand out. Lesions that are relatively fibrotic (e.g. in tissue content or scars conversely exhibit increased enhancement on delayed images).

Barium enema

This is used for evaluation of the large bowel. Increasingly, many institutions are replacing this technique with CT colonography (CTC; see topic Virtual colonos-copy) or conventional CT depending on the clinical indication. Barium is run into the colon under gravity via a tube inserted into the rectum. The column of barium is followed by air (room air or carbon dioxide) to achieve double contrast. The carbon dioxide is better tolerated and more readily absorbed. Buscopan (a smooth muscle relaxant) may be given to minimize spasm and optimize mucosal relief. Bowel preparation prior to the examination (low residue diet and aperients) is vital to ensure that there is no faecal material, which may mask mucosal abnormalities or be mistaken for small polyps. Remember the examination is uncomfortable, and requires reasonably good patient co-operation and mobility.

▶ Do not request this in frail or elderly patients unless there is a good clinical indication.

A rectal examination or sigmoidoscopy is essential to avoid abnormalities being missed.

Single vs. double contrast

If evaluation of the colonic mucosa is not the primary aim then a single contrast technique will suffice. This is applicable in children, where the patient is unco-operative and where gross pathology is being excluded, and in the evaluation of obstruction/volvulus or in the reduction of an intussusception.

Indications

Change in bowel habit, iron deficiency anaemia, abdominal pain, palpable mass of suspected colonic origin, and weight loss of unknown cause.

Contraindications

Suspected perforation, recent rectal biopsy, toxic megacolon, or pseudomembranous colitis.

Common findings

- **Solitary filling defect**: polyps are classified according to histology. The commonest are hyperplastic (no malignant potential, adenomatous polyps are premalignant with the risk of malignancy increasing with size (<5mm = 0%, >2cm = 20–40%). Also found are adenocarcinoma (increased risk in ulcerative colitis, polyposis syndromes, villous adenoma), and less commonly metastases and lymphoma.
- **Multiple filling defects**: polyps (polyposis syndromes or post-inflammatory pseudopolyps), pneumatosis coli, metastases, and lymphoma.
- **Ulceration**: inflammatory bowel disease (IBD), ischaemia, infection, radiation, and neoplasia.
- **Colonic narrowing**: neoplasms (apple core lesion), metastases, lymphoma, diverticular disease, IBD, ischaemia, and radiation.
- **Dilatation**: mechanical, e.g. proximal to neoplasm, volvulus or non-mechanical, post-operative ileus, metabolic, and toxic megacolon.

- **Diminished haustration**: cathartic colon, IBD, and scleroderma.
- **Increased haustration** (thumb printing): ischaemia, haemorrhage, neoplasm and IBD.
- **Widening of the pre-sacral space** (>1.5cm at S2): normal in up to 40%, but also seen in association with IBD, neoplasms, infection, and sacral/pelvic lipomatosis.

Colonoscopy

Remains a complementary technique, and has the advantage of being both therapeutic and diagnostic (e.g. biopsy, polypectomy, etc.). In elderly patients CT with prior bowel preparation and air insufflation is less invasive and less arduous.

Virtual colonoscopy

Helical CT images of distended colon taken during a breath hold are used to obtain 2D or 3D images of the colon. Images are acquired in the supine and prone position to assess lesional mobility (and thus distinguish stool from polyps. No intravenous contrast is administered for routine screening studies and the examination is often performed utilizing a low dose technique. Recent studies using 1° 3D interpretation, as well as national studies, such as the ACRIN II trial have shown sensitivities in the range of 94% for polyps at least 1cm in diameter and around 88% for lesions measuring at least 6mm. Current refinements in this technique include use of computer assisted detection (CAD) to improve performance as well as use of prepless techniques (i.e. the patient does not have to undergo prior bowel cleansing).

See Figs 13.23 and 13.24.

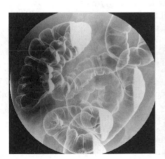

Fig. 13.23 Standard supine projection from a double contrast barium enema (DCBE) showing a normal large bowel.

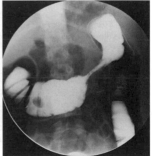

Fig. 13.24 Supine DCBE showing a tight stricture in the transverse colon in this patient with inflammatory bowel disease.

Further reading

Pickhardt PJ, Choi JR, Hwang I, *et al.* Computed tomographic virtual colonoscopy to screen for colorectal neoplasia in asymptomatic adults. *N Engl J Med* 2003; **349**, 2191–200.

Radiology of the urinary tract

Plain abdominal film

- **Look for any urinary tract calcification**: 90% stones are radio-opaque. Other causes include hyperparathyroidism, medullary sponge kidney and renal tubular acidosis.
- **Renal outline**: between T12 and L3 and 10–15cm. Left bigger and higher than the right.
- **Assess bones of spine and sacrum**: for bony metastases or spina bifida (may be relevant in enuresis).

Intravenous urogram

This provides a good overview of the urinary tract and, in particular, the pelvicalyceal anatomy. Fluid restriction and laxatives are no longer necessary and, in particular, the former is to be avoided in diabetics, renal failure, and myeloma. Following the preliminary plain film, 300mg/kg of contrast media is injected IV. The film sequence is varied according to the clinical scenario. An immediate film shows the nephrogram phase and displays the renal outlines. An increasingly dense delayed nephrogram is seen in acute obstruction, acute hypotension, acute tubular necrosis (ATN) and renal vein thrombosis. A faint persistent nephrogram is seen with acute glomerulonephritis and it may be delayed in renal artery stenosis (RAS). Later films show the pelvicalyceal systems (pyelogram), ureters, and bladder.

Common abnormalities (Fig. 13.25)

- **Loss of renal outline**: congenital absence, ectopic kidney, tumour, abscess or post-nephrectomy (look for absent 12th rib).
- **Small kidney (unilateral)**: ischaemia (RAS), radiation, or congenital hypoplasia.
- **Small kidney (bilateral)**: atheroma, papillary necrosis, or glomerulonephritis.
- **Large kidney (unilateral)**: duplex, acute pyelonephritis, tumour, or hydronephrosis.
- **Large kidney (bilateral)**: polycystic kidneys and infiltrative disease such as myeloma, amyloid, and lymphoma. Acute inflammation, such as glomerulonephritis, ATN, and collagen vascular disease.
- **Pelvicalyceal filling defect**: smoothly marginated (clot, papilloma), irregular margins (tumour, e.g. renal cell or transitional carcinoma), intraluminal (sloughed papilla, calculus, or clot), extrinsic (vascular impression or cyst), irregular renal outline (scarring, e.g. in ischaemia, TB, pyelonephritis, or reflux nephropathy).
- **Dilated ureter**: >8mm in entire length. May be due to obstruction (functional as in 1° megaureter), or mechanical stenosis as in ureteric or urethral stricture and in reflux disease.
- **Ureteric stricture**: wide differential, determine length. Differentials include tumour (TCC, metastatic), inflammatory (TB, schistosomiasis), congenital, trauma (radiation or iatrogenic).
- **Deviated ureters**: normal course of ureters in close proximity to transverse processes of vertebral bodies.

- **Lateral deviation**: seen with retroperitoneal nodes, tumours, and aortic aneurysm.
- **Medial deviation**: posterior bladder diverticulum, retroperitoneal fibrosis (can be idiopathic or related to various aetologies, including malignancy.

CT in genitourinary pathology:

CT is the preferred method for assessment of many pathologies within the genitourinary (GnU) tract including trauma, complex infections, renal and adrenal masses, neoplastic disease, retroperitoneal processes, reno-vascular hypertension, and in renal colic.

Computed tomography urography (CTU) In many institutions intravenous urogram (IVU) has been replaced by its CT counterpart. MDCT has had an impact on slice thickness and speed of scanning, such that the urinary tract mucosa can be assessed in exquisite detail. Depending on institutional protocol the examination is performed as a 2- or 3-part study. Typically it includes a non-contrast phase (to assess for stones, acute blood) and then excretory/delayed phase to assess the collecting systems and ureters. It has a high sensitivity (95%) in detecting upper urinary tract uroepithelial malignancies. Common indications for usage include:

- Haematuria (with negative cystoscopy and USS having excluded parenchymal causes).
- Unexplained hydronephrosis on USS.
- Evaluation of the upper tract in patients with known lower urinary tract TCC, or following trauma or iatrogenic ureteric injury.

Ultrasound

May be used as an alternative or complementary examination with the IVU and may be used to:

- Demonstrate or exclude hydronephrosis especially in acute renal failure (ARF).
- Evaluate renal tumours, cysts, and abscesses.
- Follow-up of transplant kidneys and chronic renal disease.
- Assess renal blood flow using Doppler.
- Serial scanning in children with recurrent urinary tract infections.
- Assess bladder morphology and volume, and the prostate.
- Provide guidance for interventional techniques, e.g. renal biopsy and nephrostomy placement.

Computed tomography and magnetic resonance imaging

CT is more accurate for staging renal tumours, assessing retroperitoneal pathology, staging bladder and prostatic tumours and for assessment of renal vascular pathology (such as renal artery stenosis). In many centres unenhanced CT is replacing IVU as a gold standard for assessment of renal stone disease. It is more accurate at depicting stone burden than IVU and precisely demonstrating the level and cause of obstruction in the acute setting.

Evaluation of ureteric pathology in the context of haematuria is also being performed with contrast enhanced CT.

MRI is valuable in staging vascular involvement by renal carcinomas. Dedicated pelvic coils and endoluminal coils show excellent results in staging pelvic and gynaecological malignancies.

Micturating cystourethrogram

Following catheterization of the bladder, contrast is introduced till bladder capacity is reached. This is the technique of choice for defining urethral anatomy and gauging the presence/degree of vesicoureteric reflux in children. It is also used if there are recurrent urinary tract infections UTIs or suspected lower urinary tract obstruction.

Ascending urethrography

Contrast is injected directly into the urethra in males in the assessment of urethral trauma, strictures, and congenital anomalies, such as hypospadias.

Retrograde pyelography

The ureters are catheterized (usually following cystoscopy in theatre) and contrast injected under X-ray screening. Of value in urothelial tumours and to define the site of obstruction, e.g. non-opaque calculi. Useful if intravenous techniques have failed to demonstrate the intra-renal collecting system, or ureters due to impaired renal function, or a high-grade obstruction.

Angiography

A femoral approach with selective catheterization of renal vessels. Main uses include haematuria (look for AVMs), hypertension (RAS), in transplant donors (to define anatomy) and in renal cell carcinoma (where embolization is being contemplated).

Nephrostomy

📖 Interventional radiology, p774.

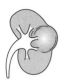

Renal cyst

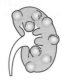

Multiple renal cysts
(elongation & distortion
of calyces – polycystic
disease)

Renal tumour

Duplex kidney with
hydronephrotic
upper, moiety.
('drooping flower')

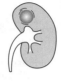

Dilatation of a
single calyx
(may be due to
vascular compression)

Fig. 13.25 Common pattern of abnormalities seen on IVU.

Breast imaging

Breast cancer is a common problem (1 in 12 women). An National Health Service (NHS) breast screening programme is in place following the Forrest report. Its aim is to use imaging to detect early clinically occult carcinomas. It screens women aged 50–64 yrs on a 3-yearly basis (the detection rate is 50 cancers for every 10,000 women screened). There are plans to extend the programme to women up to and including the age of 70. Current research estimates that by 2010 the programme will allow a 25% reduction in mortality.

Mammography

Technical factors

Breast tissue has a narrow spectrum of inherent densities and in order to display these optimally a low kilovoltage (kVp) beam is used. It enhances the differential absorption of fatty, glandular and calcific tissues. Dedicated mammographic units provide low energy X-ray beams with short exposure times. The breast is compressed to minimize motion and geometric unsharpness. High resolution is paramount in order to detect microcalcification (as small as 0.1mm). The breast is a radiosensitive organ so doses need to be kept to a minimum.

Standard projections

These are the mediolateral oblique (MLO) and craniocaudal (CC) views (Fig. 13.26). Adequacy of the lateral oblique view may be gauged by the pectoralis major muscle, which should be visible to the level of the nipple, inclusion of the axillary tail, and inclusion of the inframammary fold. The CC view detects posteromedial tumours that may be missed on the MLO view and is better at breast compression. Additional projections such as true lateral, spot compression and magnification views may be used to clarify abnormalities. These techniques provide better detail and disperse any overlapping tissue to avoid obscuration of lesions.

Mammographic signs

The breast parenchyma is made up of glandular tissue in a fibro-fatty stroma. Cooper's ligaments form a connective tissue network. The amount of glandular tissue decreases with age; as it is dense on mammography the suitability of the technique for detecting pathology increases with age.

Systematic evaluation of a mammogram
- Adequacy of study; are additional views required?
- Adequate penetration of fibroglandular tissue.
- Skin, nipple, trabecular changes.
- Presence of masses.
- Calcifications.
- Axillary nodes.
- Asymmetry (may be a normal variant).
- Architechtural distortion.

Comparison with prior imaging is imperative as changes can be subtle and progressive.

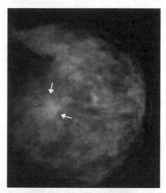

Fig. 13.26 Craniocaudal mammographic view of the breast. The arrows depict a stellate mass consistent with a carcinoma.

Primary signs of a malignancy

- A mass with ill-defined or spiculate borders (Fig. 13.27).
- Clustered, linear, or irregular calcification (which may occur in the absence of a mass).
- Secondary signs include distortion of adjacent stroma, skin thickening, and nipple retraction.

94% of breast carcinoma is ductal in origin.

Breast ultrasound

This largely forms a modality for assessment not diagnosis or detection. It can, however, be used to evaluate non-palpable masses, palpable masses not seen on mammography, to determine internal architecture (solid vs. cystic), to assess asymmetric density and as a 1° imaging modality in young women (<35 yrs). It is also used as a tool to guide intervention, i.e. drainage of cysts and biopsy of suspicious lesions.

MRI

MRI remains a problem-solving tool in breast imaging. Widespread implementation of MRI (for instance for screening) is hampered by its low specificity (37–97%). It can increase the number of benign biopsies that are performed. This clearly has resource implications, as well as generating unnecessary patient anxiety. Both MRI and ultrasound may be used to evaluate implants and their integrity, but MRI is the only modality that is sensitive in the evaluation of intracapsular implant rupture. Contrast-enhanced MRI of the breast is also a sensitive method for detection of malignancy with reported sensitivities in the region of 93%. It is especially useful to detect recurrent breast carcinoma and where conventional techniques are unable to help in the distinction from more benign lesions. Breast MRI is also being advocated for screening young patients with a family history/genetic risk of breast carcinoma.

Breast MRI is increasingly being used for staging breast carcinomas, to look for synchronous 1° lesions and to evaluate the breast in patients found to have malignant nodes in the axilla. It can also be used to evaluate tumour response to neo-adjuvant chemotherapy. In problematic mammographic patients it can be useful in distinguishing dense breast tissue or fibrosis from malignancy. In the post-operative setting it can be used in patients with positive surgical margins or to assess postoperative scar versus disease recurrence. The selection of pulse sequences and intravenous contrast administration is based on the clinical indication.

The patient lies prone on the scanner and a specialized coil surrounds the breast. The entire scan varies in duration from 20 min to 1 h. Most protocols for exclusion of malignancy rely on a dynamic enhanced sequence. Cancers typically enhance more rapidly than benign lesions.

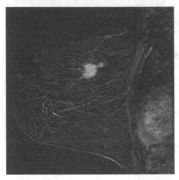

Fig. 13.27 Subtraction sagittal MR image of the breast following gadolinium showing an enhancing spiculated mass consistent with malignancy.

Ultrasound

Ultrasound is a high frequency mechanical vibration produced by piezo-electric materials, which have the property of changing thickness when a voltage is applied across them. It is an important tomographic modality and has widespread applications in the abdomen, neck, pelvis and extremities. At diagnostic levels there are no known damaging sequelae to tissues and therefore it is safe for use in obstetrics providing invaluable imaging of the developing fetus. Doppler USS is based on the principle that sound reflected by a moving target has a different frequency to the incident sound wave. The frequency shift is proportional to the velocity of the flowing material. Doppler therefore not only enables detection but quantification of velocity.

Indications

USS is cheap, readily available, and non-invasive, and has high patient acceptability. It has a wide range of applications as listed below. There are also no radiation implications. Again, advances in technology have resulted in vast improvements in the resolution of this modality such that subtle pathology is more readily identifiable.

Contraindications

None, but remember that USS is operator- and patient-dependent and should be used as a problem-orientated modality, not as a total body survey. It cannot be used to image air-containing structures or bone. The resolution of the USS image is inversely related to the depth of penetration. Therefore, image quality in obese patients is sub-optimal.

Applications

- **Head and neck**: may be used for evaluation of the salivary glands, thyroid, lymph nodes, and palpable or clinically suspected masses. Doppler is used to assess the carotid vessels and quantify degree of stenosis/occlusion.
- **Chest (excluding breast)**: the use here is limited to palpable chest wall lesions, assessment of pleural abnormalities, biopsy, and drainage of pleural effusions, and is occasionally of use in directing a biopsy of peripheral lung or mediastinal masses.
- **Abdomen & pelvis**: this is the main use of USS. Useful for assessment of solid organs, e.g. liver (Fig. 13.30), kidneys, spleen, gallbladder (Figs. 13.28 and 13.29), pancreas, uterus/adnexae, and bladder. A full bladder is used as an acoustic window in the pelvis. Retroperitoneal masses and lymph nodes may be visible depending on patient habitus. USS is useful for directing biopsy of solid organs/masses and for drainage of ascites, abscesses and collections.
- **Limbs**: musculoskeletal USS has been revolutionized by advances in high frequency probes, which enable characterization of soft tissue masses, tendon-related pathology, rotator cuff lesions, masses, effusions, and collections. It is also used for vascular assessment and the diagnosis of deep vein thrombosis.

- **Intracavitary transducers**: these place the transducer as close as possible to the area of interest. They include transvaginal, transrectal, urethral, oesophageal, and intravascular probes. They are usually high frequency transducers that produce detailed high-resolution images. Transvaginal USS is more invasive than transabdominal scanning, but is used in the routine assessment of gynaecological disorders. It can also be used for infertility monitoring, egg retrieval, and the exclusion of suspected ectopic pregnancy. Transrectal scanning is used for screening, assessment, and biopsy of suspected prostatic pathology, as well as rectal pathology including staging rectal cancers. Endo-anal probes may be used to assess morphology and characterize tears of the anal sphincter.
- **Contrast agents**: ultrasound contrast agents are available as an additional tool in diagnosis, although currently used primarily in academic centres. These are micro-bubbles, which are stable over a period of time and may be used to improve anatomical detail, assess tubal patency (hysterosalpingography), assess tumour vascularity, characterize focal masses (e.g. within the liver), and contrast enhancement.

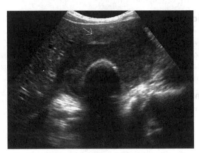

Fig. 13.28 Trans-axial view of the gallbladder on ultrasound demonstrates a soft tissue mass in the lumen suspicious for carcinoma. There is cholelithiasis, a common coexistent entity. The arrow shows an abnormal interface with the liver parenchyma suggestive of local infiltration.

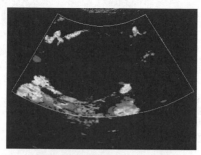

Fig. 13.29 Colour Doppler image in the same patient shows abnormal vascularity in the wall of the gallbladder. (☐ Colour plate 6.)

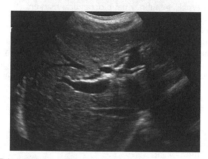

Fig. 13.30 Dilated intrahepatic ducts are seen in this axial view of the liver.

Obstetric imaging

Ultrasound is the 1° imaging modality in obstetric imaging with MRI being used for problem solving. USS is performed via both the transabdominal and transvaginal approach. Imaging is never performed in isolation and should always be performed in conjunction with clinical information, such as the patients menstrual status (including date of last menstrual period), presence/absence of pain and vaginal bleeding, as well as knowledge of biochemical parameters including serum Bhcg when available.

Role of imaging

First trimester

- Confirm a intrauterine pregnancy (IUP).
- Confirm presence of gestational sac and date pregnancy.
- Determine fetal number and placentation.
- Exclude ectopic gestation.
- If there is bleeding, assess viability of pregnancy (possible aetiologies in this scenario include a normal IUP, impending abortion (missed, incomplete or impending), ectopic pregnancy or a sub-chorionic bleed).

Second trimester
- Determine fetal number and viability.
- Locate and assess placental morphology.
- Estimate volume of placental fluid.
- Assess gestational age and evaluate growth.
- Fetal survey.
- Assess cervix and look at adnexae.

Third trimester
- Fetal presentation (cephalic, breech).
- Type of placenta.
- Assess cervix and os.
- Biophysical profile and serial growth.

Amniocentesis
Typically performed at 15–16 weeks with US guidance. Indications include advanced maternal age, abnormal biochemical markers (triple screen or α-fetoprotein (AFP)), and a history of genetic/chromosomal disorders. Chorionic villus sampling typically performed earlier 10-12 weeks) and also under imaging guidance using transabdominal or -cervical approach.

- **Gestational sac**: the product of implantation and is usually visible within the uterus at 2–3mm.
  - Normal mean sac diameter (MSD)(mms) + 30 = days of pregnancy.
  - Normal landmarks (transvaginal scan).
  - MSD > 8 mm yolk sac should be visible.
  - MSD > 16 mm heart beat should be present (CRL >5mm).
- **Other criteria** worrisome for abnormal pregnancy:
  - Irregular sac contour.
  - Decidual reaction<2mm.
  - Low position of sac.
  - Absent double decidual sac.
- *Small gestational sac* also has a high risk of subsequent pregnancy loss (>90%). MSD (mm)-Crown rump length (mm) < 5mm indicates loss of pregnancy
- **Empty sac**: one without a yolk sac or embryo. May represent a very early IUP (if MSD < 8mm) or an an embryonic pregnancy (if MSD > 8mm), or a pseudo-gestational sac as seen in ectopic pregnancy.

Table 13.8. Trans vaginal scan landmarks (accuracy +/– 0.5 week)

Age	ßHCG	Gestational sac	Yolk sac	Heart beat	Embryo (fetal pole)
5 wk	500–1000	+	–	–	–
5.5 wk	>3600	+	+	–	–
6 wk	>5400	+	+	+	–
>6 wk		+	+	+	+

A full review of obstetric imaging is beyond the scope of this chapter.

Gynaecological imaging

USS remains the modality of choice for initial assessment of pelvic pathology in females and can be used to assess uterine morphology, endometrial thickness, exclude focal uterine pathology, such as leiomyomas (fibroids), and for initial assessment of adnexal pathology.

Normal endometrium is echogenic with a surrounding hypo-echoic halo. Thickness is variable depending on stage of menstrual cycle and patient's menstrual status (e.g. pre- or post-menopausal). Typical values range from <4mm in the menstrual phase, 4–8mm in the proliferative phase (up to day 14 of cycle) to 7–14mm in the secretory phase.

The post-menopausal uterus is typically atrophic and may be modified by the administration of exogenous hormones (hormone replacement therapy (HRT)), which will also influence endometrial thickness. Normal thickness <5mm if no HRT usage.

Hysterosalpingogram

- **Indications**: for assessment of infertility, to define uterine anatomy and evaluate tubal patency as a precursor for *in vitro* fertilization or for evaluation of congenital anomalies.
- Procedure performed at days of 6–12 of menstrual cycle. Foley catheter inserted into cervical canal and contrast hand injected to define above. Complications include pain, infection. Contraindications are active infection, pregnancy, or recent uterine surgery.

Pelvic magnetic resonance imaging

Indications

Include locating and confirming presence of leiomyomas (often pre- and post-UFE, see 📖 Interventional radiology, p774), confirming presence of adenomyosis, endometriosis, in assessment of congenital uterine anomalies, as well for assessment of complex pelvic or adnexal masses.

T2W imaging of the uterus defines zonal anatomy and invaluable in staging neoplasms. MRI modality of choice for tissue characterization, and in this setting will demonstrate small quantities of blood products (as in endometriosis plaque), as well as showing tissue content such as intralesional fat (dermoids).

Computed tomography

This technique differs from conventional radiography in that it is able to visualize a vast spectrum of absorption values and, therefore, tissue densities. Furthermore, being a tomographic technique, the resultant image is essentially 2D and overcomes the problem of confusing overlap of 3D structures on plain film. The image is a grey scale representation of the density of tissues (attenuation) as depicted by X-rays. Each image is made up of a matrix of squares (pixels), which collectively represent the attenuation values of tissues within that volume (voxel). With conventional CT separate exposures are made for each slice. Current scanners can acquire data in a continuous helical or spiral fashion, shortening acquisition time and reducing artefacts caused by patient movement. This improves overall throughput and increases the likelihood of a diagnostic scan, particularly in unco-operative patients. The volumetric data that is acquired may be manipulated by image processing and displayed in a variety of techniques including 3D reformats and 'virtual' endoscopy.

The attenuation values are expressed on an arbitrary scale (Hounsfield units) with water being 0, air being −1000 units and bone +1000 units. The range of densities displayed on a particular image can be manipulated by altering the window width and level.

Prior to scanning the abdomen or pelvis dilute oral contrast is given to opacify the bowel. Intravenous contrast is given to aid the problem-solving process and differentiates vascular-enhancing lesions from surrounding tissue.

Multislice CT scanners are third generation scanners with helical capabilities and low-voltage slip rings, which acquire anywhere between 16 and 64 slices (and counting!) slices per X-ray tube rotation.

Indications

There are a wide variety as detailed below. CT is often the most diagnostic cross-sectional examination and more definitive than USS in many instances.

Contraindications

Due to the relatively high radiation dose, CT should be avoided in pregnancy. Artefact from in-dwelling, high density foreign material, e.g. hip prosthesis, dental amalgam, and barium, may limit the diagnostic quality of the examination. Claustrophobia is less of a problem compared to MRI.

Applications

- **CNS/spine**: CT remains the tool for primary diagnosis, pre-surgical assessment, treatment monitoring, and detection of relapse in many CNS disease conditions. MRI is superior in the posterior fossa and parasellar region, and for assessment in multiple sclerosis, epilepsy, and tumours. Where MRI is not available it is useful for assessment of degenerative spinal and disc disease. It is superior to MRI in the assessment of head injury. CT is also used as the primary modality in evaluation of acute stroke and in the emergency settling prior to lumbar puncture of patients suspected of CNS infection such as meningitis.

- **Orthopaedics/trauma**: uses include diagnosis and staging of bony and soft tissue neoplasms, and assessment of vertebral, pelvic, and complex extremity trauma (e.g. tibial plateau fractures). It is also used in the detection of loose bodies, assessment of acetabular dysplasia and providing an answer in joint instability (especially in shoulders, wrists, and elbows, where it may be performed as an adjunct to/in conjunction with conventional arthrography).

- **Oncology/radiotherapy**: staging of solid tumours, treatment planning, and the detection of relapse. CT is of particular value in obtaining whole body scans in oncology due to the speed and ease of use with the advent of spiral CT. CT is used for radiotherapy treatment planning to allow more precise targeting of treatment.

- **Chest**: indications include the staging of bronchogenic carcinomas, characterization of solitary nodules, diffuse infiltrative lung disease, widened mediastinum/mediastinal masses, and pleural abnormalities. With spiral CT, pulmonary angiography has advanced the diagnosis of pulmonary emboli particularly when V/Q scanning is indeterminate or equivocal. Helical CT is equivalent to formal angiography in detection of emboli within proximal arteries of <5th/6th generation. Sensitivity (80–100%, specificity 78–100%).

- **Abdomen**: applications include the diagnosis of abdominal pathology, which may be of traumatic, neoplastic, inflammatory, or infective origin (Figs. 13.31, 13.32, 13.33 and 13.35). CT is particularly useful for masses, pancreatic and hepatic disease, detection of the site and nature of obstructive jaundice and the assessment of abdominal trauma. It is also used in the pre-surgical assessment of abdominal aneurysms (Fig. 13.34) and as an aid to interventional techniques (📖 Interventional radiology, p774).

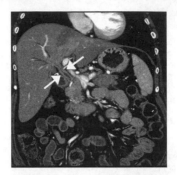

Fig. 13.31 Direct coronal reformat through the liver shows findings consistent with 1° sclerosing cholangitis. Note the markedly thickened bile duct wall (arrows).

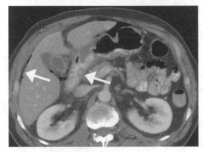

Fig. 13.32 Free intraperitoneal air secondary to perforation of a gastric ulcer. Note the thickened antrum of the stomach.

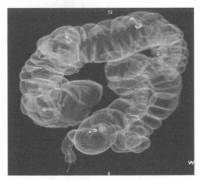

Fig. 13.33 Virtual barium enema image reconstructed from CT colonoscopy. The arrow shows the location of the polyps.

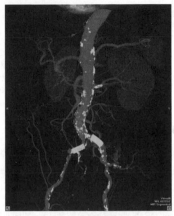

Fig. 13.34 Reformat of a CT angiogram to assess the extent of renal artery stenosis in this patient who has bilateral common iliac stents.

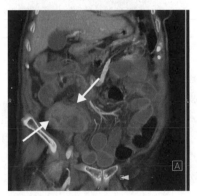

Fig. 13.35 Reformatted MIP image of an abdominal CT shows small bowel obstruction due to the presence of a caecal carcinoma (arrows).

Magnetic resonance imaging

This is a non-invasive technique, which displays internal structure, whilst avoiding the use of ionizing radiation. The nuclei of certain elements align with the magnetic force when placed in a strong magnetic field. These are usually hydrogen nuclei in water and lipid (at clinical field strengths), which resonate to produce a signal when a radiofrequency pulse is applied and display anatomical information. The I1 and I2 signal characteristics of common tissue types are seen oppotise (see Table 13.10). Further discussion of the physics is beyond the scope of this chapter.

T1-weighted images

- Contrast is due to inherent T1 relaxation.
- Provides good anatomical information.
- Fat is displayed as high signal (white).
- Distinction between cystic (black) and solid structures is possible.
- Good evaluation of marrow signal.
- The sequence of choice when evaluating enhancement, as gadolinium administration makes structures of even higher signal intensity on T1-weighted (T1W) images (Tables 13.9 & 13.10).

Table 13.9 Examples of sequences used in clinical practice

Pulse sequence	Acronyms	Clinical applications
Conventional spin echo	SE	Workhorse sequences. Therefore, integral to most protocols
Multi-spin echo	TSE, HASTE, RARE	Reduced scan time, but similar applications to SE
Inversion recovery	FLAIR, STIR	Used to suppress certain tissues by nulling their signal.
		Therefore, high net signal results in increased conspicuity of pathology, e.g. infarcts, perilesional oedema, MS plaque
		STIR invaluable in marrow imaging to show oedema, to assess optic nerves
Gradient echo	FLASH, SPGR, FISP, FIESTA many more	Uses gradient to rephase signal
		Reduced scanning time
		Useful for showing acute blood, in cardiac imaging with ECG gating.
		Can also be used in functional imaging Blood O_2 level (BOLD) dependent sequences
Echoplanar imaging	EPI	Generates multiple quantities of data (k-space) in short time so potential for real time/interventional MRI.
		Applications include cardiac, abdominal imaging

T2-weighted images
- Technique of choice for evaluating pathology.
- Fluid is of high signal and therefore optimally displays oedema.
- Improved soft tissue contrast allows evaluation of zonal anatomy of organs, such as the uterus and prostate.

Table 13.10 MR signal intensity of common tissues

Tissue or body fluid	T1 signal	T2 signal
Air	Nil	Nil
Bone or calculi	Nil	Nil
Fat	High (bright)	Medium to high
Proteinaceous fluid (e.g. abscess or complex cyst)	Medium	High
Muscle	Low	Low to medium
CSF, urine, bile, or oedema	Low	High
Blood (depends on age), hyperacute (oxyHb), chronic (haemosiderin)	Low/Low	High/Low

Magnetic resonance angiography
MRI principles are used to exploit the properties of flowing blood. Images generated display structures containing flowing blood with suppression of all other structures. These principles can be further modified so that only vessels with flow in a specific direction (i.e. arteries vs. veins are visualized). Magnetic resonance angiography (MRA) is currently being used in the evaluation of suspected cerebrovascular disease, renovascular disease, and peripheral vascular disease.

Functional imaging
MRI techniques have evolved such that diffusion imaging utilizes the diffusion of water protons in diagnosis of evolving ischaemia. This technique shows how movement of water molecules is impeded by cytotoxic oedema of ischaemic cells. These are manifested by signal changes that show early evidence of cerebral ischaemia prior to structural changes becoming apparent. Similarly, early ischaemia of the myocardium is detectable on MRI. This has great therapeutic potential as early treatment may prevent establishment of ischaemia, and result in overall improvement of ventricular function and survival. MRA is also being used to depict coronary vessel disease non-invasively.

Indications

The indications are legion and continue to grow. There are a wide variety of indications, summarized below. MR is especially useful in imaging the brain, spine, peripheral limbs and joints, neck, and pelvis. Again, improvements in scanner hard- and software have had huge impact on clinical practice. The prior limitations of long scan times have been overcome by robust sequences that can be performed in a breath-hold. This means that respiratory and peristaltic artefacts are no longer an issue when imaging in the chest and abdomen.

Contraindications

These largely apply to patients with magnetically susceptible devices or materials whose movement or loss of function can have deleterious consequences. These include cardiac pacemakers, metallic fragments, and prosthetic heart valves. Relative contraindications include pregnancy (especially the 1st trimester) and claustrophobia. MRI magnets are relatively confined and even those who are not normally claustrophobic may be provoked.

Applications

- **The spine**: MR imaging is superior to other techniques in displaying anatomy and is the technique of choice in assessing disc disease, the post-operative back, evaluating neural compression (benign or malignant), in imaging acute myelitis, infection (such as discitis or osteomyelitis), and excluding marrow infiltration. Contrast helpful in assessing the post-operative back to distinguish scar from residual herniation, as well as for confirming extruded fragments. It also helps confirm the presence of neuritis secondary to a disc herniation.
- **CNS**: imaging of the CNS is used to evaluate mass lesions, hydrocephalus, white matter disease, leptomeningeal pathology, cerebrovascular disease (Figs. 13.38–13.40), degenerative disorders, and visual and endocrine disorders, such as pituitary dysfunction. In trauma/acute haemorrhage CT is the preferred technique. See 📖 p784.
- **Paediatric**: the uses here include assessment of perinatal trauma/anoxic injury, congenital anomalies and developmental delay. Within the spine it is invaluable in the assessment of spinal dysraphism and progressive scoliosis.
- **Musculoskeletal**: along with CNS disease this is a major component of the MRI workload. It has revolutionized musculoskeletal imaging and is used to characterize meniscal pathology, ligamentous injury, degeneration and the sequelae of trauma in the knee, shoulder, wrist and ankle. Further uses include imaging mass lesions, assessing the extent of infection and diagnosing early avascular necrosis.
- **Chest/cardiac**: within the thorax MRI is useful for assessment of apical lesions such as Pancoast's tumours (Fig. 13.41), chest wall and brachial plexus lesions and mediastinal masses. Cardiac applications are legion and fast evolving; they include imaging of the great vessels to exclude congenital/acquired aortic disease (including dissection) and the diagnosis of pulmonary embolus.

- **Abdominal/pelvic MRI**: within the abdomen MR is often a problem-solving tool and can be used to more confidently characterize focal liver and pancreatic lesions, as well as assess diffuse liver disease. It is also of use in evaluating indeterminate adrenal masses. Within the pelvis, uses include the imaging of congenital anomalies, as well as staging tumours such as cervical (Figs. 13.36 and 13.37), prostate and rectal tumours. There have been rapid advances in techniques for imaging bowel-related pathology.
- **Interventional MRI**: open MRI units image the patients in large bore or C-shaped units, rather than the closed narrow tunnel used in conventional units. They can, therefore, be used for claustrophobic patients and to provide imaging guidance for interventional procedures. Disadvantages include a low magnetic field strength (0.1–0.3T vs. 1.5T) and a limited anatomical and spatial resolution due to their basic construct.

Recently, short bore magnets have been developed that combine the accuracy of a tunnel scanner and the comfort of an open MRI scan. Although they are not completely open, they are much less constrictive because of the short bore magnet (shorter tunnels), but can produce a high field.

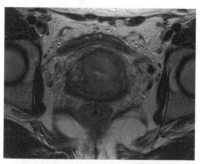

Fig. 13.36 Axial T2W sequence showing bilateral parametrial infiltration in this patient with a cervical mass.

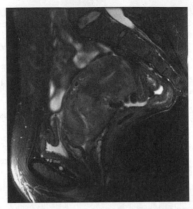

Fig. 13.37 Saggital and axial T2W images show a large cervical carcinoma. MRI is the modality of choice for local staging.

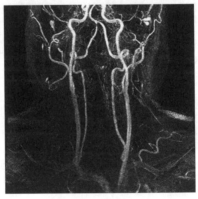

Fig. 13.38 Axial T2W shows acute infarction in the right cerebellar hemisphere.

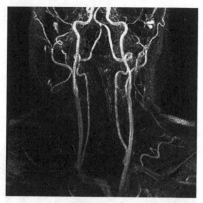

Fig. 13.39 Coronal reformatted MRI image shows a tight stenosis of the distal vertebral artery on the right.

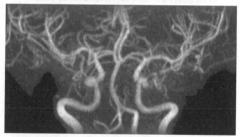

Fig. 13.40 AP coronal MRA showing mild irregularity of the carotid siphon on the left. The images are examined in multiple projections to exclude anomalies, such as stenosis or small aneurysms.

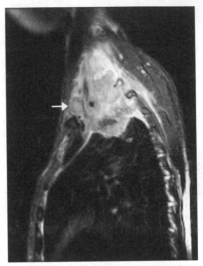

Fig. 13.41 Sagittal T2W MRI image in patient with superior sulcus (Pancoast) tumour showing invasion into the chest wall.

Spinal imaging

Basic principles of bony trauma imaging

- Obtain 2 films at right angles to one another (most commonly an AP and lateral to rule out fracture).
- Image proximal and distal joints.
- Bone scanning is more sensitive, but less specific than plain films to rule out a fracture. (*Not useful in acute setting.*)
- CT is invaluable for complex injuries (e.g. spine, calcaenus, and sacrum).
- MRI is used to assess ligaments, tendons, joint capsules, menisci, and cartilage.

In each case evaluate the following

- **Site of fracture**: assess if proximal/distal and intra vs. extra-articular.
- **Type of fracture**: simple (transverse, oblique, spiral) vs. comminuted.
- **Degree of displacement**: usually described with reference to the distal fragment.
- **Soft tissue involvement**: exclude foreign bodies, presence of gas. Open (compound) vs. closed.

Cervical spine

- **Trauma**: obtain a cross-table lateral first (this has the highest yield) and then perform the remainder of the cervical spine series (AP and open mouth peg views), if patient mobility allows and high index of suspicion. All 7 cervical vertebral bodies should be visualized (a large number of cervicothoracic injuries are missed because of inadequate views). If not seen request a specialized lateral view (swimmers) or a CT. Then sequentially evaluate:
- **Alignment**: assess the following lines (Fig. 13.41). They should be parallel with no step-offs.
- **Bones**: inspect C1 and C2. The anterior arch of C1 should be 3mm from the dens in adults (5mm in children). The vertebral bodies should be intact and they should be uniform in size and shape. Check disc spaces for any inordinate narrowing or widening which may be post-traumatic.

Cartilage

- **Soft tissues**: look for abnormal widening or a localized bulge. 50% of patients with a bony injury will have soft tissue thickening. The soft tissues should be no more than one-third of a vertebral body until C4 and a vertebral body width thereafter.
- **The peg views**: do not mistake a superimposed arch of C1 or the incisors as a fracture. Important points to remember are:
  - The lateral margins of C1 and C2 should align.
  - The spaces on either side of the peg should be equal (Fig. 13.41).

Remember: normal plain films do not exclude ligamentous injury.

In the routine setting cervical spine films are taken to exclude spondylosis (disc space narrowing and osteophytes) and atlantoaxial subluxation, which results in long tract signs and cord compression (rheumatoid arthritis, ankylosing spondylitis, Down's syndrome).

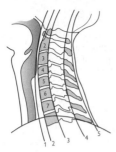

1—Soft tissue line closely applied to posterior aspect of the airway widens at level of laryngeal cartilage
2—Anterior border of vertebral bodies
3—Posterior border of vertebral bodies
4—Spino laminar line = posterior limit of spinal canal
5—Tips of the spinous processes

Fig. 13.42 Schematic diagram depicting the lines that need to be assessed when looking at a lateral film of the cervical spine.

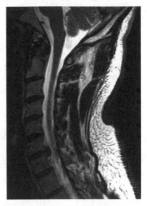

Fig. 13.43 Saggital T2W image shows a large osteophyte at the C6/7 level.

Thoracic and lumbar spine

Degenerative disease is common with disc space narrowing, end plate sclerosis, and osteophyte formation. Wedge compression fractures are common in the osteoporotic spine and need to be distinguished from the more sinister causes (absence of paraspinal mass, posterior elements spared). Multiple collapsed vertebrae are found in osteoporosis, neoplastic disease, trauma and histiocytosis X. Bone density may help narrow the differential, which includes increased (sclerotic metastases, lymphoma) and decreased (acute infection, osteoporosis)

Spondylolisthesis is the subluxation of one vertebral body on another, and may be degenerative or due to bilateral pars defects (spondylosis). This is a fracture/defect of the posterior elements of the vertebrae. On an oblique view the posterior elements form a Scottie dog (with the pars making up the collar). This may be a purely incidental finding; however, if severe it can result in neuroforaminal stenosis. Plain films are insensitive in the evaluation of disc disease. MRI is the investigation of choice for disc disease and its neurological complications.

Fractures typically occur at the thoracolumbar junction (90% at T11–L4). CT typically indicated other than in stable compression fractures, isolated spinous or transverse process fractures, and spondylolysis.

Plain film findings include paraspinal haematoma, widened interpedicular distance. An unstable injury may be accompanied by disruption of the posterior elements, widened interlaminar space, and is seen in the context of all fracture dislocations or if there is a compression fracture >50%.

Pelvis

Pelvic fractures are complex and there are many classification systems around. The pelvis should be regarded as being made up of three bony rings. The SI joints and pubic symphysis are part of the main bony ring. A fracture of one ring is frequently associated with a second ring fracture (Fig. 13.43).

- SI joints should be equal in width.
- The superior surfaces of the pubic rami should align. The joint width should be no more than 5mm.
- The sacral foramina should form a smooth arc.
- Acetabular fractures are subtle—look for symmetry.

Stable fractures (single break of pelvic ring or peripheral fractures) more common. These include avulsion injuries (e.g. ASIS, pubis, and ischial tuberosity), as well as sacral fractures and those of the ischiopubic rami.

Unstable fractures (pelvic ring interrupted in two places); less common. All require CT for clarification of extent of injury as plain film may under-estimate extent of posterior ring disruption (includes Malgaigne and bucket handle fractures).

Bone texture: The pelvis is a common site for metastatic involvement especially with urological malignancies, e.g. prostate (sclerotic metastases) and myeloma (multiple lytic lesions). Paget's disease of the pelvis may mimic sclerotic metastases, but tends to be confined to one hemi-pelvis and may expand or thicken bone.

Sacroiliitis: SI joint involvement is common in the seronegative arthropathies and is usually symmetrical in conditions, such as inflammatory bowel disease, ankylosing spondylitis, and hyperparathyroidism. More asymmetrical change is seen in Reiter's disease and rheumatoid arthritis. It is characterized by initial erosion and widening of the joint resulting in chronic sclerosis, which has a preferential involvement of the lower one-third of the joint (iliac > sacral side).

Avascular necrosis of the femoral heads is an important finding but is often advanced when plain film findings are seen. Radiographically occult avascular necrosis (AVN) may be detected on MRI or a bone scan. On plain X-ray it is characterized by sclerosis, flattening, and fragmentation of the femoral head. Subchondral crescents are pathognomonic. AVN can also be a sequel of trauma, but bilateral AVN is seen in conjunction with steroid therapy, sickle cell disease, and as part of Perthe's disease.

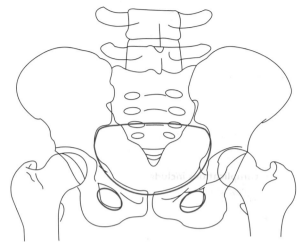

Fig. 13.44 The pelvis is made up of bony rings: the main pelvic ring and two smaller rings made up of the pubic and ischial bones.

Vascular intervention

Angiography is catheterization of a vessel followed by subsequent opacification with a water-soluble iodine-containing contrast medium. Catheterization is usually performed using the Seldinger technique.

Indications include

- Demonstration of arterial anatomy prior to surgery, where this is likely to influence surgical management.
- To elucidate the nature of arterial disease, e.g. occlusions, stenoses, thrombi, aneurysms and vascular malformations.
- To identify the source of bleeding in the gastrointestinal tract or following trauma.
- To demonstrate tumour circulation (often prior to embolization).

Potential complications include

Puncture site haematoma, infection, pseudo-aneurysm, atrioventricular (AV) fistula, dissection, thrombosis, embolic occlusion of a distal vessel.

Contrast

Volumes used are variable depending on the area being imaged. The contrast agents are iodinated, non-ionic, and of low osmolarity, resulting in reduced toxicity. Nevertheless, potential side effects include anaphylaxis, hypotension, urticaria, and bronchospasm. Patients particularly at risk include those with a history of a previous reaction, iodine allergy, and atopy. Nephrotoxicity is a potential risk and may be exacerbated by dehydration. Contrast reactions are seen in 1/1000 patients. Risk of anaphylaxis is 1/400,000. Pre-medication with corticosteroids may reduce the incidence of reactions if contrast administration is essential, but this is not universally accepted.

Specific applications

These include pulmonary angiography (gold standard for detection of pulmonary emboli), which is highly invasive and, therefore, reserved for when thrombolysis or embolectomy are being considered. Cerebral angiography is useful in the diagnosis of aneurysms, AVMs, tumour vascularity and both intra- and extracranial vascular disease. Renal angiography is selectively performed to diagnose renal artery stenosis and prior to embolization of tumours.

- **DSA (digital subtraction angiography)** is a technique whereby there is subtraction of the contrast-containing shadows from the initial plain films (mask) resulting in an image containing opacified structures only. The resulting images may be digitized and manipulated. The overall advantage is smaller doses of contrast and smaller catheters may be used.
- **Angioplasty**: PTA is a method used to fracture the vascular intima and stretch the media of a vessel by a balloon. Atherosclerotic plaques are very firm and are fractured by PTA. Healing occurs by intimal hyperplasia. Indications include claudication or rest pain
- **Intra-vascular stents**: typically metallic stents used when there has been unsuccessful PTA, or in cases of recurrent stenosis, venous

obstruction/thrombosis or as transjugular intrahepatic portosystemic stent shunt (TIPS) shunts (see 📖 Interventional radiology, Transjugular intrahepatic portosystemic stent shunt, p775). They can either be balloon expandable or self-expandable. Aortic stent grafts used to treat aortic aneurysms or dissections are typically a combination of a metallic stent with synthetic graft material. Stents can also be used in revascularization procedures when there are long segment stenoses, total occlusion or ineffective PTA.

- **Therapeutic embolization**:
  - Used to selectively occlude vessels by introducing a variety of materials via a catheter. Permanent materials used include metallic coil, balloons, and cyanoacrylate glue. Temporary embolic materials include gel foam and autologous blood clots. This technique is used at active bleeding sites and to reduce tumour vascularity pre-operatively in resectable tumours. It can also be used to treat AVM, for symptomatic uterine fibroid embolization (Figs. 13.49 and 13.50), and in varicocele embolization for infertility. Proximal occlusion of a vessel is equivalent to surgical ligation and does not compromise collateral flow.
  - Distal embolization usually infarcts tissue and is followed by necrosis.
  - Complications include post-embolization syndrome (fever, pain, elevated WBC), infection of embolized area, reflux of embolic material (non-target embolization).
- **Vascular catheterization** is also used to selectively infuse vessels as with thrombolytic treatment or rarely with cytotoxics. Vascular stenting is of increasing use in coronary and peripheral vascular disease. IVC filters (Fig. 13.45) are metallic umbrellas used to mechanically trap emboli and prevent venous thromboembolic disease. They are percutaneously placed via the femoral, jugular, or the antecubital vein. In the treatment of patients with recurrent pulmonary emboli despite anticoagulation or where anti-coagulation is contraindicated.
- **Thrombolytic therapy**:
  - Is the infusion of a fibrinolytic agent (urokinase, streptokinase, TNK, tPA) via a catheter inserted directly into a thrombus) This can restore blood flow in a vessel obstructed with a thrombus or embolus.
  - Indications include treatment of an ischaemic limb, early treatment of a myocardial infarction (MI) or stroke to reduce end organ damage, treatment of venous thrombosis (deep vein thrombosis (DVT) of leg or pulmonary embolism (PE)).
  - Contra-indications include active bleeding, recent intracranial event (CVA, tumour or recent surgery), non-viable limb and infected thrombus.

Central venous access: There are a variety of devices available—peripherally inserted central catheters (PICC), external tunnelled catheter (Hickman), subcutaneous port (Portacath™). Indications include chemotherapy, TPN, long-term antibiotics, administration of fluids and blood products, blood sampling. Potential complications are venous thrombosis, infection, and pneumothorax.

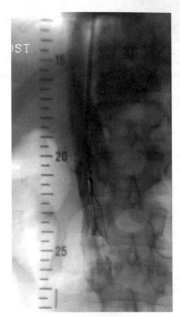

Fig. 13.45 Cavogram showing infrarenal deployment of an IVC filter (Gunther–Tulip).

Interventional radiology

Interventional radiology is a sub-speciality, where a variety of imaging modalities are used to guide percutaneous procedures. This may obviate alternative surgical procedures and consequently result in lower morbidity. Interventional procedures are usually carried out under local anaesthesia or using conscious sedation (see ☐ Interventional radiology, Concious sedation, p775), and on an outpatient basis, thereby considerably reducing bed occupancy. There is a huge range of procedures that are currently performed. The following is a limited list of some of them (See also Table 13.11.).

Percutaneous biopsy

Biopsy needle placement may be done under fluoroscopy, CT, MRI, and ultrasound. This provides a non-operative confirmation of tissue diagnosis and, in the case of a suspected malignancy, it is possible to accurately plan treatment. For histology a 14–18G needle is used. With a fine aspiration needle (20–22G) material may be obtained for cytology. Using imaging guidance, there is avoidance of damage to vital structures, such as blood vessels, solid organs, and bowel loops. With chest biopsy there is a small risk of pneumothorax.

Percutaneous drainage

With image guidance, surgical intervention may be avoided by accurate placement of a drainage catheter. Calibre varies from 8 to 14F depending on the nature of the underlying fluid. Regular irrigation of the catheter may be necessary to ensure successful drainage. Successful resolution may be impeded in the more complex and multiloculated collections.

Drainage of the urinary system

Can be via double J stents, which are placed into an obstructed collecting system with the distal catheter tip lying in the bladder. More short-term drainage is achieved via a percutaneous nephrostomy. Here, the obstructed kidney is punctured under fluoroscopic or ultrasound guidance, and a catheter placed in the renal calyx (preferably lower pole). This is the technique of choice in the acutely obstructed or infected kidney.

Biliary system drainage

Surgical outcome in patients with malignant bile duct obstruction is often poor. This may be due to carcinoma of the pancreas or cholangiocarcinoma. Biliary stenting alleviates obstruction and improves quality of life. Stenting may be performed at ERCP or percutaneously via antegrade puncture through the liver (PTC to delineate the anatomy being performed first). Other GI interventions include stenting/balloon dilatation of oesophageal strictures, stenting of obstructive colonic neoplasms (Fig. 13.46) and percutaneous gastrostomy or gastrojejunostomy insertion.

Transjugular intrahepatic portosystemic stent shunt

A procedure whereby a connection is made between the hepatic and portal veins to reduce portal pressure in patients with portal hypertension. The mortality is considerably lower than in acute shunt surgery, particularly in the context of an acute variceal bleed, which has failed to respond to sclerotherapy.

Conscious sedation

Form of sedation whereby the patient is given sedation and analgesic medication, but remains conscious and easily arousable. At all times the following are monitored—BP, pulse oximetry, ECG, and heart rate. Typical drugs used include a short-acting benzodiazepine (e.g. midazolam) and a narcotic analgesic (e.g. fentanyl), administered in small aliquots.

Table 13.11 Established and newer interventional applications

Established techniques	Newer interventional applications
Arterial and venous sampling	Arteriovenous malformation embolization
Biliary drainage, stenting, angioplasty, biopsy, and stone extraction	Chemoembolization
Diagnostic angiography	Cryoablation of liver tumours
Embolization	
Oesophageal dilatation	Endovascular repair of abdominal aortic aneurysms with stent grafts
Fallopian tube recanalization	Radiofrequency ablation of tumours
Feeding tube placement	Uterine artery embolization for symptomatic fibroids
Inferior vena cava filter placement	Varicocoele embolization
Nephrostomy placement	Vertebroplasty
Pain management (e.g. coeliac ganglion block, selective and non-selective nerve block)	
Percutaneous biopsy, cholecystostomy, and drainage of fluid collections	
Primary gastrostomy, gastrojejunostomy or jejunostomy tube placement	
Thrombolysis	
Transjugular intrahepatic portosystemic shunt insertion	
Ureteral stent placement	
Vascular angioplasty and stent placement	
Venous access and foreign body retrieval	

Endovascular repair of abdominal aortic aneurysms

With stent grafts, this is a new image-guided, catheter-based approach that provides a valuable alternative to standard open surgical repair. Radiological imaging plays an essential role in preprocedure evaluation, the procedure itself, and patient follow-up. The ultimate goal remains the same—complete exclusion of the aneurysm sac to prevent rupture. Advantages include lower blood loss, shorter ICU stay and rapid recovery. Complications include graft thrombosis, kinking, pseudoaneursym caused by graft infection and endoleak. Bifurcation grafts are used mainly for abdominal aortic aneurysms (AAA) repair and aorto-iliac occlusive disease. Tube grafts are used mainly for AAA repair.

Radiofrequency ablation

Not all patients with tumours are eligible for surgical intervention because of unfavourable location of the tumour, adverse clinical conditions or advanced disease. In addition, the cost, morbidity, and mortality associated with surgical resection have led to the search for other forms of therapy. Newer, minimally invasive treatments include intra-arterial chemoembolization, injection of ethanol, and radiofrequency ablation. Among the thermal ablative procedures, radiofrequency ablation is one of the newest and most promising. For this procedure, ultrasound, CT scanning (Figs 13.47 and 13.48) or MRI is used by the radiologist to guide percutaneous placement of long, thin (usually less than 18G), insulated needles into the tumour. The distal end (1–3cm) of each needle is not insulated and emits radio waves. Electrodes are attached to a generator and the electrical energy is converted to heat that kills cells through coagulation necrosis. The radiologist can vary the amount of current used, thereby tightly controlling the treatment radius. The entire treatment session usually lasts 1 h and can be performed in the out-patient setting. The procedure is typically performed with conscious sedation and local anaesthesia.

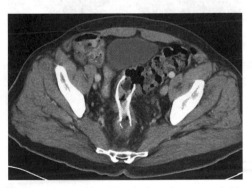

Fig. 13.46 Obstructing sigmoid carcinoma has been decompressed with a colonic stent.

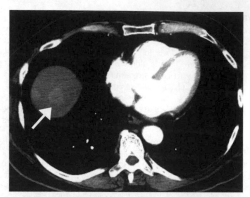

Fig. 13.47 Contrast-enhanced CT showing several high attenuation metastases overlying the dome of the liver.

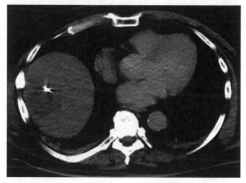

Fig. 13.48 Radiofrequency ablation of the metastasis shows the electrode *in situ*.

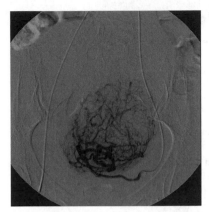

Fig. 13.49 Pre-uterine artery embolization (UFE). Selective catherization shows the supply to a large left sided fibroid.

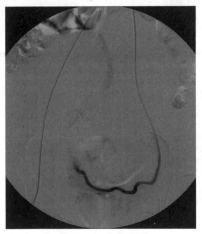

Fig. 13.50 Post-embolization with PVA shows no flow in the previously demonstrated fibroid.

Musculoskeletal imaging

Fracture terminology

Anatomical site
- In long bones, divide shaft into thirds.
- Use anatomical landmarks for description.

Pattern of fracture
- **Simple fracture**: no fragments. Describe the orientation of the fracture plane, e.g., transverse, spiral, and oblique.
- **Comminuted fracture**: more than 2 fragments: T-, V-, and Y-shaped patterns, butterfly fragments.

Apposition and alignment

Defined in relation to distal fragments

Other important descriptors include:
- Displacement (e.g. medial, lateral, anterior, posterior).
- Angulation.
- Rotation (internal *vs.* external).
- Overlap (of fragments).
- Distraction (refers to degree of separation of fragments).

Adjacent joints: are they normal? Is there dislocation, subluxation, or any intra-articular extension of the fracture line?

Magnetic resonance imaging in musculoskeletal imaging

Musculoskeletal imaging (MSK) neoplasms
Critical role in evaluating disease extent, staging, and treatment planning. Lack of mobile protons, and an acellular matrix render cortical bone, ligament, tendon, and fibrous signal of low signal intensity on all sequences. Tissues like muscle, fat, osteoid, and chondroid matrix have differing signal intensities, which can be used to differentiate tumours. Marrow involvement can be excluded by T1W and STIR sequences (see 🕮 Magnetic resonance imaging, p760). The bone involved should be imaged in its entirety to exclude skip lesions. Intravenous contrast is mandatory to assess lesional margin and assess tumour vascularity.

Joint imaging
MRI is the mainstay in assessment of joint pathology and, in particular, is excellent in depiction of ligaments, cartilage, and joint effusions. It is, therefore, the modality of choice for infection, neoplasm, trauma, and arthritis. STIR shows marrow oedema, fluid collections, and bursal inflammation. DESS is a sequence used for specific evaluation of articular cartilage. MRI is also the gold standard for marrow imaging. It is able to differentiate red from yellow marrow. T1-wighted (T1W) and STIR sequences are used for evaluating marrow pathology. Marrow oedema as well as early involvement of the marrow by pathologies, such as infection, neoplasia and subtle trauma is seen on STIR sequences when not easily evident on plain radiographs.

Hands

There are specific patterns that may be seen in the hand as an indicator of the underlying disorder. Some patterns are pathognomonic, whereas others are more non-specific.

1 **Generalized osteopenia**: osteoporosis, multiple myeloma and rheumatoid arthritis.
2 **Coarsening of the trabecular pattern**: common in haemoglobin-opathies especially thalassaemia and Gaucher's disease.
3 **Periosteal reaction**:
   (i) HPOA (hypertrophic pulmonary osteoarthropathy) associations include carcinoma of the bronchus, inflammatory bowel disease and coeliac disease.
   (ii) Thyroid acropachy, most common on the radial side of the thumbs.
   (iii) Juvenile chronic arthritis seen in about 25%.
4 **Carpal abnormalities**: include short metacarpals (Turner's syndrome, pseudo- and pseudopseudohypoparathyroidism), carpal fusion (inflammatory arthritis, RA and JCA, post-trauma), and look for syndactyly and polydactyly.
5 **Soft tissue changes**: e.g. increase in soft tissue thickness/size seen in acromegaly, localized increase seen in gouty tophi, nodes as in osteoarthritis (OA), soft tissue calcification seen in calcinosis, Raynaud's syndrome, oesophageal motility dysfunction, schlerodactyly, & telangiectasia (CREST) and scleroderma.
6 **Joint disease**: the hand X-ray above all may help in sorting out the type of arthropathy and aid rheumatological management. The ABCS approach is invaluable (see Table 13.12).

Trauma

Two views are essential for ensuring no subtle injuries are missed. On a P-A view the spaces between the carpal bones and the carpometacarpal articulations should be roughly equal (1–2mm). If a dislocation is present then there is obliteration/overlap. Common injuries include Bennett's fracture, a first metacarpal base injury extending into the joint surface with dislocation at the carpometacarpal joint. Scaphoid fractures are the most common (75–90%) of carpal injuries. Because of the blood supply there is a potential risk of osteonecrosis of the proximal pole.

Image-guided arthrography

May be performed in isolation or in conjunction with subsequent cross-sectional imaging (CT or MRI) for the following indications:
• Ligamentous and tendinous tears.
• Cartilage injuries.
• Proliferative synovitis.
• Masses and loose bodies.
• Implant loosening.

Plain films are obtained prior to the procedure. All joint fluid that is aspirated is routinely sent for culture. The contrast flows away from the needle if the tip is intra-articular.

- **Contraindications**: allergy to contrast media, concomitant infection.
- **Complications**: pain, infection, allergic reaction (to contrast), and vasovagal reaction.

When performing MR the examination is performed with dilute gadolinium.

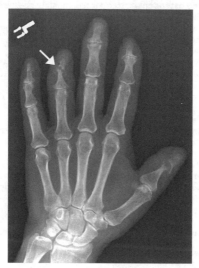

Fig. 13.51 Asymmetric oligoarthritis with dominant involvement of the DIP joints. The pencil in cup appearance is typical.

Table 13.12 An ABCS approach to interpretation of the handradiograph

A: Alignment	Subluxation/dislocation common in rheumatoid arthritis and SLE
B: Bone	*Osteoporosis*: mineralization is usually normal except in acute
	RA erosions:
	• Aggressive (i.e. no sclerosis of margins) seen in RA and psoriasis
	• Non-aggressive (with sclerotic margins) seen in gout; inflammatory erosions are marginal (OA erosions are central)
	—distinguish from subperiosteal resorption (radial border,
	—seen in hyperparathyroidism)
	Bone production: periosteal new bone formation, psoriasis
	Reiter's syndrome:
	• Ankylosis (bony bridging) in inflammatory arthropathies
	• Overhanging cortex (typical of gout)
	• Osteophyte formation, OA
	• Subchondral bone (reparative bone beneath cortex); typical of OA
C: Cartilage	Joint space has uniform narrowing in all arthritis except OA
	Eccentric narrowing: typically seen in OA, wide joint space in early arthritis, gout and PVNS
S: Soft tissue	*Swelling*:
	Symmetrical about joint seen in all inflammatory arthropathy, but most typically RA
	Asymmetric: typically due to osteophytes and seen with OA
	Lumpy swelling of soft tissues seen in gout (due to tophi)
	Swelling of entire digit; psoriasis, Reiter's
	Calcification: soft tissue; gout (calcified tophus)
	Cartilage: CPPD
	Subcutaneous tissues: scleroderma

Neuroradiology

- CT is the initial study for evaluation of neuropathology due to its speed, availability and lower cost.
- Excellent for evaluation of bony abnormality.
- Done both with and without intravenous contrast depending on clinical indication. The use of contrast delineates vascular structures and anomalies.
- Visualization of the posterior fossa is inferior to MRI.
- MRI is useful in assessing diffuse axonal injury and the sequelae of head injury.

Logical approach to interpretation

- Soft tissues.
- Bone.
- Cortical parenchyma.
- Ventricular system.
- Symmetry.
- Falx shift.

Rule out skull fracture, extradural haematoma (lentiform shape), subdural haematoma (crescentic shape), subarachnoid haemorrhage (Fig. 13.52), space occupying lesions (Fig. 13.53), hydrocephalus, and cerebral oedema. Look for target lesions (when contrast given): metastases, abscesses, and fungal infections.

Cerebral angiography

Evaluation of vascular lesions, including atherosclerotic disease, aneurysms, vascular malformations. Supplements information obtained on CT/MRI regarding tumour vascularity. Used for guidance of interventional procedures such as embolization.

CVA

Imaging may be negative in the first 6 h. Thereafter look for

- Oedema (loss of grey–white differentiation, sulcal effacement, and mass effect).
- Within 24 h there will be a low density wedge-shaped area corresponding to the vascular territory and extending to the cortical surface.
- Acute haemorrhage seen if there is haemorrhagic transformation (white = acute blood).
- Advances in MR sequences have revolutionized stroke imaging. Diffusion sequences (DWI) and perfusion weighted imaging (PWI) demonstrate acute infarction even in the context of a negative CT. Gradient echo identifies acute haemorrhage, whereas fast FLAIR can show acute subarachnoid blood. Time of flight angiography can non-invasively assess underlying vessels. If the infarct is thought to be venous (e.g. peripheral or haemorrhagic) then phase contrast MR venograms can exclude sinus thrombosis.

In the case of strokes in the posterior circulation, thin sectional axial images can exclude thrombosis or dissection within the vertebral arteries.

CT is important in the early stages of stroke evaluation to facilitate thrombolytic therapy. Highly accurate in identification of proximal occlusions in the circle of Willis and, therefore, aids triage to facilitate thrombolysis. Non-contrast CT is initially performed as haemorrhage is an absolute contraindication to thrombolytic therapy.

Multiple sclerosis

MRI is the modality of choice and is highly sensitive. There can be overlap with other entities, such as ischaemia and confluent disease may simulate neoplastic mass lesions. T2W MRI shows ovoid high signal lesions in a periventricular distribution. FLAIR sequences show lesions in a peri-ventricular distribution by suppressing (cerebrospinal fluids (CSF)) signal. Active lesions show enhancement following gadolinium. The spinal cord should also be screened to exclude involvement by multiple sclerosis (MS).

MRI in the paediatric brain

Assessing the degree of myelination is an important part of excluding structural pathology in paediatric neurological disorders. MRI is the modality of choice in brain tumours, congenital anomalies and hypoxi-ischaemic disorders (HIE). Diffusion weighted imaging is useful in acute HIE whilst spectroscopy is critical in metabolic disorders.

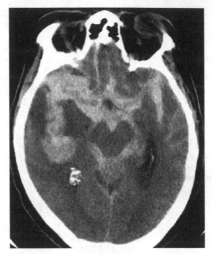

Fig. 13.52 Non-contrast CT head showing extensive subarachnoid haemorrhage in patient with underlying cerebral aneurysm (not shown).

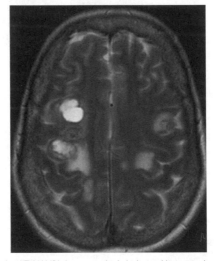

Fig. 13.53 Axial T2W MRI showing multiple high signal lesions in the deep white matter of the right frontal lobe in patient with lung carcinoma. The anterior lesion is cystic. These are consistent with metastases. Note the surrounding oedema.

Skull X-ray

Indications

The main indication is acute trauma, although skull X-ray (SXRs) are of limited use. Occasionally, the SXR is obtained as part of a skeletal survey in evaluation of metabolic bone disease, endocrine disorders, and in the assessment of metastatic disease. It is still used in assessment of sinus disease and in the evaluation of the post-operative skull.

Contraindications

None, but if there is suspicion of underlying intracranial injury plain films are unnecessary (see fractures and associated findings).

Normal findings

The bones of the skull vault have an inner and outer table of compact bone with spongy diploe between the two. Sutures are visible even after fusion and should not be mistaken for fractures. Blood vessels may cause impressions, as can small lucencies in the inner table near the vertex caused by normal arachnoid granulations which can be mistaken for small lytic lesions.

Trauma

Skull X-rays are basic, widely available, and yet potentially yield the least information in the context of trauma. The presence or absence of a skull fracture does not correlate with the presence or extent of any intracranial injury. Up to 50% of films may be technically unsatisfactory due to factors such as poor patient co-operation. With the advent of CT this is the technique of choice for evaluation in acute injury and neurological deficit. It allows a firm diagnosis to be made and excludes other alternate diagnoses.

Fractures and associated findings

Basic radiographs include a lateral projection (obtained with a horizontal beam) and a further tangential projection, depending on the site of injury.

Findings include

- **A linear fracture**: well-defined margins, no branching, and no sclerosis (cf. vascular markings or sutures that have an undulating course and sclerotic margins).
- **A depressed fracture**: increased density due to overlapping bone; those that are depressed by >5mm may lacerate the dura or cause parenchymal injury, and therefore need elevation.
- **A fluid level/pneumocephalus**: implies an associated basal skull fracture or dural tear.

Note: Pineal displacement is an inconstant finding and is not a reliable method of assessing the presence of intracranial injury.

Abnormal findings

Look for intracranial calcification, then examine the pituitary fossa, review bony density, and look for focal areas of lysis and sclerosis.

- **Intracranial calcification**: the majority is normal and of no clinical significance. However, it may be of pathological significance—causes include 1° tumours, such as meningiomas, craniopharyngiomas, arteriovenous malformations, and tuberose sclerosis, and infections, such as toxoplasmosis.
- **Raised intracranial pressure**: in practice plain film changes are only seen if the condition is long standing. These include sutural widening (diastasis) and erosion of the lamina dura of the pituitary fossa.
- **Enlargement of the pituitary fossa** (normal dimensions: height 6–11mm, length 9–16mm): expansion will result in a double floor, loss of the lamina dura, and elevation/destruction of the clinoid processes. The vast majority of the lesions will be pituitary adenomas; other causes include meningiomas and aneurysms.
- **Bone lysis**: may be diffuse as in metastasis or myeloma. Large areas of bone destruction are seen in histiocytosis X and in the active phase of Paget's disease (osteoporosis circumscripta).
- **Bone sclerosis**: may be localized as in meningiomas, depressed skull fractures, or generalized as in Paget's sclerotic metastases, myeloma, and fluorosis.
- **Sutural widening**: may be due to raised intracranial pressure, infiltration by malignancy (neuroblastoma or lymphoma), or defective ossification, as in rickets.

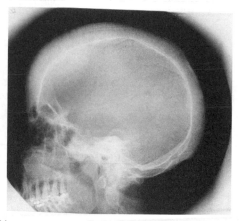

Fig. 13.54 Lateral SXR showing 'hair on end' appearance in thalassaemia major.

Reference section

Table 13.13 Abbreviations used in radiology

AP	Anteroposterior
AXR	Abdominal X-ray
CT	Computed tomography
CXR	Chest X-ray
IVU	Intravenous urogram
MRI	Magnetic resonance imaging
P-A	Posteroanterior
USS	Ultrasound scan
V/Q	Ventilation perfusion scan

Table 13.14 Management of adverse reactions to intravascular contrast agents

Symptoms	Treatment
Nausea/vomiting	Reassurance
Urticaria	Antihistamine chlorpheniramine maleate 10–20mg by slow IV injection (0.2mg/kg body weight paediatric dose)
Angio-oedema	Adrenaline (epinephrine) 1–3mL 1:10,000 IV (slowly), 0.3–0.5mL SC (1:1000) solution Protect airway and give O_2
Bronchospasm	IV hydrocortisone 100mg β2 Agonists nebulized or MDI Adrenaline (epinephrine) 0.1–0.3 mg SC (1:1000)
Hypotension	B2-agonist by nebulizer, O_2, IV access and IV fluids
Vasovagal	Atropine 0.5mg IV(up to maximum of 3mg)

Order of appearance of ossification centres of the elbow

The order of appearance is more important than the absolute age of appearance, which varies widely. Remember 'CRITOE' (Table 13.15).

Table 13.15 Order of appearance of ossification centres of the elbow

	Approximate average age (yrs)
Capitellum	1
Radial head	3–6
Internal (medial) epicondyle	4
Trochlea	8
Olecranon	9
External (lateral) epicondyle	10

Fracture healing rapid in children

- **Periosteal new bone**: 1 week.
- **Loss of fracture line**: 2–3 weeks.
- **Hard callus**: 2–4 weeks.
- **Remodelling of bone**: 12 months.
- **Types of paediatric fractures**: torus (buckle) fractures: buckled cortex only.
- **Greenstick fracture**: incomplete transverse fracture with intact periosteum on concave side (ruptured on side of convexity).
- **Complete fracture**.

Epiphyseal plate fractures: the Salter Harris classification (SALTR)

- **Type I**: epiphyseal slip separates it from physis (5–6%). S = slip of physis.
- **Type II**: fracture line extends into metaphysis (50–75%). A = above physis.
- **Type III**: the epiphysis is vertically split, i.e. the equivalent of an intra-articular fracture (8%). L = lower than physis.
- **Type IV**: fracture involves the metaphysis, epiphysis and physis (8–12%). T = through physis.
- **Type V**: crush injury with vascular compromise, i.e. poor prognosis for growth (1%). R = rammed physis.

Internet resources

National Radiological Protection Board
For issues regarding radiation safety: ✍ www.nrpb.org

Royal College of Radiologists
For information relating to radiological issues, guidelines in clinical management, training and publications: ✍ www.rcr.ac.uk

MRI safety and compatibility
✍ www.mrisafety.com

Radiological Society of North America
✍ www.rsna.org

American College of Radiology
Incorporates guidelines for use of contrast media and practice guidelines, as well as information on technical standards (e.g. teleradiology): ✍ www.acr.org

British Institute of Radiology
✍ www.bir.org

American Roentgen Ray society
✍ www.arrs.org

Also includes a image library with peer reviewed published images: ✍ http://goldminer.arrs.org/

General radiology resources
Educational website offering radiology cases, differential diagnoses, etc.: ✍ Learningradiology.com:

CT imaging/protocols: ✍ www.ctisus.com

Chapter 14

Nuclear medicine

Introduction to nuclear medicine

Nuclear medicine techniques employ a carrier molecule, selected to target the organ/tissue of interest, tagged with a gamma-emitting radioisotope. The labelled drug (radiopharmaceutical) is usually given po or IV, although it can also be administered interstitially or by inhalation. Its distribution is mapped in vivo using a gamma camera (scintigraphy) or, for non-imaging tests, biological specimens are assayed in vitro using a radiation counter. Single photon emission computed tomography (SPECT) uses images collected while rotating a gamma camera (usually multi headed) around the patient, which are then reconstructed mathematically to produce 3D images. Positron emission tomography (PET) images are obtained from a ring of detectors following administration of a positron emitting radiopharmaceutical.

Nuclear medicine procedures can detect early physiological responses to disease processes, generally before structural changes have taken place, and, thus, scintigraphy is often more sensitive than conventional radiology in early disease. Specificity varies depending on the radiopharmaceutical used and characterization of abnormalities often relies upon pattern recognition within a particular clinical setting. Anatomical detail is poor compared with conventional radiology and, increasingly, SPECT and PET images are co-registered with computed tomography (CT) images.

Nuclear medicine procedures are non-invasive and allow the whole body to be imaged during a single examination. Absorbed radiation doses depend on the radiopharmaceutical used, but are usually in the same range as diagnostic radiology. Pregnancy is an absolute contraindication to nuclear medicine examinations except where likely clinical benefit far outweighs potential risk, e.g. lung perfusion imaging. Some radiopharmaceuticals are excreted in breast milk and additional precautions may be advisable for lactating women.

Diagnostic radiopharmaceuticals are used in tracer quantities and toxicity is negligible. Individual hypersensitivity reactions are rare. The most widely used radionuclide is technetium-99m (^{99m}Tc), which can be obtained from an on-site generator, has a half life of 6 h, and is suitable for labelling a wide variety of radiopharmaceuticals.

Specific information required when requesting nuclear medicine tests includes

- Patient identification details.
- Examination requested.
- Relevant clinical history including results of other investigations.
- Pregnancy/lactation details where relevant.
- Special needs—visual/hearing/learning difficulties; needle phobia.
- Some scanning beds have a weight limit.

Bone scintigraphy: bone scan

Background

Nuclear medicine investigations supplement the anatomical information obtained from radiology. Bone scintigraphy is sensitive, with changes frequently detected earlier than on plain film, but non-specific. It plays a pivotal role in the staging of patients with malignant disease and in difficult orthopaedic cases. May be restricted to 'local views' only, e.g. loose hip prosthesis or 'whole body imaging' in metastatic screening. Can include a dynamic phase image at the time of radiopharmaceutical administration in addition to the delayed, bone phase image 2–4 h post-injection. Dynamic phase reflects blood flow to the site of interest—useful when there is concern over vascularity, infection, or recent trauma. Helps to differentiate soft-tissue from bone pathology, e.g. cellulitis *vs.* osteomyelitis.

The ^{99m}Tc-bisphosphonate complex (MDP, HDP) used to target the skeleton is renally excreted. Patients with poor renal function may need delayed imaging to improve the bone:soft tissue ratio (Fig. 14.1).

Indications

- Tumour staging—assess skeletal metastases.
- Bone pain.
- Trauma—when radiographs unhelpful.
- Prosthetic loosening, e.g. THR.
- Infection.
- Avascular necrosis (AVN).
- Paget's disease to assess extent (Fig. 14.3).
- Sports injuries.

Patient preparation

Should be well-hydrated and continent.

Procedure

Inject ^{99m}Tc-bisphosphonate complex IV. For suspected AVN or sepsis, image immediately to assess vascularity. Otherwise, image 2–4 h later. Whole body views are required for metastatic screening. Tomography improves anatomical definition and detection of small lesions, e.g. osteoid osteoma and is particularly useful in back pain. Fusion with CT images is being used increasingly.

Results

- Radiopharmaceutical uptake reflects osteoblastic activity.
- Focal ↑ uptake in sclerotic metastases, trauma or infection.
- Diffuse ↑ uptake associated with advanced metastases, Paget's and metabolic bone disease.
- ↑ uptake in acute AVN and lytic bone metastases (Fig. 14.2).

Interpretation

Sensitive, but non-specific. Interpretation relies on pattern recognition in the clinical setting.

Advantages

Sensitive—detects early changes in bone physiology, often before abnormal plain radiographs, e.g. occult trauma, metastases, and sepsis.

Pitfalls

False −ves in multiple myeloma. Artefacts due to urine contamination.

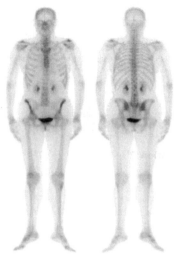

Fig. 14.1 Normal whole body ^{99m}Tc-bisphosphonate bone scan; anterior view on left, posterior view on right.

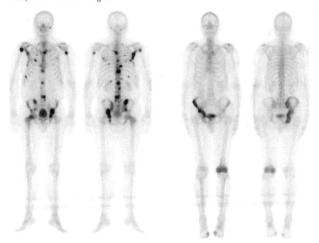

Fig. 14.2 Bone scan showing extensive metastases.

Fig. 14.3 Bone scan showing Paget's disease affecting the right hemipelvis and distal femur.

Reticuloendothelial system: bone marrow scintigraphy

Background
Largely superseded by magnetic resonance imaging (MRI). Colloid particles are cleared from the circulating blood pool by reticuloendothelial tissue—larger particles → liver and spleen; smaller particles → bone marrow. Abnormal uptake pattern where bone marrow is replaced, e.g. by tumour infiltration.

Indications
- Suspected malignant marrow infiltration.
- Equivocal conventional bone imaging.
- Osteomyelitis (rarely used).

Patient preparation
None.

Procedure
- ^{99m}Tc-nanocolloid injected IV.
- Whole body gamma camera imaging at 30–45 min.

Results
Normal marrow distribution in thoracic cage, spine, pelvis, and proximal long bones. Homogeneous uptake in liver and spleen.

Interpretation
- Focal or generalized ↓ skeletal uptake indicates marrow replacement or infiltration with marrow displacement to distal femora and humeri.
- Heterogeneous hepatic uptake is abnormal but non-specific.

Advantages
Non-invasive. Avoids sampling errors compared with bone marrow biopsy.

Pitfalls
False −ves in early malignancy. Liver and spleen uptake may obscure abnormalities in the mid spine.

Further reading
Smith FW. The skeletal system. In: Sharp PF, Gemmel HG, Smith FW (eds) *Practical Nuclear Medicine*, 2nd edn. Oxford: Oxford University Press, 1998.

Cerebral blood flow imaging

Background

Used to study acute and chronic cerebrovascular disease, dementias, and epilepsy using a radiolabelled lipophilic ^{99m}Tc complex hexamethyl-propylene-amine-oxime (exametazine, HMPAO), which crosses the blood–brain barrier, and fixes in the cerebral cortex and basal ganglia. Uptake is proportional to blood flow, with high accumulation in cortical grey matter, compared with white matter. Images reported with CT/MRI correlation to ensure appropriate interpretation, *cf.* normal variants of cerebral asymmetry.

Indications
- Dementia characterization.
- Epilepsy for localization of epileptogenic focus.

Patient preparation

Secure venous access under resting conditions. Allow the patient to relax before injection of the radiopharmaceutical. Ensure that the patient can co-operate with the imaging procedure.

Procedure
- ^{99m}Tc-HMPAO (exametazine) injected IV in quiet, darkened room, with patient's eyes closed.
- Tomographic brain imaging undertaken immediately and may be repeated 4 h later.

Results

Cortical grey matter uptake is proportional to blood flow (Fig. 14.4(a)).

Interpretation
- Characteristic patterns of abnormal uptake recognized in different dementias (Fig. 14.4b) and in cerebrovascular disease.
- ↑ Uptake at epileptogenic focus on interictal scans—often changing to ↑ uptake on ictal imaging.

Advantages

Abnormalities on functional imaging should predate structural atrophy on anatomical imaging.

Pitfalls
- Tomographic image analysis degraded by movement artefact and asymmetric positioning.
- Data processing is operator-dependent.

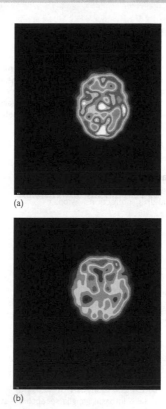

(a)

(b)

Fig. 14.4 ⁹⁹ᵐTc-HMPAO brain imaging. Transaxial tomographic slices: (a) normal and (b) dementia. (☐ Colour plate 7.)

Brain transporter imaging

Background
Reflect role of dopaminergic system in movement disorders, e.g. Parkinsonian syndromes, essential tremor. ^{123}I-Ioflupane is a cocaine analogue, which binds to dopamine transporter on pre-synaptic nerve terminal. Post-synaptic receptor imaging agents are necessary to differentiate among the various Parkinsonian syndromes (not routinely available).

Indications
Movement disorders: Distinguishes Parkinson's syndrome (PkS) from benign essential tremor.

Patient preparation
- Block thyroid—potassium iodate/iodide.
- Multiple potential drug interactions—*stop*:
  - Amphetamine.
  - Citalopram.
  - Cocaine.
  - Fluoxetine.
  - Fluvoxamine.
  - Mazindol.
  - Methylphenidate.
  - Orphenadrine.
  - Phentermine.
  - Procyclidine.
  - Sertraline.

Procedure
^{123}I-labelled radiotracer, e.g. ioflupane, injected IV. Tomographic gamma camera imaging 3–6 h later.

Results
Intense, symmetric uptake in basal ganglia receptors—striatum, caudate, and putamen (Fig. 14.5a).

Interpretation
↓ Basal ganglia uptake in PkS (Fig. 14.5b).

Advantages
Sensitive and specific for PkS, differentiating PkS from essential tremor. No other imaging technique currently available to demonstrate receptor status.

Pitfalls
Drug interactions (Patient preparation, p. 802).

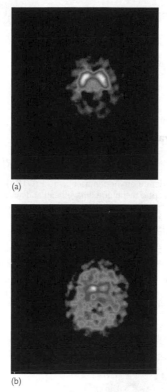

(a)

(b)

Fig. 14.5 ^{123}I-ioflupane brain transporter imaging: (a) normal dopamine transporters and (b) in Parkinson's disease. (📖 Colour plate 8.)

Further reading

Bairactaris C, Demakopoulos N, Tripsianis G, Sioka C, Farmakiotis D, Vadikolias K, Heliopoulos I, Georgoulias P, Tsongos I, Papanastasion I, Piperidou C. Imapct of dopamine transporter single photon emission computed tomography imaging using I-123 ioflupane on diagnoses of patients with parkinsonian syndromes. *J Clin Neurosci* 2009; **16**: 246–52.

CSF shunt patency

Background
Ventricular shunts are routinely used to manage hydrocephalus. Symptoms of shunt obstruction may be non-specific and do not indicate the level of obstruction. Nuclear medicine offers a straightforward means of determining shunt patency.

Indications
Suspected VP shunt obstruction.

Patient preparation
None.

Procedure
Inject ^{111}In- diethylenetriaminepentaacetic acid (DTPA) into shunt reservoir using strict aseptic technique. Image head and abdomen immediately and 30–60 min post injection. (^{99m}Tc-DTPA not recommended because difficult to ensure apyrogenicity.)

Results
Normally, rapid reservoir emptying and shunt visualization within 2–3 min of injection. Free activity within abdominal cavity by 30 min (Fig. 14.6).

Interpretation
Delayed clearance implies obstruction—level usually at reservoir/proximal shunt or due to intra-abdominal kinking.

Advantages
Sensitive, simple, rapid results.

Pitfalls
Infection risk.

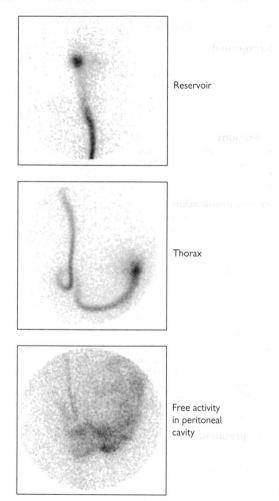

Reservoir

Thorax

Free activity
in peritoneal
cavity

Fig. 14.6 Patent ventriculoperitoneal shunt showing reservoir, shunt, and free
activity within the peritoneal cavity.

Thyroid scintigraphy

Background

Used to investigate thyrotoxicosis and thyroid ectopia. Thyroid mass or suspected malignancy should be investigated by ultrasound/CT and fine needle aspiration cytology. Imaging is undertaken using ^{99m}Tc-pertechnetate, which is trapped by the thyroid by the same transporter mechanism as iodine, but unlike iodine, is not organified. ^{123}I is more sensitive and specific for the investigation of congenital hypothyroidism.

Indications

- Characterization of thyrotoxicosis—diffuse toxic goitre (Graves' disease), toxic multinodular goitre (Plummer's disease).
- Solitary autonomous nodule.
- Acute thyroiditis.

Patient preparation

Thyroxine and iodine rich preparations, e.g. iodine supplements, contrast media, amiodarone will block tracer uptake by the thyroid for up to 9 months. T4 should be withdrawn for 6 weeks; T3 for 2 weeks. Antithyroid drugs can be continued.

Procedure

Inject ^{99m}Tc-pertechnetate IV. Image after 15–30 min. Include anterior thorax views if retrosternal extension is suspected. Neck palpation essential to assess function in discrete thyroid nodules. ^{123}I may be administered either orally or IV. Imaging is carried out at 2 h.

Results

- Uptake reflects function of the thyroid iodine trap.
- Diffuse ↑ uptake in Graves' disease (Fig. 14.7(a)).
- Heterogeneous uptake with suppressed background activity indicates toxic multinodular change (Fig. 14.7(b)).
- Solitary autonomous nodules show intense increased uptake with complete suppression of the remainder of the gland.
- Acute thyroiditis is characterized by absent tracer uptake.

Interpretation

Sensitive and specific for hyperthyroidism.

Advantages

Simple, cheap, and non-invasive. Essential to planning therapy in hyperthyroidism.

Pitfalls

Anatomical definition inferior to ultrasound, CT, etc. Superseded by ultrasound guided fine needle aspirate (FNA) for diagnosis of thyroid mass lesions.

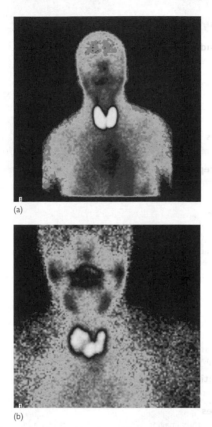

(a)

(b)

Fig. 14.7 Thyroid scintigraphy: (a) in Graves' disease and (b) in toxic multi-nodular goitre.

Parathyroid scintigraphy

Background

Hyperparathyroidism may be primary, i.e. functioning adenoma; secondary, where there is hypocalcaemia from chronic lowering of serum calcium, e.g. renal insufficiency, or tertiary, i.e. hypersecretion of PTH in the presence of either normal or elevated levels of calcium. Nuclear medicine is of value in localizing parathyroid adenomas, particularly following previous surgery.

Indications

Localization of parathyroid adenoma in proven hyperparathyroidism.

Patient preparation

Withdraw thyroxine or iodine containing compounds (*cf.* thyroid imaging).

Procedure

3 different techniques are available
1 ^{123}I-iodide IV followed by ^{99m}Tc-sestamibi, *or*
2 ^{99m}Tc-sestamibi IV 5min and 4h delayed images, *or*
3 ^{99m}Tc-pertechnetate followed by ^{201}Tl-thallous chloride.

Image anterior neck and mediastinum after each administration.

Results

Normal thyroid concentrates ^{123}I, ^{99m}Tc-pertechnetate, ^{99m}Tc-sestamibi (initially), and ^{210}Tl, whereas parathyroid only concentrates ^{99m}Tc-sestamibi and ^{201}Tl (Fig. 14.8).

Computer assisted image subtraction [(thyroid + parathyroid) – thyroid] identifies abnormal parathyroid tissue.

Interpretation

Parathyroid adenoma shown as hyperfunctioning nodule(s).

Advantages

Good when other imaging fails, particularly ectopic adenomas and after unsuccessful neck exploration.

Pitfalls

Multinodular thyroid prevents subtraction analysis. False –ves in multiple parathyroid adenomata or hyperplasia. Many surgeons still prefer intraoperative blue dye.

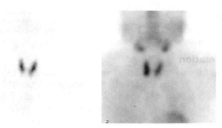

Fig. 14.8 Parathyroid scintigraphy showing images obtained with both ^{123}I-iodide and ^{99m}Tc-sestamibi.

Metaiodobenzylguanidine imaging

Background

Neuroendocrine tumours are rare. Symptoms reflect hormone hyper-secretion, but intermittent secretory patterns can result in false negative screening tests, e.g. 24 h urine collections. MIBG is concentrated by adrenergic tissue via the noradrenaline reuptake mechanism. Virtually all phaeochromocytomas and neuroblastomas will be demonstrated using ^{123}I-MIBG scintigraphy. The sensitivity for other neuroendocrine tumours is variable. High dose ^{131}I-MIBG therapy is a useful treatment for MIBG +ve neuroendocrine tumours.

Indications

- Localization, staging, and response monitoring of neuroectodermal tumours.
- Phaeochromocytoma (imaging investigation of choice).
- Neuroblastoma.
- Carcinoid tumours.
- Medullary thyroid cancer.

Patient preparation

- **Multiple known and theoretical drug interactions**: *Stop for >48 h:*
  - Antidepressants—tricyclics, tetracyclics, MAOIs, serotonin reuptake inhibitors.
  - Phenothiazines.
  - Labetalol*.
  - L-dopa, dopamine agonists.
  - Sympathomimetics—including OTC nasal decongestants.
- **Block thyroid**: potassium iodate/iodide; perchlorate.

Procedure

Inject ^{123}I-MIBG slowly IV with blood pressure monitoring. Image posterior abdomen at 5 min to identify renal outlines, then whole body imaging at 18–24 h. Tomographic imaging may improve tumour localization—not always required.

Results

Physiological uptake at 24 h in salivary glands, myocardium, liver, and normal adrenals with gut and renal excretion.

Interpretation

- Intense ↑ uptake in phaeochromocytomas, with suppressed activity in the contralateral, normal adrenal, and myocardium. Whole body imaging identifies extra adrenal and metastatic disease (Fig. 14.9a).
- Diffuse bone marrow uptake common in stage IV neuroblastoma (Fig. 14.9b).

Advantages

Sensitive, non-invasive tumour localization pre-operatively excludes multi-focal and extra-adrenal tumours. Non-invasive treatment response monitoring in neuroblastoma—avoids sampling errors compared with bone marrow biopsy.

Pitfalls

Drug interactions causing false −ve results. Dilated renal pelvis sometimes confused with tumour uptake. Check with 5 min renal image if in doubt.

*No interaction with any other α- or β-blocker or antihypertensive.

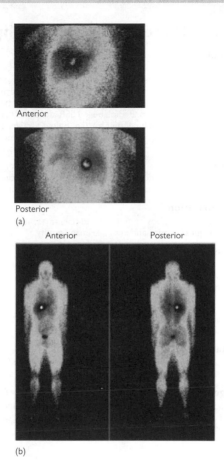

Fig. 14.9 ¹²³I-MIBG scan: (a) right intra-adrenal phaeochromocytoma; (b) whole body scan—right intra-adrenal phaeochromocytoma. Excludes multifocal, ectopic and malignant tumour. (☐ Colour plate 9.)

Somatostatin receptor scintigraphy

Background

Somatostatin receptor (SSR) imaging identifies neuroendocrine tumours including gastroenteropancreatic tumours e.g. carcinoids, gastrinomas, insulinomas. Many other common neoplasms also express surface somatostatin receptors. Somatostatin analogues, e.g. octreotide, bind to cell surface somatostatin receptors. Radiolabelled SSR analogues demonstrate receptor positive disease. Sub-centimetre (i.e. below the limits of cross-sectional radiology) hyperfunctioning 1° tumours can be detected. High-dose radiolabelled SSR therapy is used to treat multi-site disease.

Indications

Localize and stage neuroendocrine tumours (NETs), e.g. carcinoid, insulinoma, gastrinoma, phaeochromocytoma, and medullary thyroid cancer.

Patient preparation

None. Prophylactic laxatives at time of radiopharmaceutical administration accelerate gut clearance and improve image quality.

Procedure

Inject ^{111}In or ^{99m}Tc labelled SSR analogue (octreotide or lanreotide) IV. Whole body gamma camera imaging at 4 and 24 h (±48 h), with tomography if necessary.

Results

Normal uptake in thyroid, liver, spleen, kidneys, and RE system with gut and renal excretion.

Interpretation

↑ Uptake in tumours expressing surface somatostatin receptors. Tomography improves detection of small pancreatic and intrahepatic tumours (Fig. 14.10).

Advantages

Tumour uptake predicts symptom response to somatostatin analogue therapy. Image co-registration with CT or MRI improves localization of occult pancreatic NETs.

Pitfalls

Interpretation often hindered by gut excretion.

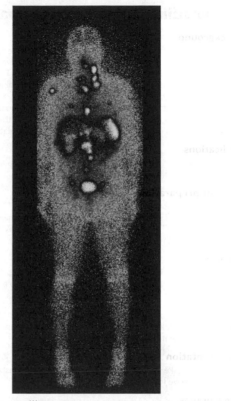

Fig. 14.10 Whole body ^{111}In-octreotide scan showing neuroectodermal tumour with hepatic metastases. (See also 📖 Colour plate 10.)

Radioiodine thyroid cancer imaging

Background
The 1° treatment for thyroid carcinoma is total thyroidectomy with lymph node dissection, depending on tumour stage. Radioactive iodine is administered postoperatively to ablate the thyroid remnant. Thyroglobulin (Tg) can then be used as a tumour marker—Tg is undetectable in the absence of functioning thyroid tissue. Rising Tg following ^{131}I ablation indicates recurrence. If Tg rises, a diagnostic ^{131}I imaging study localizes the site of relapse and assess the feasibility of further radio iodine therapy. The sensitivity of imaging is increased by recombinant TSH stimulation.

Indications
Routine differentiated follicular thyroid cancer follow up, after surgery and ^{131}I thyroid remnant ablation.

Patient preparation
Need high TSH drive to stimulate ^{131}I uptake—stop T3/T4 replacement for minimum 2 (T3) or 6 weeks (T4) or give recombinant thyroid stimulating hormone (TSH). Avoid iodine administration, IV contrast media, amiodarone (*cf.* thyroid imaging).

Procedure
Give ^{131}I sodium iodide po/IV. Obtain blood samples for Tg and TSH at the time of ^{131}I administration. Whole body gamma camera imaging 2–5 days later.

Results
Physiological uptake in salivary glands. Occasional stomach and gastrointestinal (GI) retention. Renal excretion.

Interpretation
Abnormal uptake indicates functioning thyroid metastasis. Anatomical markers improve localization (Fig. 14.11).

Advantages
Detects residual tumour and identifies patients likely to benefit from ^{131}I therapy.

Pitfalls
False −ves without significant TSH drive—aim for TSH >50mU/L; undifferentiated and papillary tumours may be ^{131}I negative.

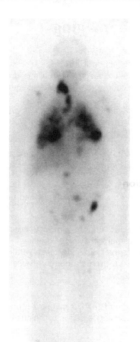

Fig. 14.11 Anterior whole body ¹³¹I image showing local tumour recurrence in the thyroid bed and mediastinum.

Sentinel node imaging

Background

Regional lymph node dissection is performed for cancer staging, to determine the need for adjuvant therapy. Lymphatic drainage can be demonstrated by radiolabelled colloid imaging, which identifies the first or 'sentinel' draining node. Staging based on the excision and histological examination of this node for evidence of metastasis is as reliable as that obtained from block dissection and avoids the morbidity of extended lymph node dissection.

Indications

Pre-operative assessment in breast cancer and melanoma. May have applications in head and neck, vulval and penile cancer staging.

Patient preparation

None. Usually undertaken within 24 h of planned surgery.

Procedure

Intradermal, subcutaneous, or intratumoural injection of ^{99m}Tc labelled nanocolloid. Gamma camera imaging of draining lymph nodes to identify sentinel node. Where surgery is undertaken within 24 h, an intra-operative gamma probe can be used to identify the sentinel node for staging excision biopsy.

Results

Sentinel node usually identifiable 15 min to 2 h post-injection, depending on the 1° tumour location and injection technique used.

Interpretation

The sentinel node is the first lymph node identified on gamma imaging or the node with the highest radioactive count rate using the gamma probe (Fig. 14.12).

Advantages

Accurate sentinel node identification avoids block node dissection, where this is undertaken solely for tumour staging.

Pitfalls

May fail if local lymphatic channels have been disrupted by previous surgery.

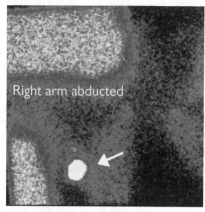

Fig. 14.12 ⁹⁹ᵐTc-nanocolloid sentinel node study—anterior thorax, right arm abducted. Peri-tumoural, subcutaneous injection right breast and sentinel node (arrow). (📖 Colour plate 11.)

Scintimammography

Breast cancer diagnosis relies on accurate localization (ultrasound ± mammography) and tissue biopsy (FNA) or core biopsy. Where mammography is non-diagnostic MRI, CT, or ^{18}F-FDG PET/CT are useful. Nuclear medicine scintimammography is as sensitive, but more specific than MRI and mammography in palpable lesions.

Indications

Investigation of suspicious breast lesions, in difficult-to-interpret mammograms, e.g. dense or lumpy breast tissue, calcification, breast implants, previous surgery.

Patient preparation

None.

Procedure

^{99m}Tc-sestamibi administered IV ideally into contralateral foot, with early (5–10 min) imaging post-injection. Patient is imaged prone, with breast fully dependent, with prone and lateral views of each breast, to include axillae.

Results

Normal distribution of ^{99m}Tc-sestamibi is to the myocardium, liver, and occasionally thyroid.

Interpretation

Focal accumulation in breast and/or axilla implies the presence of tumour. Findings should be interpreted in conjunction with other tests.

Advantages

Can demonstrate multifocal, multicentric disease, both ipsilateral and contralateral axillary spread. May be used to identify most suitable site for guided biopsy.

Pitfalls

Not reliable in small (<1cm) lesions; extravasation of injection in upper limbs may result in false-positive axillary uptake.

Poor injection technique will lead to errors in analysis. The camera and supporting software require high count rate capability, and the technique require expertise in data analysis to ensure reliable, reproducible results. Close liaison with referring clinician is essential to maximize value of the investigation.

Further reading

Buscombe J, Hill J, Parbhoo S. *Scintimammography. A Guide to Good Practice.* Gibbs Associates Ltd., Birmingham, UK 1998
Taillefer R. Clinical applications of 99mTc-sestamibi scintimammography. *Semin Nucl Med*, 2005; **35**: 100–15.

Positron emission tomography

PET is expanding rapidly. Tomographic PET images are acquired using a dedicated PET scanner after administration of positron emitting radiopharmaceuticals. Spatial resolution (5–7mm) is significantly superior to conventional nuclear medicine imaging.

PET images biologically important molecules such as radiolabelled water, ammonia, amino acids or glucose derivatives—the glucose analogue ^{18}F-fluorodeoxyglucose (^{18}F-FDG) is used for most clinical PET studies, particularly in oncology. Malignant cells have both a higher glycolytic rate and over expression of membrane glucose transporters leading to high ^{18}F-FDG uptake compared to normal tissues. ^{18}F-FDG is trapped within metabolically active cells so that abnormalities are detected by metabolic differences rather than anatomical size i.e. inherently more sensitive than structure based imaging.

The main indications for PET imaging are in oncology where ^{18}F-FDG PET is used for diagnosis, staging and monitoring treatment response. Low grade uptake occurs in granulomatous disease, inflammation, and sepsis.

PET allows radioactive concentrations within tissues to be measured accurately so that physiological processes can be expressed in absolute units. The standardized uptake value (SUV) measures the concentration of tracer within a tumour compared to the injected activity, normalized to body weight. Serial SUV measurements allow ^{18}F-FDG uptake to be followed as a marker of treatment response and may be of prognostic value.

Other major applications include nuclear cardiology, where patterns of myocardial ^{18}F-FDG uptake are used to detect myocardial hibernation. In neurosciences, PET remains a largely research tool for the investigation of movement disorders, dementia and degenerative disease.

Other tracers that are available for clinical use include ^{11}C-methionine, measuring tumour amino acid transport and protein synthesis and H_2^{15}O water for blood flow measurements. ^{68}Ga-labelled somatostatin peptides are used to image neuroendocrine tumours. Future developments will include labelled thymidine analogues (e.g. ^{18}F-FLT) to measure proliferation, hypoxic markers, and tracers capable of detecting apoptosis and angiogenesis.

The main limitation of PET imaging in oncology is limited anatomical definition. To improve attenuation correction and tomographic localization, PET imaging is usually combined with CT. The combination of functional and anatomical data in fused images significantly improves the sensitivity and specificity of imaging. Future developments may involve combined PET/magnetic resonance imaging.

Indications

- **Tumour diagnosis**: solitary pulmonary nodule characterization, location of carcinoma of unknown primary origin.
- **Tumour staging**: non-small cell lung cancer; lymphoma; oesophageal cancer; colorectal cancer; head and neck cancer; melanoma.
- **Response assessment/relapse detection**: as above.

Patient preparation
- Cellular ^{18}F-FDG uptake is glucose-dependent.
  - Non-diabetic patients—6 h fast.
  - Aim for blood glucose <7mmol/L.
  - Insulin-dependent diabetic patients—allow normal diet and insulin.
  - Avoid hyperglycaemia—use sliding scale if necessary or defer investigation.
- **Patients should be rested**: to avoid skeletal muscle uptake.
- **Diazepam administration**: 5mg po reduces physiological brown fat uptake in young patients.
- Patients with head and neck cancer should be silent during injection and until completion of imaging to prevent vocal chord uptake.

Procedure
- ^{18}F-FDG injected IV supine in restful surroundings.
- Whole body or half body (base of skull to proximal femora) imaging undertaken 60–90 min post-injection.

Results
The normal distribution of ^{18}F-FDG is to the brain and myocardium. with GI and renal excretion (Fig. 14.13).

Interpretation
Abnormal uptake should be correlated with cross-sectional imaging for precise anatomical localization (Figs. 14.14, 14.15). SUV (see 📖 p. 956) measurement helpful in serial studies.

Advantages
- Discriminates between viable and necrotic/scar tissue, where a residual mass may persist on anatomical imaging post-therapy (Figs. 14.16, 14.17).
- Non-invasive, whole body, 3D imaging.

Pitfalls
- Sensitivity lower in more indolent tumours—lung carcinoid, alveolar cell carcinoma, neuroendocrine tumours, depending on proliferative index and, occasionally, in pancreatic tumours.
- Limited availability—specialist centres only.
- Relatively expensive.

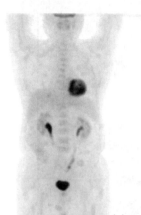

Fig. 14.13 Normal ^{18}F-FDG PET scan—coronal tomogram.

0 deg

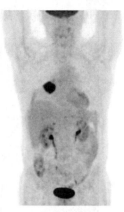

Fig. 14.14 ^{18}F-FDG PET scan—non-small cell lung cancer right lung. Whole body coronal.

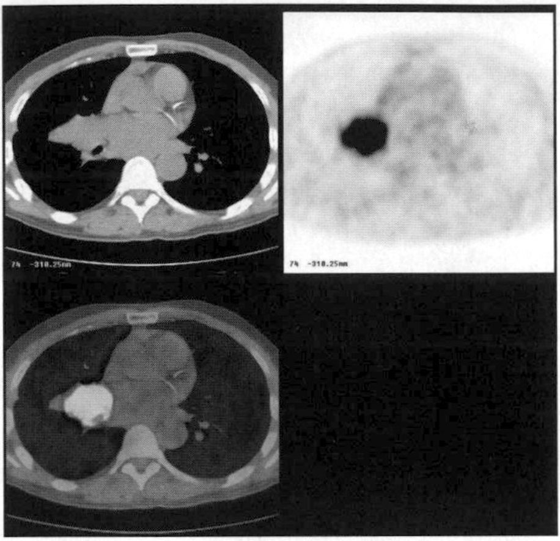

Fig. 14.15 ^{18}F-FDG PET scan—transaxial views showing CT (top left) correlation with PET (top right). The image fusion is shown bottom left. (📖 Colour plate 12.)

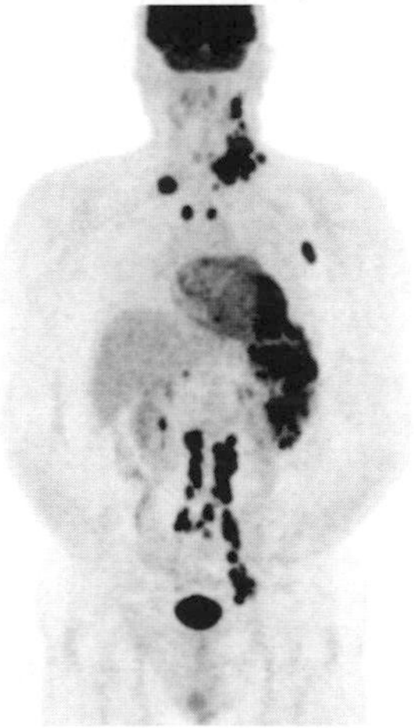

Fig. 14.16 ^{18}F-FDG PET scan—non-Hodgkin's lymphoma. Whole body coronal view of patient pretreatment showing extensive FDG avid adenopathy.

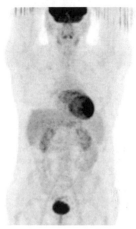

Fig. 14.17 ^{18}F-FDG PET scan—non-Hodgkin's lymphoma. Post-treatment showing complete metabolic response.

Myocardial perfusion imaging

Background

MPI reflects regional blood flow during stress (increased demand) and at rest providing prognostically significant information that, both in isolation and in conjunction with coronary angiography, can be used to optimize patient management.[1]

Originally performed using ^{201}Tl-thallous chloride, but now based on ^{99m}Tc labelled tracers—sestamibi (methoxy-isobutylisonitrile) or tetrofosmin. Exercise or pharmacological stress are used to challenge coronary artery reserve. Exercise is performed by treadmill or bicycle, while pharmacological stressors are either adenosine/dipyridamole infusion, which increases coronary artery blood flow by vasodilatation, or dobutamine infusion with both inotropic and chronotropic activity.

Indications

Ischaemic heart disease

Pre-angiography
- When conventional stress testing fails, e.g. bundle branch block.
- Left ventricular hypertrophy.
- Atypical chest pain.
- Recurrent chest pain post-intervention. Good prognostic indicator.

Post-angiography
- Assess functional significance of known stenoses.
- Identify critical vascular territory for intervention.

Patient preparation

- Stop β-blockers 24 h prior to stress study.
- Sometimes helpful to withdraw all anti-anginal medication.
- Assess optimal stress technique for individual patient, i.e. exercise or pharmacological.
- Attach 12-lead ECG.
- Insert IV cannula.
- Check baseline blood pressure.

Procedure

2-part investigation comparing myocardial perfusion during stress and at rest

Stress test
- Treadmill or bicycle exercise to >85% maximum predicted heart rate or adenosine 140µg/kg/min IVI for 6min—sometimes with submaximal exercise *or*, Dobutamine 5–40µg/kg/min in 5µg/kg/min increments over 16min

1 Marcassa C, Bar JJ, Bengel F, Hesse B, Petersen CL, Reyes E, Underwood R on behalf of the European Council of Nuclear Cardiology (ECNC), the European Society of Cardiology Working Group 9 (Nuclear Cardiology and Cardiac CT), and the European Association of Nuclear Medicine Cardiovascualr Committee. Clinical value, cost-effectiveness, and safety of myocardial perfusion scintigraphy: a position statement. *Eur Heart J* 2008; **29**: 557–63.

- Inject radiopharmaceutical (^{201}Tl-thallous chloride, ^{99m}Tc-sestamibi or ^{99m}Tc-tetrofosmin) at peak stress.
- Tomographic imaging immediately (^{201}Tl) or 15–60min post-injection (^{99m}Tc compounds). Images generally acquired with ECG gating.

Rest study
- 2nd ^{99m}Tc radiopharmaceutical injection under resting conditions.
- Tomographic imaging as before.
- With ^{201}Tl, 2nd injection not necessary, since tracer redistributes into ischaemic areas over 4 h, but top-up dose sometimes given.

Results
Myocardial uptake reflects radiopharmaceutical delivery and myocyte function (Fig. 14.18).

Interpretation
Infarction causes matched perfusion defects during stress and rest. Inducible ischaemia creates a perfusion defect at stress, which reperfuses at rest = reversible ischaemia (Fig. 14.19). The severity, extent, and number of reversible defects are prognostically significant. A normal MPI study implies risk of an adverse cardiac event <0.5% per annum.

Advantages
Non-invasive; relatively inexpensive compared with angiography.

Pitfalls
Less sensitive in multiple small vessel coronary disease, e.g. diabetes mellitus. Sensitivity depends on stress test quality.

Stress   Rest

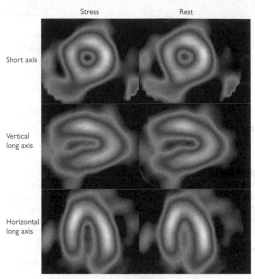

Short axis

Vertical
long axis

Horizontal
long axis

Fig. 14.18 Normal myocardial perfusion scan. (📖 Colour plate 13.)

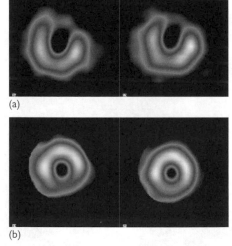

(a)

(b)

Fig. 14.19 Myocardial perfusion scan: (a) in fixed perfusion loss (anterolateral infarction) and (b) in inferior stress-induced (reversible) ischaemia. (📖 Colour plate 14.)

Radionuclide ventriculography: MUGA scans

Background

Increasingly replaced by transthoracic echocardiography (TTE), trans-oesophageal echocardiography (TOE) and contrast ventriculography at time of cardiac catheterization. MUGA scans are less operator-dependent than either TTE or TOE which may be important if serial assessment is required. The cardiac blood pool is imaged dynamically after injection of radiolabelled red blood cells. From this, wall motion, synchronicity of ventricular contraction and ejection fraction are measured (Fig. 14.20). The estimated ejection fraction is unreliable in the presence of dysrrhythmias—the acquisition requires a relatively regular heart rate.

Indications

- Left ventricle (LV) ejection fraction measurement, e.g. unechogenic patients (Fig. 14.21a).
- Monitor anthracycline cardiotoxicity.

Patient preparation

None.

Procedure

Radiolabel red cells (*in vivo* or *in vitro*) using ^{99m}Tc-pertechnetate. Image patient supine in anterior and left anterior oblique projections. Camera acquisition gated to cardiac cycle. Imaging sometimes combined with low impact exercise/pharmacological stress to assess cardiac reserve.

Results

Visual image of 300–400 summated cardiac cycles. Computer generated images used to assess regional wall motion and synchronous contraction (Fig. 14.21b). Computer generated ejection fraction calculation. Normal EF 60–70%, ↓ with age.

Interpretation

EF used to monitor treatment response in cardiac failure, cardiomyopathy.

Advantages

Good for serial measurement during anthracycline chemotherapy. Reliable in unechogenic subjects.

Disadvantage

Moderately high radiation dose: echocardiography preferable in most patients.

Pitfalls

Cardiac dysrrhythmias interfere with gating e.g. atrial fibrillation.

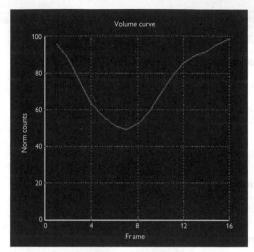

Fig. 14.20 Computer-generated ejection fraction 40%.

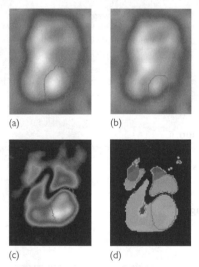

Fig. 14.21 MUGA scan showing (a) LV regions of interest at end diastole and (b) end systole for ejection fraction calculation; (c) amplitude image showing relative anteroseptal hypokinesis, but (d) synchronous LV contraction. (📖 Colour plate 15.)

Radionuclide first pass cardiac studies

Background

Nuclear medicine can assess simple shunts, e.g. left-to-right shunts (ventricular and atrial septal defects), but has no place in bi-directional shunting or multiple sources of pulmonary blood flow (e.g. patent ductus arteriosus). First pass studies quantify shunt severity both pre- and post-surgical correction. Complementary to cardiac catheterization and colour Doppler flow echocardiography. Dynamic imaging of a small bolus of IV radioactivity, usually ^{99m}Tc-DTPA, outlines cardiac venous return, pulmonary circulation, left heart, and the systemic circulation. Largely superseded by angiography and MRI.

Indications

Measurement of simple left-to-right cardiac shunts.

Patient preparation

None.

Procedure

- ^{99m}Tc-DTPA administered IV as a bolus into a right antecubital vein with shoulder abducted.
- Images are obtained immediately, as a dynamic acquisition over 60 s.

Results

Normal circulation will demonstrate sequential appearance of right heart, pulmonary outflow tract, lungs, left heart, and aorta.

Interpretation

Variation in the normal sequence implies cardiac shunting. Interpretation must be performed in conjunction with definitive knowledge of patient's anatomy, e.g. echocardiography with Doppler colour flow.

Advantages

Relatively non-invasive technique for serial follow-up of congenital heart disease. Mathematical analysis of the data allows quantification of shunt size, and is important for consideration and timing of corrective surgery.

Lung scan: ventilation/ perfusion imaging

Background

One of the most widely requested nuclear medicine studies. Sensitivity and specificity reduced in co-existing lung disease, when computed tomographic pulmonary angiography (CTPA) is more useful. All patients should have had a chest radiograph within 24 h to aid V/Q interpretation and exclude other causes of pleuritic chest pain and hypoxia, e.g. pneumothorax.

Lung perfusion shown by injection of tiny ^{99m}Tc particles which are trapped by the pulmonary capillary bed. Ventilation shown using radio-labelled gases or aerosols.

Indications

- Suspected pulmonary embolism.
- Pre-operative lung function assessment.

Patient preparation

None. Relative contraindication in right left intracardiac shunts; caution in severe pulmonary hypertension.

Procedure

- Lie patient supine and inject ^{99m}Tc-macroaggregated albumin (MAA) IV.
- Obtain gamma camera perfusion images in 4 views.
- Ventilation images are obtained in same projections by continuous breathing of ^{81m}Kr gas or using ^{99m}Tc aerosol or ^{133}xenon gas.

Results

Homogeneous, matched ventilation and perfusion patterns (Fig. 14.22).

Interpretation

Four abnormal patterns recognized

1 **Segmental perfusion loss with preserved ventilation**: pulmonary embolism (Fig. 14.23b).
2 **Segmental matched perfusion and ventilation loss**: pulmonary infarction/infection.
3 **Segmental/subsegmental ventilation loss with preserved perfusion**: infection.
4 **Non-segmental, patchy, matched perfusion, and ventilation loss**: COPD (Fig. 14.23a).

Advantages

Quick, non-invasive. Normal scan virtually excludes PE.

Pitfalls

Specificity reduced in underlying lung disease—chronic obstructive pulmonary disease (COPD), asthma giving indeterminate results. False +ves with tumour, bullae, vasculitides, fibrotic lung disease, and old, unresolved pulmonary embolism (PE).

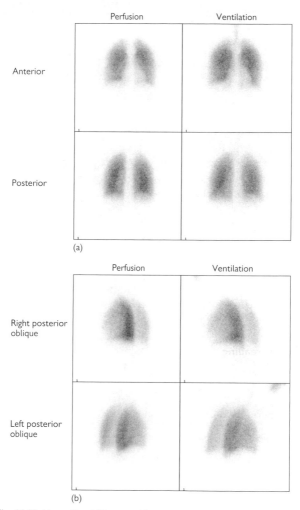

Fig. 14.22 Normal lung V/Q images: (a) anterior and posterior views; (b) oblique views.

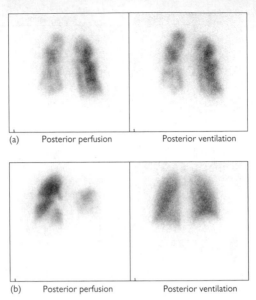

Fig. 14.23 Lung scans: (a) showing matched, non-segmental V/Q defects in COPD; and (b) showing segmental V/Q mismatch—extensive bilateral pulmonary thromboembolism and unmatched perfusion loss.

Further reading

Worsley DF, Alavi A. Comprehensive analysis of the results of the PIOPED study. *J Nucl Med* 1995; **36**: 2380–7.

Lung shunt studies

Background
Largely research procedure.

Indications
Suspected pulmonary AV shunting.

Patient preparation
None.

Procedure
Inject ^{99m}Tc-nanocolloid IV. Gamma camera lung, abdomen, and head imaging. Calculate relative uptake in lungs, kidneys, and brain. Express as fraction of cardiac output to quantify shunt fraction.

Results
Kidneys and brain not normally visible on lung perfusion imaging.

Interpretation
Abnormal extrapulmonary activity implies degree of shunting. Intensity of uptake rises with shunt severity.

Advantages
Non-invasive, quantitative. Can be used to monitor response to intervention.

Pitfalls
Injection extravasation invalidates shunt calculation.

Lung permeability studies

Background

Altered alveolar permeability affects gas exchange. Also shown by lung transfer factor measurement.

Indications

- *Pneumocystis carinii* **(PCP) infection**: rapid screening in high risk patients with normal CXR.
- Monitor treatment response in cryptogenic fibrosing alveolitis.

Patient preparation

None.

Procedure

Patient breathes ^{99m}Tc-DTPA aerosol. Gamma camera images of thorax over 1 h. Computer data analysis generates lung clearance curves reflecting integrity of alveolar cell barrier.

Results

Clearance curves used to calculate permeability index. Individual results compared with centre defined normal range.

Interpretation

Accelerated clearance in PCP, which ↓ with successful treatment.

Advantages

Non-invasive. Allows rapid PCP diagnosis.

Pitfalls

Non-specific, e.g. accelerated clearance in smokers.

Lymphoscintigraphy

Background

Lymphoedema can be congenital or acquired. The lymphatic system normally drains subcutaneous tissues → local lymphatic channels and regional nodes. Lymphatic channels can be imaged using radiolabelled colloid particles (🕮 Sentinel node imaging, p816).

Indication

Unexplained limb swelling, e.g. lymphatic hypoplasia.

Patient preparation

None.

Procedure

^{99m}Tc-nanocolloid injection subcutaneously into finger or toe webspace on affected and contralateral limb. Regional gamma camera imaging at 10 min intervals over next hour.

Results

Normally rapid clearance via lymphatic channels to regional nodes (Fig. 14.24).

Interpretation

Slow clearance and failed regional node uptake in hypoplastic systems or metastatic regional node infiltration, depending on clinical context.

Advantages

Much easier than conventional (contrast) lymphography—avoids lymphatic channel cannulation.

Pitfalls

Lymphatic drainage may be disrupted by surgery or radiotherapy.

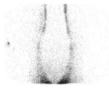
Feet/ankles

Pelvis/abdomen

Fig. 14.24 Normal lymphoscintigrams.

Static cortical renography: dimercaptosuccinic acid imaging

Background

Dimercaptosuccinic acid (DMSA) is concentrated by the proximal convoluted tubules in the renal cortex. ^{99m}Tc-DMSA provides good definition of functioning renal parenchyma. It should be used in conjunction with anatomical imaging, e.g. ultrasonography, to differentiate between scarring, cysts, or calculi.

Indications

- Urinary tract infection: 'gold standard' for renal scarring.
- Measurement of relative renal function.
- Renal duplication assessment.
- Ectopic kidney localization.
- Renal trauma.
- Renal vein thrombosis.
- Pre-biopsy.

Patient preparation

None, but avoid dehydration.

Procedure

^{99m}Tc-DMSA injected IV. Static anterior, posterior, and posterior oblique images acquired 2–4h later.

Results

Visual image evaluation, assessing integrity of cortical outlines for scarring (Fig. 14.25a). Quantitative computer image analysis is used to measure relative renal function, i.e. the contribution of each kidney to overall glomerular filtration rate (GFR).

Interpretation

Cortical scars distort renal outline (Fig. 14.25b). Duplication may result in non-functioning upper moiety, usually due to obstruction, or scarred lower moiety, secondary to vesicoureteric reflux. Relative renal function is usually 50:50 ± 5%.

Advantages

Sensitive for renal scarring. Superior to ultrasound. Non-invasive.

Pitfalls

False +ves during or immediately after acute pyelonephritis. May give cortical defects that do not progress to scarring. Splenic impression at left upper pole may be mistaken for scarring.

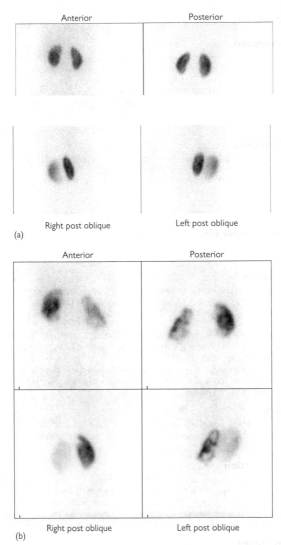

Fig. 14.25 DMSA static renogram: (a) normal and (b) showing extensive bilateral cortical scarring.

Dynamic renography

Background

Nuclear medicine offers unique 'real time' imaging of renal function, i.e. visualization of uptake, drainage and bladder emptying. Available radio-pharmaceuticals: ^{99m}Tc-DTPA, cleared by glomerular filtration, and ^{99m}Tc-mercaptoacetyltriglycine (MAG3), cleared by glomerular filtration and tubular secretion. ^{99m}Tc-MAG3 preferred particularly in the presence of renal impairment and in the immature kidney. ^{99m}Tc-DTPA reserved for assessment of acute tubular necrosis, post-transplant viability, etc.

Indications

- **Assessment of renal drainage**: discrimination between renal dilatation and outflow obstruction.
- Measurement of relative renal function.
- Loin pain.
- Post-pyeloplasty follow-up.
- Renal artery stenosis (📖 Captopril renography, p839).

Patient preparation

Good hydration essential. Empty bladder immediately before undertaking study.

Procedure

1 Position patient supine or seated erect, with the camera behind.
2 Obtain good peripheral venous access. Bolus radiopharmaceutical injection ^{99m}Tc-MAG3 or ^{99m}Tc-DTPA followed by 10–20mL saline flush.
3 Image immediately acquiring real time dynamic data for 20–30 min.
4 Diuretic administration is essential to distinguish dilatation from outflow obstruction.
5 Post-voiding images are always required to assess the completeness of bladder emptying and may improve drainage of the upper renal tracts in high pressure systems.

Results

Visual inspection of renal size, perfusion, function, and drainage (Fig. 14.26a). Quantitative computer image analysis measures relative function, transit times, and generates drainage graphs.

Interpretation

Uptake and excretion of activity normally rapid. Dilated systems show progressive pooling in the renal pelvis that empties following diuretic challenge. Obstructed systems show progressive tracer accumulation with no diuretic response, often associated with ? function on the affected side (Fig. 14.26b).

Advantages

Sensitive, non-invasive, quantitative renal function assessment. Anatomical imaging, e.g. intravenous urogram (IVU), better for renal morphology, stones, etc.

Pitfalls

Movement artefact, chronic renal failure, and dehydration reduce data reliability. Renal drainage may be gravity dependent—always complete study with an erect image. Drainage curves invalidated by radiopharmaceutical extravasation.

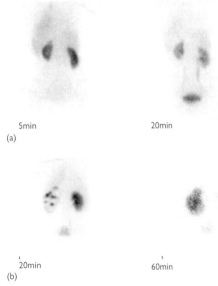

5min   20min
(a)

¹20min   ¹60min
(b)

Fig. 14.26 Dynamic renogram posterior images: (a) normal, showing an early parenchymal image and later symmetrical excretion with bladder filling; (b) outflow obstruction: early image shows left hydronephrosis secondary to pelviureteric junction obstruction, with poor drainage at 60 min.

Captopril renography

Background

Renal artery stenosis is a rare (<2%) cause of hypertension. Suspected in young adults presenting with hypertension, usually due to fibromuscular dysplasia. In patients >50 years, the most common cause is atherosclerosis. Perfusion pressure is maintained by angiotensin II in renal artery stenosis. Captopril is an angiotensin converting enzyme inhibitor (ACEI), which blocks the conversion of angiotensin I to angiotensin II. Captopril reduces perfusion pressure leading to fall in relative function and delayed tracer uptake on affected side. Captopril administration is contraindicated in the presence of a solitary kidney.

Indications
Diagnosis of renal artery stenosis (RAS; especially fibromuscular dysplasia) and prediction of response to revascularization.

Patient preparation
Well-hydrated. Baseline blood pressure. IV access. Stop angiotensin converting enyme (ACE) inhibitors for 48 h prior to test.

Procedure
- Perform standard dynamic renogram using ^{99m}Tc-MAG3.
- Repeat renogram 1h after oral captopril 25mg single dose po.
- Monitor blood pressure—beware hypotension.

Results
Quantitative evaluation of R:L renal function and time to peak activity in each kidney.

Interpretation
RAS due to fibromuscular dysplasia—fall in relative renal function and delayed time to peak renal activity >10 min.

Advantages
Distinguishes generalized atherosclerosis (often poor blood pressure outcome following angioplasty) from fibromuscular hyperplasia (good angioplasty response).

Pitfalls
- ↓ Reliability in the presence of renal impairment.
- Severe hypotension.

Gastrointestinal bleeding: labelled red cell imaging

Background
The source of gastrointestinal blood loss is usually identified by GI endoscopy, but may be difficult to localize. Labelled red cell studies are useful when there is evidence of ongoing bleeding (typically falling Hb of 1g/L/day). The patient must be actively bleeding at the time of the study. This is a time-consuming investigation, with serial imaging beyond 24 h often performed.

Indications
Localize source of active GI haemorrhage when other techniques (e.g. endoscopy or angiography) have failed.

Patient preparation
No recent contrast barium studies. Fasting during first 2 h of imaging.

Procedure
Label red cells (*in vitro* or *in vivo*) using ^{99m}Tc-pertechnetate. Abdominal γ camera blood pool imaging immediately and at intervals for up to 36 h post-injection or until bleeding source is identified.

Results

Activity normally restricted to vascular compartment.

Interpretation

Any activity in gut lumen implies active haemorrhage. Serial images helpful (Fig. 14.27).

Advantages

More sensitive and less invasive than angiography for intermittent bleeding.

Pitfalls

- **Poor red cell label**: degrades image quality, could lead to false +ve.
- **Limits of detection**: 0.5mL/min blood loss.

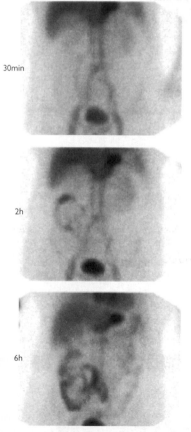

Fig. 14.27 Anterior abdominal images showing increasing red cell haemorrhage into the distal ileum.

Gastric emptying studies

Background

The diagnosis of dysfunctional gastric emptying can be difficult. In children, delayed gastric emptying may contribute to gastro-oesophageal reflux. In adults, both gastric stasis and 'dumping' syndromes occur, sometimes following previous surgery. Imaging following ingestion of radiolabelled solids or liquids demonstrates timing and pattern of gastric emptying.

Indications

Altered GI motility—delayed or accelerated gastric emptying.

Patient preparation

Fast for 4 h. Stop drugs likely to influence GI motility, e.g. domperidone, metoclopramide.

Procedure

Milk study

- Give radiolabelled (^{99m}Tc-DTPA) milk drink orally.
- Image anterior abdomen immediately and at 10min intervals for 1 h. Generate computer derived clearance curves to calculate emptying half time.
- Delayed thoracic image helpful to exclude lung aspiration if clearance significantly delayed.

Dual isotope method

- Give ^{99m}Tc-labelled standard meal (e.g. porridge, egg) with ^{111}In-DTPA in water.
- Anterior abdomen gamma camera imaging as before using dual isotope settings.
- Generate solid and liquid phase clearance curves.

Results

Normal gastric emptying half time (milk = 20 min). Normal range for solids is centre-specific, depending on standard meal composition (Fig. 14.28).

Interpretation

Visual image evaluation and half time calculation.

Advantages

Non-invasive and quantitative.

Pitfalls

Vomiting during study invalidates emptying time calculations.

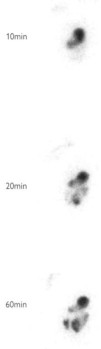

Fig. 14.28 Normal gastric emptying study: anterior images showing clearance of ^{99m}Tc-labelled milk into the proximal small intestine.

Meckel's scan: ectopic gastric mucosa localization

Background

Meckel's diverticulum is the commonest congenital anomaly of the GI tract, occurring in ~2% of the population. <10% contain ectopic gastric mucosa, which may bleed, but diverticuli can also cause obstruction or become inflamed. Typically, childhood presentation. Nuclear medicine provides a straightforward imaging technique that targets gastric mucosal cells, which normally take up ^{99m}Tc-pertechnetate.

Indications

Unexplained abdominal pain or GI haemorrhage—after endoscopy/contrast radiology.

Patient preparation

- Fast for 4 h.
- H_2 antagonist administration may improve specificity.
- No recent barium studies.

Procedure

Inject ^{99m}Tc pertechnetate IV. Immediate and serial abdominal imaging over 1 h.

Results

Normal uptake in gastric mucosa.

Interpretation

Focal abnormal uptake appearing at the same time as the stomach implies ectopic gastric mucosa (Meckel's diverticulum) or, occasionally, duplication cyst. Commonest site— right iliac fossa (RIF).

Advantages

Non-invasive.

Pitfalls

False +ves due to activity in renal tract—lateral images usually help.

Hepatobiliary scintigraphy

Background

Iminodiacetic acid (IDA) compounds are cleared from the circulation by the hepatocytes and secreted into the bile in the same way as bilirubin. ^{99m}Tc-labelled IDA compounds show biliary excretion through the biliary tree and gallbladder → duodenum. Useful in acute/chronic acalculous cholecystitis and to diagnose biliary atresia.

Indications

- Acute cholecystitis.
- Trauma.
- Post-operative leak detection.
- Bile duct/stent patency.
- Gallbladder emptying.
- Bile reflux.
- Neonatal biliary atresia.

Patient preparation

- **Adults**: fast for 6 h.
- **Neonates**: phenobarbitone 5mg/kg/day po for 3days prior to study (enzyme induction).

Procedure

- **Adults**: IV injection ^{99m}Tc-labelled IDA complex (mebrofenin, disofenin). Gamma camera imaging over 1 h.
- **Neonates**: IV injection ^{99m}Tc-IDA. Immediate dynamic imaging for 5 min then serial static images for up to 24 h or until activity reaches small bowel lumen.

Results

Gallbladder and biliary tree normally shown with tracer excretion via common bile duct into duodenum by 30 min post-injection. Cholecystokinin 0.5unit/kg IV sometimes administered to stimulate gallbladder emptying.

Interpretation

- **Acute cholecystitis**: absent gallbladder.
- Obstruction, leak, or reflux assessed visually.
- **Neonates**: passage of activity into gut lumen excludes biliary atresia.
- Quantification of T0 to T10 min images improves specificity for atresia diagnosis.

Advantages

Non-invasive. Straightforward pattern recognition.

Pitfalls

Delayed IDA excretion in severe jaundice: bilirubin >300µmol/L.

Splenunculus detection: heat-damaged red cell imaging

Background
Splenectomy may be indicated in haemolytic syndromes and in refractory haemorrhagic tendencies [e.g. idiopathic thrombocytopenic purpura (ITP)] if associated with hypersplenic thrombocytopenia. Remnant splenic tissue or 'splenunculi' can give rise to recurrent thrombocytopenia—difficult to detect on anatomical imaging. As the spleen removes abnormal red cells from the circulating blood pool, radiolabelled heat damaged red cells can be used to localize ectopic splenic tissue.

Indications
Recurrent thrombocytopenia post-splenectomy.

Patient preparation
None.

Procedure
- Obtain venous blood sample.
- Radiolabel red cells *in vitro* using ^{99m}Tc-pertechnetate.
- Heat to 49.5°C for 20–30 min.
- Cool and re-inject IV.
- Image anterior abdomen 30 min later.

Results & interpretation
Damaged red cells taken up by splenic remnants (Fig. 14.29).

Advantages
Investigation of choice for splenunculus detection.

Pitfalls
Enlarged left lobe of liver may obscure small splenic remnant.

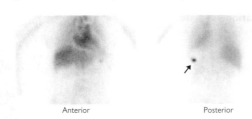

Anterior   Posterior

Fig. 14.29 Post-splenectomy. Intense uptake in splenunculus lying in splenic bed.

Hepatosplenic scintigraphy

Background

Largely superseded by ultrasonography and cross-sectional imaging. Maps reticuloendothelial tissue within the liver (Kupffer cells) and spleen, to identify space occupying lesions, and confirm the presence or absence of functioning splenic tissue.

Indications

Liver space occupying lesions—now largely replaced by ultrasound, CT, or MRI.

Patient preparation

None.

Procedure

^{99m}Tc-colloid injected IV. Abdominal gamma camera images 30 min post-injection.

Results

Normal, homogeneous liver and spleen uptake.

Interpretation

Focal ↓ uptake in space occupying lesions. ↑ Spleen and bone activity in portal hypertension. Focal ↑ uptake in caudate lobe pathognomonic of Budd–Chiari syndrome.

Advantages

Cheap.

Pitfalls

Non-specific. Largely superseded by anatomical imaging.

Labelled leucocyte imaging

Background

Localization and assessment of acute or chronic infection/inflammation can be difficult. Nuclear medicine techniques show inflammation, but do not differentiate infective from non-infective causes. Radiolabelled leucocytes are injected and imaged. The normal distribution includes liver and spleen making peri-diaphragmatic collections difficult to identify. Delayed imaging useful in chronic low grade infection, e.g. osteomyelitis, where cell migration to the site of inflammation is slow.

Indications

- Sepsis localization.
- Inflammatory bowel disease to determine disease activity, extent, severity.

Patient preparation

None. Avoid recent barium contrast radiology.

Procedure

- Obtain 40–60mL blood sample.
- Separate white cell layer and radiolabel *in vitro* using ^{99m}Tc-exametazime (HMPAO) or ^{111}In-oxine.
- Re-inject labelled cells IV.
- Image 1 and 3 h later (inflammatory bowel disease) or 2, 4, and 24 h for intra-abdominal sepsis/osteomyelitis.

Results

Physiological uptake in reticuloendothelial system. Variable GI and renal excretion, depending on radiopharmaceutical used (Fig. 14.30a).

Interpretation

Focal ↑ uptake indicates sepsis. Diffuse ↑ gut uptake reflects extent and activity of inflammatory bowel disease (Fig. 14.30b).

Advantages

Very sensitive in inflammatory bowel disease. Non-invasive, useful in sick patients, e.g. acute exacerbation of inflammatory bowel disease.

Pitfalls

- **False –ves**: leucopenia and poor white cell label, perihepatic and perisplenic collections obscured by normal liver and spleen uptake.
- **False +ves**: physiological gut and renal activity.
- Damaged white cells during labelling causing lung sequestration.
- ^{99m}Tc-exametazime (HMPAO) preferred for routine imaging and inflammatory bowel disease—lower radiation dose and earlier result than ^{111}In-oxine label.
- Reserve ^{111}In-oxine for low grade bone sepsis localization.
- Requires aseptic facilities and trained personnel.
- Risk to staff (blood handling) and patient (contamination, re-injection into wrong patient).

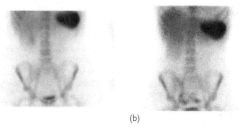

(a) (b)

Fig. 14.30 Labelled leucocyte imaging: (a) normal, and (b) acute inflammatory bowel disease—intense uptake in small and large bowel loops (Crohn's disease).

Gallium scintigraphy

Background

Previously used to diagnose and monitor sarcoid and lymphoma, but increasingly superseded by ^{18}F-FDG PET ([Labelled leucocyte imaging, p847) and cross-sectional imaging. Sometimes useful in 'pyrexia of unknown origin', pyrexia of unknown origin (PUO), e.g. immunocompromised patient where there is a suspicion of *Pneumocystis carinii* infection cf. lung permeability studies.

Indications

- PUO and infection localization, especially in acquired immunodeficiency syndrome (AIDS).
- Lymphoma follow-up.
- Sarcoidosis follow-up.

Patient preparation

None.

Procedure

- Inject ^{67}Ga-citrate IV. Gamma camera imaging at 48–96 h with tomography.
- Non-specific gut retention reduced by laxative administration.

Results

Normal uptake in lacrimal glands, nasal mucosa, blood pool, liver, spleen, testes, female perineum, breast.

Interpretation

- Focal lymph node uptake in lymphoma and sarcoid distinguishes active disease from post-therapy scarring/fibrosis.
- In AIDS, ↑ lung uptake indicates infection—*Pneumocystis jirovecii* pneumonia (PCP), cytomegalovirus (CMV), mycobacterium—chest radiograph correlation essential.
- ↑ activity in inflammatory bowel disease and focal sepsis; largely superseded by white blood cell (WBC) imaging.

Advantages

Excellent, non-invasive marker of disease activity in lymphoma—but likely to be superseded by ^{18}F-FDG.

Pitfalls

Poor specificity. High radiation dose often difficult to justify when alternative techniques available. Prolonged test (48–96 h).

Dacroscintigraphy

Background

Epiphora may arise from excessive tear production or inadequate drainage due to lower lid ectropion or nasolacrimal obstruction, i.e. nasal puncti, lacrimal sac, nasolacrimal ducts. Straightforward technique to assess function of the nasolacrimal apparatus.

Indications

Epiphora.

Patient preparation

None.

Procedure

1–2 drops ^{99m}Tc-labelled DTPA or pertechnetate instilled into outer canthus of each eye. Immediate dynamic gamma camera imaging for 20 min with delayed static scans as required.

Results

Normal rapid radiopharmaceutical clearance through nasolacrimal apparatus.

Interpretation

Delayed clearance implies obstruction—level of dysfunction usually identified, i.e. punctum, lacrimal sac, nasolacrimal duct (Fig. 14.31).

Advantages

Non-invasive. Avoids nasolacrimal duct cannulation (*cf.* dacrocystography).

Pitfalls

Obstructed systems result in excess radiolabelled tears on cheek altering drainage times.

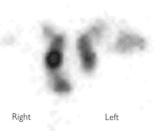

Right   Left

Fig. 14.31 Dacroscintigram (lacrimal drainage) showing normal lacrimal drainage on the right and on the left obstructed drainage at the proximal nasolacrimal duct.

Glomerular filtration rate measurement

Background

In many instances, GFR estimation from creatinine clearance (CrC) is adequate, but accurate measurement is essential in renal impairment or to monitor nephrotoxic drug therapy. Glomerular compensation prevents early renal damage detection by CrC measurements—60% of filtration activity can be lost before CrC falls.

Indications

Accurate GFR to monitor renal failure, cytotoxic chemotherapy, immunosuppression, e.g. cyclosporin.

Patient preparation

Well-hydrated.

Procedure

- IV injection ^{51}Cr- ethylenediaminetetra-acetic acid (EDTA) or ^{99m}Tc-DTPA.
- Venous sampling 2 and 4 h later.
- Count plasma sample radioactivity and known standards in gamma counter. Correct for height and weight.

Results

Normal GFR = 125mL/min (age-dependent).

Interpretation

↓ Values in CRF.

Advantages

More reliable and reproducible than CrC—avoids need for urine collection.

Pitfalls

Accuracy depends on accurate measurement of dose and good injection technique—avoid any extravasation. Unreliable results in severe peripheral oedema.

Urea breath test

Background

Helicobacter pylori infection is associated with duodenal ulceration. Eradication therapy reduces ulcer recurrence. *H. pylori* produces urease which converts labelled urea → labelled CO_2, detected in breath samples.

Indications

Helicobacter pylori detection—diagnosis and confirmation of eradication.

Patient preparation

Stop antibiotics, H_2 antagonists, proton pump inhibitors for 2–4 weeks.

Procedure

- Patient swallows urea drink labelled with ^{13}carbon (stable isotope) or ^{14}carbon (radioactive isotope).
- Breath samples (CO_2) collected over next 30 min.
- Labelled CO_2 measured by mass spectroscopy (^{13}C) or liquid scintillation counting (^{14}C).

Results

Normal range varies according to local protocol.

Interpretation

↑ Exhaled CO_2 levels imply abnormal urea breakdown by urease-producing bacteria in stomach, e.g. *H. pylori*.

Advantages

- Very sensitive marker of active *H. pylori* infection (*cf.* serology).
- Non-invasive (*cf.* endoscopy) and avoids sampling errors.
- Good for non-invasive monitoring of recurrent symptoms.

Pitfalls

Occasional false +ves in oral *H. pylori* infection.

Red cell survival studies

Background

Although infrequently performed, provides evidence of abnormal red cell survival and localizes sites of red cell destruction. The investigation is prolonged, with initial *in vitro* red cell labelling and daily activity measurements over target organs—spleen, liver, and heart for 14 days.

Indications

- Haemolytic anaemia (to confirm ↓ red blood cell (RBC) survival, i.e. active haemolysis).
- Localize abnormal red cell sequestration.
- Predict response to splenectomy.

Patient preparation

None. Avoid blood transfusion during study.

Procedure

- Obtain venous blood sample and label patient's red cells with ^{51}Cr-chromate.
- Re-inject cells and measure blood activity over 14 days using gamma counter.
- Measure activity over liver, spleen and heart using gamma probe daily for 14 days.

Results

- Normal red cell half-life >24 days.
- Equal fall in heart, liver and spleen counts with time.

Interpretation

Short red cell life confirms abnormal destruction. Ratio of counts in liver: spleen indicates site of red cell destruction.

Advantages

Only available technique.

Pitfalls

Lengthy and labour-intensive. Sensitivity reduced by blood transfusion during 14 days measurement period. Consistent probe positioning essential for accurate organ sequestration curves.

Red cell volume/plasma volume measurement

Background

Polycythaemia is suspected when haemoglobin and haematocrit are raised. Routine laboratory screening does not differentiate true polycythaemia, i.e. elevated red cell mass, from apparent, stress or pseudo-polycythaemia, i.e. reduced plasma volume. Radiolabelled red cells can be used to measure red cell mass. Plasma volume can be calculated from the haematocrit or measured independently using radiolabelled human serum albumin.

Indications

Polycythaemia, to distinguish between true polycythaemia (↑ RBC mass) from apparent polycythaemia (↓ plasma volume).

Patient preparation

Avoid recent therapeutic venesection. Less sensitive in patients already receiving myelosuppressive therapy.

Procedure

- Obtain 10mL venous blood.
- Radiolabel red cells using ^{99m}Tc or ^{51}Cr.
- Re-inject radiolabelled blood and, if required, ^{125}I-albumin.
- Obtain venous samples at 15 and 30 min.
- Count activity in blood samples compared with known standards using gamma counter to establish plasma and red cell volumes.

Results

Compare measured red cell mass and plasma volume with predicted values for height and weight.

Interpretation

Distinguish relative polycythaemia (due to ↓ plasma volume) from genuine elevation of red cell mass.

Advantages

Only technique available.

Pitfalls

Recent venesection or myelosuppressive therapy reduces test reliability. Plasma volume measurement unreliable in severe peripheral oedema.

Bile salt deconjugation studies

Background

Bile salts are synthesized and stored in the liver and are essential for adequate GI absorption. They are excreted into the gut as conjugated, water soluble bile salts and recycled by the enterohepatic circulation with terminal ileal reabsorption. Bile salt deconjugation products are insoluble and cannot enter the enterohepatic circulation, leading to bile salt malabsorption. Bacterial overgrowth after small bowel surgery or terminal ileal disease can ↑ deconjugation.

^{14}C-labelled synthetic bile acid, glycocholine, is administered po. Rapid transit into the large bowel will result in breakdown of the label by the normal large bowel flora and a rise in detected exhaled $^{14}CO_2$. Small bowel bacterial overgrowth, e.g. due to a 'blind loop', will also result in increased liberation of $^{14}CO_2$.

Indications

- Bacterial overgrowth.
- Bile salt malabsorption.

Patient preparation

- Starve overnight.
- Avoid antibiotics for one month before study.

Procedure

- Give oral ^{14}C-labelled glycocholic acid in water.
- Count $^{14}CO_2$ activity in breath samples over 6 h using β liquid scintillation counter.

Results

Glycocholate is deconjugated into ^{14}C glycine and cholic acid by small intestine bacteria releasing expired $^{14}CO_2$. Correct result for age-related variations in endogenous $^{14}CO_2$ production.

Interpretation

↑ $^{14}CO_2$ levels imply bacterial colonization or bile salt malabsorption.

Advantages

Accurate. Only available test.

Pitfalls

False −ves (unusual).

Bile salt deconjugation studies

Background

Indications

Patient preparation

Procedure

Interpretation

advantages

Results

Index

Notes: Page numbers in **bold** indicate the main discussion of a topic. Subjects are indexed in their unabbreviated form: a list of abbreviations appears on pp. xxix–xl.